Handbook of Developmental Psychiatry

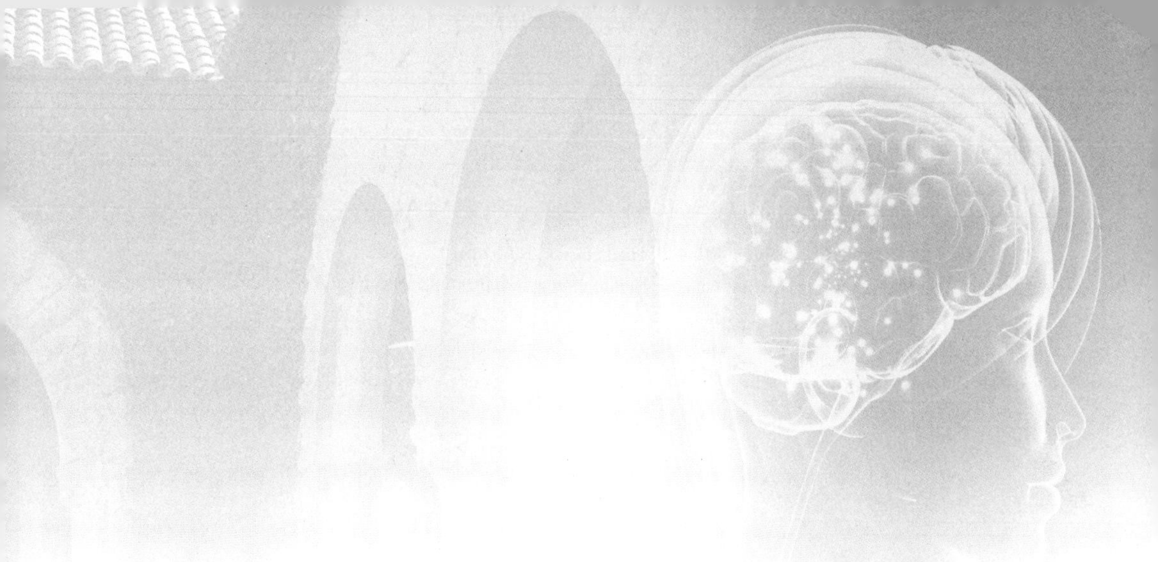

Handbook of Developmental Psychiatry

edited by

Hans Steiner

Stanford University, USA

World Scientific

NEW JERSEY • LONDON • SINGAPORE • BEIJING • SHANGHAI • HONG KONG • TAIPEI • CHENNAI

Published by

World Scientific Publishing Co. Pte. Ltd.
5 Toh Tuck Link, Singapore 596224
USA office: 27 Warren Street, Suite 401-402, Hackensack, NJ 07601
UK office: 57 Shelton Street, Covent Garden, London WC2H 9HE

British Library Cataloguing-in-Publication Data
A catalogue record for this book is available from the British Library.

HANDBOOK OF DEVELOPMENTAL PSYCHIATRY

ISBN-13 978-981-4324-81-6
ISBN-10 981-4324-81-7

Typeset by Stallion Press
Email: enquiries@stallionpress.com

Printed in Singapore by B & Jo Enterprise Pte Ltd

Dedication

To all of you whose teacher I have been, whether you were in high school, undergraduates, graduate, or postgraduate students or were already practicing child psychiatrists, adult psychiatrists, psychologists, social workers, pediatricians, or neuroscientists and the public. Teaching you is how I have learned the most. And to my father, Johann Steiner, whose teaching under extreme adversity, has always been an inspiration to me.

Hans Steiner, May 16, 2010

Lieber Vati: Dir ist dieses Buch gewidmet. Ohne Deine Zusage zur Unterstuetzung waere ich ja ein Auto-Mechaniker geworden. Und ich bin dann doch in Deine Fussstapfen getreten: Ich lehrte alle, so wie Du es getan hast, mit Energie und Zuneigung, und grosser Hingabe an das was gelehrt werden musste.

Dein Sohn Hans, 16.Mai 2010

Contents

Contributors

Richard D. Abbey, Ph.D.
President, Abbey Psychology and Psychiatry Associates
366 S. California Ave, Palo Alto, CA, 94301, USA
Tel: (650)-614-0014
drrichardabbey@gmail.com

Mary E. Bancroft, M.S.
Psychology Department
University of New Mexico
1 University of New Mexico
MSC03 2220
Albuquerque, NM 87131-0001, USA
meb29@unm.edu

Rebecca S. Bernard, Ph.D.
Program Manager, Children's Wellness Program
San Diego Center for Children
3002 Armstrong Street
San Diego, CA 92111, USA
Tel: (858) 569-2142
rbernard@centerforchildren.org

Michael H. Bloch, M.D., M.S.
Assistant Professor,
Room I-375, Sterling Hall of Medicine
Child Study Center, Yale University School of Medicine
P.O. Box 7900230
New Haven, CT 06520-7900
Tel: (203) 974-7551
Fax: (203) 785-7611
michael.bloch@yale.edu

Victor G. Carrion, M.D.
Associate Professor of Psychiatry
Director, Stanford Early Life Stress Research Program
401 Quarry Road, Stanford, California, 94305, USA
vcarrion@stanford.edu
http://pbpl.stanford.edu/

Kiki D. Chang, M.D.
Associate Professor
Director, Pediatric Bipolar Disorders Program
Division of Child and Adolescent Psychiatry
Department of Psychiatry and Behavioral Sciences
Stanford University School of Medicine
Lucile Packard Children's Hospital
Tel: (650) 725-0956
Fax: (650) 723-5531
kchang88@stanford.edu
http://pediatricbipolar.stanford.edu/

Graham J. Emslie, M.D.
Professor of Psychiatry
Chief of Child and Adolescent Psychiatry, University of Texas Southwestern Medical Center
5323 Harry Hines Blvd., Dallas, TX 75390-8589, USA
graham.emslie@utsouthwestern.edu

Sarah J. Erickson, Ph.D.
Associate Professor of Psychology and Pediatrics, UNM
Department of Psychology, Logan Hall, University of New Mexico, Albuquerque, NM 87131, USA
erickson@unm.edu
www.unm.edu/~psych/faculty/sm_erickson.html

Carl Feinstein, M.D.
Professor of Psychiatry and Behavioral Sciences
Director, Division of Child and Adolescent Psychiatry
Endowed Director of Psychiatry, Lucile Packard Children's Hospital
Stanford University School of Medicine
401 Quarry Road, Stanford, CA 94305-5719, USA
Tel: 650-498-5246
Fax: 650-724-7389
carlf@stanford.edu

Rebecca Hall
Research Consultant
Stanford University, School of Medicine
401 Quarry Road, Stanford, CA, 94305, USA
Becky.e.hall@gmail.com

Antonio Hardan, M.D.
Associate Professor of Psychiatry and Behavioral Sciences
Child and Adolescent Psychiatry and Child Development
Stanford University, School of Medicine
401 Quarry Road, Stanford, CA, 94305, USA
hardanay@stanford.edu

Chris Hayward, M.D., M.P.H
Professor of Psychiatry and Behavioral Sciences
Stanford University, School of Medicine
401 Quarry Road, Stanford, CA, 94305, USA
hayward@stanford.edu

George Hexter, M.D.
Formerly Clinical Professor
Stanford University, School of Medicine
401 Quarry Road, Stanford, CA, 94305, USA

Kyle Hinman, M.D.
Clinical Instructor of Child & Adolescent Psychiatry
Lucile Packard Children's Hospital at Stanford,
Division of Child & Adolescent Psychiatry,
401 Quarry Rd, Stanford, CA 94305, USA
khinman@stanford.edu

Julia Huemer, M.D.
Department of Child and Adolescent Psychiatry
Medical University of Vienna
Waehringer Guertel 18-20, 1090 Vienna, Austria, Europe
julia.huemer@meduniwien.ac.at

Shashank V. Joshi, M.D.
Assistant Professor of Psychiatry and Behavioral Sciences
Child and Adolescent Psychiatry and Child Development
Stanford University, School of Medicine
401 Quarry Road, Stanford, CA, 94305, USA
svjoshi@stanford.edu

Niranjan Karnik, M.D., Ph.D.
Assistant Professor of Psychiatry & Behavioral Neuroscience
University of Chicago Pritzker School of Medicine
5841 South Maryland Avenue, MC 3077
Chicago, Illinois 60637, USA
nskarnik@uchicago.edu

Leena A. Khanzode, M.D.
Child & Adolescent and Adult Psychiatrist
Bay Area Children's Association
20380 Town Center Lane
Cupertino, CA- 95014, USA
docleeno@yahoo.com

James F. Leckman, M.D.
Neison Harris Professor of Child Psychiatry, Psychology & Pediatrics
Room I-383, Sterling Hall of Medicine
Child Study Center, Yale University School of Medicine
P.O. Box 7900
New Haven, CT 06520-7900, USA
Tel: (203) 785-7971
Fax: (203) 785-7611
james.leckman@yale.edu
http://childstudycenter.yale.edu/faculty_people/james_leckman.profile

Anna Lembke, M.D.
Assistant Professor and Chief, Stanford Addiction Psychiatry Initiative
Department of Psychiatry and Behavioral Sciences, Stanford University
401 Quarry Road, Stanford, CA, 94305-5723, USA
alembke@stanford.edu

James Lock, M.D., Ph.D.
Professor of Psychiatry and Behavioral Sciences and by courtesy, of Pediatrics
Child and Adolescent Psychiatry and Child Development
401 Quarry Road
Stanford, CA, 94305, USA
jimlock@stanford.edu

Rudolf Moos, Ph.D.
Professor Emeritus, Department of Psychiatry, Stanford University
Research Health Science Specialist, Department of Veterans Affairs
VA Health Care System, 705 Willow Road, Menlo Park
California, 94025, USA
rmoos@stanford.edu

Paresh D. Patel, M.D., Ph.D.
Assistant Professor of Psychiatry
Research Assistant Scientist, Molecular and Behavioral Neuroscience Institute
5053 Biomedical Sciences Research Building
University of Michigan Medical Center
Ann Arbor, MI 48109-2200, USA
pdpatel@umich.edu

Rafael Pelayo, M.D.
Associate Professor of Psychiatry and Behavioral Sciences Assistant Professor of Psychiatry and Behavioral Sciences
Sleep Center
Stanford University, School of Medicine
401 Quarry Road, Stanford, CA, 94305, USA
pelayo@stanford.edu

Jennifer M. Phillips, Ph.D.
Clinical Associate Professor of Psychiatry and Behavioral Sciences
401 Quarry Road, Stanford, California, 94305-5719, USA
jennifer.phillips@stanford.edu

Belinda Plattner, M.D.
Assistant Medical Direktor
Department of Child and Adolescent Psychiatry, Division of Child and Adolescent Forensic Psychiatry,
University of Zurich, Switzerland
Neptunstrasse 60, 8032 Zurich, Switzerland,
Tel: +41 43 556 40 43
Fax: +41 43 556 40 41
Belinda.Plattner@kjpdzh.ch

Claire Remy
Former Academic Training Coordinator
Department of Psychiatry and Behavioral Sciences
Stanford University, School of Medicine
15, rue du Général Leclerc
78430 Louveciennes, France
claire6remy@yahoo.com

Alan F. Schatzberg, M.D.
Kenneth T. Norris, Jr., Professor
Department of Psychiatry and Behavioral Sciences
Stanford University School of Medicine
401 Quarry Road
Stanford, California 94305-5797, USA
afschatz@stanford.edu

Richard Shaw, M.B.B.S
Professor of Psychiatry and Pediatrics
Stanford University School of Medicine
Medical Director, Pediatric Psychosomatic Medicine Service, Lucile Packard Children's Hospital at Stanford
401 Quarry Road, Stanford, California, 94305, USA
rjshaw@stanford.edu
http://med.stanford.edu/profiles/Richard_Shaw/

Doctor medicinae universalis (Dr. med. univ.) Hans Steiner
Professor Emeritus of Psychiatry
Founding Member, *The Pegasus Physicians at Stanford*
Stanford University, School of Medicine
401 Quarry Road, Room 3324
Stanford, CA, 94305
USA
A-1060 Wien
Brueckengasse 10-12, Stiege 2, Tuer 35
Oesterreich, Europe
steiner@stanford.edu
drhanssteiner@gmail.com
Private website: www.hanssteiner.com
Tel: (650)-303-2638
Fax: (650)-723-5531

Pascale G. Stemmle, M.S.
Doctoral Candidate, PGSP-Stanford Psy.D. Consortium
Stanford University, School of Medicine
401 Quarry Road, Stanford, CA, 94305, USA
pascale@gmail.com

Margo Thienemann, M.D.
Clinical Associate Professor of Psychiatry
Stanford University School of Medicine, Stanford California
401 Quarry Road, Stanford, CA, 94305, USA
mthiene@gmail.com

Vishal Madaan, M.D.
Resident in Psychiatry
Creighton Nebraska Psychiatry Program
3528. Dodge Street, Omaha, NE 68131
vishalmadaan@creighton.edu

Charles O. Walton, M.D.
Formerly Clinical Professor
Stanford University, School of Medicine
401 Quarry Road, Stanford, CA, 94305, USA

Marina Zelenko, M.D.
Clinical Associate Professor
Stanford University, School of Medicine
401 Quarry Road, Stanford, CA, 94305, USA
Marina.Zelenko@kp.org

Chapter 1

Introduction

Hans Steiner and Alan Schatzberg

> What do we know: Mental disorders are brain disorders. Mental disorders are developmental disorders.
>
> *Thomas Insel, Director, NIMH, April 27, Stanford University, 2007*
>
> *Die Luft der Freiheit weht. Stanford Motto*

We are very pleased to present this *Handbook of Developmental Psychiatry for Children and Adolescents*, representing the state of the art and of the science of developmental psychiatry for mental health clinicians and trainees. It provides a detailed description of diagnosis and treatment of mental disorders in the Stanford University, School of Medicine, Division of Child and Adolescent Psychiatry and Human Development. Most of the authors of this volume are or at some point in their career have been members of our faculty and trainee pool and represent the distinct practice of psychiatry in our center. The handbook approaches clinical problems from a combination of evidence-based medicine and practice-based rationale utilizing current diagnostic and treatment algorithms in Stanford clinics.[1] Each chapter provides a summary of the pertinent knowledge base and ends with a description of our clinical practices. While evidence-based medicine is the ultimate goal of medical practice, it may not always be attainable or perhaps desirable, because either the knowledge base is too restricted or the practice is self–evidently effective.[2] This book is intended for the serious student of psychopathology from all levels of professional development, whether they are practitioners, teachers, or researchers. By offering a concise summary of the basic sciences of the field, alongside the evidence base and complementing both with how our faculty copes with all the unknowns, it should be helpful to those who seek to establish or further their professional development and careers.

The Stanford University, School of Medicine, has many characteristics that help shape the departments and the faculty within them. I quote from the Dean's Newsletter of February 13, 2007[3]

> "*Size and Connectivity* — I have previously noted that Stanford is one of the smallest Schools of Medicine among our peers — about 40% the size of UCSF and less than 10% the faculty of Harvard Medical School. I see our small size largely as an advantage, since it forces us to make strategic choices and to appoint the highest quality faculty we can find. So, an obvious challenge stands before us in sustaining excellence and meeting programmatic needs in the context of our current Provostial cap. It is part of our culture to value excellence and a relatively small size."

The implication here is that the School requires faculty who are specialists, but also conversant with broader aspects of their disciplines, especially as they relate to the scientific underpinnings of the practice.

> "*Depth and Breadth* — Our small size may limit our depth and breadth compared to peer institutions.... At the same time, it imposes a challenge to individual faculty, who, because of our small size, have multiple demands and expectations. While this is true for virtually everyone, there are additional pressures for clinical faculty, who are expected to demonstrate excellence and leadership in academic pursuits as well as in clinical care."

The implication here is that medical practitioners also need to be educated in research, oriented toward evidence-based practice, and engaged in research in either a leadership or a supportive role. Thomas Insel, the Director of the NIMH, on the occasion of a recent keynote address at the *10th Annual Stanford Symposium on Developmental Approaches to Psychopathology*, reemphasized this important connection between progress in the basic sciences and improvement of medical outcomes (Fig. 1).

Using heart disease and stroke as examples, he showed that significant reductions in morbidity and mortality occurred only after some decades of concerted basic research efforts, around 25 years. The point can be made that in mental health, we are just at the beginning of the phase of professional development where we will reap the benefits of two decades of progress in the neurosciences. We must have a cadre of physicians ready to receive and translate this information into clinical action. He proposed that following the Decade of the Brain (1990–2000), we are now in a position to have a Decade of Discovery (2000–2010).

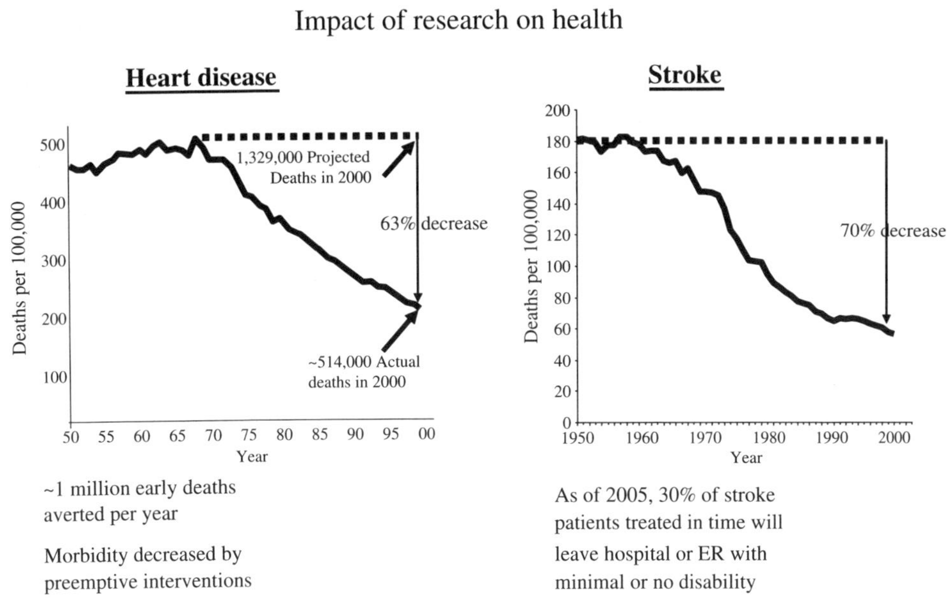

Fig. 1: Insel T (Director, National Institute of Mental Health). Stanford University, April 27, 2007.

> "*Disciplinary and Interdisciplinary* — Academic medical centers, including Stanford, are built on a foundation of disciplines in the form of departments — both basic and clinical. Many of these disciplines were formulated during the 20th century, and a number have evolved dramatically — or will do so in the future.... Most medical schools have evolved to more interdisciplinary areas of focus — and at Stanford, these more traditional departments or disciplines have been supplanted by new departments and programs. At the same time, most clinical departments have retained their traditional components."

The implication here is that there is constant cross-fertilization between basic research fields and fields of medical practice, which informs either end of this medical school spectrum. In all of these aspects, Child & Adolescent Psychiatry and Human Development at Stanford is a reflection of the school's profile, as will become evident throughout this volume. Additionally, because of its relatively small size, the division resembles many community clinics and practices in its configuration and the demands placed on the faculty. We would like to suggest that this makes the solutions found in our practice as we diagnose and treat patients with a wide range of problems with relatively limited resources particularly applicable to community practices and clinics.

During the past 25 years, the Division of Child & Adolescent Psychiatry and Human Development has become one of the premier clinical, research, and educational facilities in the United States Stanford faculty members are and have been for some time leading the field in several key domains of psychopathology in basic and clinical research. The faculty's approach is distinct. It is informed by the principles of developmental psychopathology and results in an emphasis on integrated treatment packages. The faculty has always maintained close ties with pediatrics, ever since the days of our inception as a medical subspecialty (see appendix for a more detailed discussion and timeline). We value and carefully develop the physician's ability to communicate and collaborate with primary care physicians, within our own system and in the community. Many disorders (such as eating disorders, somatoform disorders, and a range of neuropsychiatric syndromes) are collaboratively diagnosed, treated, and followed by interdisciplinary teams. These teams have been carefully assembled in many years of collegial collaborations.[4]

Another major influence on our practices has been the close proximity to superb basic scientists from all backgrounds. This is yet another instance where our relatively small size works to our advantage, leading to relatively facile and frequent contacts that often turn into close collaborations. The fact that we share a campus with the psychology department ranked as number one in the United States, and probably the world, further expands the intellectual resources that we can bring to bear. It is this special mix of proximity to both primary care and basic science, which has decisively shaped our practices into a unique blend. Because we are small and the medical school's size was limited by the university founders, we need to become experts, but remain conversant with many adjacent fields.

During a National Board Examination Review Course in 2004, chaired by Dr. Steiner for the American Academy of Child and Adolescent Psychiatry and staffed almost exclusively with our own faculty, it became clear to the audience and the faculty how distinct our approach to patients is compared to other highly regarded programs in the country. The course was such a success that it was repeated in the spring of 2008, at the request of the academy. Let us list the distinctive elements.

1. The physician's relationship to the patient and the family and its sophisticated management is considered essential to good practice. We practice patient-centered medicine. The relationship provides the platform from which we deliver many different interventions. We carefully examine the physician–patient relationship in the course of treatment and manage it to optimize its positive effects. Such management is informed by interpersonal and dynamic principles that have stood the test of time.
2. We are treating patient and family with the full range of available interventions, from environmental manipulation (sociotherapy) to psychotherapy and pharmacotherapy. We have illustrated this comprehensive and integrated

approach to treatment in a previous volume.[5] The decision about which treatment elements apply in a particular case is based on the strength of the empirical and practical evidence rather than on an *a priori* reductionistic assumption that pharmacotherapy, for instance, is always the best approach.

3. Different treatments are carefully integrated and matched to pathogenic processes in an effort to disrupt the causal loops creating the problem.

The *Handbook of Developmental Psychiatry* reflects this integrated developmental approach to diagnosis and treatment. While the specific techniques used to deal with different problem areas will vary due to the nature of the problem, the developmental basis and the integrated approach is common to all the areas of practice. The challenge we have posed all our authors is to convey the special Stanford brand of Developmental Psychiatry, while avoiding being parochial.

The *Handbook of Developmental Psychiatry* is distinct from our previously published *Handbook for Mental Health Interventions in Children and Adolescents*.[5] In the previous volume, we focused on highly detailed summaries of specific treatments in three sub domains: sociotherapy or environmental manipulation, psychotherapy, and pharmacotherapy; thus making readers expert in a range of techniques of interventions, across diagnoses. This current volume adds assessment tools needed to start treatment; making the readers experts in the identification and delineation of psychopathological clusters. The current volume also discusses treatment, but from a less detailed perspective. The two volumes are complementary and ideally should sit next to each other on the clinician's bookshelf. This current volume helps identify the problem and initiates treatment; the previous volume offers an expert/specialist view on a range of treatments employed.

This *Handbook of Developmental Psychiatry* invites the scientist/practitioner to go beyond the current DSM or ICD taxonomy in several important ways: (1) Use the phenomenology of the DSM or ICD as a point of departure, but eliminate multiple diagnoses as much as is possible. Diagnosis is a rigorous exercise, not a mindless listing of criteria met. (2) Establish a principal diagnosis (as per the ICD), based on the pattern of the unfolding of symptoms in the patient's history. Such an approach is increasingly possible and desirable now because we are accumulating basic science knowledge allowing the definition of underlying pathogenetic pathways. We realize that this may not always be easy to do, but every effort should be made to select a primary disorder. (3) Differential diagnosis remains an important tool of medicine. Our knowledge base in developmental psychiatry has matured, so that we can focus on pathogenic processes that need to be disrupted in order to bring about symptom control, renewed progress in development, and potential healing. Description is a beginning, but not an end point, of infinite recess and untested splitting into smaller and smaller categories, with sometimes spurious significance. (4) Instead of following the committee-driven splitting procedures invited by the DSM and to a lesser extent the ICD process, we invite the scientist practitioner to think of clusters of systems of regulation as the units of disorder. Eating, sleeping, attachment, impulse control, affect, mood, attention, appetitive behaviors, cognition, and monitoring of intactness are all examples of such complex systems that have survival value and common underlying networks and can be manifestly disordered in somewhat distinct but also related ways. The chapters of this book are organized along this principle; clustering disorders that probably share systems of self-regulation and thus are potentially treated by related interventions. These diagnostic clusters are based on a model of psychopathology rooted in development and evolutionary thinking, in contradistinction to a simple (and probably outdated) medical disease model underlying the prevalent descriptive phenomenological approach.

Psychopathology in children and adolescents is manifestly less differentiated than in adults and seems to aggregate in larger and less distinct categories. In the DSM system, the disorders of youth are very often NOS — not otherwise specified — as many core criteria are missing. Highly distinct and separate disorders, from a developmental perspective, are developmental "achievements."[6] For instance, anxiety and mood disorders are found to overlap to a high degree, having some authorities comment that they perhaps are not distinct at all in most cases, but developmentally linked: anxiety antedates depression, and as subjects age and become more chronically ill, more depression appears relative to anxiety (see the chapters on anxiety disorders and depression). Rather than regarding this fact as a problem of precision, we see it as an opportunity to expand our thinking regarding the nature of psychopathology: childhood syndromes, just like children, are works in progress, *formes frustes*. Still, they are of clinical significance, as they prevent normal development from proceeding. They also offer the unique opportunity of early and preventive interventions.

Because of progress in the basic and clinical sciences, we can more effectively handle the fact that the phenomenology of symptoms can be similar across different diagnoses, yet the underlying pathogenic processes are quite distinct, requiring quite different interventions. The fact that disturbances in multiple domains can be driven by a single pathogenic process is most likely explained by the high degree of interconnectivity of the brain, the complex role of most neurotransmitters in neural networks, and the relative immaturity of the juvenile central nervous system (CNS) of our patients. In order to become better psychiatrists, we have to go below the phenomenological surface, as Nobel Prize-winning psychiatrist Eric Kandel reminded us all on the occasion of his Baxter Lecture at Stanford University on May 10, 2006.

After establishing a diagnosis, we look to identify causal pathogenic processes that can be the target of specific interventions. True co-morbidity (*i.e.* the independent co-existence of two separate disorders) is the psychopathology that remains after the principal disorder has been treated as well as one can. There are many clinical examples to illustrate the advantages of our thinking. For example, aggressive behavior frequently occurs in the context of a mood disorder. In such cases, we will not assign a new diagnosis, such as oppositional defiant disorder, but will expect that by treating the principal disorder, *i.e.* the disturbance of mood, the problems with aggression will recede. The same logic applies to attention problems in the context of bipolar disorder. As a logical first step, before starting a stimulant to treat the attention problem, we will assess the effects of mood stabilizers on attention.[7]

Our approach insists on parsimony as a first principle. A diagnosis is more akin to a scientific hypothesis that gets tested against the success or failure of the selected interventions. By contrast, the prevalent descriptive DSM taxonomy practiced in other centers gives license to, or even encourages, the diagnosis of multiple-disease states based on phenomenology alone. This often leads to irrational situations in which patients receive as many as 10 supposedly distinct diagnoses and a correspondingly large number of psychopharmacological agents. It becomes increasingly impossible to know when one is wrong, and seemingly one is always right.

Finally, the *Handbook of Developmental Psychiatry* differs from standard child psychiatry textbooks because it insists that syndromes and syndrome clusters are a starting point to formulate treatment, not an end point. We have discussed our distinct approach in several of our previous publications.[4,5,8,9] After diagnosing, we expand our vision to examine the entire range of developmental domains in order to gain a fuller picture of a given patient's problems. Strengths and weaknesses are plotted and used in designing successful intervention strategies. Disorders are always seen in the whole person in his or her social context, a stance more akin to humanistic psychology.[10] Our treatment plans reflect this understanding, drawing on all available resources in a particular case and not limiting ourselves to DSM and ICD symptom lists, because we might lose the patient and the person in the process. Neither the DSM nor the ICD was ever meant to be exclusionary and complete.[11] The formulation of a case always was encouraged to include other sources of information, as we will discuss in greater detail in Chap. 2. In the past few years, however, some have taken it upon themselves to limit psychiatric practice to just that, bringing a stultifying narrowness to our field that ultimately may lead to the rapid demise of the phenomenological enterprise.

The Structure of this Volume

Any textbook, however, comprehensive it aims to be, represents a snapshot of a given field in time and is selective by necessity. We have outlined how we see developmental psychiatry as a distinct field in some detail above. Added to that vision is the considerable data base generated by multidimensional systems of assessments, such as Achenbach.[12] The final structure of this book also takes into account how the clinician needs to prepare to approach the patient to optimize data gathering and interventions. Thus, this volume is divided in four parts and 17 chapters.

Part I defines the *domain of clinical developmental psychiatry*. It begins with a brief historical account of how the field originated and maps the development of our division onto the development of the field. A core chapter is Chap. 3, where we outline the entire knowledge base that we require clinicians to consider as they formulate a given case.

Part II (Dr. med. Julia Huemer, assistant editor) groups disorders and syndromes that manifest predominantly with internalizing symptoms, *i.e.* symptoms that are experienced by the patient as bothersome, ego dystonic, and problematic, making it relatively easy to establish a working alliance with patients.[13] Attachment, anxiety, psychiatric trauma, mood, and bipolar disorders are discussed.

Part III (Niranjan S. Karnik, M.D., Ph.D., assistant editor) groups externalizing disorders, *i.e.* syndromes that are usually experienced as ego syntonic and predominantly lead to problems with people and systems around the patient (problems with learning, aggression and impulse control, attention, and substance and alcohol abuse). It tends to be more difficult to establish a working alliance and engage patients in treatment, as they very often do not see that they have a problem, and if they do, very often blame others for their difficulties.

Part IV (Richard J. Shaw, M.B., B.S., assistant editor) groups psychosomatic and neuropsychiatric syndromes that are difficult for mental health specialists to manage because they manifest with complex combinations of other medical symptoms concurrently (somatoform disorders, eating disorders, pervasive developmental disorders, intellectual disability, and sleep disorders). Very often, patients and their parents insist that their difficulties lie exclusively in a domain of medicine other than psychiatry. Mental health specialists need to be very skilled in establishing a working alliance with these patients and throughout treatment work in close consultation with pain medicine, neurology, adolescent medicine, and pediatrics to be maximally effective.

Certain disorders, although part of other textbooks, were no longer included in this volume: Elimination disorders are currently mostly managed within primary care settings. They at times have psychiatric co-morbidities that fall into one of the groupings above and should be treated along the principles outlined in these chapters. There is a vigorous debate as to how to best classify and approach sexual disorders in psychiatry. In the absence of decisive data, we have chosen to refer clinicians to volumes on sexual development that might be helpful.[14–16] Finally, we will not discuss personality disorders, taking seriously the fact that most systems classify these only if the patient is older than 18, with some rare and serious exceptions.

Each chapter contains information regarding the importance, evolution, diagnosis, differential diagnosis and co-morbid conditions, importance of the condition in primary care, the basic science underpinnings, the evidence-based treatments, the practice-based evidence from our clinics, and a brief section on the immediate future developments for a given diagnostic spectrum. The quality of data supporting each of these sections in the respective chapters varies, as our field is in rapid and uneven development. Some diagnoses are extremely well studied (*e.g.* ADHD), some are less so. In the latter, we rely more on clinical algorithms and use cases to illustrate our approach.

Peer-reviewed papers are some of the scientific building blocks for evidence-based practice. The other stream of information supporting this book is the cogent and careful practice in our consulting rooms (practice-based evidence). Both these streams will be integrated in each of the content areas. Change occurs with rapid pace, and at the second writing of this volume, we expect to see a different landscape. We have asked that all the authors conclude their chapter with a snapshot of the future: what lines of evidence concerning each domain can be expected to alter our diagnostic and therapeutic practices? What lines of investigation and practice should practitioners and trainees heed especially, as they prepare to embark on clinical, teaching, and research careers?

Developmental psychiatry, as it applies to children and adolescents, has become a solidly established discipline in the medical pantheon since we entered it some decades ago. Our profession is vibrant; child psychiatrists are known experts and contributors to research, teaching, and clinical care, much sought after and in short supply. There is an increasing neuroscience and social science database supporting more sophisticated formulations of problems and interventions. We are on the threshold of a better and more useful taxonomy because of progress in the sciences underpinning our practices.

Some problems remain and require our attention. We need to pursue improved diagnostic instruments that free us from symptom counts and historical data. We need clinical trials of integrated treatments. Much needed are naturalistic efficiency studies reaching very complex and difficult to study populations to bring in the large base of wisdom generated in our practices.

The rapid progress in the neurosciences and psychopharmacology has also given rise to a programmatic biological reductionism that threatens the integrity of our practices and the welfare of our patients.[17] The most concrete expression of this is in the abandonment in many programs of the physician–patient relationship as a vehicle for treatment and delivery of treatments, the emergence of pseudoscientific "comorbidity" diagnoses, and the overuse of medications in extensive and irrational combinations to treat children and adolescents with psychopathology. Our group provides a strong antidote to this phenomenon.

In assembling books such as this one, we always owe a great deal of gratitude to many. I, Hans Steiner, would like to thank my many students and mentees. It is well known that the teacher learns a great deal from those whom he or she has taught. The chapters in this volume are an excellent illustration of this point. I had the good fortune to identify, recruit, and train most of the authors in their specialty. Together, we published papers based on research that we designed and completed jointly. It is with great pride that I witness their very promising careers. Claire Remy deserves special mention as well. As the longtime administrative assistant of the child and adolescent psychiatry training program, she brought to it all her excellent preparation, her transcultural perspective, her French love for paradox, enjoyment of working with complex situations, and never flagging energy and dedication. We would like to thank all the patients that have provided us with their support and willingness to be studied and treated. We thank our assistant editors (Drs. Huemer, Karnik, and Shaw) and editors of World Scientific and Imperial College Press, who were patient and insistent at the same time, helping us complete the necessary steps toward finalization of this book.

References

1. Margison FR, Barkham M, Evans C, *et. al.* Measurement and psychotherapy: evidence based practice and practice based evidence, *Br J Psychiatry* 2000; **177**: 123–130.
2. Smith GCS, Pell JP. Parachute use to prevent death and major trauma related to gravitational challenge: systematic review of randomized controlled trials, *Br Med J* 2003; **327**: 1459–1461.
3. Pizzo P. Dean's newsletter [letter]. *Stanford University School of Medicine.* February 13, 2007.
4. Steiner H, Sanders M, Canning E, Litt I. The Department of Pediatric Psychiatry at Children's Hospital at Stanford: A model for managing clinical and personnel issues in C-L psychiatry, *Psychosomatics* 1994; **35**(1): 73–79.
5. Steiner H, Ed. *Handbook of Mental Health Interventions in Children and Adolescents: An Integrated Developmental Approach.* San Francisco, CA: Wiley/Jossey-Bass, 2004.

6. Sroufe LA, Rutter M. The domain of developmental psychopathology, *Child Dev* 1984; **55**: 17–29.
7. Steiner H, Karnik NS. Integrated treatment of aggression in the context of ADHD in children refractory to stimulant monotherapy: a window into the future of child psychopharmacology, *Am J Psychiatry* 2009; **166**(12): 1392–401.
8. Steiner H, Shaw R. Psychiatric assessment and management of the medically ill children. In: Stoudemire A, Fogel B, Greenberg D, Eds. *The Psychiatric Care of the Medical Patient*. New York, NY: Oxford University Press, 2000; pp. 1097–1110.
9. Steiner H. Developmental approaches to consultation liaison psychiatry, *Clin Child Psychol Psychiatry* 1999; **4**: 309–324.
10. Schneider KJ, Bugental JFT, Pierson JF, Eds. *The Handbook of Humanistic Psychology: Leading Edges in Theory, Research, and Practice*. Thousand Oaks, CA: Sage Publications, 2001.
11. Andreasen N. DSM and the death of phenomenology in America: an example of unintended consequences, *Schizophr Bull* 2007; **33**: 108–112.
12. Ivanova MY, Achenbach TM, Rescorla LA, *et al*. The generalizability of the youth self-report syndrome structure in 23 societies, *J Consult Clin Psychol* 2007; **75**(5): 729–38.
13. Achenbach TM, Howell CT, Quay HC, Conners CK. National survey of problems and competencies among four- to sixteen-year-olds: parents' reports for normative and clinical samples, *Monogr Soc Res Child Dev* 1991; **56**(3): 1–131.
14. Huegel, K. *GLBTQ: The Survival Guide for Queer and Questioning Teens*. Minneapolis, MN: Free Spirit Publishing, 2003.
15. Parents, Families, and Friends of Lesbians and Gays Web site. www.pflag.org. Accessed on May 22, 2010.
16. Hetrick-Martin Institute Web site. http://www.hmi.org. Accessed on May 22, 2010.
17. Steiner H, Leckman J, Gabbard G. Quo Vadimus? [overview]. *Perspectives in Biology and Medicine*, 2011; submitted.

Chapter 2

The Development of Child and Adolescent Psychiatry: A Brief History

Claire Remy, Julia Huemer, Charles O. Walton, and George Hexter

The antecedents of child psychiatry date back to the late 19th century in Europe (Table 1). In this context, the social recognition of childhood as a particular phase of life with its inherent developmental stages represented an important prerequisite. In 1887, Emminghaus, a German psychiatrist, pioneered child and adolescent psychiatry, particularly by defining important cornerstones of developmental psychopathology in his publication on childhood mental illness titled "*Die psychischen Störungen des Kindesalters*" [*The Mental Disorders of Childhood*].[1] In 1899, the term "psychiatrie infantile" [child psychiatry] was used as a subtitle in Manheimer's monograph "*Les Troubles Mentaux de L'Enfance*" [*The Mental Problems of Childhood*].[2] Moritz Tramer (1882–1963), a Swiss psychiatrist, contributed to the definition of diagnosis and treatment of childhood phenomena in his textbook on *Child and Adolescent Psychiatry*.

Sigmund Freud's attempts to understand the underlying patterns of neurosis, soon led him to the analysis of early childhood development. This approach became particularly evident in "*Drei Abhandlungen zur Sexualtheorie*" [*Three Contributions to the Theory of Sexuality*] (1905)[3] and "*Traumdeutung*" [*The Interpretation of Dreams*] (1900).[4] The writing "*Analyse der Phobie eines fuenfjaehrigen Knaben; Der kleine Hans*" (1905) [*Analysis of a Phobia in a Five-Year-Old Boy; Little Hans*][5] represented the beginning of child psychotherapy. Soon after, rules of adult psychoanalysis were not merely transformed into child and adolescent psychoanalysis but amended by particular methods, such as play therapy. Anna Freud, Sigmund Freud's daughter, has left a lasting mark on the definition of key theories of child psychotherapy. The Second World War gave Anna

Table 1: Cornerstones in the History of Child and Adolescent Psychiatry

19th century Europe	Social recognition of childhood as a particular phase of life with its inherent developmental stages: Emminghaus, 1887: "*Die psychischen Störungen des Kindesalters*" [*The Mental Disorders of Childhood*]. Manheimer, 1899: "Psychiatrie Infantile" [*Child Psychiatry*] in "*Les Troubles Mentaux de L'Enfance*" [*The Mental Problems of Childhood*].
Sigmund Freud	"*Drei Abhandlungen zur Sexualtheorie*" [*Three Contributions to the Theory of Sex*] (*1905*), "*Traumdeutung*" [*The Interpretation of Dreams*] (*1900*); "*Analyse der Phobie eines fuenfjaehrigen Knaben; Der kleine Hans*" (*1905*) [*Analysis of a Phobia in a Five-Year-Old Boy; Little Hans*]: beginning of child psychotherapy.
"Das Rote Wien" [Red Vienna]	Changes in social and health-related policies (Julius Tandler, August Aichhorn). The first child guidance clinic was created in 1919 by Alfred Adler with government support. Shortly thereafter, a number of child guidance clinics started in Vienna and in several other European countries. In 1926, Alfred Adler moved to the United States and opened clinics at various places, especially in New York and Chicago.
Charlotte Buehler	First woman to hold a professorship in psychology in Europe. She introduced concepts of developmental psychology in her book "*Das Seelenleben des Jugendlichen*" [*Psychology of Adolescence*] (1922).
Leo Kanner	Established the first American academic child psychiatry department at the Johns Hopkins Hospital in Baltimore in 1930; first textbook of child psychiatry was written by him in 1935.
Arnold Gesell	Importance of both nature and nurture, by stating that many aspects of human behavior were heritable; use of medication in child psychiatry.
Anna Freud	WW II: Center for young war victims, named "The Hampstead War Nursery," in London. Research on the effects of stress on children and their relationships; importance of a developmental psychopathology perspective on child and adolescent psychiatry; child psychotherapy.
Recognition as medical speciality, United States	1953: Founding of the American Academy of Child Psychiatry (now American Academy of Child and Adolescent Psychiatry, AACAP). Establishment of a board-certified medical speciality in 1959.
Michael Rutter	First comprehensive population survey of 9- to 11-year-olds which was carried out in London and the Isle of Wight.
1960s, 1970s—today	Classification of child and adolescent psychiatric disorders. DSM-IV and ICD-10 have distinguished certain symptomatologies into "childhood" and "adult" disorders. Reconciling aspects of biological and social psychiatry.

Freud the opportunity to analyze the impacts of deprivation of parental care on children. She established a center for young war victims, named "The Hampstead War Nursery," in London. In her research, she described the effects of stress on children and their relationships, and reinforced the importance of a developmental psychopathology perspective on child and adolescent psychiatry.[6]

The beginning of the 20th century took place in, what was called, "Das Rote Wien" [Red Vienna],[7] referring to the fact that Social-Democrats, such as Julius Tandler, who were the ruling party between 1918 and 1934, had initiated important changes in social-and health-related policies. These changes gave rise to a health care system for youth from all different social ranks. Moreover, an innovative program to support families (establishment of the first day-care centers for children, kindergartens, etc.) was introduced on a broad national scale. August Aichhorn, the founder of psychoanalytical pedagogy, cleared the way for some of these social breakthroughs by his advocacy and research. In this context, child guidance actually found its origin in the Vienna socialist movement after WWI. The first child guidance clinic was opened in 1919 by Alfred Adler with government support, as an activity helping the promotion of standards of living, especially among socially lower classes. Shortly thereafter, a number of child guidance clinics started in Vienna and in several other European countries. For most of them, some connection with public schools was established.

In 1926, Alfred Adler moved to the United States and he and his trainees opened clinics at various places, especially in New York and Chicago. Child guidance clinics were part of general hospitals or psychiatric departments. Alexandra Adler in her *handbook of Child Guidance*[8] gives an example of Alfred Adler's work: "A special feature of the Viennese guidance clinics were the school guidance clinics, eleven of which were being conducted by 1928. The class teacher of the child gave the case history and described in detail the problems which the child presented. Alfred Adler or one of his pupils then interpreted the case. The audience consisted of the teachers and superintendents of schools in the district. They participated in the discussion that followed. Then, the individual psychologist spoke to the child and to the parents and relatives. This was usually done before the same audience, although the procedure varied in the individual cases. The teacher was then entrusted with the further handling of the child. Eventually, the case was discussed again before the same audience."

Charlotte Buehler, who was the first woman to hold a professorship in psychology in Europe, introduced concepts of developmental psychology in her book "*Das Seelenleben des Jugendlichen*" [*Psychology of Adolescence*] (1922).[9] In 1934, Tramer founded the "*Zeitschrift für Kinderpsychiatrie*" [*Journal of Child Psychiatry*], which later became "*Acta Paedopsychiatria*," the first publication devoted entirely to the study of childhood psychopathology.

Under the direction of Adolf Meyer, Leo Kanner, an Austrian-American, established the first American academic child psychiatry department at the Johns Hopkins Hospital in Baltimore in 1930. Leo Kanner, the psychiatrist who coined the term "infantile autism," wrote the first textbook of child psychiatry in 1935.[10] Kanner's seminal paper, "Autistic Disturbances of Affective Contact," together with the work of Hans Asperger, represents the basis of the modern study of autism.[11]

The use of medication in the treatment of childhood psychopathology also began in the 1930s. Arnold Gesell (1880–1961), professor at Yale University and author of several books on child psychiatry, emphasized the importance of both nature and nurture, by stating that many aspects of human behavior were heritable. Additionally, he made use of latest advancements in video and photography, and integrated them into his research methods.

In 1937, the first international conference for child and adolescent psychiatry was held in Paris. In the United States, child and adolescent psychiatry was recognized as a medical speciality in 1953 with the founding of the American Academy of Child Psychiatry (now American Academy of Child and Adolescent Psychiatry, AACAP) by a group of analytically trained child psychiatrists. It was later established as a Board-certified medical specialty in 1959. In 1959, the new medical sub-specialty of child psychiatry was officially recognized by the American Board of Psychiatry and Neurology (ABPN). In 1986, the ABPN piloted a triple board residency program that offered five-year combined training in adult psychiatry, child and adolescent psychiatry (CAP), and pediatrics. This program was intended to recruit medical students who were interested in both pediatrics and CAP directly from medical school rater than *via* general psychiatry training. In the 1970s, child psychiatry witnessed major theoretical and intervention breakthroughs in terms of a paradigm shifts toward a socio-therapeutically orientated pedagogy. Much of this was driven by the pathbreaking scholarship of Sir Michael Rutter.[12] He completed the first comprehensive population survey of 9- to 11-year-olds which was carried out in London and the Isle of Wight. He raised issues which have not lost their relevance: for instance, the prevalence of psychiatric disorders among youth, gene–environment interactions, social impacts on children's adjustment, *etc.*

Since the 1960s and 1970s, particular attention has been paid to the classification of child and adolescent psychiatric disorders. As a consequence, DSM-IV[13] and ICD-10[14] have distinguished certain symptomatologies into "childhood" and "adult" disorders. Today, child and adolescent psychiatry particularly faces the challenge of reconciling aspects of biological and social psychiatry.

The Division of Child and Adolescent Psychiatry and Child Development at the Stanford University School of Medicine parallels in its growth the maturation of the field. At Stanford University, it was not until 1939 that the Commonwealth Fund began supporting an enlarged clinical program under the direction of a full-time pediatric psychiatrist (Dr. Hale Shirley) (For further details regarding the history of the department at stanford, please refer to http://elane.stanford.edu/wilson — John Wilson, 1998). The Commonwealth Fund of New York completely supported the clinic for three years and partially supported for three more years a full-time pediatrician and a psychiatrist, a full-time psychiatric social worker, and a secretary were added to the staff. It was called the Pediatric Psychiatric Clinic and was made a unit of the Medical School, its management and procedures being under the direction of executives of the Department of Pediatrics, the executive of the Division of Neuropsychiatry and the executive director of the unit. From January 1, 1940 to January 1, 1959, 4383 children were seen in the clinic and at least 21 psychiatry residents, 6 residents, 4 pediatric residents, 8 psychiatric social workers, and 14 psychologists were given training in the service. Until July 2, 1955, psychiatry at Stanford was a Division of the Department of Medicine. At that time, the department of psychiatry was established and the division of child psychiatry became part of that department. In 1959, child psychiatry became organized as a division of the Department of Psychiatry maintaining, however, liaison relationship with the Department of Pediatrics. In 1960, there was the creation of a formal child psychiatry fellow training program. In 1977, child psychiatry was referred to for the first time as a division, but was not formally established as such until 1997. Existing training and clinical programs were expanded and a formal research training supported by national grants was added. In 1978, the program moved into the Lucile Salter Packard Children's Hospital at Stanford with the creation of the first coordinated psychosomatic inpatient treatment program, an expanded consultation liaison program to pediatrics along with the intensification of collaboration with the Children's Health Council in providing coordinated outpatient services. The period between 1990 and 1995 saw the first NIMH-supported Institutional Research Training grant in child psychiatry (Roland Ciaranello, M.D. and Hans Steiner, M.D., principal investigators). A significant expansion of trainee pool occurred making the Stanford Program the largest program west of the Mississippi. The year 1997 saw the formal creation of a Child Psychiatry Division, the expansion of existing outpatient clinics to a full range of tertiary care portfolio and a significant expansion of faculty to provide expanded services and research.

Initially, child psychiatry, a relatively young branch of medicine, has provided its expert medical care to a small proportion of emotionally disturbed children. The limited access problem has not improved much despite the opening of new training programs in the 1960s and 1970s and by the triple boards programs in the 1980s and 1990s. It is believed that 7 to 12 million children and adolescents in the United States suffer from diagnosable psychiatric conditions, and about seven million of them exhibit severe to extreme functional impairments due to their psychiatric conditions. Several commissions by government agencies (including Presidential commissions) and professional organizations have reviewed the status of CAP work force in the last four decades. All of these commissions have recognized a marked shortage of child and adolescent psychiatrists. It is estimated that in order to provide adequate care to the population in the United States, we would need a cohort of approximately 20,000 child psychiatrists; currently, there are 7400 AACAP members. In the last four decades, various recruitment ideas have been proposed to expand the field to meet the needs of the nation's children and adolescents.

References

1. Emminghaus H. Die *Psychischen Störungen des Kindesalter* [*The psychic Disturbances of Childhood*]. Tuebingen: Verlag der H. Laupp'schen Buchhandlung, 1887.
2. Manheimer M. *Les Troubles mentaux de l'Enfance: Par le Dr. Marcel Manheimer.* Paris: Société d'Éditions Scientifiques, 1900.
3. Freud S. *Drei Abhandlungen zur Sexualtheorie* (*1905*). Frankfurt am Main: Studienausgabe Bd. 5. Fischer Taschenbuch Verlag, 1982.
4. Freud S. *Die Traumdeutung.* Frankfurt am Main: S. Fischer Verlag, 1999.
5. Freud S. *Analyse der Phobie eines fünfjährigen Knaben* (*"Der kleine Hans"*) (*1909*). Frankfurt am Main: S. Fischer Verlag, 1995.
6. Freud A. *Einfuehrung in die Technik der Kinderanalyse.* Muenchen: Reinhardt, Ernst, 1995.
7. Gardner S, Stevens G. *Red Vienna and the Golden Age of Psychology, 1918–1938.* New York, NY: Praeger Publishers, 1992.
8. Harms E. *Handbook of Child Guidance.* New York: Child Care Publications, 1947.
9. Buehler C. *Das Seelenleben des Jugendlichen.* Jena: Gustav Fischer, 1927.
10. Kanner L. *Child Psychiatry.* Springfield, Illinois: C.C. Thomas, 1935.
11. Kanner L. Autistic disturbances of affective contact, *Nerv Child* 1943; **2**: 217–250. Reprint. *Acta Paedopsychiatr* 1968; **35**(4): 100–136.
12. Rutter M, Tizard J, Whitemore P. *Education, Health and Behavior*. London, England: Longman Group, 1970.
13. American Psychiatric Association. *Diagnostic and Statistical Manual of Mental Disorders — DSM-IV.* Washington, DC: American Psychiatric Association Press, 2008.
14. International Statistical Classification of Diseases and Related Health Problems. http://apps.who.int/classifications/apps/icd/icd10online/. Accessed on March 30, 2010.

Chapter 3

Psychiatric Diagnosis, Case Formulation, and Treatment Planning Along the Principles of Developmental Psychiatry

Hans Steiner, Julia Huemer, Pascale G. Stemmle, Rebecca E. Hall, and R. Chris Hayward

Panta chorei kai ouden menei (Everything changes and nothing stays the same)

Heraklitus of Ephesus, circa 540–475 BC

"Consciousness is really only a net of communication between human beings; it is only as such that it had to develop; a solitary human being who lived as a beast of prey would not have needed it."

Friedrich Nietzsche, Die Froehliche Wissenschaft, 1887

1. Introduction

All clinicians treating disorder and illness need a system of classification that enables them to act swiftly, decisively, and effectively. Diagnoses identify the nature of a disorder,[1] and allow clinicians to quickly and reliably communicate complex sets of facts to other colleagues. In these aspects, psychiatry is similar to all other medical specialties. However, as psychiatry deals with the mind/brain system, which is arguably the most complex organ in the universe, it faces several special challenges. The existence of conscious and unconscious states, which are inaccessible to external observers, the ensuing necessity of relying on subjective reports, and the extreme dependence of humans on social contexts all pose special challenges to the psychiatrist. Psychiatry, a discipline that straddles the social, psychological, and biological sciences[2] challenges the reductionist approach which has been so successful in other branches of medicine. This chapter reviews these challenges and offers some solutions from a developmental perspective.

Our premise is that descriptive taxonomies (whether they be DSM or ICD) are starting points in the process of identifying mental disorders, but are insufficient to capture the complexity of a disordered brain/mind/person system. We also propose that in most of the disorders described in this volume, we have sufficient information regarding proximate and distal causes to go beyond the descriptive surface. The descriptive framework has to be enriched considerably to capture the entire person and to enable more comprehensive and accurate communication about all the relevant factors in a particular case. Only by considering all relevant factors (be they social, psychological, or biological in nature), can we arrive at an adequately in-depth understanding of pathology which enables us to assign the best possible treatment. This is the essence of the developmental approach to diagnosis, formulation, and treatment planning.

2. Definitions

In psychiatry, we deal with mental disorders. There has been considerable debate in the literature and among our faculty regarding the basic definition of a mental disorder.[3–5] Suffice it to say, we currently have no uniformly agreed upon definition of either mental or disorder. The entire issue could be solved rather pragmatically by saying "mental disorders are those treated by psychiatrists and related mental health professionals." However, that is too unprincipled and expedient for researchers, scientists, and clinicians alike. We therefore propose the following definition, modeled after the pluralist views described by Reznek (1991), and Spitzer and Endicott (1978)[6]:

A disorder is "mental" when it involves the mind/brain system, and the key symptoms operating within the disorder must be understood in psychological terms. Examples are cognition, perception, emotion, motives, self-regulation and coping, self-observation, and attachment.

Stedman defines disorder as "a disturbance of function, structure, or both, resulting from a genetic or embryologic failure in development or from exogenous factors such as poison, trauma, or disease."[1] To this, we would like to add the criterion proposed by Wakefield, relevant in the context of developing organisms, that the failure involves a deviance from the original function for which this particular mental process was designed. It should be apparent that in this definition (as in the DSM or ICD) there are no indications given as to the etiology of this problem. Both descriptive systems were deliberately designed this way to avoid the premature reference to causes and orthodoxy.

It is difficult to imagine clinical practice without a phenomenological taxonomy that defines the domains of disorder. However, it is also clear that, in clinical practice with patients of all ages, but especially with children and adolescents, additional steps need to be taken to enrich the existing system. In psychiatry, as in other branches of medicine, it is essential to treat the person, not just the disease, because in the larger context of the individual and his/her social network we encounter causal loops maintaining the disorder. We also encounter domains of undisturbed functioning; individual assets which can be utilized to positively impact treatment and outcome. Such an expanded, holistic, humanistic point of view is especially important in psychiatric practice with children and adolescents, where we know developmental forces to be very active. In youth and humans of all ages there are, in addition to defects and disorders, normative forces pushing toward organization, reorganization, differentiation, complexity, and spontaneous healing. Change is directional and, in optimal conditions, proceeds in the direction of differentiation and complexity.[7] The developmentally oriented clinician has great respect for the homeopathy of human development as a force toward normalization in even the most disturbed individuals. As Magnusson[8] states: "An individual functions and develops as a total, integrated and, complex adaptive system. This (makes) the individual the organizing principle for psychological inquiry."

3. Using Developmental Theory to Expand the Phenomenology of Mental Disorders

In the past 100 years, several domain-specific developmental theories have informed and influenced clinical practice and research. They are discussed in some detail and critiqued in an excellent compendium by Miller.[9] The major theories deal with cognition and information processing (Piaget); psychopathology and the human life cycle (Freud, Erikson); behaviorism and social learning theory (Bandura); and adjustment and adaptation (Bowlby, Lorenz, and Tinbergen). From these theories, we can distill certain characteristics that are central to a developmental approach to diagnosis and treatment.

3.1. *Change*

Central to developmental theory is the contention that humans, disordered or not, change as a function of time. Change is not random, but directional: especially in the early phases of life, humans spontaneously progress toward increasing differentiation, complexity, and capability. Such change occurs automatically in cases of both health and disorder. Change will shape the presentation, or phenomenology, of the disorder. Disorders can present differently at different ages because disorders are shaped by the interaction of normal development with disordered function. Consequently, a developmental clinician has to look below the phenomenological surface because descriptors of the same psychopathology can manifest in dramatically different ways at different ages or stages of life.

Inherent in the concept of developmental change is the concept of several key developmental phases which define age-relative (normative) functioning. These standards are used in defining symptoms of disorders as well as age-appropriate attainments.[7] This age-driven relativism is one of the defining hallmarks of developmental thinking. The divisions of developmental phases into infancy, preschool, school age, early adolescent, late adolescent, and young adult, still have considerable clinical utility, despite an extensive scholarly debate as to whether such phases are clearly discernable and helpful.[10]

What is considered pathological at one age may not be at another one. This age-relative definition of diagnostic criteria is dealt within the descriptive classifications by listing disorders by age groups. However, the assumption that disorders are age specific may not always be correct, particularly if we encounter certain disorders that are present across the life span. Based upon recent data on the early manifestations of mental disorders, we may be better off to assume that disorders are present from very early on, but do not manifest in the same way in children or adolescents as they do in adulthood. Disorders can be isomorphic or nonsisomorphic. The basic assumption in descriptive systems is the stability of diagnoses and types. The basic assumption in the developmental model is that there are no guarantees in this regard.

3.2. *Continuity or discontinuity?*

Another question that becomes relevant in the developmental model is at what rate change occurs. Does it proceed in large quantum leaps or in slowly accumulating doses?[11] Is it continuous or discontinuous? Quantum leaps can be mistaken for psychopathology, as the new state appears suddenly and may be qualitatively different from the pre-existing state. The change in an adolescent's capacity for abstract thinking is a good example of this paradigm. Early adolescents frequently challenge both parental demands and the assumptions underlying parental control. In part, this behavior is related to their newly acquired cognitive skills, which enable them to view situations more broadly, and to identify alternative views and countervailing arguments. Such behavior may emerge suddenly and may appear as a manifestation of an externalizing disorder, such as oppositional defiant disorder. Another example is the appearance of sexual behavior with the onset of pubertal maturation. Interest in sex, sexual partners, and the mechanics of sexual activity is usually not a sign of paraphilia or perversion, as some parents fear, but rather part of a developmentally normative maturational process.

3.3. *History: Pathways into and out of disorder*

The concept of a developmental trajectory directs the clinician to an individual's history. In traditional medicine, the history of a chief complaint is an effort to reconstruct the unfolding of pathology over time. This is an important enterprise, because in many disorders this temporal unfolding guides the clinician's thinking about what kind of diagnosis he/she is dealing with. Acute, versus subacute, versus chronic trajectories have direct implications for diagnosis and treatment. The developmental clinician expands this view to include information from all domains of functioning over time. For one, caseness is determined by deviance from functioning. But for another, it is essential to place as much emphasis on developmental progress and attainment as upon deviance. Progress achieved in various domains of functioning (grouped as psychological, interpersonal, academic-vocational, recreational, and basic needs) is charted.

The reconstruction of these pathways in the clinical setting is almost always retrospective and based upon the accounts of patient and parents. This has obvious weaknesses, as multiple distortions, based primarily on faulty recollections, are prevalent.[12] Ideally, we would have prospective data available, but this will be the exception rather than the rule in the clinical setting. Nevertheless, sources such as pediatric developmental records, baby books, and home movies can provide snapshots of development which go beyond mere patient and parent recollections. Another potential safeguard to distortion is the use of multiple informants (with the patient's consent) who have intimate knowledge of the patient and their life trajectory.

The patient's narrative, with all its distortions and faulty memories, can nonetheless be used to fine tune our empathic stance with him or her in preparation for building a strong working alliance. The patient's historical report of growing up does not just contain facts, but facts from his or her perspective. It is a synthesized recollection of historical details, remembered and told, a coherent (or sometimes disjointed) narration. Through the patient's account we might glimpse how they see themselves in this world in dealing with adversity, as well as their own view of their strengths and weaknesses. How do they see him/herself: active or passive; a victim of circumstance or a perpetrator of bad deeds; a person challenged by, struggling with or overwhelmed by adversity. At times, such beliefs are self-fulfilling prophecies. Additionally, they very often color the therapeutic alliance. Someone who takes pride in taking on challenges might not be inclined to rely upon expert advice. Someone who sees himself as a permanent victim may make excessive demands for attention and support.

3.4. *Complexity: From simplicity to complexity with increasing age*

The developmental model explicitly embraces the notion that functioning becomes more diversified, capable, and complex as we mature. Thought, emotion, action, judgment, insight, and self-regulation change as we learn. Learned skills go from effortful and conscious control, to automatic effortless, and reflexive, as they shift from being encoded in explicit to implicit memory.[13] Learning and interaction with the environment ultimately leaves permanent traces. Thought processes become more differentiated and abstract.[10] Emotions proceed from simple startle and distress states in early infancy[14] to basic forms of emotions during childhood[15] including fear, anger, sadness disgust, contempt, happiness, interest, and surprise. Secondary elaborations of these basic emotions appear later, such as guilt, shame, and concern, until we see in adolescence the full and complex range of emotions.[16] Self-control begins with simple inhibitions, then progresses to restraint, responsibility, consideration for others, and thoughtful ethical constraints on human behavior.[17] Human relationships diversify as well, expanding outside the nuclear family to include peer groups, neighbors, teachers, tutors, and finally partners, friends, and mates.[18]

The emphasis on directional growth toward complexity means that the manifestations of disorder can appear anywhere along the continuum of differentiation. Symptoms can be simple deficits, but can also involve a lack of progression and differentiation (a developmental arrest, or a "fixation" in psychoanalytical language), the appearance of a function prior to what is expected for the individual's age (precocity), or a temporary loss of complexity under duress (regression). To some extent, this thinking is contained in the fifth axis of the DSM diagnostic system, but the developmental model calls for a more fine-grained view of these processes.

Complexity also allows us to deal effectively with emergent structures of the brain-mind system, such as consciousness, unconsciousness, and subjective mental states. Our intentions, motives, attitudes, and beliefs constitute parts of our psychiatric disorders and can bring about changes in our biology. Eating disorders are an excellent illustration of this point: what you think of your body shape in relation to a cultural ideal of beauty leads through a cascade of events to profound alterations in your cardiac, hormonal, and osseous systems. As another example, willful efforts can directly stop symptoms, such as tics, or impulsive behavior; such efficacy of will[19] adds a whole new dimension to our treatment tool box. By using patients' effortful rational thought, we can assist patients in changing highly irrational behaviors, such as by asking a phobic patient to handle a snake or transverse a bridge. The pathogenesis of many syndromes discussed in this book can be effectively described in mentalistic and non-reductionistic terms, leaving open the possibility for multiple avenues of psychosocial intervention with proven efficacy, shown to be comparable in effect size as medications in the treatment of some disorders (see Chaps. 5, 6, and 14 of this volume). The conceptual map of the developmental clinician is truly biopsychosocial in character. Individuals are both top-down, self-directed, and driven by bottom-up causality.

3.5. *Context*

Complementary to the notion that individuals are self-directed and self-organizing is the notion that humans are also exquisitely context dependent. This is especially true for children and adolescents, who function as part of a family system for a prolonged period of time. This dependence on context shapes both normative functioning and symptom expression. Also, some of the most potent interventions regarding symptom control consist of simple environmental manipulation. The developmental clinician is always assessing the many orbits of social circles as part of their assessment of normal and abnormal functioning.

Bronfenbrenner and others have elegantly described a schema for the systematic description of psychosocial contexts. Social learning theory[20] deserves credit for calling our attention to the fact that maladaptive behavior can be precipitated by factors in the psychosocial environment (such as maltreatment and abuse),[21] but can also be maintained by the environment. It is not just the individual who needs to be changed in order to allow a child to return to normal functioning. Functioning in sick social groups can negate and nullify even the most potent biological and psychological interventions (see Chaps. 11, 12, and 14 in particular of this volume). A useful synopsis of the psychosocial context in relationship to interventions is provided by Karnik[18] in our previous volume on *Mental Health Interventions for Children and Adolescents*.

3.6. *Adaptation*

The developmental approach carefully considers the adaptive status and outcome of each patient, going beyond the single judgment required by the descriptive systems on Axis V to assign a past and current global assessment of functioning score.[22] The GAF combines an assessment of symptoms and functioning that is serviceable, but not ideal. The GAF's comingling of symptoms and adjustment obscures the fact that sometimes people can be symptomatic, yet function well, and conversely, function poorly but not fulfill psychiatric diagnostic criteria.

Function and syndrome overlap but are also distinct. Within a developmental framework, we assess positive adaptive functioning in several domains and compare it to age-appropriate norms, keeping it separate from symptoms' tallies. Simple symptom counts overestimate the prevalence of psychopathology in non-clinical populations.[23]

The developmental model takes the evaluation of adaptive functioning one step further. Even psychopathology itself is considered a developmental achievement, an end result of the interplay between positive and negative forces.[24] This position raises the important question as to whether a particular syndrome also enables the patient to adjust to an abnormal situation. Is there perhaps a positive, adaptive, valence to certain symptoms or even syndromes? Despite all the suffering and dysfunction generated by the syndrome, does the patient stand to gain from certain problems? The positive dimension of pathological symptoms is readily understood when dealing with disorders which are addictive (see Chap. 12) or where personal gain is involved (see Chapter 13). However, even aggression and eating disorders serve a homeostatic purpose: aggression aids survival in extreme social adversity, while the semistarvational states in eating disorders often achieve emotional numbing in the face of overwhelming anxiety.[25] Even in the most severe forms of psychopathology, such as autism, we can see the positive, adaptive value of certain symptoms. The gaze avoidance in autism serves partially to downregulate threat detection related emotions in interpersonal encounters. Furthermore, the social and emotional withdrawal associated with depression may function as a means to "buy time out," in order to reset one's cognitive expectations after significant loss.[26]

3.7. *Synthesis*

The last characteristic of the developmental model to be discussed is the fact that any assessment aims at a final synthesis, describing the entire person, not just a disorder. The entire assessment summarizes all aspects of the person: this includes strengths and weaknesses in addition to symptoms, signs, and deficiencies. This synthesis is achieved in the formulation of the case, which goes beyond the diagnosis and draws upon the entire clinical knowledge base regarding this person's past and present symptoms and habitual functioning.

4. Establishing a Developmentally Informed Diagnosis

What are the implications of the developmental model for clinical practice? We suggest that successful clinical practice is based on a blend of evidence-based medicine, consensus clinical judgment (such as the guidelines outlined in practice parameters), and practice-based evidence. In addition, we also expect that some practices are self-evidently effective — *e.g.* social control of violent individuals.[27] The remainder of the chapter specifies the steps necessary to produce a comprehensive case formulation, which includes diagnosis, profiles both normal and disturbed areas of functioning, and addresses each of the biopsychosocial domains.

4.1. *What are the sources of information?*

Using the child as an informant in obtaining the history, or even symptom description, is perfectly admissible when the patient is older than 11 but becomes increasingly problematic with younger children. A young child's capacity to self-observe and report on his/her own bodily and mental functioning, behavior, or inner state is quite limited because of cognitive factors. In fact, pre-schoolers are extremely vulnerable to suggestion and lead questioning.[28] As such, parental report is absolutely necessary when dealing with pre-schoolers, and is highly recommended when working with school-aged children. However, rarely if ever are the child's parents dispassionate observers and accurate reporters of problem behaviors. A great deal of interference can be generated by parental guilt (whether right or wrong), their own desire to appear competent (or at times incompetent) in the eyes of the clinician, and frequently, by a parent's own mental health symptoms. In many cases, contact with other collateral sources is helpful, such as school administrators, teachers, and primary care physicians. This is explicitly required in some diagnoses (such as disruptive behavior disorder and ADHD), but is good clinical practice in most cases.

In adolescents, a similar divergence between self and parental report occurs, but for very different reasons. The adolescent possesses all the cognitive equipment necessary to accurately report symptoms and functioning. However, there are motivational factors which may augment the wish to conceal (or minimize) what might be deemed risky and/or pathological behavior. As we develop into adolescents, we gain new and more effective ways of deceiving others as well as ourselves.[29]

4.2. *Descriptive phenomenology, symptoms, signs, and tests*

As a first step we always elicit chief complaints, symptoms, and signs. Most clinics use initial paper and pencil screening instruments[30–32] to help clinicians focus on the subsequent clinical inquiry, supplemented by some developmental history forms. Usually, these instruments are completed before the actual clinical encounter takes place.

Most sessions begin with parents and patient in the clinician's office. The first initial question to be answered is what each party's understanding is regarding the purpose of the office visit and what roles people have within the family system. Then, we ask parents and child to separate and conduct our clinical examination. Further instruments can be completed at this time, expanding our view of the patient's adaptive status and habitual functioning. The exact scales utilized will vary by age and specific diagnosis.

After careful rapport building with parents and patient, we allow time for a more free flowing assessment period where patients describe to the best of their abilities the problem, their developmental history, and their strengths, and assets. We facilitate the flow of information and save probing questions for later while taking great care to note specific points of interest to be explored in greater detail. We then proceed to either use portions of or complete structured interviews, depending on the presenting problem and our relative level of certainty that we are capturing the essentials of the case. These interviews tend to be tiring, tedious, and lengthy. We allow for sufficient time and breaks to maintain everyone's good will and cooperation.[33–36] At times, we employ simplified and less time-consuming structured interviews, such as the MINI.[37] We usually add self-report scales, and structured or semi-structured interviews which can give greater details to specific areas of dysfunction or determine caseness.[38–42] These scales often are used to track core symptoms over time, as is now suggested as basic clinical practice in several practice parameters.[43–45]

This initial part of the assessment elicits mostly symptoms, or subjective reports of distress and dysfunction by patient and parent. As we proceed into the structured interview, we gradually shift into eliciting signs of disorder, as they are observable by us. This begins with a formal and age appropriate mental status exam.[46]

The question of a physical exam is a complicated one that requires careful consideration. It is good medical practice to have a physical exam available. Whether it is wise to obtain such as a psychiatrist very much depends on the case in question and what types of exams are conducted. When issues of abuse and sexual abuse are being considered, it is not wise to conduct this investigation as a treating psychiatrist. To do so is fraught with potential problems, as a recent case in California vividly illustrates.[47] Furthermore, in cases of eating disorders or oppositional defiant disorders, where there is a great deal of defensiveness and fear of medical intrusion, physicals are not an innocuous procedure. At the very minimum, we require that the child has a recent (within the past six months) physical on file from their primary care physician. We usually obtain weight, height, body mass index, blood pressure, and resting heart rate with the child fully clothed in a semiprivate area. Any child requiring a more detailed assessment is referred to our pediatric colleagues, who are then asked to comment on specific problems, *e.g.* if there are any cardiac contraindications for the treatment of ADHD. In many cases (such as eating disorders and somatoform disorders), the pediatrician is an active member of the multidisciplinary treatment team.

As the basic sciences provide us with new insights regarding pathogenesis and syndromes, we can anticipate that laboratory findings, imaging, genetic investigations, and pharmacogenetic profiles will increasingly find their way into standard psychiatric practice. Currently, there is no standard set of tests that we obtain across all diagnostic groupings. Each diagnosis has, at the time of this writing, several biophysical investigations that are of interest. We discuss these as appropriate in the various chapters. In general, our attitude tends to be conservative regarding these investigations, as they are costly, invasive, and potentially hurtful. Inasmuch as they help us prevent diagnostic uncertainty and track adverse side effects of medications, we will not hesitate to use them after appropriate preparation of parent and child.

Detailed psychological assessment (personality, intelligence, learning, adaptation, education, vocation, neuropsychology) is available to all of us, but is not part of any standard assessment package across all diagnostic groupings. Such assessments are part of the core assessment of neuropsychiatric syndromes, such as mental retardation and pervasive developmental disorders. They should strongly be considered in evaluating disorders of aggression, social behavior, and attention; otherwise, we tailor our assessment to the problem areas at hand.

4.3. *Developmental history*

The developmental diagnostic approach relies heavily on an extensive developmental history. Such a history includes, but is not limited to, the cataloging of maturational milestones. Additionally, we are also always concerned with the child's successful mastery of crucial tasks at different key phases of development.[7] The longitudinal cataloguing of competencies, adaptive successes and failures goes beyond the history of symptom development. It addresses all domains and reports on functions that are not necessarily contained in diagnostic algorithms.

The concept of phases is helpful for scientists and practitioners to understand normal and abnormal from the developmental perspective.[48,49] Phases are circumscribed periods in a person's life that are characterized by groupings of certain capacities, tasks, and achievements. Erikson (1970) provided an initial template for phases from the point of view of global psychological adjustment.[50] Most recently, this progression has been updated and refined by Sroufe and Rutter (1989).[51] Table 1 outlines a progression of developmental tasks by domains of functioning that we have found quite useful in our practice. Note that as tasks are

Table 1: Key Components of the Developmental Assessment

1. Chief complaint: A summary of what ails the patient, predominantly in their view and as much as possible in their words.
2. History of present illness: The initial development of a timeline of difficulties where the clinician looks for links to life events and normative and non-normative stressors.
3. Current life circumstance: An assessment of how much all these problems interfere with the five major domains of life — psychological, recreational, academic/vocational, interpersonal, and basic biological.
4. Family history: A tally of disorders in the family of origin.
5. Medical history: Associated general health status of the patient.
6. Mental status exam: An assessment of the patient's mental faculties at the present time — orientation, memory, thought, speech, attention, affect, mood, sleep, appetite, intellect, education, judgment, insight, and the presence of symptoms as observed by the clinician.
7. Descriptive diagnosis: An initial tally of disorders defined by the clustering algorithms of the DSM or ICD system.
8. Temporal context: Patient's present phase of development, along with a tally of what tasks s/he faces currently.
9. Social context: A description of the social network the patient is embedded in (micro-, endo-, meso-, and exosystemic) and the patient's relationship to it: pre- or postconformist or conformist.[83]
10. Developmental and maturational history and timeline: An extended investigation of the patient's maturation with special attention to temporal sequences and intercurrent events in his/her life, as well as alterations in the social network.
11. Adaptive history: Mastery of previous developmental tasks (infancy, preschool, school age, preadolescence, adolescence, young adulthood, middle adulthood, late adulthood, early senescence, senescence), along with a tally of unresolved issues.
12. Self-regulation: Ways of coping, defense reactions under stress, locus of control in self-efficacy, self-image (real and ideal), and the hierarchical ordering of states of mind.
13. Vulnerabilities: A tally of risk factors this patient has for specific disorders.
14. Resilience: A tally of protective factors and strengths that are not impacted by the disorder at hand.
15. Residua of previous disorders: Leftover symptoms of previous problems, isomorphic to symptoms experienced previously, but of a lesser degree.
16. Sequelae of previous disorders: Leftover dysfunctions, not necessarily part of the earlier disorder.
17. Positive impact of current disorder on patient, their social context, or other domains.

achieved in each phase and domain, subsequent developments build on this achievement. The reader is referred to a more complete discussion of this model in Patricia Miller's book.[9]

It is useful to think of these phases in humans as less rigidly defined than in lower-level organisms. Still, they are helpful to construct a template for expectations of what is normative and what types of interventions might be helpful. Thus, the clinician can chart dysfunction in a more comprehensive yet age-specific way, divided into five subcategories: psychological (*e.g.* self-esteem, self-regulation), basic biological (sleep, eating, fitness, hygiene); interpersonal (family, friends, superiors, peers, younger siblings); academic/vocational (grades, jobs); and interests, hobbies, and recreational (how they spend their free time and recharge their batteries).

Having established a descriptive diagnosis, the developmental clinician adds continuous variables in these domains to the categories to obtain a more fine-grained picture. An adolescent with anorexia nervosa whose functioning in the domains of school and recreation is relatively unimpaired differs significantly from another patient where this is not the case in terms of need for intervention and prognosis.[52] A child with somatoform disorder whose family is implicated in outright abuse has a very different prognosis from a child where somatoform disorder occurs in the context of a chronic illness and a supportive (if overinvolved) family. By their descriptive diagnosis alone, both of these children would appear the same. The descriptive system's Axis IV and V are too rudimentary to be helpful to the developmental clinician.

5. Special Consideration of the Conscious/Unconscious Mind and its Relationship to Symptoms, Syndromes, and Clinical Practice

In eliciting the core descriptive symptoms of syndromes and the reconstruction of a person's developmental history, we are brought face-to-face with a very elementary fact that differentiates psychiatric practice from the rest of medicine: we are habitually dealing with phenomena that have special ontological status. Mental states, such as are described in almost all syndromes in the descriptive diagnostic systems, are subjective, private. Patients have unique access to them.[53] But unlike most of the rest of medicine, we cannot relinquish our study of these states. For the pediatrician, in most cases, the complaint of a painful stomach can sooner or later be replaced by the results of a series of investigations, laboratory tests, X-rays, and physical findings that supplant the necessity for them to take into account the patient's subjective experience of pain, other than for compassionate reasons. The diagnosis of an inflamed appendix, and the tracking of response to subsequent treatment can all be made without any further reference to the patient's subjective report of either his/her pain or his/her affective state with respect to this illness.

In psychiatric practice this is not so, not now, and most likely not ever. Subjective Mental states are at the core of psychiatric diagnoses, with rare exceptions. They are ontologically irreducible to brain functioning. At the same time, they powerfully influence behavior, physiology, and hormones.[2] They do so in generating pathology, and restoring health. We have termed this "top-down" efficacy.[54] While we do not now,[53] and maybe never will,[55] understand how this is possible, the clinician must be aware of this fact, as it has several crucial implications for practice.

The descriptive diagnostic system deals with this reality by ignoring the differences in ontological status between its components of diagnoses. By putting anhedonia and sleep and appetite disturbance (in the case of major depression), or body image, distortions, weight loss, and amennorhea (in the case of anorexia) on the same definitional plane, the system pretends there are no differences between these symptoms. However, there is a critical and crucial difference that is overlooked by DSM. We can definitively establish the presence or absence of sleep or menses and the loss of weight and/or appetite without relying any further on the patient's report. This is impossible with anhedonia, body image distortion, fear of social contacts, flashbacks of PTSD, dissociative experiences, and countless other symptoms.

The developmental model is in a position to deal with this issue in a more realistic fashion, because it has built into its structure the assumption of evolving complexity. Private mental states simply become a matter of biological emergentism.[53] While these states may require special methods of assessment, these can be tested as reliable and valid.[56] Facing this reality is more principled and intellectually honest, allowing for more creative solutions. At the same time, this approach avoids an unrealistic methodological reductionism which holds out the false hope that one of these days we will not have to refer to any of these states,[2] because we will have imaging, hormones, or genetics take their place.

What are the crucial implications of this simple fact that our brain generates private, privileged states that form the core of psychopathology? There are several, which are outlined below.

1. To obtain a report on mental activity, the clinician needs to get a subjective report from the patient. This can be supplemented by observations from family and others about behavior, but one does not replace the other.

2. Because of developmental limitations, the patient's capacity to self-observe may vary. Generally speaking, the capacity to offer detailed introspective reports is a relatively late achievement (beginning around ages 7–8 and culminating in adolescence).

3. Because the patient has privileged access to these states, they may withhold or deliberately distort reports in order to protect themselves or others from embarrassment, harm, or other negative consequences. This greatly limits the value of structured diagnostic interviews which proceed in an algorithmic fashion, largely

ignoring this fact. A good example occurred in an interview of a 12-year-old boy in the same room with his mother. As the interviewer, a very senior child psychiatric researcher, reached the module on bipolar disorder, he asked the boy: "Did you have any unusual sexual experiences lately?" The boy turned bright red, looked back at his mother, then laughed uncomfortably and answered with a long, drawn out "NOOOOO." The response was coded as negative by the researcher. Needless to say, the reliability of this response would be very much questioned by a developmental clinician.

4. Because most of our mental activity is unattended to and runs automatically, inquiries into special domains may need a skillful refocusing of the patient on such domains. A good example would be one's thoughts about one's identity. Rarely do we reflect about who we think we are as we are engaged in activities of daily living. But questions about what we hope to be in a few years will quickly bring to the fore problems in this area. Another complexity which is reintroduced by the explicit acknowledgement of the special ontological status of mental states is the fact that humans can be mistaken about them when we question them about how they are feeling and what problems they are experiencing. This can come about in a variety of ways, which call for different styles of intervention. For one, patients could simply be preoccupied with other matters and not paying attention to the fine fabric of their mental life. Calling their attention to simple incongruencies should correct the problem. On the other hand, we also know that patients sometimes have highly motivated ways of withholding or disguising mental states from others and even from themselves. Patients may respond defensively in order to protect certain impressions (*e.g.* that they are reputable, honorable people); they might find it difficult to face the negative impact of the mental state in question (*e.g.* facing the pain of grieving a lost one); or, perhaps, the state in question would call for a reappraisal of who they are (*e.g.* admitting to oneself that they are capable of lustful or vengeful acts).

5. Subjective reports can be defensively distorted. In contradistinction to conscious dissimulation, defensive distortion involves deception of oneself and others. The defensive patient gives an answer that he/she believes in but that is at variance with the facts. Defensive withholding and distortion can be an important part of the clinical picture for diagnosis and treatment. Establishing a diagnosis of depression or post-traumatic stress disorder in someone who is deeply vested in appearing invulnerable and strong (like in soldiers exposed to loss and extreme threat; or hardened juvenile delinquents who have to appear tough to survive in a world of extreme threat) can be challenging.

In a recent study, we found that the defensiveness of patients leads to symptom minimization on self-report, as always, but also influences interviewers on structured interviews so that they underreport symptoms.[57] Girls and boys high in defensiveness were much less likely to be diagnosed with multiple comorbid conditions than their less defensive counterparts. Additionally, adolescent subjects characterized by a repressive adaptive style were usually assigned higher GAF scores by objective raters. At the very least, we must assess unconscious and preconscious mental states when we examine patients and attempt to arrive at a complete diagnostic picture, especially in those individuals who have a high need to avoid negative self-representation.

We are aware that this complex layering we are describing creates some difficulty for the clinician in deciding what problems they are encountering. Mental states must not only be described and collected, but also a decision must be made as to whether the description we obtain is truthful. If it is not, then we have to be prepared to see what deception is taking place: conscious or unconscious/automatic. By contrast, the current medical disease model makes no such complex assumptions. If the clinician queries the patient about a symptom, the answer is assumed to be given in earnest. As noted above, this stance is perhaps overly optimistic and naïve, and may lead to inaccurate assessment and flawed treatment.

More recently, increasingly sophisticated ways of measuring different aspects of the distortion of mental states have become available. These include analysis of facial expressions and gestures, which can be contrasted to verbal expressions of emotion and behavior: any discrepancies between the two are noted[15]; examination of paralinguistic properties in speech that may indicate emotional perturbance and conflict[58]; and characterization of narrative forms of relaying negative events that may indicate an avoidance of emotionally charged material.[59] These new methodologies enhance the clinician's ability to identify disavowed, avoided, unattended, and barely articulated mental states, which may have bearing on the diagnosis of psychopathology.

At the same time, we have also acquired increasingly psychometrically sophisticated methods of characterizing normative defensive processes which effect special layers of conscious and unconscious thoughts.[60] We can now successfully track mental states that are conflicted, and processes that distort mental states and their content.

The "unconscious" we are describing here is different than the original description by Freud, which was a hydraulic model of instincts driving the mental apparatus. It is also different than the unconscious process posited by modern cognitive psychology, which refers to the mechanistic underpinnings of mental operations, which are not accessible to conscious examination.[53] By contrast, our definition of unconscious refers to the existence of a network of dispositions, motives, attitudes, and beliefs that operate outside of one's awareness and have significance for diagnosis and treatment. These unconscious dispositions can be made conscious by giving them the appropriate attention. One example would be the patient who professes to want to be in treatment, but regularly comes late for his/her appointments and even forgets some altogether. An appropriate intervention would be to focus on the discrepancy between professed motive and actual behavior. Such a discussion might lead to a whole set of conflicting emotions and attitudes about dependency and reliance on authority figures, or financial problems which require the containment of other pleasurable activities in exchange for being able to pay for treatment. Self-deception is most commonly found in cases of long-term mental states (dispositions), such as beliefs, attitudes, and emotional states, all of which form the backbone of many mental disorders. Anhedonia may be just that or it may be the expression of significant conflicts about enjoyment for fear of appearing wanton and reckless. Thinking that one is overweight despite all evidence to the contrary may disguise a profound sense of self-hatred.

6. Social Environment

As we briefly discussed above, contextual factors shape the internal program in normal and abnormal development. The developmental model is inherently interactionist, and emphasizes the interplay between internal, intraindividual variables and external forces in the causation, precipitation, and maintenance of psychopathology, as well as its treatment. The following gives some practical hints as to how to approach the assessment of this important aspect of a person's life. For clinical purposes, Bronfenbrenner's distinctions of micro-, meso-, exo-, and macrosystemic components, derived from his Ecological Systems Theory[61] can be helpful to clarify this point.

Microsytems are defined as those that are immediately present and influential (*e.g.* the mother for infants, the family for preschoolers, the classroom for school-age children). The mesosystem consists of two microsystems interacting (*e.g.* family and classroom), and the exosytem is the external environment, which indirectly influences the child (*e.g.* parental work place). Finally, the macrosystem refers to the larger sociocultural influences that shape the family and child (*e.g.* being part of the Latino Community in California).

Importantly, the relative configuration and power of the psychosocial context will vary with the age of the patient. The younger the child, the more potent the direct influence of micro- and mesosystems; the influence of exo- and macrosystems would be filtered through the parents. In older children, and for certain late adolescents, exo- and macrosystems have major direct influences of the child, as is all too evident in eating disorders and disorders of aggression. Parental microsystems and their mesosystemic interactions with the child's social environment recede in importance. Other finer distinctions of the characterization of social context have been made in research (*e.g.* shared and nonshared)[18] and can also be used for clinical purposes.

The patterns of interactions with the social context are also important to consider. On the one hand, there are the familiar traumatic life events that strike, usually without warning, and leave a devastating impact. These are particularly important in the discussion of psychiatric trauma (Chapter 8). However, it is important to recognize that traumatic events do not have to be outside of ordinary human experience: the death of a grandparent to a teenager is a normative event, one that is to be expected to occur in this age group, yet depending on the circumstance, can be traumatic or evoke only mild grief. The distinction between normative and non-normative stressors is an important one, as we assess the allostatic load generated by life events.[62] We should expect that normative stressors should not lead to a major decompensation. If psychopathology occurs in the wake of such an event, it should alert us to the possibility of a special vulnerability or risk in this patient. Isolated normative traumatic events can also exert potent negative influences because they permanently alter the conditions under which children and adolescents live. Two examples are parental loss at an early age and the children of divorced parents.[63]

Another pattern of importance is the slow accumulation of adversities over long spans of time, such as are found in the pathogenesis of disruptive behavior disorders[64] and under the impact of chronic pediatric illness, that can have devastating effects which are barely noticed initially, but become fully evident in adolescence.[65]

The precise nature of disorder determines the relative importance of social context for pathogenesis. The influence is paramount in the pathogenesis and treatment of disorders of aggression, psychiatric trauma, and eating. On the other hand, in profound neuropsychiatric disorders such as autism, mental retardation, and Rett syndrome, psychosocial contextual influences are relatively minor in terms of pathogenesis. Contextual factors may be important for precipitation of behavioral crises and maintenance of pathological adjustment.

At the same time, even in cases where there is an overwhelming role for environmental events in the precipitation and maintenance of psychopathology, the developmental model is still interested in individual vulnerabilities, which may contribute to adverse outcomes.[66,67] Simple, univariate causal models are usually not considered as possessing enough explanatory force to account for the pathogenesis of psychopathology. An array of interactions between an individual and his/her environment are thought to be the most useful models to consider.

Context can be important in more subtle and complicated ways by maintaining existing maladaptation. These are the insights of the social learning theory model, proposed by Bandura.[20] Sometimes patients seek out social contexts that accommodate and perpetuate their psychopathology. This is the case in an antisocial child, who associates with antisocial peers rather than giving up antisocial exploits. Having grown up in lawless and unstructured circumstances, which either reinforced and or modeled aggressive behavior, the antisocial child has come to enjoy the advantages of his maladaptive aggression. Humans carry the results of our deficient interactions with the environment within us in the form of perceptual distortions, misinterpretations, and misguided expectancies. These contribute to humans' appetitively seeking out environments which reinforce existing patterns of thinking, feeling, and behavior. One of the strongest predictors of relapse in substance-abusing adolescents is their affiliation with substance-abusing peers (see Chapter 12 of this volume). The avoidance of traumatogenic environments prevents the mastery of what has happened. Avoidance of exposure to phobic stimuli prevents deconditioning. Most forms of psychopathology have a self-perpetuating quality that needs to be expected, assessed, factored into our treatment plans, and counteracted by specific interventions. Psychopathology can also be adaptive, however strange this may seem. To ask a patient to improve is in most cases to ask them to step out of a familiar and perhaps more or less comfortable ecological niche. Our invitation may not be met with the enthusiasm we expect.

7. Dysfunction Beyond Syndromes

Because of its process orientation, the developmental model also seeks to capture the *forms frustes* of disorders. Prodromes, residuals, and sequelae of disorder are important targets of diagnosis and intervention, especially if they interfere with developmental progression. Presence of a prodrome might lead to preventive interventions in the absence of fully syndromal illness, while careful tracking of residual problems or sequelae of disorder is important as the patient transverses nodal points in development.

Because of this special attention to factors that promote disorder, a developmental approach to psychopathology has an important link to other sciences. For example, epidemiology, the study of diseases and risk factors in populations, is important to define the abnormal and normal. Epidemiology also helps to characterize specific risk and protective factors, which hinder normal development and adaptation. Epidemiology provides information about the possibilities for early intervention and prevention. The link to public health is an important one, and may point to interventions in the environment rather than the individual. Sometimes these interventions are with family or friends of the patient. At other times, the clinician will actively consult with broader systems, such as the school.

The ability to influence these systems is a vital component of a developmentally based practice.

Change in response to intervention is also more complex in a developmental model than in a simple disease model. Because there are internal organizational forces that may influence adjustment in a certain direction, the response to intervention may not be rapid or uncomplicated. The individual has his or her own internal set of processes that equilibrate adjustment to change. These processes can be cognitive, emotional, or otherwise, and may change the direction of adjustment toward or away from treatment goals. Progress in treatment will often not be linear, but more like a series of equilibrating steps. Repeated applications of interventions are required to move an individual along the path toward healing. In the process of recovery, we would expect to encounter relapse, although not necessarily to levels encountered at baseline, followed by continued healing and growth.

8. Case Formulation: A Brief History

The endpoint of a developmental assessment is the case formulation, where an attempt is made to coalesce all that is known into a coherent picture, which will guide future intervention and practice. As the developmental clinician formulates a case he/she seeks to establish special strengths and protective factors in addition to establishing symptoms, risks, and vulnerabilities. An assessment includes a careful weighing of those factors in a patient's life which will promote development and allow for spontaneous recovery. We have shown in two prospective outcome studies with conduct and eating disordered adolescents[68–70] that such subtyping beyond comorbidities leads to significant predictions of prospective outcome 4.5 and 6 years after the establishment of diagnoses in both internalizing and externalizing disorders.

Throughout the history of medicine, psychiatry, and psychology, two different schools of thought have dominated the clinician's approach to a case formulation. Both schools are equally important in understanding the concept of the psychiatric case formulation that we outline in this chapter, which integrates components from both historical approaches and defines new concepts that are important for today's clinicians.

The psychoanalytic or psychodynamic approach is rooted in the theories of Sigmund Freud, which were the mainstay of American psychiatric and psychological thinking in the early half of the 20th century. It is based on the idea that individuals are often unaware of the unobservable, unconscious factors that influence their emotions and behavior. Freud was the first to recognize and define the role of the dynamic unconscious in influencing both normal and abnormal behavior. This was a revolutionary idea during a time when positivism, the idea that people could ascertain real knowledge about themselves and their environment and exert judicious control over both, was the dominant ideology.

The concept of a psychiatric case formulation was originally developed for use in psychodynamic approaches.[71] The seminal work of Perry *et al.*[72] introduced the psychodynamic case formulation. In their model, the clinician organized his formulation into four categories: summarizing statement, description of non-dynamic factors, psychodynamic explanation of central conflicts, and predicting responses to therapeutic intervention. In 1989, Theodore Shapiro argued for the use of a clinical case formulation approach in the evaluations of children and adolescents. In his article, he debunked the myths that clinical case formulations are only useful for long-term treatments, that they were only useful for psychodynamic therapy, that they were primarily training devices and not useful in actual clinical practice, and that the case formulation must be all-inclusive, lengthy, and elaborate.[73]

The biopsychosocial approach, on the other hand, has its origins in the work of Meyer and Engel. From the early 1900s until his death in 1950, Swiss neuropathologist and psychiatrist Meyer was responsible for shaping many key issues in the practice of American psychiatry. Meyer taught what was called a psychobiological approach, which required the clinician to research and note all biological, psychological, and social factors relevant to a case. He strongly emphasized the need to collect detailed case histories of patients, paid special attention to the social and environmental background to a patient's upbringing, and was well-known for constructing timelines of major events in a patient's life. In Meyer's view, causes of disease operated in a summative, rather than linear fashion.[74] As such, diagnosis of illness or disease was secondary to a humanistic assessment of the patient as a person.

Despite the work of both Freud and Meyer, medicine became increasingly biomedical during the 20th century, and this approach was extended to psychiatric illnesses. Engel's great insight was to point out that the reductionist, biomedical approach, "left no room for the social, psychological, and behavioral dimensions of illness."[75] Influenced by the general systems theory pioneered in the 1950s by von Bertalanffy, Engel called instead for the adoption of an inclusive, systems-based framework that took into account "the patient, the social context in which he lives, and the complementary system devised by society to deal with the disruptive effects of illness, that is, the physician role and the health care system." The third edition of the DSM, published in 1980, drew heavily from Engel's biopsychosocial paradigm to introduce a system of five axes for comprehensive assessment of a patient's mental and emotional health. This system of multiple axes was designed to "promote the application of the biopsychosocial model in clinical, educational, and research setting."[76]

A review of the current literature indicates that of late there has been a renewed interest in encouraging the usage of psychiatric case formulations.[77–81] Formulations can be psychodynamic, cognitive-behavioral, interpersonal, emotion-focused, or stemming from any other theoretical orientation. The interested reader is referred to Eells[82] for a synthesis of the many different approaches to case formulation. Regardless of theoretical orientation, case formulations must always be informed by culturally specific knowledge about the patient,[79–81] as cultural factors can impact the expression of symptoms, the patient's understanding of and beliefs about mental health treatment, and the emerging therapeutic alliance. This chapter describes an integrative approach to case formulation, incorporating components of psychodynamic, systems, and developmental schools of thought to provide a comprehensive description of the patient in context.

9. Components of the Developmental Assessment

We now discuss each of the items from Table 1 in detail.

1. Chief complaint: It is crucial to obtain this information at the beginning of the encounter. As discussed above, standardized screening tools can be utilized, but should not take the place of a narrative self-report of symptoms. As a rule, we allow for the first 10 min of the evaluation to have the patient report uninterruptedly; this is done in order to facilitate the formation of a therapeutic alliance, and also because much can be gleaned by the manner in which a patient presents himself/herself and his/her difficulties. While the patient proceeds to describe their dilemmas, we start forming an initial map of where to probe and go next. We also note the particular illness patterns and templates that emerge and seem relevant, holding them in abeyance until we can probe details. Ultimately we need a tally of problems, how severe and chronic they are and how much they interfere with function in all the domains in the patient's life, what helps the patient tolerate the symptoms and what appears to make them worse.

2. History of present illness: This is a fairly standard psychiatric procedure. After knowing about all that is wrong, we now explore the time patterns of all that is wrong. This is actually the beginning of a developmental timeline: we try to assess when signs and symptoms appear and disappear, whether that seems to occur entirely independent of life events, and whether the events which precipitate the problem can be judged to be within or outside of the range of normal human experience.

3. Current life circumstance: An assessment of several domains of functioning, including psychological, recreational, academic, relational, and basic biologic. In the domain of psychological functioning, we assess the patient's mood and affect, ability to think and express themselves, attend to tasks and demonstrate persistence, how they see themselves and how realistic this seems to be, how they are able to judge complex situations, especially social ones, how well they understand what is happening to them, and how idiosyncratic such an understanding is. We probe their self-esteem, their identity, and their predominant modes of self-regulation and handling of stressful events. We attempt to chart what their interests and passions are, and whether they are future, present, or past.

In the domain of recreation, do we see evidence that there is a regular pattern of play and unstructured enjoyment? Are the activities chosen more intellectual, physical, or both? Is there a history of athletic achievement, and in what phase of that process is the person now? Do we see evidence for high risk taking or impulsive behavior? Is alcohol or drugs a large part of the recreational process? Are the recreational endeavors lonely pursuits or do they involve people, especially family? Do others find these activities enjoyable? How open is this person to novel experiences?

In the academic and vocational domain we inquire about status, success, and failure. We want to know about imminent and distant goals and how realistic they seem to be. We want to assess educational attainment, difficulties with such and considerations to remedy missed educational opportunities. We try and see how the interests of the person map onto the job they are engaged in. We try and assess how much the person sees their work as a career and hopes to actively grow in the job, influence the field, or, alternatively, how much they see it as a means to an end. Is there a balance between this domain and other ones in their life? What is the ordering of importance of the domains? Does the job always come first?

Interpersonally, we assess the whole range of relationships the person is involved in, both intimate and superficial: peer relations and relations with superiors and inferiors, familial and extra-familial interactions, friends and foes, longevity of relationships and legal transitions (marriage, divorce, separations). In all these, a good entrée is the question of how satisfied the person is with their interpersonal orbit and how much the symptom they just reported seems to impact the domain. As we show in this progression from infancy to adulthood, the endosystemic (familial) component of a person is predominant in infancy, but then progressively contracts in scope and importance over the next two decades. What takes its place is the expansion of the extra-familial relationships and ultimately one's involvement in community and society.

Finally, we are very interested in assessing the impact of what ails the patient on their domain of basic biological functioning. We inquire about weight and height and plot these on growth curves. We are interested in the regular circadian interplay between appetite and satiety, dietary intake, and balance of meals. Sleep is carefully assessed, plotting time to fall asleep, repeated awakenings, final wakening, as well as quality of sleep; is it restful, deep, or shallow? Is it disrupted by nightmares and dreams? We measure pulse and blood pressure as basic indicators of levels of arousal and autonomic responsivity. We inquire about health habits, medical problems, and current medications, as well as adherence to physician's recommendations. We attempt to get some feel for physical fitness, by asking about exercise and ability to do sit-ups. We inquire about sexual habits and expression of sexual needs. We are interested in hygiene and standards for appearance. We try and assess the degree to which a day is fairly well predictable and structured in its various activities.

The expectation is that not all areas are going to be equally affected, and preserved functioning in some will ultimately be useful to exploit in promoting the patient's recovery. Thus, an eating disorder patient with preserved ability to do well in school, handle stress maturely and to face adversity proactively when it occurs will ultimately have a different outcome from those whose functioning in these areas is impaired.

It is important not only just to ask about the various symptom interferences with these functions, but also to develop some understanding of the positive aspects of each domain. Such a profile of preserved and perhaps even better than average levels of functioning in all those domains gives us a more realistic picture of the pervasiveness of disturbances, their severity, and impact on a person's life and the set of preserved skills and strengths which we can use to develop a more realistic treatment plan.

4. Family history: We are now in a position to appreciate the familial clustering of certain disorders in mental health. Eating, mood, anxiety, schizophrenia, substance abuse, and conduct problems are among the many problems that present in familial clusters. While it is premature at this point to point to any firmly established genetic factors in the genesis of most psychopathology, (except for certain forms of mental retardation), we have other interests in documenting familial medical and psychiatric disorder. There is fairly good evidence that children from families with at least one psychiatrically ill adult are at higher risk for disorder themselves, although the specific link between disorders is not always established. We are seeking to appreciate the characteristics of the patient's family which might pose special problems altogether. Such an understanding is particularly important in those patients where we have some reason to believe that the family is overreacting to the child's illness or perhaps even inducing it. Second, the treatment of another family member may provide an important lead as to what might be effective with our patient. This is particularly true for psychopharmacological interventions.

5. Medical history: One of the most difficult aspects of mental health assessment is the fact that many psychiatric disorders can be brought on secondarily by medical disorders that are not immediately diagnosed, but cause many of the symptoms. While a detailed discussion of medical history is beyond the scope of this book, there are certain systems of bodily functioning that are notorious in generating psychiatric symptoms. The central and peripheral nervous system are obviously prime candidates, and primary disease processes of an inflammatory, neoplastic, degenerative, or traumatic nature need to be included in our thinking. Other systems commonly associated with psychiatric symptoms include the endocrine system (which is well known to mimic psychosis, depression, eating disorders, and anxiety states in particular), the digestive system (depression and eating problems), the kidneys, and the reproductive system. In any case, no matter how seemingly psychiatric the disorder before us, a quick review of systems should also be part of any good developmental assessment, if only to tally the bodily functions which seem to be affected by the primary disorder.

6. Mental status exam: This exam is the major parallel to the physical examination performed by any physician as s/he assesses a disorder. The goal of the exam is to personally create an inventory of mental functioning at the present time and map it onto the problems described by the patient in the previous part of the exam. Attention is paid to discordance or concordance of symptoms found here and reported by the patients. The mental status is clearly an "expert exam" of the patient's faculties, and thus is best performed toward the end of the first encounter, after a certain amount of working alliance has been established. It should be introduced by some qualifying remarks about its intrusive nature and the testing of faculties that are usually presumed to be intact (*e.g.* memory). Each practitioner usually has a staple of pet procedures to examine sensorium, thought, reasoning, judgment, memory, orientation, affect, mood, *etc.*, and there are some standardized versions of the exam available.[46] More detailed exams may be necessary and may best be administered *via* standardized psychometric tests.

7. Descriptive diagnosis: As much as is possible, the clinician will now decide on what are the most likely diagnoses that generate problems. More often than not, the clinician will find considerable overlap between multiple diagnoses, all presenting at the same time. Some effort should be made to assign primacy to some of them, keep the number of diagnoses to a reasonable minimum, and establish which deserve the predominant attention in treatment.

8. Temporal context: Although we previously noted the patient's chronological age, we now make an attempt to assign a developmental phase to this patient, which informs us as to where in the life cycle the patient fits and what general developmental tasks need to be accomplished. Erikson's schema of developmental phases

and their core tasks is still a very valuable tool.[50] We also note, however, whether the patient has embraced this phase as relevant, whether they have "leftover" or unresolved issues from previous stages, and we note how these issues will affect the mastery of the current stage.

9. Social context: The description of the patient's social network is of great importance, especially when dealing with extremely young, infirm, or dysfunctional patients. The examination of social context relates directly to the domain of interpersonal functioning. Relationships with parents, peers, significant others, and subordinates are important to assess, as well as how much the present disturbance is influencing each one of these subdomains. Much developmental research has focused on the study of the relationship to the primary caretaker, as it was thought that this relationship was paradigmatic for all future relationships. While it has become quite clear that patterns of attachment relate to adjustment and choice of partners,[84] it also has become clear that most humans show a great capacity for flexibility in this regard. Relationships are usually quite complex and not rigidly modeled after relationships with primary caregivers. There also is little evidence for a critical sensitive period, such as that exists in ducks or geese.[85] Nevertheless, a close and exacting examination of the patient's primary relationships is still important, as we know that such relationships form the first internalized templates of how one navigates in the interpersonal world, and thus we can derive considerable knowledge from these templates about the patient's expectancies and their future relationship to us as we prepare to treat them. An abused child most likely will expect to be hurt and exploited; a conduct-disordered child will see the world and its rules as unfair, capricious, and unjust. A depressed person who lost his/her mother will see the world as full of disappointments, while an anxious person raised by a hypercritical mother or father will expect attack and criticism every step of the way.

10. Developmental and maturational history and timeline: We begin by creating a longitudinal plot of the patient's life early in assessment, and we advocate that information gathered in treatment or at later follow-up sessions be added to the timeline as appropriate. Usually, timelines by year are most serviceable, but in very young and in very old patients, we may change the scale to reflect their short and long lives (*e.g.* months or decades). The goal of this timeline is multifold. First, we wish to chart major events and life transitions (moves, illnesses, graduations, deaths, births). Next, we want to plot the emergence of symptoms in relation to these life events, recognizing that this is retrospective and difficult, but usually worthwhile, especially if we rely on collateral informants. Finally, we want to add developmental and maturational progressions and regressions in order to keep track of unresolved issues which may emerge in another form later on in life, or which will make transitions into new periods of development impossible (to marry without having dated will not work too well in cultures which emphasize mate

self-selection; expecting to be pregnant without ovulatory periods will usually result in disappointment).

As much as is possible, we will also keep track of early manifestations of psychopathology — not necessarily in the "classic" forms we have come to expect from the DSM. For instance, evidence from bipolar offspring suggests that is quite possible for certain disturbances to make their appearance very much earlier than was previously thought, if one takes into account the possibility that disorders may manifest themselves in nonisomorphisms: the most common forerunner of bipolar disorder (BD) in children of bipolar parents is not classic BD, but ADHD.[86] Similarly, we may expect that eating disorders would show more difficulty with mood, self-regulation, and anxious affect and attachment[87–89] rather than classic dieting in preschool. The link between these states would not be through their phenomenology, but through the underlying processes which must be detailed and described.

11. Adaptive history: As we chart the developmental and maturational progress of the patient, it should also become quite clear what their adaptive history has been up to this point.[7] Which developmental tasks have been resolved? How successfully? Which continue to create problems? Were there certain periods in the patient's life which were more successfully dealt with, while others were quite difficult? Was the difficulty created by external problems, internal problems, or a combination of both?

12. Self-regulation: In the course of examining the various phases of life tasks, we should become aware of the patient's particular and habitual way of handling problems in terms of self-regulation. We have come to appreciate that ways of handling oneself in adverse circumstances are somewhat independent of psychopathology, and appreciating the way in which a particular person conducts himself under duress will actually add to our ability to predict how well they will do in the long run. Moreover, this also contributes to our overall understanding of how to best work with this particular patient.

The ultimate goal of self-regulation is to maintain a positive image of oneself as one negotiates difficult situations where they may not always be victorious. The person needs a certain sense of self-efficacy, which allows them to digest disappointments and frustrations without falling into a pessimistic and defeated stance. Very often, such self-regulatory maneuvers involve illusory assumptions of self-control, which can be quite efficacious if the situation allows for control on the part of the person. However, if the situation does not allow for the assumption of control on part of the individual, then increasingly frantic attempts to assume such can be extremely counterproductive.

Coping implies a conscious and effortful way of dealing with a situation.[90] Most coping can be taught and learned and has important links to health risks[91] that are established as early as adolescence.

Defenses, by contrast, are generally more primitive ways of handling situations that are conflicted. Defenses constitute a kind of mental immune system, which preserves ability to function under conditions of immediate threat and challenge. They buy time for more suitable responses, but because of their more or less appropriate nature they also can lead to complications and adverse outcomes. Defenses operate outside of a person's awareness, are reflexive and quick, and usually result only in temporary solutions to problems. Defenses are probably not learned phenomena, but are most likely based on temperamental characteristics, which become refined in the process of socialization. As a child becomes aware of his/her habitual and reactive ways of handling problems, he/she develops suitable "cognitive tags" that identify the particular reaction. It is this package of reaction and cognitive tag that becomes a defense pattern. The cognitive tag enables us to "get a hold" of the defense, identify it, and analyze its appropriateness in certain contexts. Once this pattern is understood by the patient, we can then work on substituting more useful responses.

They are most often evoked in times of threat when the person is not completely in charge and unable to rationally prepare. There is a fair amount of evidence suggesting that defenses are distinct from coping,[91] thereby making their own independent contributions to adjustment. They also cluster in predictable ways, resulting in more adaptive and a less adaptive continuum (immature and mature have been the traditional labels applied to these defense structures). Prospective and cross-sectional research supports the notion that defenses present specific risk for short- and long-term health, possibly by mediation of high- and low-health risk behaviors. Defense profiles provide useful information about aspects of personality functioning which are important to consider across different diagnoses. They are a proxy for assessing individual strengths and weaknesses in addition to symptoms. These defenses also provide information about a person's psychological maturity which in turn has implications for stress management and the way they utilize interventions.

13. Vulnerabilities: As we approach the end of the assessment, we want to make special notes regarding the presence of risk factors. These are factors that are not part of the specific symptom cluster of the descriptive diagnosis, but we want to keep track of in order to assess the antecedents that are present and have resulted in this particular diagnosis. In addition, it is useful to keep track of these risks, should we not be able to fully diagnose the patient. The DSM actually provides a category of diagnoses for those patients who do not have full-fledged syndromes. For instance, eating disorder NOS allows us to diagnose and treat a patient who is lacking some of the cardinal symptoms of Anorexia Nervosa (and recent research shows that many patients with clinically significant disturbances in eating may fit into the category of eating disorder NOS, which provides a

further critique of the limitations of the existing DSM diagnostic system). To further detail the picture, we can add a tally of all the present risks in order to form an impression of how close the patient actually is to becoming syndromally ill. Such a tally also opens the door for preventive intervention, if the patient is judged to be at extremely high risk for early deterioration. Thus, a young woman who has lost 15% of her weight, but denies a desire for thinness, will be treated differently if she comes from a lower class family, is outgoing and popular, comes from a family that is not particularly diet and health and fitness conscious, has a boyfriend, and is sexually active. By contrast, an upper class girl who manifests the same weight loss, but who has just become menstrual, is habitually inhibited and anxious, excels in school, and whose mother is a former model who currently runs a fitness firm would deserve much more of our attention and tracking.

14. Resilience: Comparatively speaking, we know much less in regards to protective factors and resilience than risk and vulnerability, because the field has been so busy developing criteria for pathology. Having now a much better way of assessing syndromes than ever before, it is equally important to devote attention to those factors in the case which offer protection and help, and which constitute islands of preserved functioning on which we may build certain aspects of treatment. Most commonly, diverse coping, social connectedness, academic achievement, even temperament, high levels of impulse control, humor, and other higher level defenses such as altruism, ability to distance oneself from a charged situation, seek out council and advice of others, and access to good schools and education have all been identified with good outcomes in the face of chronic adversity.

We prefer to tally risk and protective factors on a balance beam, ordering individual factors according to ecological, constitutional, endosystemic, mesosystemic, or exosystemic and achievement domains. The profile adds to our understanding of what forces are impacting the case and which ones we can rely on, strengthen or weaken by our interventions.

15. Residua of previous disorders: If there are symptoms present, we also attempt to see if they can be attributed to an unresolved episode of illness, which was perhaps not diagnosed or fully treated. Presumably, the patient will be more likely to relapse if there has been a time of full syndromal illness at some point, or we also can explore why this particular symptom was not fully treated and therefore remains active. We would then contemplate new approaches to help matters. The persistent absence of menses after weight restoration in anorexia nervosa is a good example. Amenorrhea is clearly part of the original diagnosis, yet correction of the menstrual absence might in fact trigger a recurrence of the disorder. To help the patient with the problem we might have to consider hormone substitution, an intervention that is usually not part of the original treatment.

16. Sequelae of previous disorders: Sequelae are dysfunctions based on previous disorders, which do not necessarily form part of the original symptom complex. While brought on by the disorder, they constitute deficits left behind after the original disorder has receded. As they are not part of the original problem, we would not necessarily expect the disorder to be present, or even easily induced, but we might have to consider new treatment to correct this dysfunction. Osteoporosis after a bout of anorexia nervosa is such a problem. Although it was not part of the original disorder, it was clearly caused by the prolonged absence of menstrual cycling in these patients, and as such, requires whole new treatments for its correction.

17. Positive valence and importance of the current disorder for the patient, their social context, or other domains: A surprising, unique, and complex part of the developmental assessment is the consideration of the positive adaptive value of the current disorder. In all but the most profound disturbances of the nervous system we can find some positive adaptive value to the patient. Temporal and social contexts have to be considered in order to establish the positive ecological values of problems. Life circumstances may not necessarily be relevant any longer, but symptoms may persist because behaviors that have positive adaptive value are very difficult to change, especially if symptoms arose during a developmental period in which there was pronounced dependency. For instance, if it was important to suppress emotional upset because of mother's depression, which rendered her unable to deal with regressive tantrums, and such an inability was combined with a constant and real threat of abandonment by the parent, stoic acceptance of stressful circumstances would have a high adaptive value, as would precocious functioning in a variety of domains.

Questions about positive adaptive value arise for several different reasons. Most of these reasons reflect the developmental understanding that mental health symptoms stand in a special relationship to the environment, unlike other simple disease processes. They are intentional — they have mental content, which is generated by the patient's life, either past or present. Many mental health symptoms are not simply expressions of an existing deficit, as the DSM proposes. They are at the same time expressions of a problem and an attempt to adjust to, cope with, and finally, to neutralize the problem. Because so much of psychopathology involves diverse aspects of the emotional system, which has the task of signaling problems of the commerce between the person and the environment, symptoms of disturbance cannot just be eradicated without creating new problems. Thus, depression is not just simply the powerful emotion of sadness, it is also emotion triggered by significant loss, and signals to the person to withdraw, reassess one's situation, and redirect one's attachment efforts in order to lead a happier life again.

Similarly, anxiety is not a simple release of noradrenergic discharge, but a signal of threat to one's integrity, and an invitation to flee and get to safety. Anger is not aggressive arousal, but a reaction to injustice, harm, and injury, and also a signal to attack and to set things straight, and so on. To take away a person's emotional reactivity — even if it were possible to do so — would handicap them in their efforts of daily living. To leave them without emotions would leave them without an important navigation device. Although we need to treat exaggerated and distorted expressions of emotionality, or reactions which are based on predominantly past but not current life circumstances, we also need to be aware that this navigational device is important to the patient, fulfills meaningful and needed functions in their lives, and cannot be treated as a useless artifact.

Additionally, some symptoms are means of symbolic expression and communication, which serve to as an indirect way of letting others know that something is profoundly wrong. Psychoanalysis termed this aspect of symptoms their "primary gain," referring to the fact that such symbolic expressions neutralized anxiety about certain conflicts and was particularly interested in this aspect of symptoms, and at times has grossly overestimated the importance of this aspect. Somatoform symptoms and conversion symptoms brought on by sexual abuse are in this category: we sometimes express symbolically how we were wronged, without running the risk of direct communication and exposure of the perpetrators on whom we are dependent. The symptom gives us access to resources without directly asking for them. By the same token, the vomiting up of precious food prepared by a loving mother is an angry gesture of rejection. The emaciation of anorexia is a symbol of the emotional starvation the patient experiences in a family, which seems to provide for everything while not providing for basic emotional needs.

Finally, some psychiatric symptoms grant the sufferer all the advantages of the traditional sick role: protection, succor and sustenance, the delay of demands, and even pecuniary gain. Such gains are often concentrated in the patient–therapist relationship, which is often idealized and experienced as a correction of all past emotional wrongs. There it needs to be dealt with in a transference/countertransference paradigm.

Such positive valence probably leads to surprising resistance when we begin to "heal" the patient. Unless we are prepared to encounter such resistance to letting go of what appear to be problematic behaviors and thoughts we will not be effective in dealing with these extremely complex pictures. However destructive the symptoms appear to be, we always should ask ourselves what positive role they have in the patient's life. It could be that the adaptive value was in a past phase of development, with primary attachment objects or other persons on which the person stood in a long relationship of dependency. Ultimately, we will have to deal with these positive aspects of disorder, to help the patient move into a definite phase of recovery and independence, and they will have to find substitutes for the gains the illness affords them.

10. A Concrete Example of the Developmental Diagnostic and Treatment Planning Process

Emily is a 17-year-old girl, referred for a second opinion for the treatment of her alcohol and drug abuse. She is comorbidly depressed. She has some past diagnoses, which are not active and only have some isolated symptoms (nightmares, but not full blown PTSD; some preoccupation with weight, but no drive for thinness, weight loss, or absence of menses; some periodic overeating and even purging which does, however, not cluster frequently enough to give her the diagnosis of bulimia). She is on antidepressants and involved in a rehabilitation program that uses a relapse prevention approach. She is not responding very well, having had three relapses within the past two months.

From a descriptive diagnostic perspective, we would not concern ourselves with the partial diagnoses of anorexia, bulimia, or PTSD, as she does not fulfill criteria at the present time. We would watch for a worsening of these symptoms, and/or their potential clustering into syndromes, but that would be the end of our interest in that cluster of problems. Our immediate course of action would be to consider intensification of her rehabilitation program, a change in medication, and potential consideration of Bipolar Disorder (she reported episodes of flighty speech and increased activity in her sales job, but as these were induced by the illicit use of amphetamines, she does not qualify for a diagnosis of bipolar disorder at this time). We would consider augmentation strategies. All these considerations would take us to point number 7 in Table 1.

The developmental approach would expand this vision considerably. To begin with, we would put the mentioned syndromes into a timeline, matching them up with potentially triggering external and internal events. We would appreciate that Emily was a reasonably happy girl until age 10, when her maternal grandfather died. She had a prolonged phase of mourning, which ultimately led to PTSD: Emily experienced nightmares, had intrusive visions of him returning, avoided places where he and she used to be together, and had difficulty with arousal, which manifested itself in disturbed and shallow sleep. This was not diagnosed or treated. The family did not discuss it, and the symptoms worsened at the onset of menarche. She turned from a happy, confident girl into a moody, anxious, and withdrawn one. Boys frequently teased her: she was taller than most and developing quite early. In her class, she was among the first to menstruate. She gained some weight, and then lost a good deal due to an intercurrent GI infection around age 13. She never gained that back, in fact she lost better than 15% of her weight altogether, and her menses stopped, much to her relief. In order to keep her weight low, she had to be on a highly restrictive diet regimen, despite her being extremely active in three sports at an elite level. Her dietary restrictions and weight loss were never diagnosed either, but did draw her parents intrusive attention. Consequently, Emily began overeating and purging after reading about such practices in teen magazines. This solved several problems: it diffused everyone's concern about her weight and eating, as she appeared to be eating normally. It kept her menses from recurring, which is not unusual in very active athletes. It dealt somewhat successfully with her ravenous hunger during her periods of restriction. At age 14, Emily began experimenting with drugs. She started with marijuana, but to her horror discovered that it greatly stimulated her already difficult to control appetite. She then sought out appetite suppressants and found that amphetamines fit the bill. They eliminated her appetite, kept her weight low, and temporarily picked up her irritable and depressed mood. To counteract the "wired" feeling she developed on amphetamines, she began using alcohol. The net effect of this whole cascade was that she became increasingly inefficient at her sport and in school. For a while the coaching staff ignored the obvious fact that she had multiple problems both physically and academically, because she was a star athlete. As her performance declined, she lost that status, became just another expendable teammate, and was suspended.

Expanding our vision even further, and including a view of her social and temporal context, we can refine our understanding of the case further. Her difficulties started in a phase of development which deals with the beginnings of separation from the family of origin. The problems culminated during a phase of development where Emily was expected to step out, define her education and career, and begin looking for a mate. She does not seem prepared to take these steps. Why?

Examining her social context, beginning with her family, we note that she is the youngest of four children. Her mother is an accountant, her father a teacher. Her mother's family history is unremarkable, but her father's is highly significant, as he came from a severely disordered background. His father had severe alcohol addiction, as did his two older sisters. He was the sole survivor of his nuclear family. His mother died when he was nine due to cancer, and father and sisters died of the consequences of their alcoholism when he was a young adult. Emily's father was a distant and severe figure, determined not to have similar problems occur in his family. His grim determination made him quite unforgiving and unapproachable, and difficult for a child such as Emily to relate to, especially in times of need and transgression. Emily's maternal grandfather took the place of the nurturer in this young woman's life. His death when Emily was 10 years old was devastating, as there was no ready substitute. Mother was an anxious and inhibited woman, playing second fiddle in the family and unable to provide much comfort and support. The young woman's scholastic and sports success by far surpassed her parents' achievements. Father's pride in her was solidly tied to her achievements, and any deviation from that pattern was simply not tolerated. As Emily began to feel the dual pressure of academic and athletic demands, she felt increasingly less able to meet them and unconsciously sought a way out of her dilemma without losing her one line of connection to father. The weight loss induced by her GI illness was a blessing, but to her horror, it did not relieve her from her role. Neither did any of the other developing symptoms, as coaches and parents ignored what was obvious. Emily had to become quite severely compromised for people to take note.

From this description, it should be quite clear why the original treatment plan was not successful. It addressed only the end phase of a process which began years ago and addressed only a part of the disturbances in multiple domains, while not opening up to exploration and examination of the processes leading to this patient's worsened state. It is very difficult to see how a treatment package with just medication and relapse prevention of drug abuse would do the job. Family sessions, explorative sessions attempting to link events and symptoms (which would not be obvious to the patient initially), planning for alternate role definitions, and nutritional and vocational advice all would play a role in the care of this patient. Exploration of her feelings about becoming a woman would be a core component of Emily's treatment plan. Her considerable strengths (such as her athletic ability, determination, and leadership skills) should be tallied and called upon. Her partial symptoms would be used to plot residual concerns, Vulnerabilities and risks that could be exacerbated in times of stress (such as when she moves out to attend college). Only then can we anticipate a good outcome for Emily.

11. Outcomes of Patients Treated in an Academic Practice with the Developmental Psychiatry Approach

In examining how this approach to the patient might be helpful, we had the opportunity to report on a 20-year follow-up on 34 patients who were treated with this approach by a senior clinician with 38 years of experience in the field (H.S.). The preliminary results of this naturalistic outcome were presented at the symposium "*Integrated Treatment: Psychotherapy and Psychopharmacology*" (Annual Meeting of the American Psychiatric Association, San Francisco, California, 2003.)

The patient cohort described was referred to this professor's private clinic. He provided all the treatment methods utilized, and collated treatments as per his formulation of each case.

The total patient sample comprised 34 patients (18 women, 16 men). Their mean current age was 30 with a standard deviation of 6 years (their ages ranged on follow up from 23 to 42). Their SES by Hollingshead Redlich 2 factor index was a mode of 2, with a range of 1–4, indicating upper middle class. Their mean age at the onset of disorder was mid-adolescence (M = 14; SD = 6, range = 12–18).

Their diagnoses at baseline were established by structured interviews (MINI). Established principal diagnoses at baseline were: major depressive disorder (10 patients); eating disorders (6 patients); generalized anxiety disorder (4 patients); oppositional defiant disorder (6 patients); attention deficit disorder (3 patients); substance use disorder (1 patient). Their NIMH CGI SEVERITY (CGI-S) score was 4.5 (SD = 0.9).

The follow-up period comprised 20 years with a 100% retention rate (range = 6–25 years). At that time, only 26.47% had an active diagnosis (4 anxiety, 3 mood and 2 ADHD). The remainder were diagnosis free. Their NIMH-CGS-S was 1.5 (SD = 0.5). 30% had a CGI-S score of 0. Their CGI-improvement (CGI-I) score mean was 1.6 (SD = 0.9), indicating very much improved. The worst patient showed no change (CGI-I = 4).

All patients were treated with integrated treatment packages. The mean doses of interventions were as follows: there was a mean of 28 days of sociotherapeutic treatment in inpatient, day treatment, or residential care. All patients received a mean of 20 family therapy sessions. Patients were treated an average of 40 months with medications (ranging from tranquilizers to SSRIs to atypicals and mood stabilizers at age appropriate dosages). The bulk of treatment consisted of 110 individual psychotherapy sessions with medication management. These interventions tended to cluster in the patterns illustrated in Fig. 1.

In terms of measures of habitual functioning, all patients completed the Response Evaluation Measure (REM-71)[92] and the Weinberger Adjustment Inventory (WAI)[11] on diagnosis and on final visit. These measures provided an enriching additional source of information about patients.

The CGI-S and CGI-I scores were the primary measures of outcome. Diagnoses established at baseline did not predict the CGI outcomes. However, all the subscales on the measure of habitual functioning did (all values $p < 0.05$). REM-71 factor 1 (immature defenses) predicted CGI-S on follow up; REM-71 factor 2 (mature defenses) predicted CGI-I on follow-up. The Weinberger Distress and Repression Score predicted positively the CGI-S score on follow-up. The Weinberger Restraint and Denial of Distress Score predicted positively the CGI-Improvement score. When entered into a simultaneous regression equation, the defense subscales were the more powerful predictors of the CGI-S and CGI-I scales. This means that automatic, unconscious self-regulation is more important than symptom counts and conscious personality variables in predicting outcomes. Thirty years after the inception of integrated treatment, immature

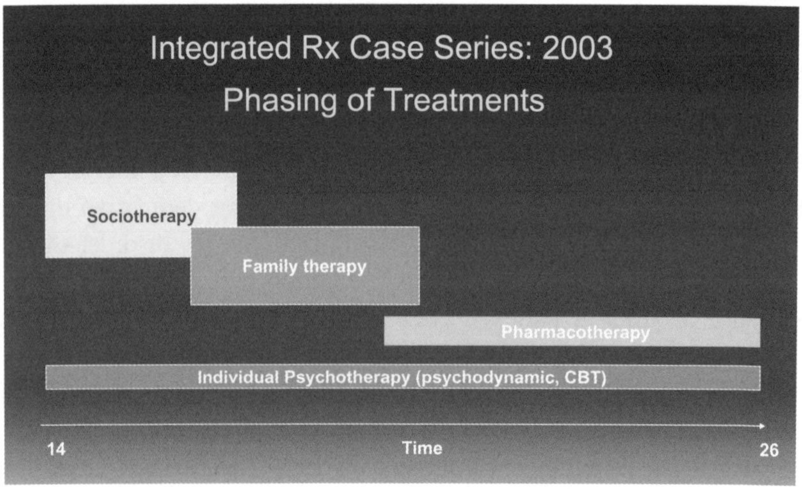

Fig. 1:

defense mechanisms predicted severity of symptom persistence at follow-up. Mature defense mechanisms predicted improvement after 30 years. This phenomenon occurred across diagnoses, genders, and ages. The Weinberger subscales of distress and restraint showed a similar pattern, but this correlation was weaker than the automatic self-regulators. Finally, denial of distress and repressive defensiveness also repeated this pattern: denial predicted improvement, while repression predicted symptom severity at follow-up.

Finally and most encouragingly, cohorts were classified as being in or out of developmental phase with their chronological age at baseline assessment (based upon Erikson's phases, 1970). On follow-up, we found that all patients now operated in one of the two phases closest to their chronological age: they either predominantly struggled with identity versus role confusion (Eriksonian phase 5 from age 12 to 20) or intimacy versus isolation (Eriksonian stage 6, ages 21–35). Two-thirds were age-matched with their appropriate phase, while one-third was in an adjacent phase. By all standards, this cohort did quite well. Even those patients who still had diagnoses, were not impaired by their symptom clusters in the activities of their daily living or in their developmental progression.

These findings are encouraging. While it may seem that our proposed integrated treatment packages are elaborate and perhaps costly by today's treatment standards, they also provided excellent treatment for a wide range of diagnoses. There were no suicides, homicides, or deaths in this cohort and no further hospitalizations after the conclusion of treatment. Studies and careers were pursued or concluded and families were built. Indicators of happiness in the cohort were on par with age-matched norms.

This type of naturalistic trial and its follow up provides a complimentary database to clinical trials. In this cohort, we treated all comers and some patients presenting with extremely severe symptoms. We treated them with all the tools of psychiatry — environment, family, psychotherapy, and medications. These treatments were carefully blended according to our case formulations and amended when new information emerged that changed our knowledge of causal loops. We propose that this type of study would be an excellent addition to psychiatry's emerging database of practice-based information. This cohort was truer to life, and much truer to clinical practice than what can be found in clinical trials (which by necessity are tightly controlled — weeding out complex, sick patients — and are of short duration, due to limited funding and problems with sample retention). We hope to stimulate practitioners from all kind of backgrounds to emulate this model and to contribute significantly to enriching our database from the angle of practice-based evidence.

References

1. *Stedman's Medical Dictionary*. 28th edition. New York, NY: Lippincott Williams & Wilkins, 2005.
2. Steiner H, Leckman J, Gabbard G. Quo Vadimus? [overview], *Br J Psychiatry* 2010 (submitted).
3. Brülde B, Radovic F. What is mental about mental disorder? *Philos Psychiatr Psychol* 2006; **13**(2): 99–116.
4. Gipps R. Mental disorder and intentional order, *Philos Psychiatr Psychol* 2006; **13**(2): 117–121.
5. Wakefield JC. What makes a mental disorder? *Philos Psychiatr Psychol* 2006; **13**(2): 123–131.
6. Fulford B, Thornton T, Graham G, Eds. *Oxford Textbook of Philosophy of Psychiatry. (International Perspectives in Philosophy and Psychiatry)*. New York, NY: Oxford University Press, 2006.
7. Feldman RS. *Child Development*. 5th edition. Upper Saddle River, NJ: Prentice Hall, 2009.
8. Magnusson, D. Individual development: Toward a developmental science, *Proc Am Philos Soc* 1999; **143**: 86–96.
9. Miller, PH. *Theories of Developmental Psychology*. 5th edition. New York, NY: Worth Publishers, 2009.
10. Remmel E, Flavell JH. Recent progress in cognitive developmental research: Implications for clinical practice. In: Steiner H, Ed. *Handbook of Mental Health*

Interventions in Children and Adolescents: An Integrated Developmental Approach. New York, NY: Jossey-Bass, 2004, pp. 73–97.

11. Kagan J, Lamb S. *The Emergence of Morality in Young Children*. Chicago, IL: University of Chicago Press, 1990.
12. Luby JL, Steiner. Concordance of parent-child temperament ratings in a clinical sample of adolescent girls, *Child Psychiatry Human Dev* 1993; **23**(4): 297–305.
13. Kandel, E. *In Search of Memory: The Emergence of a New Science of Mind*. New York, NY: W. W. Norton, 2006.
14. Sroufe LA. *Emotional Development: The Organization of Emotional Life in the Early Years*. New York, NY: Cambridge University Press, 1996.
15. Ekman, P. *Emotions Revealed: Recognizing Faces and Feelings to Improve Communication and Emotional Life*. 2nd edition. New York, NY: Holt Paperbacks, 2007.
16. Damasio A. *Looking for Spinoza: Joy, Sorrow, and the Feeling Brain*. New York, NY: *Harvest Books/Harcourt Inc*, 2003.
17. Gross JJ, Ed. *Handbook of Emotion Regulation*. New York, NY: Guilford Press, 2007.
18. Karnik, NS. The social environment. In: Steiner H. *Handbook of Mental Health Interventions in Children and Adolescents: An Integrated Developmental Approach*. San Francisco, CA: Jossey-Bass, 2004.
19. Swain JE, Scahill L, Lombroso PJ, King RA, Leckman JF. Tourette syndrome and tic disorders: A decade of progress, *J Am Acad Child Adolesc Psychiatry* 2007; **46**(8): 947–968.
20. Bandura A. *Self-Efficacy: The Exercise of Control*. New York, NY: Freeman, 1997.
21. Cicchetti D, Toth SL. The past achievements and future promises of developmental psychopathology: The coming of age of a discipline, *J Child Psychol Psychiatry* 2009; **50**(1–2): 16–25.
22. Tungström S, Söderberg P, Armelius BA. Relationship between the global assessment of functioning and other DSM axes in routine clinical work, *Psychiatr Serv* 2005; **56**(4): 439–443.
23. Bird HR, Canino GJ, Davies M, *et al*. The brief impairment scale (BIS): A multi-dimensional scale of functional impairment for children and adolescents, *J Am Acad Child Adolesc Psychiatry* 2005; **44**(7): 699–707.
24. Rutter M, Sroufe LA. Developmental psychopathology: Concepts and challenges, *Dev Psychopathol* 2000; **12**(3): 265–296.
25. Miller SP, Erickson SJ, Branom C, Steiner H. Habitual response to stress in recovering adolescent anorexic patients, *Child Psychiatry Hum Dev* 2009; **40**(1): 43–54.
26. Nesse RM. Is depression an adaptation? *Arch Gen Psychiatry* 2000; **57**(1): 14–20.
27. Smith GCS, Pell JP. Parachute use to prevent death and major trauma related to gravitational challenge: Systematic review of randomized controlled trials, *Br Med J* 2003; **327**: 1459–1461.

28. Remmel E, Flavell JH. Recent progress in cognitive developmental research: Implications for clinical practice. In: Steiner H. *Handbook of Mental Health Interventions in Children and Adolescents: An Integrated Developmental Approach.* San Francisco, CA: Jossey-Bass, 2004.
29. Araujo KB, Medic S, Yasnovsky J, Steiner H. Assessing defense structure in school-age children using the Response Evaluation Measure-71-Youth version (REM-Y-71), *Child Psychiatry Hum Dev* 2006; **36**(4): 427–436.
30. Achenbach TM, Howell CT, Quay HC, Conners CK. National survey of problems and competencies among four- to sixteen-year-olds: Parents' reports for normative and clinical samples, *Monogr Soc Res Child Dev* 1991; **56**(3): 1–131.
31. Hayes MA, McReynolds LS, Wasserman GA. Paper and voice MAYSI-2: Format comparability and concordance with the voice DISC-IV, *Assessment* 2005; **12**(4): 395–403.
32. Jackson, C. The general health questionnaire, *Occup Med* 2007; **57**: 79.
33. Ambrosini PJ. Historical development and present status of the schedule for affective disorders and schizophrenia for school-age children (K-SADS), *J Am Acad Child Adolesc Psychiatry* 2000; **39**(1): 49–58.
34. Shaffer D, Fisher P, Lucas CP, Dulcan MK, Schwab-Stone ME. NIMH diagnostic interview schedule for children Version IV (NIMH DISC-IV): Description, differences from previous versions, and reliability of some common diagnoses, *J Am Acad Child Adolesc Psychiatry* 2000; **39**(1): 28–38.
35. Reich W. Diagnostic interview for children and adolescents (DICA), *J Am Acad Child Adolesc Psychiatry* 2000; **39**(1): 59–66.
36. Jane JS, Pagan JL, Turkheimer E, Fiedler ER, Oltmanns TF. The interrater reliability of the structured interview for DSM-IV personality, *Compr Psychiatry* 2006; **47**(5): 368–375.
37. Sheehan DV, Lecrubier Y, Sheehan KH, *et al.* The mini-international neuropsychiatric interview (M.I.N.I.): The development and validation of a structured diagnostic psychiatric interview for DSM-IV and ICD-10, *J Clin Psychiatry* 1998; **59**(Suppl. 20): 22–33.
38. Saxena K, Mora L, Torres E, *et al.* Divalproex sodium-ER in outpatients with disruptive behavior disorders: A three month open label study, *Child Psychiatry Hum Dev* 2010; **41**(3): 274–284.
39. Nader K, Kriegler JA, Blake DD, Pynoos RS, Newman E, Weathers FW. Clinician Administered PTSD Scale, Child and Adolescent Version. *White River Junction, VT: National Center for PTSD, 1996.*
40. Young RC, Biggs JT, Ziegler VE, Meyer DA. A rating scale for mania: Reliability, validity and sensitivity, *Br J Psychiatry* 1978; **133**: 429–435.
41. Erickson SJ, Steiner H. Predicting adolescents' global functioning from personality typologies, *Child Psychiatry Hum Dev* 2003; **34**(1): 63–80.

42. Steiner H, Araujo K, Koopman C. The Response Evaluation Measure (REM-71): A new instrument for the measurement of defenses in adults and adolescents, *Am J Psychiatry* 2001; **158**: 467–473.
43. Karnik NS, McMullin MA, Steiner H. Disruptive behaviors: Conduct and oppositional disorders in adolescents, *Adolesc Med Clin* 2006; **17**(1): 97–114.
44. Steiner H, Remsing L. Practice parameter for the assessment and treatment of children and adolescents with oppositional defiant disorder, *J Am Acad Child Adolesc Psychiatry* 2007; **46**(1): 126–141.
45. Pliszka S, AACAP Work Group on Quality Issues. Practice parameter for the assessment and treatment of children and adolescents with attention-deficit/hyperactivity disorder, *J Am Acad Child Adolesc Psychiatry* 2007; **46**(7): 894–921.
46. Folstein MF, Folstein SE, McHugh PR. "Mini-mental state". A practical method for grading the cognitive state of patients for the clinician, *J Psychiat Res* 1975; **12**(3): 189–198.
47. Williamson K. Child Psychiatrist charged with molesting patients. *The Examiner*. April 6, 2007. http://www.examiner.com/a-659821~Child_20psychiatrist_20charged_20with_20molesting_20patients.html.
48. Mash, EJ. *Child Psychopathology*, 2nd edition. New York, NY: The Guilford Press, 2002.
49. Wakefield JC, First M. Clarifying the distinction between disorder and non-disorder: Confronting the over diagnosis ("false positives") problem in DSM-V. In: Phillips KA, First MB, Pincus HA, Eds. *Advancing DSM: Dilemmas in Psychiatric Diagnosis.* Washington, DC: American Psychiatric Press, 2003, pp. 23–56.
50. Erikson, E. *Childhood and Society*. New York, NY: W. W. Norton & Company, 1993.
51. Sroufe LA, Rutter M. The domain of developmental psychopathology, *Child Dev* 1984; **55**: 17–29.
52. Smith C, Feldman SS, Nasserbakht A, Steiner H. Psychological characteristics and DSM-III diagnoses at 6-year follow-up of adolescent anorexia nervosa, *J Am Acad Child Adolesc Psychiatry* 1993; **32**(6): 1237–1245.
53. Searle J. *Mind.* New York, NY: Oxford University Press, 2004.
54. Steiner H. *Handbook of Mental Health Interventions in Children and Adolescents: An Integrated Developmental Approach.* San Francisco, CA: Jossey-Bass, 2004.
55. McGinn C. *The Mysterious Flame: Conscious Minds in a Material World.* New York, NY: New York Basic Books, 1999.
56. Searle J. *Rationality in Action.* Cambridge, MA: The MIT Press, 2001.
57. Delizonna L, Haapanen R, Silvermann M, Redlich A, Steiner H. Defensiveness and structured interview detection of DSM-IV diagnoses in incarcerated youth. *Poster Presentation at Annual Convention of Association for the Advancement of Behavior Therapy*, November 2003.

58. Weintraub W. *Verbal Behavior in Everyday Life*. New York, NY: Springer Pub Co, 1989.
59. Nelson KL, Bein E, Ryst E, Hall R, Huemer J, Steiner H. Listening for avoidance: Narrative form and defensiveness in adolescent memories, *Child Psychiatry Hum Dev* 2009; **40**(4): 561–573.
60. Nelson K, Moskovitz D, Steiner H. Narration and vividness as measures of event specificity in autobiographical memory, *Discourse Process* 2008; **45**: 1–15.
61. Bronfenbrenner, U. *The Ecology of Human Development: Experiments by Nature and Design*. Cambridge, MA: Harvard University Press, 1979.
62. McEwen BS, Dhabhar F. Stress in adolescent females: Relationship to autoimmune diseases, *J Adolesc Health* 2002; **30**(Suppl. 4): 30–36.
63. Lehmkuhl U. The problem of divorce in adolescence, *Z Kinder Jugendpsychiatr* 1990; **18**(4): 192–197.
64. Loeber R, Green SM, Lahey BB, Frick PJ, McBurnett K. Findings on disruptive behavior disorders from the first decade of the developmental trends study, *Clin Child Fam Psychol Rev* 2000; **3**(1): 37–60.
65. Danese A, Moffitt TE, Harrington H, *et al.* Adverse childhood experiences and adult risk factors for age-related disease: Depression, inflammation, and clustering of metabolic risk markers, *Arch Pediatr Adolesc Med* 2009; **163**(12): 1135–1143.
66. Caspi A, Hariri AR, Holmes A, Uher R, Moffitt TE. Genetic sensitivity to the environment: The case of the serotonin transporter gene and its implications for studying complex diseases and traits, *Am J Psychiatry* 2010; **167**(5): 509–527.
67. Caspi A, Sugden K, Moffitt TE, *et al.* Influence of life stress on depression: Moderation by a polymorphism in the 5-HTT gene, *Science* 2003; **301**(5631): 386–389.
68. Smith C, Nasserbakht A, Feldman S, Steiner H. Psychological characteristics and DSM-III-R diagnoses at six-year follow-up of adolescent anorexia nervosa, *J Am Acad Child Adolesc Psychiatry* 1993; **32**(6): 1237–1245.
69. Steiner H, Cauffman E, Duxbury E. Personality traits in juvenile delinquents: Relation to criminal behavior and recidivism, *J Am Acad Child Adolesc Psychiatry* 1999; **38**(3): 256–262.
70. Steiner H, Lock J. Anorexia nervosa and bulimia nervosa in children and adolescents: A review of the past 10 years, *J Am Acad Child Adolesc Psychiatry* 1998; **37**(4): 352–359.
71. Luborsky L, Barrett MS. The history and empirical status of key psychoanalytic concepts, *Annu Rev Clin Psychol* 2006; **2**: 1–19.
72. Perry S, Cooper AM, Michels R. The psychodynamic formulation: Its purpose, structure, and clinical application, *Am J Psychiatry* 1987; **144**: 543–550.
73. Connor DF. *Aggression and Anti-Social Behavior in Children and Adolescents: Research and Treatment*. New York, NY: Guilford Press, 2002.

74. Neill JR. Adolf Meyer and American psychiatry today. *Am J Psychiatry* 1980; **137**(4): 460–464.
75. Engel GL. The need for a new medical model: A challenge for biomedicine, *Science* 1977; **196**(4286): 129–136.
76. American Psychiatric Association. *Diagnostic and Statistical Manual of Mental Disorders*, 4th edition. Text Revision. Washington, DC: American Psychiatric Association, 2000.
77. Summers RF. The psychodynamic formulation updated, *Am J Psychotherapy* 2003; **57**: 39–51.
78. Sim K, Gwee KP, Bateman A. Case formulation in psychotherapy: Revitalizing its usefulness as a clinical tool, *Acad Psychiatry* 2005; **29**: 289–292.
79. Butler G. Clinical formulation. In: Bellack AS, Hersen ME, Eds. *Comprehensive Clinical Psychology.* New York, NY: Pergammon Press, 1998, pp. 1–23.
80. Cipani E, Golden JA. Differentiating behavioral and traditional case formulations for children with severe behavioral and emotional problems, *Int J Behav Consult Ther* 2007; **3**(4): 537–545.
81. Pine DS, Costello JE, Dahl R. Increasing the Developmental Focus in DSM-V: Broad Issues and Specific Potential Applications in Anxiety. *Proposed Draft Revisions to DSM Disorders and Criteria*. American Psychiatric Association, 2010.
82. Eells T. *Handbook of Psychotherapy Case Formulation.* 2nd edition. New York, NY: Guilford Press, 2006.
83. Loevinger J. Confessions of an iconoclast: At home on the fringe, *J Pers Assess* 2002; **78**(2): 195–208.
84. Erwin PG, Salter K, Purves DG. Attachment style, family and romantic relationships, *Psychol Rep* 2001; **883**(2): 1251–1252.
85. Lorenz K. *King Solomon's Ring: New Light on Animal Ways.* 2nd edition. New York, NY: Routledge, 2002.
86. Chang K, Steiner H, Dienes K, Adleman N, Ketter T. Bipolar offspring: A window into bipolar disorder evolution, *Biol Psychiatry* 2003; **53**(11): 945–951.
87. Feldman S, Araujo K, Steiner H. Defense mechanisms in adolescents as a function of age, gender and mental health status, *J Am Acad Child Adolesc Psychiatry* 1996; **35**:1344–1354.
88. Schur E, Sanders M, Steiner H. Socio-cultural influences on body dissatisfaction and dieting in young children, *Int J Eat Disord* 2000; **27**: 74–82.
89. Sharpe T, Ryst E, Hinshaw S, Steiner H. Reports of stress: A comparison between eating disorders and normal adolescents, *Child Psychiatry Hum Dev* 1998; **28**(2): 117–132.
90. Erickson S, Feldman S, Steiner H. Defense mechanisms and adjustment in normal adolescents, *Am J Psychiatry* 1996; **153**(6): 826–828.

91. Steiner H, Erickson S, Pavelski R, Hernandez N. Coping and health risks: Findings in a high school population, *J Adolesc Health* 2002; **30**(5): 326–355.
92. Steiner H, Araujo K, Koopman C. The Response Evaluation Measure (REM-71): A new instrument for the measurement of defenses in adults and adolescents, *Am J Psychiatry* 2001; **158**: 467–473.

Chapter 4

Attachment and Related Psychopathology

Marina Zelenko and Sarah J. Erickson

1. Introduction

This chapter reviews contemporary understanding of attachment-related psychopathology. Before we begin this chapter, it may be helpful to the reader to review the basic concepts of attachment.

There are two general ways by which attachment is associated with early childhood psychopathology. One refers to attachment operating as a risk or protective factor, *i.e.* either increasing risk or buffering the effects of other risk factors. The second way in which attachment may be associated with psychopathology refers to the abnormalities in the formation or functioning of the primary attachment relationship itself. These conditions are called "attachment disorders."

Attachment disorders are clinical syndromes characterized by abnormalities of the child's attachment behaviors. These abnormalities may affect the child's socioemotional development and future significant relationships. They develop as a result of the child's absent or untoward attachment experiences which are considered causal in the development of attachment disorders.

2. Epidemiology of Attachment Disorders

Negative attachment experiences do not automatically lead to the development of attachment disorders. Many children who experience neglect and attachment disruption do not exhibit symptoms of attachment disorders, even if the deprivation was prolonged and severe.[17,20,21] This implies that other biological and/or environmental factors may affect the brain plasticity and resilience and influence the child's predisposition to the development of attachment disorder. Further, adverse attachment experiences are not specific antecedents to attachment disorder only, but rather may be causal or contributing factors for a host of other childhood psychopathological disorders.

The prevalence of attachment disorders in the general population is unknown. Perhaps attachment disorders are more common in general clinical practice than is currently appreciated.[22] The current lack of agreed upon, validated diagnostic criteria and the relatively infrequent occurrence of attachment disorder in general clinical practice make it difficult to conduct epidemiological studies. However, in spite of the challenging clinical presentation and frequent psychiatric comorbidity, attachment disorders have been shown to index a distinct set of behaviors related to the attachment domain.[21,23]

Clinical observation suggests that attachment disorders are more prevalent among adopted children and children from orphanages and foster care since most of these children experienced multiple changes in caregiving environment and disruptions of attachment. Thus, the studies of attachment disorders usually are conducted in these specific populations which often include childhood survivors of maltreatment, domestic violence, or war.[16] One study estimated the prevalence rate of attachment disorders at about 40% in a sample of maltreated toddlers.[24]

3. Diagnosis of Attachment Disorder

3.1. *DSM criteria for reactive attachment disorder*

The initial DSM-III definition of attachment disorder (reactive attachment disorder)[25] was developed based on early research with institutionalized children. The reactive attachment disorder (RAD) in the DSM-III described social withdrawal and physiological shutdown as the primary features in young children who were separated from their primary caregivers. This definition emphasized grossly impaired social relatedness and the child's failure to gain weight as the core features of the attachment disorder.

The current DSM-IV[26] criteria maintain general "inappropriate social relatedness" as the core feature of attachment disorder (Table 1). However, the disorder no longer includes a causal link between problematic attachment and the child's weight loss previously suggested in the DSM-III. The DSM-IV criteria present two types of attachment disorder. Both types describe maladaptive attachment relationships and deficits in general social functioning as a result of pathogenic care. The inhibited type describes a withdrawn child whose social interactions are mostly inhibited, unresponsive, and/or hypervigilant, while the disinhibited type describes a child who exhibits marked inability to develop appropriate selective attachments and displays indiscriminate sociability that is considered "diffuse" attachment.

Table 1: DSM-IV Criteria for Reactive Attachment Disorder of Infancy or Early Childhood

A. Markedly disturbed and developmentally inappropriate social relatedness in most contexts, beginning before age of five years, as evidenced by either (1) or (2):

(1) Persistent failure to initiate or respond in a developmentally appropriate fashion to most social interactions, as manifest by excessively inhibited, hypervigilant, or highly ambivalent and contradictory responses
(2) Diffuse attachment as manifest by indiscriminate sociability with marked inability to exhibit appropriate selective attachments

B. The disturbance is not accounted for solely by mental retardation and does not meet criteria for a pervasive developmental disorder

C. Pathogenic care as evidenced by at least one of the following:

(1) Persistent disregard of the child's basic emotional needs for comfort, stimulation, and affection
(2) Persistent disregard of the child' basic physical needs
(3) Repeated changes of primary caregiver that prevent formation of stable attachments

D. There is a presumption that the care is responsible for the disturbed behavior

Specify type: *Inhibited Type:* If criterion A. (1) predominates *Disinhibited Type:* If criterion A. (2) predominates

In a sample of maltreated toddlers, Zeanah and colleagues were able to reliably identify both types of the disorder. Moreover, the two types were moderately convergent, with some children demonstrating features of both types.[24] As expected, the disinhibited type was identified in children who did not have a consistent attachment figure. It is not clear how two different patterns of the disorder arise from similar adverse caregiving environments. Perhaps children's temperamental differences contribute to the different manifestations of attachment disorder.[27]

ICD-10[28] criteria for Reactive Attachment Disorder are similar to those of the DSM-IV.[26] ICD-10 also maintains the focus on diffuse abnormalities of social relatedness across contexts, suggests the etiological link to adverse caregiving experiences, and describes two subtypes — inhibited and uninhibited. However, ICD-10 allows for relationship variability and the "capacity for normal social relatedness with non-deviant adult caregivers."

Although the DSM-IV concept of attachment disorder represents a substantial advance compared to the earlier definitions, it fails to reflect several clinically, developmentally, and theoretically salient issues. First, considering that attachment is a selective affectional bond that the child develops with the primary caregiver,[29] a disorder of attachment should describe the disordered quality of this primary relationship rather than general "social relatedness in most contexts."

Inappropriate, especially indiscriminate, social behavior is indeed a common finding in previously institutionalized children and a frequent complaint of their adoptive parents.[30] However, these behaviors in institutionalized children may represent a learned adaptive strategy in the environment lacking a consistent caregiver. In children who were never institutionalized or who had a preferred caregiver in an orphanage, indiscriminate social behaviors are found much less frequently.[31] Thus, indiscriminate social relatedness may be a specific feature associated with the experience of institutionalization and lack of a consistent caregiver rather than a core feature of attachment disorder.[32] The indiscriminate behavior is considered problematic or maladaptive when, in previously institutionalized children, these behaviors persist even after the children were adopted and developed attachments to their new caregivers.[33] This persistence of inappropriate social relatedness is thought to be related to the absence of selective inhibition of affiliative behaviors by 9 months of age in institutionalized children.[32]

Second, the DSM-IV criteria of attachment disorder do not reflect the fact that behavior in infancy is often relationship-specific and, thus, the child may display signs of attachment disorder in some relationship contexts but not in others.[34] Third, the criteria do not take into consideration developmental and age differences. For example, although conceptualizations of attachment disorder in early childhood are relatively clear, it is not clear whether they can be applied to attachment disorder-related behavior in middle childhood and beyond and if not, what are the manifestations of the disorder in older children.[22] Fourth, the presence of pathogenic care as a diagnostic criterion sometimes is difficult to confirm in clinical practice because of often deficient past history and lack of collateral information. Finally, the DSM-IV criteria do not allow for a dimensional approach to assessment and classification, thereby limiting the description of symptom severity.

3.2. *Alternative diagnostic criteria for attachment disorders*

To address these issues, Zeanah and colleagues suggested alternative diagnostic criteria for attachment disorder in infancy and early childhood.[2] The classification reflects three possible problematic scenarios in the attachment domain (Table 2).

The first category is non-attachment, wherein the child did not have an opportunity to develop a selective attachment relationship due to the physical absence of a consistent caregiver. This child displays either no attachment behaviors at all or lack of preference in directing attachment behaviors, *i.e.* the child directs the attachment behaviors nonselectively toward various people. The former is parallel to the inhibited type of attachment disorder described in the DSM-IV, while the

Table 2: Alternative Criteria for Attachment Disorders (Zeanah *et al.*, 2000)[2]

I. Attachment disorder: Disorders of nonattachment

1. Lack of evidence of a preferred caregiver as evidenced by:
   - (a) Lack of differentiation among adults or
   - (b) Seeking comfort preferentially from unfamiliar adults rather than from familiar caregivers or
   - (c) Failure to seek or respond to comfort from caregivers when hurt or distressed or
   - (d) Lack of emotional responsiveness to and reciprocity with familiar caregivers
2. Child has a mental age of at least 10 months
3. Does not meet criteria for PDD
   Associated features may include:
   - (a) Poorly organized emotions with dampened positive affect, irritability, or sadness
   - (b) Failure to check back with caregiver after venturing away, especially in unfamiliar settings
   - (c) Absence of usual social reticence with unfamiliar adults
   - (d) Willingness to go off readily with relative strangers

II. Attachment disorder: Secure base distortions. The child has a discriminated attachment figure, but the relationship is disturbed or disordered as indicated by one or more of the following:

- (a) Self-endangering, risk-taking, and/or aggressive behavior that is worse in the presence of the attachment figure rather than other caregivers
- (b) Inhibition of exploration and excessive clinging that occurs in the presence of the attachment figure and less familiar adults
- (c) Excessive vigilance and anxious hypercompliance directed toward the attachment figure
- (d) Inverted caregiving in which the child is preoccupied by and seems to feel responsible for the attachment figure's emotional well-being

III. Attachment Disorder: Disrupted Attachment. The child experienced prolonged separation from a discriminated attachment figure

- (a) Emotional withdrawal; sleep and eating disturbance; refusal to accept comfort from others; and regression

Note: Disturbed attachment should be indicated if signs are only somewhat or sometimes present. Disordered attachment should be noted if signs are usually or often present.

latter is similar to the DSM-IV's disinhibited type. The features associated with nonattachment may include poorly organized emotions, absence of reticence with unfamiliar adults, and willingness to go off with strangers. These features are analogous to the "inadequate social relatedness" described in the DSM-IV, but are considered associated features rather than core symptoms of attachment disorder.

The second category is called secure base distortions. The notion of the secure base[28] refers to the child's ability to consistently rely on the caregiver for safety, comfort, and support. The category describes a child who has a primary caregiver, but the relationship and the child's attachment behaviors are disturbed such that the child is unable to use the relationship with the primary caregiver as a secure base. Formulation of the secure base distortions has advanced the concept of attachment disorders by delineating existing, nondisrupted, but yet seriously problematic attachment relationships.

Four types of secure base distortions have been identified.[23] Attachment disorder with self-endangerment refers to a child who engages in a variety of dangerous behaviors in the presence of the specific caregiver. Attachment disorder with clinging/inhibition is suggested when the child clings to the caregiver and is reluctant to explore away from the caregiver, as if the child is afraid to leave the caregiver. Attachment disorder with vigilance/hypercompliance is characterized by the child's emotional restriction, vigilance of the caregiver, and hypercompliance with the caregiver's requests as well as by inhibition of exploration. It appears as if the child is afraid to displease the caregiver, especially if the caregiver demonstrates anger or frustration. Attachment disorder with role reversal involves an inversion of the caregiving relationship; *i.e.* the child appears to attempt to take care of the caregiver and ensure the caregiver's emotional well-being.

Finally, the disrupted attachment category refers to a child who had a primary caregiver in the past, but the attachment relationship was disrupted due to loss of the caregiver. The children present with emotional withdrawal, sleep- and eating disturbance, refusal to accept comfort from others, and developmental and behavioral regression.

This alternative diagnostic system defines the age (at least 10 months of mental age) by which a child is expected to develop an attachment relationship with a primary caregiver and therefore, an assessment of various departures in this process may occur. The alternative diagnostic criteria also allow a dimensional approach to the diagnosis by suggesting two degrees of severity and frequency of the problematic behavior (yielding a diagnosis of disturbance versus disorder). Although these diagnostic criteria have not yet been fully validated, results of the emerging research on their reliability and validity are promising.[20]

3.3. *Clinical assessment of attachment*

Attachment history

Considering the role of attachment in the child's socioemotional development and its possible contribution to the child's psychopathology, assessment of attachment should be a regular part of mental health evaluations with all children under the age of five.[35,36] Along with assessments of other areas of the child's and the family's functioning, attachment assessment contributes to the understanding of the child's clinical presentation and guides interventions that may include improvement of the attachment relationship. Evaluating for possible attachment disorder, the clinician should be particularly focused on the child's attachment history, attachment behaviors, and the caregiving environment. At this point, there are still no validated standardized instruments to diagnose attachment disorders.

The interview with a primary caregiver in attachment assessment usually starts with a general description of the caregiving environment and discussion about all involved caregivers and their role in the child's life since birth. Inquiry about all disruptions in the primary relationships during the first three years of life, including prolonged separations from the primary caregivers, hospitalizations, and alternative placements, should include a detailed time-line and description of the child's concurrent reactions and consequent emotional and behavioral changes.

Specific questions about the child's attachment behaviors serve to form a preliminary understanding of the child's attachment strategies. By asking open-ended and focused questions regarding the child's behaviors when the child is distressed, the evaluator can establish the presence or absence of a preferred caregiver. Specific questions about how the child uses the relationship with the caregiver when distressed and how the child behaves during separations and reunions with the caregiver help to evaluate the child's secure base behavior.[31]

A significant part of the attachment assessment history pertains to the caregivers, their own attachment history, and current psychosocial functioning. Gathering this sensitive information requires an established rapport between the clinician and the caregivers. Although caregivers usually recognize the presence of the problem, they often tend to see it as residing within the child and, especially in the beginning, may not be ready to consider their own contribution to the problematic relationship. Thus, it is advisable to begin the interview with the focus on the child's developmental and behavioral issues and then proceed to the caregivers' history.

The caregiver's history includes inquiry about caregivers' individual difficulties that could potentially contribute to the attachment problems. Presence of psychiatric illness, especially depression and substance use, can substantially compromise the caregiver's ability to provide adequate care and may increase the risk for attachment problems. Inquiring about the caregiver's own past attachment experiences provides valuable information because the caregiver's perceptions and attitudes regarding the child may be distorted by the caregiver's own unresolved attachment-related feelings.[37]

It is essential to evaluate the caregiver's social situation and support system, including housing, vocational, and financial issues. The quality of support the caregiver receives from the rest of the family and the community affects the caregiver's well-being and therefore, influences the caregiving environment.

The evaluator should always explore the possibility of child abuse and neglect. Questioning about discipline techniques and child welfare authority

Table 3: Attachment Assessment: Outline for History

Caregiving history	General description of the caregiving environment, list of important caregivers
	History of child abuse and neglect, CPS involvement, techniques for discipline
	History of other risk factors for attachment disorder (caregivers' depression, substance use, failure to thrive, etc.)
Disruptions of caregiver–infant relationship	Prolonged separations from the primary caregivers in the first three years of life with detailed time line, including all placements, hospitalizations, absences of the caregivers
	Description of the child's behaviors during these separations and upon reunions, the child's reactions to new caregivers
Attachment behaviors	The presence or absence of a preferred caregiver
	The child's secure base behaviors
Caregiver's history	Past and present psychosocial functioning
	Past and present psychiatric history, including substance use
	Caregiver's own attachment history
	Current social support system, family, and cultural influences

involvement and gathering collateral information from other family members, daycare and medical care providers helps to clarify this sensitive issue. The outline for the history for conducting attachment assessment is presented in Table 3.

Observation in attachment assessment

At this point, there are no validated observational protocols to diagnose attachment disorders. The parent–child early relational assessment (PCERA)[38] is among the few standardized protocols that may be used to assess the affective and behavioral quality of child–parent interactions. The PCERA includes child–parent interactions that are videotaped, rated, and reviewed with the parents. Although this semistructured protocol is not designed specifically to diagnose attachment disorders, it reliably identifies strengths and concerns in the parent–child relationships.

In attachment assessment, observation of the child's and caregiver's behavior is focused on attachment salient relationship domains and other relevant behaviors.[39] The child domains include emotion regulation; affection towards caregiver; trust and security; balance between attachment and exploratory behaviors; reunion responses; comfort seeking; vigilance and self-protection; reliance for help; and cooperation and compliance. The caregiver domains include emotional availability, sensitivity, provision of comfort, and protection. The relationship domains include interactions between the caregiver's emotional availability and child's emotion regulation, caregiver's sensitivity and child's trust and security, caregiver's protection and child' vigilance and self-protection, and caregiver's provision of comfort and child's comfort seeking.

Other foci of observation of the child–caregiver interaction include the amount and extent of physical and eye contact; the quality and quantity of verbal exchange; the presence or absence of shared interests; imitation and attuned exchanges; the level of pleasure and harmony; and mutual engagement during play. As we discussed earlier, it is helpful to conduct separate observation sessions with different caregivers or family members in order to observe the range of the child's interactive behaviors in different relationship contexts. The child's capacity for and interest in interpersonal relatedness with people other than the caregivers and the family, and the manner and extent to which the child engages in or initiates interactions with unfamiliar people, *i.e.* the evaluator(s), should also be noted.[40]

In order to asses these attachment-relevant areas, semistructured observational formats include, along with free play and other structured tasks, a brief separation of the child from the caregiver and a subsequent reunion.[36] As per the evaluator's request, the caregiver leaves the playroom while the child stays there with the evaluator. The length of the separation may vary depending on the child's age and his or her discomfort in the caregiver's absence: the separation may last from several seconds to several minutes. If the child becomes upset, the evaluator asks the caregiver to come back to the playroom. This procedure allows assessing the child's reaction to the separation from the caregiver (*e.g.* the level of distress, coping behaviors, and responses to the evaluator in the caregiver's absence) as well as reunion behavior when the caregiver comes back (*e.g.* the child's seeking comfort from the caregiver, and ability to use the relationship with the caregiver to cope with the distress of separation). It also provides useful information regarding the child's interactions with the evaluator.

For children aged three years and older, particularly if they regularly attend group settings and are used to daily separations from their caregivers, the separation paradigm may not be as informative as for younger children. Considering the relatively advanced verbal skills and symbolic play skills of children older than three years, the clinician may use the attachment story stems,[41] a story telling technique with doll figures.

Among clinicians, there may be some confusion between attachment disorders and attachment insecurity as defined by the strange situation paradigm[42] and other research measures. It is important to keep in mind that attachment disorder is a clinical psychiatric diagnosis while attachment insecurity is a research category developed in a normative sample. Although insecure attachment, as we discussed in the beginning of this chapter, suggests a suboptimal infant–caregiver relationship and may predict poorer outcomes, it is not diagnostic of attachment disorder. The insecure-disorganized attachment pattern, which has been shown to be prevalent in maltreated children, theoretically appears the most relevant to attachment disorders. However, at this point there is no research data supporting this association.[20]

3.4. *Differential diagnosis*

Due to complex clinical presentation and the lack of valid diagnostic criteria, differential diagnosis of attachment disorders presents a significant challenge.[43] In the differential diagnosis process, it is important to consider the entire constellation of the clinical features taken in the context of the early caregiving history.

Many of the attachment disorder symptoms are not specific to attachment disorder. Children with adverse attachment history may present with apathy, social withdrawal, aggressive behaviors, inattention and hyperactivity, failure to thrive, various developmental delays and regressions, and autistic-like behaviors.[44–46] Some of these clinical symptoms may represent true disturbances of the attachment relationship while some may be the consequences of other environmental influences, such as inadequate nutrition or emotional or cognitive understimulation. For example, as we discussed earlier, indiscriminate sociability seems to be a result of institutionalization rather than a specific characteristic of attachment disorder. Aggressive behaviors and other psychosocial difficulties also appear to be non-essential features of the disorder.[47]

Differentiation between attachment disorder, inhibited type and pervasive developmental disorder PDD may be challenging because social withdrawal and restricted interests are characteristic of both conditions. Moreover, children with a history of severe early neglect may present with global developmental and language delays and stereotypic behaviors similar to those of children with PDD.[46] The differentiation between the two conditions sometimes is possible only after the children are placed in a normal caregiving environment. Children with attachment disorder are more likely to show a catch up in development and remission in social relatedness compared to children with PDD.

Social behaviors of children with attachment disorder, inhibited type may also appear similar to those of temperamentally inhibited children. However, children with attachment disorder would be expected to manifest significant variability in social inhibition across different relationships, whereas in children with a temperamental attribute, the social inhibition would be more pervasive and would not show relationship-specificity.[48] In older children with adverse attachment history who present with disinhibited social behaviors and other behavioral problems, distinguishing between attachment disorder, inhibited type, conduct disorder, and impulse control disorders may present another challenge.[44]

3.5. *Comorbidity*

Considering that disordered attachment relationship itself increases the risk for childhood psychopathology, it is not surprising that clinical features concomitant with attachment disorder may be signs of various comorbid conditions.

These comorbidities may include such conditions as post-traumatic stress disorder, separation anxiety disorder, and other anxiety disorders: depression, or sleep disorder. Environmental understimulation and physical neglect, prenatal adversities, such as intrauterine undernourishment and prenatal exposure to drugs and alcohol, physical illness and trauma, malnutrition, developmental disorders, and behavioral disorders including attention deficit hyperactivity should be considered as well.

Because the same adverse early experiences may contribute to both attachment disorder and other psychopathological conditions, true comorbidity of attachment disorders with other emotional, behavioral, and developmental problems is likely to be high. The comorbid conditions need to be evaluated and diagnosed separately and may require separate psychotherapeutic or psychopharmocological interventions.

4. Pathogenesis of Attachment-Related Psychopathology

The pathogenesis of attachment disorders is thought to be related to the structural and functional effects of negative attachment experiences on the developing brain of the child. The effects of negative attachment experiences have thus been repeatedly observed in children who either lost their primary caregivers or were abandoned by them and, as a result, were raised in orphanages or foster homes.[16] These disturbances of attachment have also been described in children who were maltreated and neglected[17] or were separated from their primary caregivers due to prolonged hospitalization.[18]

The research on early trauma and attachment suggests that untoward environmental experiences may trigger neuropathological mechanisms underlying behavioral changes in children with attachment problems.[19] This notion is in accord with the finding that the presence of attachment disorder behaviors is positively correlated with duration of early caregiving deprivation.[17]

Childhood mental disorders are multidetermined: they are unlikely to be caused by a single factor and usually are associated with multiple risk factors in different combinations. The effect of a particular risk factor depends on its timing, a number of other risk factors, and the relationship among them. Further, risk factors for childhood mental disorders are usually not disorder-specific but are related to a variety of maladaptive outcomes.[1] The quality of attachment and attachment disruptions, as could be expected, are more influential in early childhood. Effects of attachment on the child's development and functioning are the most prominent in the social adaptation domain, with intermediate effects in the behavioral functioning domain, and lesser effects in the cognitive domain.[2]

The quality of attachment is more likely to affect the child's mental health when attachment difficulties are combined with other risk factors, such as poverty, family violence, and parental psychopathology. The combination of early insecure attachment with other risk factors is known to be associated with a variety of children's behavioral and mental health problems.[3] For example, children in high social-risk environments who had early insecure attachments are significantly more likely to show poor peer relations, moodiness, and symptoms of depression and aggression than children who had early secure attachments.[4,5] Similarly, children who had early secure attachments have been shown to be less dependent, more ego resilient, more socially competent, and more likely to develop friendships.[6,7]

The studies demonstrated some links between particular patterns of infant insecure attachment and later psychopathology. For example, children who had early insecure-resistant attachment have been shown to be a higher risk for the development of anxiety disorders.[8] Children who showed early insecure-avoidant attachment have been shown to be at a higher risk for the development of aggressive behaviors.[9] The insecure-disorganized attachment, which often is associated with child maltreatment and severe caregiver's psychopathology, has shown the strongest association with later child behavioral and mental health problems such as aggression and dissociative disorders.[10,11]

The contribution of the quality of attachment to the later social adaptation and behavioral and psychological functioning can be understood from several points of view. A securely attached child feels confident about the availability of the attachment figure and is more likely to feel safe and secure. Thus, this child is more likely to engage in exploratory and sociable behaviors, which enhance the child's knowledge and competence of the world and the relationships and facilitate adaptation. An insecurely attached child, on the other hand, is often unsure about the availability of the attachment figure, is more likely to worry about the attachment relationship, and thus, is less likely to engage in advantageous exploratory and sociable behaviors.

Consistently sensitive caregiving, which contributes to the development of secure attachment, helps the infants to develop a positive sense of self and others and generally positive expectations of the relationships. These positive internal working models facilitate the children's social interactions and adaptation. Insensitive and inconsistent caregiving that contributes to the formation of insecure attachment may also lead to the child's negative internal working models of self, others, and relationships, which in turn make social adaptation more difficult.

Another approach to the role of attachment in later adaptation and psychopathology is to consider the role of attachment in the child's affective and behavioral regulation. While the child's strong self-regulatory abilities may serve as a protective factor, the deficient affective and behavioral regulation is likely to be a risk factor in the development of psychopathology.[12] The development of infant regulatory capacity is dependent upon regulatory input from the attachment figure. Caregiver–infant affective and behavioral attunement, or synchrony, has been proposed as an important contributor to the development of the child's self-regulation.[13]

Consistently responsive care entails appropriate affective stimulation and interventions to keep arousal within reasonable bounds. Thus, consistently responsive care facilitates the development of the child's own arousal regulation and helps the child to learn to modulate emotional expression and to maintain organized behavior.[12] On a psychophysiological level, it has been shown that consistently responsive care supports the development of the child's emotional regulation and behavioral flexibility through facilitation of tuning and balancing of the excitatory and inhibitory systems in the child's central nervous system.[14] On the other hand, maternal insensitivity and unresponsiveness to the child's signals potentially leads to the child's affective regulatory problems which in turn may put the child at higher risk for psychopathology.[15]

5. Relevance to Primary Care

Although attachment disorders appear to be relatively infrequent in the general population, perhaps they are more common in general clinical practice than is currently appreciated.[22] Pediatricians are more likely to encounter attachment disorders among young adopted children and children from orphanages and foster care since most of these children experienced multiple changes in caregiving environment and disruptions of attachment. Young children presenting with malnutrition, severe environmental understimulation, and other signs of neglect, as well as with physical traumas suggestive of physical abuse, are at high risk for attachment disorders. In addition to addressing medical and nutritional issues and involving child protective services, the primary care providers should consider referral to child psychiatry for assessment of attachment.

6. Interventions for Attachment Disorders

A treatment plan should be individually tailored according to the particular child and caregiver's situation. Depending on the child's previous attachment experiences, needs of the current caregiving environment, and the child's clinical presentation, treatment may include social, psychotherapeutic, educational, and biological interventions. Frequently, collaborative effort of several institutions, including social, mental health, educational, and medical agencies, is needed. A comprehensive coordinated multidisciplinary treatment approach is often necessary to help the child and the caregiver overcome the consequences of the early untoward attachment experiences and to optimize the child's socio-emotional and behavioral development.

Considering that the diagnosis of the attachment disorder is still problematic, there have been no formal efforts to evaluate interventions for attachment disorders.

6.1. *Social interventions*

If the child did not have a consistent attachment figure due to multiple placements, every effort should be taken to arrange as soon as possible for a caregiving situation in which at least one selective attachment relationship can develop. Permanent placement with caring and nurturing caregivers is ideal. Recent research has shown that even children who experienced severe neglect and previously did not have attachment figures are capable of forming attachment relationships once they are placed in more normative environments.[21,31,33]

In case of child maltreatment, the first vital task is to ensure the child's safety. Appropriate social interventions may also include assistance with financial, housing, and respite needs, and assuring availability of medical care. If the child has lost a primary attachment figure, a new attachment figure and an optimal placement should be identified as soon as possible.

6.2. *Caregiver education*

It is essential to help the caregiver understand the meaning of the child's behaviors and the caregiver's role in the child's recovery. By definition, children with attachment disorders have a history of attachment trauma. Thus, the clinician should educate the caregiver regarding clinical presentations of trauma and loss in young children and guide the caregiver to perceive the child's behaviors as non-pathological and to be more attuned to the child's emotional state.

Supporting the formation of the new attachment is a critical clinical task which may be especially complicated in children coming from institutions or multiple prior placements. It is important to educate new caregivers about this process that may take much time and effort.[50] The discussion about attachment behaviors and the importance of consistent and sensitive caregiving in the development of attachment should be tailored to the caregiver's level of sophistication and general education.

Caregivers adopting a previously institutionalized child should also be educated about the specific deficits and behaviors frequently seen in these children, such as the tendency not to seek comfort from a caregiver but rather to engage in non-interactive self-soothing behaviors including rocking or headbanging.

Educating the caregiver regarding the child's developmental strengths and delays is yet another important part of the therapeutic work. This helps the new caregiver develop a realistic view of the child's current capacities and reasonable expectations regarding the child's future development. Helping the caregiver to build upon strengths and address weaknesses in a supportive way will optimize the child's development and enhance the caregiver's sensitivity and acceptance of the child and, thus, contribute to the development of the new attachment relationship.

6.3. *Psychotherapy*

The primary therapeutic goal in treatment of attachment disorders is the development of a strong healthy attachment between the child and primary caregivers. The focus of therapy may differ depending on the type of the disorder. For example, work with the secure base disturbances focuses on improving the existing relationship, while work with the disrupted attachment includes addressing the loss and the development of a new attachment, which is also essential in nonattachment. Promoting parental behaviors known to facilitate secure attachments, such as emotional availability and sensitive responsiveness, has been a consistent component of all psychotherapy approaches.[23,51,52]

Psychotherapeutic interventions may include individual therapy for the child, individual therapy for the caregiver, family or marital counseling, and child–caregiver (dyadic) psychotherapy. At this time, there is no convincing data to suggest that one particular modality of psychotherapy is more efficient in treatment of attachment disorders than any other. For more detailed discussion of psychotherapy approaches in early childhood, we refer the reader to the *Handbook of Mental Health Interventions in Children and Adolescents*.[53]

Dyadic infant–parents therapy[37] is frequently used in the treatment of young children with attachment disorders. This therapy is focused on the child–caregiver relationships and interactions rather than on individual issues. This approach, which integrates crisis intervention, developmental guidance, social support, and dyadic psychotherapy, is perhaps the most tailored for attachment problems.

With pre-school children, play therapy is helpful in eliciting the child's inner experiences, feelings, and fantasies. The development of a supportive and dependable relationship between the child and the therapist is critical to provide a safe place for the child and help the child develop a positive relationship model. Issues of safety, separation, and abandonment require particular attention in therapeutic work with children with attachment problems.

The caregiver's participation in the treatment process is essential. Depressed, drug abusing or otherwise disturbed caregivers may not be able to participate in the process. Addressing the caregiver's individual problems is an important part of the treatment plan and may necessitate separate treatment.

6.4. *Biological interventions*

Perhaps the most important biological intervention in treatment of attachment disorders is an adequate management of the young child's medical condition(s). A mental health clinician should always keep in mind the importance of the child's physical condition and ensure appropriate involvement the medical care providers. The interventions may include normalization of the child's basic physiologic functions such as sleep and feeding, medical management of the child's physical trauma, and pain management in case of physical child abuse, and correction of the child's nutritional status in case of malnutrition and growth failure. Psychiatric medications may be considered to address severe psychiatric conditions that often are associated with attachment disorder, such as post-traumatic stress disorder, anxiety, depression, or insomnia.

7. Course and Outcome of Attachment Disorders

The natural course of attachment disorders is unknown. The English and Romanian adoptees (ERA) Study, which followed Romanian orphans who were adopted into the United Kingdom homes,[21] and other studies of orphans present the most relevant data on the prognosis of attachment disorder behaviors when the previously severely deprived children were ultimately placed in more favorable environments. The ERA study has demonstrated a close association between the duration of severe institutional deprivation and the severity of attachment disorder behaviors. Children who stayed in the orphanage after the age of 6 months were more likely to exhibit attachment disorder behaviors than children who left the orphanage and were adopted before the age of 6 months.

The ERA study also showed a 2-year stability of attachment disorder and related behaviors in the adopted children, suggesting that severe early deprivation has profound and lasting negative effects on the child's functioning and the recovery may be incomplete.[21,30] As we discussed, the ERA and other studies showed that indiscriminate social behaviors may persist after the children were placed in more favorable environments and even after new and healthier attachment relationships had developed with adoptive caregivers.[21,33] Over the years, the children in the ERA study have demonstrated significant heterogeneity in outcome. While some children showed adequate catching up in physical growth, cognitive development, and development of attachment, others, especially children adopted after the age of six months, continued to show notable deficits. The marked heterogeneity of individual outcomes suggests that the outcome is a function of numerous factors, including the length of deprivation, the level of functioning at the time of adoption, individual temperament, early biological programming effects of deprivation on the brain, and possible neural deficits.[49]

8. Clinical Practice

In our clinic, we recommend therapeutic guidelines which we find helpful in the treatment of trauma in young children following the loss of a mother.[50] The guidelines have been developed based on attachment theory and theories of grief and bereavement. The young child who lost a mother in a traumatic event, in addition to the effect of the traumatic event itself, is going through the dramatic process of permanent loss of a primary attachment figure. This implies that along with the general therapeutic approaches to trauma in young children, issues of attachment and loss should be incorporated in the treatment as well. The following clinical vignette illustrates the application of the guidelines.

8.1. *Case vignette*

Mitchell, a 3-year-old Hispanic boy, was brought to the clinic by his maternal aunt Mayra. Mayra was concerned about Mitchell's unstable, often sad mood, frequent tantrums, and angry outbursts. Mitchell had nightmares 2–3 times per night and was afraid to sleep alone. These behaviors, as well as fear of darkness, sirens, police and ambulance cars, clinginess to Mayra and resistance to separations from her, developed after a car accident. During the accident, which resulted from the father's falling asleep and losing control of the car, Mitchell sustained minor injuries while his mother was instantly killed. Given the father's low functioning due to his psychiatric and substance abuse history, after the accident the court placed the child temporarily with Mayra. After a several-month custody contest between Mitchell's father and Mayra, the boy's placement with Mayra was finalized.

Mitchell, an attractive well-developed boy with bright eyes, was somewhat slow to warm up during the initial evaluation. He stayed in close proximity to Mayra in the room and was reluctant to explore the new toys. Gradually, he became interested in small cars, which were the only toys that attracted his attention. Mitchell's play was repetitive and monotonous. The play involved car crashes and a mother and the baby being killed. Again and again, he threw a car on the floor or bumped one car to another and yelled, "they all are killed!" When Mayra had to leave the office for a few minutes, Mitchell became obviously distressed, tried to follow her out the door, and did not calm down until she came back.

Mitchell's clinical presentation met criteria for PTSD.[26] In addition to the trauma, he presented with salient attachment-related problems. In this discussion, we focus on therapeutic approaches to these attachment issues.

8.2. *Attachment-related therapeutic issues*

Identification of a new caregiver and formation of the new attachment bond

Bowlby[54] suggested that the quality of caregiving from a new caregiver, "mothering care from a substitute mother" upon separation from the mother, is one of the most important factors in a child's adjustment to the loss. The ability of other people to adapt to the absence of the mother and, if needed, to assume a new role is an important factor in the child's overall adaptation to change. If the mother was the only primary caregiver, one of the therapist's first tasks is to help the family reorganize and identify a new caregiver(s). Support for the formation of the new attachment relationship may be the most urgent initial focus in therapy before the trauma itself can be processed. The therapist should also help the new caregiver understand that the formation of the new attachment bond may take time.

After the accident, Mitchell stayed mostly with Mayra but several times a week he visited his maternal grandmother and stayed overnight in her house. Mayra and the grandmother were unsure which one of them should be considered Mitchell's primary caregiver. At the time of the evaluation, the father was visiting with Mitchell twice a week. The father believed that he was a competent caregiver and should have custody of the child. Mayra and the grandmother felt that the father was not able to provide necessary structure and support for the boy.

The therapist's effort was directed at bringing the families together in accepting Mayra as a primary caregiver. This work focused on:

- Helping the father understand that in present circumstances, Mayra had been providing the most optimal environment for Mitchell. The therapist emphasized that Mitchell would attain a more stable emotional state if the father would support the boy's relationships with Mayra rather than contest it. At the same time, the therapist encouraged the father to pursue his own relationship with Mitchell.

- Helping Mayra and the grandmother recognize that Mayra might be a more appropriate primary caregiver than her elderly sick mother. The therapist encouraged the women to make clear to Mitchell through everyday conversations, bedroom and sleeping arrangements, that now he permanently lived at Mayra's house but would visit with his grandmother.
- Helping Mayra, who did not have her own children and felt somewhat anxious whether she would be a good enough mother, alleviate anxiety regarding her new role and accept the new identity. The therapist consistently reassured Mayra and formally endorsed her as a competent primary caregiver in the court procedure. The therapist also helped the father to accept this development in Mitchell's relationship with Mayra.

New caregiver's understanding of the process of separation and loss in young children

Observing behaviors of young children recently separated from their mothers, Bowlby[54] described initial active protest as a reaction to perceived danger of loss; then agitation and search for the mother as a reaction to loss that already occurred; and finally, despair, depression, or withdrawal as a way of dealing with the pain of loss. It is important to discuss this bereavement process in young children with the new caregiver. With this understanding, the new caregiver is able to perceive these behaviors as non-pathological, to be more attuned to the child's emotional state and validate it, and thus to relieve some of the pain and facilitate healing. The caregiver should also know that the child may experience recurrence of distress when something reminds him about the loss. The child may be particularly sensitive and vulnerable around holidays and at the time of anniversaries of the loss; this could be due to reminders and also could be a result of the child's perceiving distress that is experienced by the adults at those times. Understanding of this process and awareness that the reappearance of symptoms is temporary helps the caregiver to be more tolerant and patient should the child's distress recur.

Neither Mayra, the grandmother, nor the father were aware of the process of grieving Mitchell had been going through since his mother's death. The adults, who were grieving themselves, thought that Mitchell was "too young to understand" and chose not to talk with him about it. Mayra noticed that when Mitchell saw his mother's pictures, he often would sulk and start crying. Not wanting to upset him, Mayra took the pictures away. The adults were not sure how to respond when Mitchell looked at the sky and yelled for his mother, which he did frequently. Around the first anniversary of the mother's death, the adults noticed that Mitchell became more tearful and sad and he also became more aggressive in daycare.

The therapist:

- Explained that some of the Mitchell's symptoms were a part of a normal grieving process.
- Helped Mayra understand that Mitchell would benefit more if she recognized his feelings and joined him in his grief.
- Suggested that when Mitchell cried and called for his mother, Mayra would not try to distract him with a toy as she used to do, but rather acknowledge his search for his mother and talk with the boy about his mother while physically comforting him.
- Explained to the adults that their emotional states powerfully influenced Mitchell. The therapist suggested to the caregivers to discuss their own feelings with the boy in an appropriate way rather than try to hide the negative emotions which he sensed anyway. The adults were also advised that they seek help with their own bereavement.

Reorganization of the child's life

The death of a mother should not be viewed as a single stressful event, but as a traumatic reorganization of the child's life. The impact of the death pervades most aspects of the child's life; thus, the child is dealing not only with the death of the mother, but with the death of a way of life.[55] These great disruptions and changes in the child's day-to-day life can be seen as concomitant losses for the child. With an understanding that the family will never be the same, attempts should be made to maintain the routine of the child's previous life as much as possible. The presence of familiar people and surroundings, including familiar toys and other personal items in the child's new life, may bring some continuity and thus, help mitigate the effect of the loss.[54]

Mitchell's life with his parents was notably lacking structure. During the day, Mitchell used to eat numerous snacks; he almost never ate at the table. He would fall asleep on the floor at irregular times during the day or night. After the accident, Mitchell's life drastically changed. The new daily routine in Mayra's care was a difficult change which Mitchell tried to resist. The adults noticed that Mitchell insisted on wearing the same shirt (which was already getting small) and a few other things bought by his mother. The grandmother resentfully stated that new clothes that she bought for Mitchell were "wasted." Mayra and the grandmother threw out some old items and hid the shirt from Mitchell hoping to help him "forget and start anew." The therapeutic work focused on:

- Supporting Mayra in her efforts to establish routines for Mitchell and, at the same time, emphasizing the importance of keeping in his new life any positive elements of Mitchell's life with his mother.
- Helping the caregivers understand that the old clothes, toys, and other items from the mother's house brought Mitchell a comforting sense of stability and continuity in his life.

New caregiver's awareness of the child's heightened anxiety regarding separation experiences

Many young children separated from primary caregivers develop unusual clinginess to their new caregiver and resistance to separation from them.[54] Any seemingly insignificant short separation from a new caregiver may be perceived by the traumatized hypersensitive child as a threat of yet another permanent loss. Being aware of this, the new caregiver can preventatively discuss the separation with the child and help the child to handle new transitions (*i.e.* to daycare or other caregivers). By being calm and supportive, keeping promises, and being back on time, the caregiver can reassure the child that another permanent separation will not happen.

Initially, Mitchell was very distressed when Mayra was leaving for work in the mornings. He would cry and try to hold onto her. The grandmother stated that at her house, because of Mitchell's distress on even short separations, she "could not do anything without him, not even go to the bathroom." Both Mayra and the grandmother were concerned that when Mitchell needed to go from one house to another, he became very upset and sometimes refused to go. Often he would refuse to leave Mayra's house when his father came to pick him up, then later he would refuse to leave the father and go back to Mayra. The adults suggested different interpretations of these behaviors. The grandmother sometimes thought that Mitchell did not like her or her husband; the father suspected that the other family members had turned Mitchell against him. The therapist:

- Helped the adults to learn that most likely Mitchell's behavior was a reflection of his intense fear of losing a caregiver again rather than an expression of a personal attitude toward a particular person.
- Explained to the caregivers that, in the light of his loss, Mitchell was very sensitive to any transitions and needed a lot of support and reassurance during those times.

- Advised Mayra to leave her small personal items with Mitchell in the morning so he could feel more connected with her while she was away and to telephone Mitchell during the day to reassure him that she would come back.
- Explained to the father, who was late sometimes or missed the visits with Mitchell, that this could be quite traumatic to Mitchell who needed stability and consistency in his relationships in order to start feeling more secure.

Acceptance of the loss through continuous maternal presence in the child's life

Sometimes new caregivers choose not to talk with the child about the loss. This might occur because the caregivers are mourning their own loss. Also, the caregivers may mistakenly assume that the young child does not remember the trauma; they may worry that talking about it will remind the child about the loss and unnecessarily disturb the child. The caregivers need help in learning that reflecting and remembering and thus, maintaining a sense of the lost mother in the child's current life, is an important part of the bereavement process and may be critical to the accommodation the child makes to the loss over time.[55] One task for the new caregiver in the early phase of bereavement is to develop a language that will allow the child to talk about the dead mother and to maintain a place for her in the child's life. This includes conversations about the mother and reminiscing of past events and mutual experiences with the deceased. The connection with the deceased through play, talking, personal belongings, and pictures helps the child accept a new reality.

Mitchell's relatives felt uncomfortable when he asked about his mother. Mitchell seemed to accept the explanation that his mother went to "heaven" but had a lot of questions about it. When he brought up the topic, the adults tried to distract him or offered answers that would close the discussion. For example, when he repeatedly asked where the mother's car went, they usually answered that it went to a garbage can. The therapist:

- Encouraged the caregivers to develop a dialogue about the loss. Observing the therapist talking with Mitchell about the accident and exploring the boy's thoughts and feelings about his mother's death through play helped the adults to overcome their hesitancy and start doing it at home.
- Supported the idea of an anniversary family picnic. Although the family initially did not want Mitchell to participate in the family picnic, with the therapist's support they decided to include Mitchell. This poignant event seemed to bring some relief to all of the family. Although Mitchell was sad during the picnic, he seemed to enjoy the family time devoted to his mother.

- Encouraged the adults to participate in Mitchell's play and help him to restructure the story. By observing the therapist playing with Mitchell, the caregivers learned to be active participants in the play and thus be able to redirect the content of the play and moderate the affect.

Over the six-month treatment, Mitchell's' symptoms significantly improved. His mood became positive and stable. The bouts of agitation and depression became less frequent and Mitchell became more responsive to comforting efforts of the adults. The tantrums and aggressive behaviors disappeared. The boy started falling asleep in his bed without protest and the nightmares stopped. He was not distressed anymore on separation from Mayra and the grandmother.

Gradually, the loss seemed to become less painful to Mitchell. He started bringing his mother's death up in a more positive, accepting vein. For example, he asked to buy several air balloons and let them go, "sent to heaven" to his mother. The boy became less interested in cars and started playing "house" where he "resided: with" Mayra, her husband, the grandmother, and himself. His new toy "family" had a positive, structured life: together they watched TV, went shopping, and had dinner. Finally, Mitchell started calling Mayra "Mama Mayra" and Mayra's house "home."

9. Areas for Future Investigations

Although some studies suggest that attachment disorders may be reliably identified,[24] sufficiently validated diagnostic criteria of attachment disorders are still lacking. Validation of the diagnostic criteria of attachment disorders is currently a truly critical area of research. Valid diagnostic criteria are essential to advance our understanding of this condition and to develop valid diagnostic instruments and focused effective interventions. Further, there is still no adequate validation of the two types of attachment disorder. No discriminate validity studies have been conducted: it is possible that mixed or other types of attachment disorder also exist.[24, 32]

Another promising area of future research is the identification of risk and protective factors for attachment disorders. This may potentially influence the development of interventions as well as foster care and adoption practices, thereby improving children's outcomes. Genetic studies and imaging studies, which are lacking at this point, may also be helpful in the study of risk and protective factors for attachment disorder.

Further study of the relationship between insecurity of attachment and attachment disorders is warranted, especially considering that existing interventions to increase security of attachment have been shown to be effective.[51,52]

The major methodological difficulty in studying attachment disorders is that prospective designs are difficult to apply early enough in the life of children at risk for attachment problems. The retrospective designs, on the other hand, often involve deficient information about the child's attachment experiences and the child's functioning prior to the development of an attachment disorder.

Acknowledgment

The authors thank Anneliese Korner, Ph.D. for her ongoing support and inspiration.

References

1. Greenberg MT. Attachment and psychopathology in childhood. In: Cassidy J, Shaver PR, Eds. *Handbook of Attachment: Theory, Research, and Clinical Applications*. New York: Guilford Press, 1999, pp. 469–496.
2. Zeanah CH, Boris NW, Lieberman AF. Attachment disorders in infancy. In: Sameroff AJ, Lewis M, Miler SM, Eds. *Handbook of Developmental Psychopathology*. Dordrecht, Netherlands: Kluwer, 2000.
3. Carlson EA, Sampson MC, Sroufe LA. Implications of attachment theory and research for developmental-behavioral pediatrics, *J Dev Behav Pediatr* 2003; **24**: 364–379.
4. Sroufe LA. Pathways to adaptation and maladaptation: Psychopathology as developmental deviation. In: Cicchetti D, Ed. *Rochester Symposium on Developmental Psychopathology: The Emergence of Discipline*. Vol. 1. Hillsdale, NJ:, Erlbaum, 1990, pp. 13–40.
5. Urban J, Carlson E, Egeland B, Sroufe LA. Patterns of individual adaptation across childhood, *Dev Psychopathol* 1991; **3**: 445–460.
6. Boris NW, Zeanah CH. Disturbances and disorders of attachment in infancy and early childhood: An overview, *Infant Ment Health J* 1999; **20**: 1–9.
7. Sroufe A, Egeland B, Carlson E, Collins WA. Placing early attachment experiences in developmental context: The Minnesota Longitudinal Study. In: Grossmann KE, Grossmann K, Waters E, Eds. *Attachment from Infancy to Adulthood: The Major Longitudinal Studies*. New York: Guilford Publications, Inc., 2005, pp. 48–70.
8. Warren SL, Huston L, Egeland B, Sroufe LA. Child and adolescent anxiety disorders and early attachment, *J Am Acad Child Adolesc Psychiatry* 1997; **36**: 637–644.
9. Shaw DS, Owens EB, Giovannelli J, Winslow EB. Infant and toddler pathways leading to early externalizing disorders, *J Am Acad Child Adolesc Psychiatry* 2001; **40**: 36–43.
10. Lyons-Ruth K, Alpern L, Repacholi B. Disorganized infant attachment classification and maternal psychosocial problems as predictors of hostile-aggressive behavior in the preschool classroom, *Child Dev* 1993; **64**: 572–585.

11. Ogawa JR, Sroufe LA, Weinfield NS, Carlson EA, Egeland B. Development and the fragmented self: Longitudinal study of dissociative symptomatology in a non-clinical sample, *Dev Psychopathol* 1997; **9**: 855–879.
12. Sroufe LA. Psychopathology as an outcome of development, *Dev Psychopathol* 1997; **9**: 251–268.
13. Feldman R, Greenbaum CW, Yirmiya N. Mother-infant affect synchrony as an antecedent of the emergence of self-control, *Dev Psychol* 1999; **35**: 223–231.
14. Schore AN. Effects of a secure attachment relationship on right brain development, affect regulation, and infant mental health, *Infant Ment Health J* 2001; **22**: 7–66.
15. Sroufe LA, Carlson EA, Levy AK, Egeland B. Implications of attachment theory for developmental psychopathology. In: Hertzig ME, Farber EA, Eds. *Annual Progress in Child Psychiatry and Child Development: 2000–2001*. New York: Brunner-Routledge, 2003, pp. 43–61.
16. Rutter ML, Kreppner JM, O'Connor TG. English and Romanian adoptees study team. Specificity and heterogeneity in children's responses to profound institutional privation, *Br J Psychiatry* 2001; **179**: 97–103.
17. O'Connor TG, Bredenkamp D, Rutter M. English and Romanian adoptees study team. Attachment disturbances and disorders in children exposed to early severe deprivation, *Infant Ment Health J* 1999; **20**: 10–29.
18. Minde K. Mediating attachment patterns during a serious medical illness, *Infant Ment Health J* 1999; **20**: 105–122.
19. Schore AN. The effects of early relational trauma on right brain development, affect regulation, and infant mental health, *Infant Ment Health J* 2001; **22**: 201–269.
20. Boris NW, Hinshaw-Fuselier SS, Smyke AT, Scheeringa MS, Heller SS, Zeanah CH. Comparing criteria for attachment disorders: Establishing reliability and validity in high-risk samples, *J Am Acad Child Adolesc Psychiatry* 2004; **43**: 568–577.
21. O'Connor TG, Rutter M. English and Romanian adoptees study team. Attachment disorder behavior following early severe deprivation: Extension and longitudinal follow-up, *J Am Acad Child Adolesc Psychiatry* 2001; **39**: 703–712.
22. O'Connor TG, Zeanah CH. Current perspectives on attachment disorders: Rejoinder and synthesis, *Attach Hum Dev* 2003; **5**: 321–326.
23. Zeanah CH, Boris NW. Disturbances and disorders of attachment in early childhood. In: Zeanah CH, Ed. *Handbook of Infant Mental Health*, 2nd edition. New York: Guilford Press, 2000, pp. 353–368.
24. Zeanah CH, Scheeringa M, Boris NW, Heller SS, Smyke AT, Trapani J. Reactive attachment disorder in maltreated toddlers, *Child Abuse Negl* 2004; **28**: 877–888.
25. American Psychiatric Association. *Diagnostic and Statistical Manual of Mental Disorders*. 3rd edition. Washington, DC: American Psychiatric Association, 1980.
26. American Psychiatric Association. *Diagnostic and Statistical Manual of Mental Disorders*. 4th edition. Washington, DC: American Psychiatric Association, 1994.

27. Zeanah CH, Fox NA. Temperament and attachment disorders, *J Clin Child Adolesc Psychol* 2004; **33**: 32–41.
28. The ICD-10 classification of mental and behavioural disorders: Clinical descriptions and diagnostic guidelines. Geneva: World Health Organization, 1992.
29. Bowlby J. *Attachment and Loss* Vol. 1, *Attachment*. New York: Basic Books, 1969.
30. O'Conner TG, Marvin RS, Rutter M, Olrick JT, Brittner PA. The English and Romanian adoptees (ERA) study team. Child-parent attachment following severe early institutional deprivation, *Dev Psychopathol* 2003; **15**: 19–38.
31. Smyke AT, Dumitrescu A, Zeanah CH. Attachment disturbances in young children I: The continuum of caretaking casualty, *J Am Acad Child Adolesc Psychiatry* 2002; **41**: 972–982.
32. Zeanah CH, Smyke AT, Dumitrescu A. Attachment disturbances in young children II: Indiscriminate behavior and institutionalized care, *J Am Acad Child Adolesc Psychiatry* 2002; **41**: 983–986.
33. Chisholm K. A three-year follow-up of attachment and indiscriminate friendliness in children adopted from Romanian orphanages, *Child Dev* 1998; **69**: 1092–1106.
34. Stafford B, Zeanah CH, Scheeringa M. Exploring psychopathology in early childhood: PTSD and attachment disorders in DC: 0-3 and DSM-IV, *Infant Ment Health J* 2003; **24**: 398–409.
35. American Academy of Child and Adolescent Psychiatry. Practice parameters for the psychiatric assessment of infants and toddlers (0–36 months), *J Am Acad Child Adolesc Psychiatry* 1997; **36**: 215–365.
36. Boris NW, Fueyo M, Zeanah CH. The clinical assessment of attachment in children under five, *J Am Acad Child Adolesc Psychiatry* 1997; **36**: 291–293.
37. Fraiberg S. *Clinical Studies in Infant Mental Health*. New York: Basic Books, 1980.
38. Clark R. *The parent-child early relational assessment: Instrument and manual*. Madison: University of Wisconsin Medical School, Department of Psychiatry, 1985.
39. Zeanah CH, Larrieu JA, Heller SS, Valliere J. Infant-parent relationship assessment. In: Zeanah CH, Ed. *Handbook of Infant Mental Health*, 2nd edition. New York: Guilford Press, 2000, pp. 222–235.
40. O'Connor TG, Zeanah CH. Attachment disorders: Assessment strategies and treatment approaches, *Attach Hum Dev* 2003; **5**: 223–244.
41. Bretherton I, Ridgeway D, Cassidy J. Assessing internal working models of the attachment relationship: An attachment story completion task for 3-year-olds. In: Greenberg MT, Cicchetti D, Cummings EM, Eds. *Attachment in the Preschool Years: Theory, Research, and Intervention*. Chicago: University of Chicago Press, 1990, pp. 273–308.
42. Ainsworth MDS, Blehar MC, Waters E, Wall S. *Patterns of Attachment: A Psychological Study of the Strange Situation*. Hillsdale, NJ: Erlbaum, 1978.

43. Zilberstein K. Clarifying core characteristics of attachment disorders: A review of current research and theory, *Am J Orthopsychiatry* 2006; **76**: 55–64.
44. Kreppner JM, O'Connor TG, Rutter M, *et al.* Can inattention/overactivity be an institutional deprivation syndrome? *J Abnorm Child Psychol* 2001; **29**: 513–528.
45. O'Connor TG, Rutter M, Beckett C, Keaveney L, Kreppner JM. English and Romanian adoptees study team. The effects of global severe privation on cognitive competence: Extension and longitudinal follow-up, *Child Dev* 2000; **71**: 376–390.
46. Rutter M, Anderson-Wood L, Beckett C, *et al.* Quasi-autistic patterns following severe early global privation, *J Child Psychol Psychiatry* 1999; **40**: 537–549.
47. Minde K. Assessment and treatment of attachment disorders, *Curr Opin Psychiatry* 2003; **16**: 377–381.
48. Kagan J, Snidman N. Temperamental factors in human development, *Am Psychol* 1991; **46**: 856–862.
49. Rutter M, O'Connor TG. English and Romanian adoptees study team Are there biological programming effects for psychological development? Findings from a study of Romanian adoptees. *Dev Psychol* 2004; **40**: 81–94.
50. Zelenko M, Benham A. Attachment theory, loss, and trauma: A case study, *J Cl Child Psychol Psychiatry* 2002; **7**: 199–209.
51. Brisch KH, Bechinger D, Betzler S, Heinemann H. Early preventive attachment-oriented psychotherapeutic intervention program with parents of a very low birth weight premature infant: Results of attachment and neurological development, *Attach Hum Dev* 2003; **5**: 120–135.
52. Cicchetti D, Rogosh FA, Toth SL. Fostering secure attachment in infants in maltreating families through preventive interventions, *Dev Psychopath* 2006; **18**: 623–649.
53. Zelenko M. Psychotherapeutic interventions in infancy and early childhood. In: Steiner H, Ed. *Handbook of Mental Health Interventions in Child Adolescence,* San Francisco: Jossey-Bass, 2004, pp. 557–585.
54. Bowlby J. *Attachment and Loss,* Vol. 2, *Separation*. New York: Basic Books, 1973.
55. Silverman PR, Worden JW. Children's reactions in the early months after the death of a parent, *Am J Orthopsychiatry* 1992; **62**: 93–104.

Chapter 5

Anxiety and Special Impulse Control Disorders

Margo Thienemann, Kyle Hinman, Michael Bloch, and James Leckman

A Clinician's View: Case 1

Diana, a 16-year-old high school junior who was referred by her high school counselor for evaluation of school nonattendance, reluctantly came to the Stanford Pediatric Clinic. She had stopped attending school altogether three months prior to evaluation. In the previous semester, she had missed approximately 40% of school days. Even though she was working one-on-one with an independent study tutor from the school district, her parents and the school counselor felt that she was too isolated and needed to return to school.

While she preferred to be interviewed with her parents in the room, she did agree to speak alone with the clinic psychiatrist. During that conversation she raised many concerns. She told the psychiatrist that she could not bear to show her face at school after having been gone so long. She remarked that she would be so far behind in her work, she would not know how to answer questions in class and if the teacher called on her, she would probably blush and everyone would laugh.

When the psychiatrist asked about her mood, she reported that she felt tired, irritable, and could not sleep well. This report of sleep disturbance, irritability, and fatigue led the clinician to ask about other mood symptoms. She did not feel optimistic, nor did she feel like socializing. Her appetite was fine, but concentration was poor. While she did not think about her own death, she found herself thinking about what would happen if her parents died, and what would happen to the earth due to global warming. Once these thoughts occurred to her, she could not get them out of her mind.

1. Introduction

Like many children who suffer from anxiety, this young woman experienced physical symptoms that limited her activities. Her family members, affected by her behavior, spent time and money trying to help. Many children, like this girl, suffer feelings of anxiety and fear. They cry and cling to their parents when separating, or when meeting unfamiliar people or faced with a big barking dog. For parents, the question of whether these behaviors are "just a phase" or a serious problem is often hard to answer. Anxiety causes anguish, and it is costly. In 1990, medical services for anxiety disorders cost 42.3 billion dollars and in 1999 the estimated cost was 63.1 billion dollars. Short-term and long-term consequences include poor social skills, depression, low self-esteem, and achievement below ability level in school. Childhood anxiety disorders have been linked to adult mental health issues such as substance abuse, anxiety, and depression.

As many as 20% of children suffer from anxiety symptoms that significantly interfere with school, social interaction, quality of life, and maintaining their developmental trajectory. This chapter presents the neuropsychological model of anxiety, describes the forms excessive anxiety takes in school-aged children through adolescence, discusses pathways thought to lead to anxiety disorders, and reviews the most recent therapeutic interventions.

2. A Neuropsychological Model of Anxiety

When humans sense threat, the central nervous system is activated. The alarm warning begins in the medial temporal lobe's amygdala, where both direct and indirect cortico-striato-thalamic pathways relay neural information about the perceived danger and prepare a person to react. When threatened, humans may respond immediately and reflexively or with a flexible, better thought-out response. Before conscious thought, the autonomic nervous system, stimulated *via* the direct pathway, results in uncomfortable physical sensations. The heart beats faster and harder, breathing becomes shallower, muscles tense, and sweat glands and the gastrointestinal systems are activated. Humans behave as other threatened animals do: freezing, fleeing, or fighting to avoid harm. Meanwhile, the indirect pathway processes threat on a cognitive level, registering the immediate circumstance, comparing it to past experience, assessing the risk, noting available resources, and choosing a response designed for survival. Each past experience with a specific threat shapes a person's thoughts, feelings, and behaviors when encountering a new threat. Humans feel the physiologic concomitants of anxiety in anticipation of and during subsequent exposures to situations that remind them of other, threatening ones. These physical sensations lead them to think and plan ways to cope with the next threatening stimuli. If repeated reencounters with the stimuli are safe, the severity of the anxious feelings, thoughts, and behaviors attenuate, allowing a person to get on without dysfunctional anxiety. Though reexposure to a conditioned threatening stimulus can extinguish the fear response, the extinction is not permanent. The original fear reemerges when exposure to the initial stimulus is dangerous. Human survival has depended on this alarm system. However, when the alarm system is activated in low-risk situations, it causes excessive, inappropriate anxiety. For a number of individuals, this excessive anxiety begins in childhood and may interfere with normal development.

3. Childhood Fears

Every child experiences fears, worries, and frightening dreams. Babies experience fear of strangers. Toddlers experience fear of separation from parents and primary caregivers. Children aged between 4 and 6 years tend to be afraid of fantastical creatures such as monsters. Children in mid-childhood often fear being hurt physically or experiencing natural disasters. When surveyed across age, gender, and culture, children most commonly fear being hit by a car, not being able to breathe, being attacked by bombs or burned by fire, falling from a high place, burglars breaking into the house, earthquakes, death, poor grades, and snakes. As children age, one fear can replace another. Where a nine year old may be terrified of bees and unwilling to join in a family picnic, an older child may worry more about school and the unknown.

Although fearful and anxious behavior, such as waking in the middle of the night or hiding from new houseguests may trouble parents, many childhood fears serve a functional purpose. Learning to adapt to new situations or stimuli and learning healthy ways to cope with frightening experiences prepares children to deal with the disturbing and potentially threatening events. However, severe anxiety can also be associated with somatic symptoms such as complaints of stomach aches or headaches without cause. Trouble in getting to sleep and nightmares also may indicate pathological underlying anxiety. At times, the child's efforts to avoid situations that can make him/her anxious can also lead to impulsive, distracted, or even oppositional behavior. About 23% of children who report experiencing fears and worries have sufficient impairment to qualify for the diagnosis of an anxiety disorder. When the degree of emotional suffering and activity avoidance caused by anxiety interferes with normal functions (failing to make any friends for fear of rejection, nonattendance at school, and/or family unable to sleep because child awakens them repeatedly in the night), these symptoms qualify for a clinical diagnosis of an anxiety disorder.

4. Childhood Anxiety Disorders

The DSM-IV-TR defines two anxiety disorders specific to childhood: separation anxiety disorder and selective mutism. The five other anxiety disorders described below occur in both children and adults. The disorders share numerous risk factors and symptoms. Research continues to clarify whether and which diagnoses represent etiologically distinct disorders. Based on the course of illness, physiologic findings and heritability, some diagnoses appear to stand as distinct entities while others may be manifestations of an anxiety diathesis presenting differently at different developmental stages. Some may represent manifestations of a yet-undefined anxiety-depression disorder. Finally, Obsessive compulsive disorder (OCD) stands apart as a distinct unrelated neuropsychiatric entity.

The standard diagnostic tool used to determine these disorders in the United States is the *Diagnostic and Statistical Manual of Mental Disorders, DSM-IV* (American Psychiatric Association). In European countries, clinicians use the Composite International Diagnostic Interview (CIDI, World Health Organization).[1,2] In the 1990s, the World Health Organization (WHO) worked to correlate the different tools to facilitate reliable crossnational comparable analysis of risks factors, consequences, treatments, or barriers to seeking treatments.

4.1. *Separation anxiety disorder*

Toddlers, preschoolers and healthy individuals of any age feel distress at separation from people on whom they depend. Intense, dysfunctional discomfort upon separation from primary caretaker(s) troubles as many as 4% of children. When anticipating separation, children with separation anxiety disorder complain of physical symptoms, especially stomach aches. They worry that separation will be permanent and fear that they or their parent will be harmed. They resist and protest separation, cry, scream, cling, and tantrum when parting. They may refuse to sleep alone. Up to 75% may refuse to attend school.

The intensity of separation anxiety symptoms may increase insidiously or begin precipitously after a stressor such as illness in a parent. The age of onset peaks between seven and nine years. Separation anxiety usually worsens after a period of spending extensive time with the caretaker, such as following a school vacation or illness. Its course may be chronic or symptoms may abate with time, with prevalence rates falling in adolescence. Later in life, children with separation anxiety disorder, social phobia, and specific phobia experience panic disorder and major depression at an increased rate.

4.2. *Selective mutism*

Children with selective mutism can speak, but either do not choose to speak in the presence of others or are selective about to whom they speak. This rare disorder with an incidence of less that 1/1000 occurs primarily in girls. It typically begins at between three and six years of age, with most children being referred for treatment during kindergarten, when the children must interact with the public. For the diagnosis to be made, symptoms must persist after the first month of school.

Selectively mute children may be experienced by others as stubborn and oppositional. However, a study of 50 children with selective mutism found no evidence of an externalizing disorder in the absence of a primary anxiety disorder. All met criteria for avoidant disorder or social anxiety disorder and half met criteria for an additional anxiety disorder. In another study, 69% of those with selective mutism versus 15% of controls met criteria for a concomitant developmental problem, including speech disorder or delay.

4.3. *Generalized anxiety disorder*

Most children worry about a variety of things from time to time. However, about 5% of children aged from 8 to 13 meet criteria for Generalized anxiety disorder (GAD), when prominent somatic symptoms and excessive anxiety and worry interfere with functioning and quality of life. Emotional symptoms of GAD include edginess and irritability. Concentration may be diminished. Somatic symptoms include restlessness, fatigue, muscle tenseness, and sleep disturbance. Worry may focus on upcoming situations, concerns about behavior in past situations, war, disasters, others' health, money and divorce, or be "free floating." Having GAD carries significant risk for future psychopathology such as depression and substance abuse.

4.4. *Specific phobia*

Four percent of children suffer from specific phobias. Phobic children fear an object or a situation so much that they avoid contact with it, or, if they must encounter it, they endure it only with extreme distress. If the fear or avoidance interferes significantly with functioning in areas of academic, social, or family life, symptoms qualify for the diagnosis of specific phobia. Common phobic stimuli include heights, small animals, doctors, dentists, darkness, loud noises, and storms. Interestingly, phobias causing vaso-vagal reactions, such as fear of needles or blood, have a strong heritability. Children with specific phobias avoid the feared stimuli by refusing to go places, fleeing, clinging, screaming, crying, and disobeying. Physiologic reactions to exposure or the thought of exposure may include increased heart rate, shakiness, upset stomach, and intrusive thoughts. Over the period of several years, most phobias improve without treatment.

4.5. *School refusal*

While not a DSM-IV-TR diagnosis, the extent of clinical impairment and ongoing research on school refusal justifies its inclusion for discussion. Children with school refusal avoid attending school or have difficulty remaining in school for the entire school day, causing youth to get behind in their schoolwork and homework, become less involved with friends and after school activities and stressing parents as their children remain at home all day. Extensive absence from school may initiate a cascade of problems for the patient, limiting opportunities for attending schools of higher education and gaining suitable employment.

Approximately 5% of girls and boys are school refusers. Symptoms most commonly occur between the ages of 5 and 11 years around academic transition points, such as transfer to another school or change of classroom. These children often miss school on Mondays and after vacation days. Unlike truancy, associated with antisocial conduct, school refusal is associated with some form of anxiety. Children may have school refusal on the basis of separation anxiety (38%), social anxiety (30%), and phobic avoidance of other specific situations such as tests (22%). Sometimes, children who will not attend school fear actual risks, such as bullies or crime. Comorbid depression and language and learning disorders are common. Families may reinforce school refusal by making children comfortable staying home, causing the avoidance behavior to become further entrenched by reinforcing it. The longer school refusal continues, the more difficult it is to return to school.

4.6. *Social anxiety disorder*

Many young children feel wary or shy when meeting strangers. When the fear of embarrassment or humiliation in social settings causes functional impairment, the diagnosis is social anxiety disorder. Approximately 4 to 6% of children and adolescents suffer from social anxiety disorder. It affects an equal number of boys and girls and usually begins early in school. Socially anxious children and adults most commonly fear performing in front of others (performance type), but may also fear reading aloud in class, joining a conversation, being observed, and speaking to adults (generalized type). Children with social anxiety disorder may become socially isolated, fail to meet their potential academically, and become depressed in adulthood.

4.7. *Panic disorder*

Panic disorder rarely starts before adolescence. Episodes of physical and cognitive symptoms not precipitated by a discernable cause define panic disorder. Adolescents with panic disorder feel symptoms of shortness of breath, heart palpitations and forceful beats, dizziness, tremulousness, sweating, abdominal cramps, need to urinate or defecate, and muscular weakness. During the attacks, which last for about 20 to 40 min, patients may feel that they will die or are going crazy. Panic disorder may occur alone or with agoraphobia — the avoidance of specific circumstances associated with a fear of experiencing a panic attack. The time onset is associated more closely with the level of pubertal development than with age. Having panic disorder increases the risk for depression. In a four-year study of more than 2000 high school students, having panic disorder predicted the development of major depression and having depression predicted the development of panic disorder.

4.8. *Obsessive compulsive disorder (OCD)*

While classified as an anxiety disorder, OCD stands apart from the other anxiety disorders in its comorbidity, neuropsychiatric findings, and precipitants. Plagued by uneasy feelings that something is wrong, patients with OCD experience fears, worries, thoughts, urges, and images that can be ignored only with great effort and practice. In response to those thoughts, they perform rituals to relieve the uncomfortable feelings. The thoughts and rituals may take hours per day and interfere with school, extra-curricular activities, and family life. The disorder presents similarly in childhood and adulthood, except that children may not realize that the content of the obsessions and the compulsive response are not rational.

Common obsessive concerns include fears of contamination, harmful circumstances, religious or moral misdeeds, unwanted sexual thoughts, and need to know or remember something. Common rituals include needing to clean and wash, checking things repeatedly, and asking the same questions again and again. Only one-fourth of children with OCD display this disorder alone. Secondary depression, other anxiety disorders, and tic disorders are common. Those with comorbid tics and Tourette's syndrome are different from those without, in that they are most likely to feel the need to do things "just right" or symmetrically, to be male, and have onset before age 11.

A subset of children with OCD has been identified whose disorder has been precipitated or exacerbated by streptococcal infection or other immune-response eliciting insult. These children have been labeled with the diagnoses of PANDAS (pediatric auto-immune neuro-psychiatric disorders associated with streptococcal infection).[3] In addition to obsessive-compulsive symptoms, these children experience movement disorders, separation anxiety, mood lability, and attention deficit hyperactivity symptoms. While experimental treatments are being tested, current standard care addresses manifest symptoms and maintains vigilance about infections. On the whole, OCD affects 1 to 2% of children and adolescents. The incidence of PANDAS has not been determined.

5. Epidemiology

5.1. *Overall prevalence*

Anxiety disorders rank as the most common childhood psychiatric diagnoses, with prevalence rates estimated at 6–15% for US school-aged children and 20% in a survey of German adolescents. In that study, specific phobia occurred most commonly. Less than 2% of adolescents reported OCD and less than 1% reported panic disorder or generalized anxiety disorder. While many identified themselves as being psychosocially impaired by anxiety, few sought treatment. Reported anxiety disorder incidence was higher in girls than boys and increased with age. Other epidemiological studies indicate that anxiety disorders, with the exception of social anxiety disorder and OCD, manifest at least twice as commonly in females. This difference in sex distribution offers support to the validity of social phobia and OCD as separate diagnoses.

5.2. *Prevalence and age*

In children and adults, anxiety disorders begin at an average age of 11, but the age of onset of the various disorders varies systematically. Separation anxiety and specific phobias begin in young children, while selective mutism, generalized anxiety disorder, and separation anxiety disorder occur most in middle or late childhood. Generalized anxiety disorder begins early in adolescence. Some individuals may carry a diathesis toward separation and generalized anxiety disorders manifesting with symptomatic presentation changes with developmental stage such that during early school years, when children are preoccupied with control of aggressive urges in themselves and others, they depend on others for protection and care. In these years, anxiety about separation from these protectors occurs. Adolescents care about conforming to socially desirable standards for appearance, behavior and achievements. It makes sense, then, that generalized anxiety disorder in teens concerns the appropriateness of one's own behavior and the adequacy of one's achievements. This developmental theory about separation anxiety and generalized anxiety is supported by a prospective study demonstrating a one-way sequence of developing separation anxiety disorder and overanxious disorder. Hormonal factors may play a role in the onset of anxiety disorders. The time of onset for panic disorder is most closely linked to level of sexual development. The OCD symptoms may increase in peripubertal boys.

5.3. *Comorbidity*

Forty percent of children with anxiety disorders have at least another psychiatric diagnosis. A study using a structured interview in an anxiety clinic found that only 33% of subjects had only one anxiety diagnosis, 50% two or more anxiety diagnoses, and 67% had two or more diagnoses of any type. Depression and anxiety manifest together in 33 to 44% of anxiety-disordered children and adolescents. That incidence increases in those adolescents with more severe anxiety. This common comorbidity (and response to similar treatments) has led some to speculate that the diagnoses represent different manifestations of a single diathesis. Cognitively, in anxiety, one fears bad things will happen, in depression, they already have.

Having an internalizing anxiety disorder does not protect children from having an externalizing disorder. Thirty-four percent of the 879 subjects in the Multi-center Treatment Study of Attention Deficit Hyperactivity Disorder had an anxiety disorder in addition to ADHD.[4] Thirty percent of youth with conduct disorder also have an anxiety disorder. The presence of a comorbid anxiety disorder in delinquents with severe conduct disorder does not temper the severity of their behaviors. Developmental and learning problems may be associated with anxiety. The majority of children with pervasive developmental disorders qualify for a diagnosis of an anxiety disorder and have ritualistic behaviors.

6. Etiology and Pathogenesis

A Clinician's View: Case 2

Chris was a 14-year-old high-school freshman who came to the Stanford Clinic because habits were taking too much time away from his schoolwork and recreational time and because his family was frustrated by his falling grades, angry attitude, and his tying up the bathroom, making everyone late in the morning.

Chris's troubles began, as his parents recall, at about age seven. After a bad cold with a sore throat, he would hesitate whenever he crossed a threshold, touching the sides four times before going through. At that time, he was clingier at home and more restless in class and developed a habit of blinking his eyes. After a time, things returned to normal until a few years later, in November, he had a few months during which he asked his parents the same questions over and over again: questions like "When are we going to sign me up for spring softball?" or "What did you say in the car?" At that time, too, he was irritable and anxious. Within months, questions abated and mood improved.

As Chris's puberty began, symptoms of excessive hand washing and showering disrupted Chris's and his family's life. He had a hard time going anywhere or starting anything without an extended (30 min) grooming session in the bathroom. These activities took so much time that he did not finish his homework until midnight or later. He felt dejected, listless, and irritable. Even at going to bed at midnight, he had trouble going to sleep for at least an hour.

Current thinking about anxiety disorders posits that anxiety disorders develop when an individual with a biological diathesis toward excessive anxiety encounters sufficient environmental, biological, or developmental stress to tip them into a symptomatic pathological state. This section discusses evidence for biological predisposition and environmental risk factors. Studies have begun to focus on the relevance of a child's temperament to the development of an anxiety disorder. Anxious children and shy or inhibited children share characteristics of having overly sensitive danger detection systems, pronounced attentional bias to threat, avoidant coping style, and over-reactive amygdala.

6.1. *Genetic/family history*

Childhood anxiety develops under heritable influences. The strongest evidence of genetic influence comes from twin studies where examination of large samples found that both the cognitive symptoms — fear of negative evaluation (central to social anxiety) and fear of anxiety-related physical sensations (anxiety sensitivity central to panic disorder) are heritable. Seven-year-old monozygotic twins correlate more closely than dizygotic twins in reports of physiological anxiety symptoms and fear of negative evaluation. A study of Australian child twin pairs found that genetic influences contributed significantly to the development of separation anxiety disorder. In studies of adult twins, panic disorder and generalized anxiety disorder were found to have heritability rates of approximately 40%.

Studies of relatives of children with anxiety disorders confound the influences of genes with the influence of environment, but do lend support for genetic transmission. If a parent has depression, an anxiety disorder, or both, a child has a four to eight times higher relative risk of having an anxiety disorder and a five to six times higher risk of having any psychiatric disorder. Children of depressed parents are at increased risk for depression and overanxious disorder. First-degree relatives of children with separation anxiety disorder-caused school refusal have more panic disorder and agoraphobia than controls, while first degree relatives of school refusers with specific or social phobia have more simple and social phobia.

6.2. *Behaviorally inhibited temperament*

Approximately 10% of toddlers withdraw or freeze when faced with novel stimuli, a reaction observed as early as in the newborn nursery. Individuals with this temperamental tendency approach new situations with more restraint, avoidance, and distress than others do. They demonstrate a low threshold for sympathetic arousal as measured by reduced heart rate variability, increased systolic blood pressure response to stress, and a higher resting cortisol. So far, this temperamental quality has been shown to persist in some individuals from age 21 months to adolescence.

Behavioral inhibition to the unfamiliar is a risk factor for later anxiety disorders. While most children with behavior inhibition do not develop anxiety disorders, children with behavioral inhibition develop anxiety disorders more frequently than behaviorally uninhibited or typical children. Classification as behaviorally inhibited at age two increases the risk of generalized social anxiety disorder in adolescence, especially in girls. Development of social anxiety — the most frequent anxiety diagnosis in behaviorally inhibited adolescents — may stem from fear of negative appraisal especially in unfamiliar contexts. This fear may be an adolescent derivative of the caution exhibited by the behaviorally inhibited in new settings.

6.3. *Physiological concomitants*

Anxious children differ from normal children in physiologic sympathetic nervous system responsiveness when challenged. When yohimbine, an alpha-adrenergic antagonist that increases the release of norepinephrine, is administered to anxiety-disordered child subjects and controls, the anxious subjects feel more anxious and demonstrate a blunted growth hormone output. When challenged with the alpha-adrenergic agonist, clonidine, children with elevated self-rated anxiety differ in growth hormone response compared to controls and to anxious adults. These findings suggest that children with anxiety disorders have excessive noradrenergic activity. Over time, that chronic overactivity may change receptor sensitivity in adulthood.

Those with panic disorder may feel a sense of suffocation with lower provocation. When children and adolescents with separation anxiety disorder, social anxiety disorder, and overanxious disorder, and control subjects breathe 3 to 5% carbon dioxide for 15 min in an escapable canopy, panic or near panic and enhanced respiratory rate are significantly more frequent in those with anxiety, especially separation anxiety disorder. Breathing room air, those with anxiety disorders demonstrate increased respiratory variability compared to controls, as well.

Neuroimaging is shedding light on differences between anxiety-disordered and other children. When presented with images of fearful faces, children with generalized anxiety disorder or panic disorder show an exaggerated amygdala activation compared with depressed and healthy children. During adolescence, functional magnetic resonance imaging has shown that amygdala activity appears to be related to social and interpersonal fears more than non-social anxiety types.

6.4. *Attachment*

Bowlby[5] contributed to the field of psychiatry by describing attachment — a concept important to the development of anxiety in some individuals. Attachment is a system of adaptive behaviors and mental schema that protects infants by prompting caretaker proximity. Researchers in attachment identify the quality of the attachment of the child to the caretaker as secure or insecure based on the child's confidence that the attachment figure will be available in times of trouble. If the child feels that he/she will be helped and protected by his or her caretaker, he/she demonstrates a secure attachment. An insecurely avoidantly attached child perceives the caretaker as unavailable and rejecting. If the caretaker is experienced as inconsistent and intrusive, children are considered insecurely and anxiously attached and may act angry, resistant, and ambivalent around the caretaker.

If an individual feels that he/she (and his/her resources) cannot successfully withstand a stressful situation, he/she will experience anxiety and distress. For young children especially, confidence that they can cope in a stressful situation depends on the availability of the attachment figure. Some evidence substantiates disordered or insecure attachment as a risk factor for development of anxiety disorders. A comparison of attachment status at age 1 with results of a structured diagnostic interview at age 17.5 showed that adolescents who had been classified as anxiously attached in infancy had a twofold increased risk of having an anxiety disorder over non-anxiously attached infants. Attachment status correlated with the presence of anxiety disorders in adolescent subjects even more than with behavioral inhibition observed in the nursery. Children who perceive their parents as (more) rejecting and anxious describe themselves as more avoidantly or ambivalently attached than do typical children. Attachment status of mothers to their own mothers relates to anxiety disorders in offspring. Anxiety-disordered children's mothers are more likely to be insecurely attached, have decreased social support, and be anxious. Their children have insecure attachment and more anxiety disorders than others. One's attachment type is a risk factor that initiates a developmental interpersonal relationship pathway which may increase vulnerability to later anxiety disorder in oneself or one's progeny.

6.5. *Parenting practice*

Parents may add to children's anxiety. Anxious children may shape parents' behaviors. Those interested in learning theory suggest that some child-rearing practices promote the development of anxiety disorders. Mothers of anxious children have been described as anxious acting, over protective, less warm, and less positive toward their children and more critical and catastrophic in predicting outcomes of situations. A study of 9- to-12-year olds found that anxiety symptoms were associated with parental rejection, anxious rearing, and parental control. Anxiety of the child, rather than maternal anxiety, predicted how much of autonomy and criticism parents gave to their children. In addition, anxious mothers do think in more catastrophic ways and act less warmly toward their anxious children. In these interactions, mothers interpret situations more negatively, possibly teaching children to interpret situations as out of one's control. In everyday life, parents frequently need to help their children take appropriate risks. Lack of maternal warmth and encouragement could lead to children avoiding taking the risks necessary to master developmentally appropriate tasks thereby increasing the risk of dysfunctional anxiety.

6.6. *Animal models*

Some researchers have examined animal models hoping to further understand human anxiety. In the model of subordination stress, animals were placed in a confined environment with a dominant individual appearing anxious. They spend more time alone and fearfully scan their social environment, somewhat like humans with social anxiety disorder. These animals display excessive hypothalamic–pituitary–adrenal (HPA) axis activation, impaired serotonergic function and dopamine neurotransmission, and hypercortisolemia. Human subjects with social anxiety disorder differ from primates exposed to subordination stress in that they do not typically develop social anxiety *de novo* as a response to environmental manipulations, nor do they show evidence of HPA axis disturbance.

Another anxiety disorder paradigm experimentally induces an unstable attachment pattern *via* a variable foraging demand model. In this model, simian mothers with infants spend unpredictable periods of time away from their babies to gather food. The infants reared with disrupted contact with their attachment figures act timid and avoid both friendly and unfriendly contact from others. Physiologically, the infants appear similar to humans with acute post-traumatic stress disorder.

They had increased corticotrophin releasing factor, homovanillic acid, and 5HIAA (5-hydroxy indole acetic acid).

Two varieties of voles demonstrate differing levels of social affiliation and comfort in social situations. The prairie vole spends the majority of its time in physical contact with its family while the montane vole contacts others for reproductive necessities only. The voles differ in their argenine vasopressin brain receptors. It is intriguing to wonder whether any parallels exist for those with social anxiety symptoms.

7. Differential Diagnosis

In traditional psychiatric interviews, clinicians pick up a thread in the tangle of complaints and follow it, testing hypotheses that will lead to diagnoses. The weaving together of pieces of information about a patient's temperament, family history, social history, psychiatric history, and developmental history to form a diagnosis calls upon a combination of clinician experience and knowledge, choice of diagnostic tools, disclosure from patient and parents, and additional information from school personnel or pediatricians. Other diagnostic methods exist, as well.

A Clinician's View: Case 2 continued

Interviewing Chris, the clinician would likely query about the presence of intrusive thoughts and images, and about other repetitive behaviors Chris may have or his family may report. Returning to the chief complaint, the clinician could investigate the reason for falling grades. Are they due to OCD symptoms interrupting thoughts or causing avoidance or precipitating repetitive rituals that interfere with school work? Does Chris have an undiagnosed learning disorder? Does depression secondary to the OCD sap Chris's motivation? Is Chris attending class? Using drugs? Following educated hunches, much can be learned. Then, any missing information (developmental, social, medical, and family histories, mental status exam) may be gathered more systematically.

Alternatively, the interviewer may systematically visit each diagnostic category to find symptom clusters consistent with DSM (*Diagnostic and Statistical Manual of Mental Disorders*). Using a structured interview such as the Diagnostic Interview Schedule for Children (DISC) or having the patient and family complete the computerized Voice DISC can be a good starting point.[6] At least one study has shown better outcome in adult inpatients when a structured interview was used at admission. Diagnostic results differ by method and informant. Parents are better reporters of overt behavior and children and adolescents of their own behaviors.

Externalizing disorders (attention deficit disorder with hyperactivity, oppositional defiant disorder, conduct disorder) are more reliably diagnosed than internalizing disorders (anxiety and depression). To date, no gold standard diagnostic system exists. Clinically, we interview the family together and separately and clinically reconcile findings. As well, we integrate semistructured interviews and paper and pencil measures. We used the Children's Yale-Brown Obsessive Compulsive Scale (CY-BOCS) checklist.[7] To quantify the severity, we asked him about the time symptoms took, how much they interfered with life and his control over them. To rule out other anxiety disorders, we used the semistructured Anxiety Disorders Interview Schedule for Parents and Children (ADIS-CP) and used the Child Depression Inventory (CDI) to quantify the degree of depression.[8,9]

In this case, many more OCD symptoms were reported by parents and Chris than in the spontaneous report. Chris did not meet clinical criteria for other diagnoses according to the ADIS-CP, but we learned that Chris had subclinical social anxiety. His results on the CDI did not meet the cutoff for clinical significance.

Currently, symptomatic presentations rather than laboratory findings lead to diagnoses of childhood anxiety. Symptoms of anxiety disorders, such as restlessness, inattention, and social withdrawal may appear in other childhood conditions. To appropriately diagnose an anxiety disorder, the constellation of symptoms, information from multiple informants, family history, developmental age of onset, and history of stressors should be considered.

Children's classroom behaviors which may appear to parents or teachers to be caused by anxiety stem from reactions to academic issues. Children with unidentified or inadequately addressed learning disorders often look inattentive and feel anxious in the classroom. When attempting homework that demands too much, children with learning disorders may feel inadequate and appear anxious, lazy, and oppositional. Attention deficit hyperactivity disorder and anxiety share symptoms, including inattention, difficulty sitting still, and failure to finish schoolwork. The clinician must consider other concomitant symptoms, the course of illness, and family history to distinguish the two disorders. The largest study of attention deficit hyperactivity disorder to date, the multisite treatment study of attention deficit disorder found that one-third of subjects with attention deficit disorder also had a comorbid anxiety disorder, suggesting that both disorders may often be present.[4]

Mood disorders also share symptoms with anxiety disorders. Children with mood disorders may appear inattentive, socially withdrawn, avoidant of participation in activities, and restless. Like children with OCD, depressed children may suffer from inability to get unpleasant ideas out of their mind.

When anxious children are backed into a situation beyond their ability to remain calm, they may hit, kick, scream, swear, and destroy things in an attempt to communicate their upset and to avoid doing whatever it is they are being pushed to do. If the adult does not understand that the child is anxious, then the behavior will be misinterpreted as oppositional defiant behavior.

Both overlap of symptoms and comorbidity can confuse the diagnosis of anxiety disorders in pervasive developmental disorders and learning disorders. Children with pervasive developmental disorders become anxious when a social situation obviously requires some response from them, but they do not know what to do. They may become distressed when routines are changed or when required to desist from a familiar, perseverative, and calming pursuit. Repetitive behaviors of those with pervasive developmental disorders may be misidentified with the compulsive behavior of those with OCD.

8. Clinical Instruments and Methods

A Clinician's View: Case 1

After meeting with school-refusing Diana, the clinician began to weave together various threads of information to provide a diagnosis. First, she reviewed the patient's psychiatric history. Diana had not been evaluated by a psychiatrist in the past. She had worked with the school counselor to strategize catching up on her schoolwork and had once seen a peer counselor.

Second, the clinician looked at the patient's developmental history. The mother's pregnancy and delivery were normal. After Diana's birth, her mother suffered her second bout of post-partum depression, which responded to medication. When Diana's parents enrolled her in preschool, she suffered significant separation anxiety, so much that her parents did not send her to school again until kindergarten. Because she was so anxious, Diana's mother stayed in the classroom or on campus until Thanksgiving. The girl, always reluctant to leave home or to have her parents go out without her, avoided going to slumber parties or had her parents pick her up at bedtime. When her school had overnight trips, she would not attend. Even in her parents' presence at familiar relatives' homes, she would not interact. Her teachers commented on her good effort on school work, but noted that she would only interact with a few close friends in unstructured time and did not volunteer to answer questions in class. When she did approach the teacher, it was when other students could not hear. She would attend summer camp only if a close friend (from early childhood) went with her.

Despite school nonattendance, Diana maintained a B average. Any social contact Diana had shrunk to the friends she saw at church, which she attended with her family. She did not participate in extra-curricular activities. Family history was significant in that Diana's mother had suffered post-partum depression and panic disorder. Her maternal uncle also had panic disorder and her paternal grandmother may have had depression.

To accurately diagnose childhood anxiety disorders, information should be obtained from the child — the authority about the child's internal experience — and from the observers of the child's behaviors — parents, therapists, and school staff.

Clinical interviews: The Anxiety Disorders Interview Schedule for Children (ADIS-C/P 4) provides differential diagnosis among anxiety disorders using DSM-IV criteria and severity ratings of each particular diagnoses.[8] The semi-structured interview may be given to the child and/or parent. The semistructured format allows for complete coverage of the anxiety disorders and most other childhood diagnoses (not bipolar mood disorder) and for opportunity to expand information gathering when relevant. Within the interview, specific symptoms are rated on distress and interference, which helps direct therapy. Its test-retest reliability within 7–14 days is reported to be excellent for primary anxiety disorders and good to excellent for comorbid anxiety disorders. In the author's clinic, introduction of this interview into the standard evaluation lead to the elimination of non-specific diagnoses and was acceptable to patients. The ADIS-C/P is used as both a diagnostic measure and outcome measure in much of child anxiety disorder research.

Frequently used self-report measures with substantiated reliability and validity include the Revised Children's Manifest Anxiety Scale (RCMAS), State-Trait Anxiety Inventory for Children (STAIC), the Fear Survey Schedule for Children-Revised (FSSC-R), the Revised Screen for Child Anxiety Related Emotional Disorders (SCARED-R), and the Multidimensional Anxiety Scale for Children (MASC).[10–14] The RCMAS is a 37-item scale designed for children 6 to 19 years. It includes a lie scale and describes three factors: physiological manifestations of anxiety, worry and sensitivity, and fear/concentration. Scores on the RCMAS correlate closely with those of the STAIC. The STAIC has two, 20-item questionnaires assessing anxiety in the present state and enduring anxiety and is a good screening instrument. The FSSC-R identifies sources and severity of phobic fear and may be used to track treatment effects. The 66-item self-report questionnaire: Revised Screen for Child Anxiety Related Emotional Disorders (SCARED-R) measures the spectrum of DSM-defined anxiety disorder symptoms in children. It is reported to have reliable internal consistency, validity, and ability to discriminate between anxious and disruptive children. The MASC is a 39-item scale that contains four factors: physical symptoms, social anxiety, harm avoidance, and separation anxiety in children 8 to 19 years old.

The Child Behavior Checklist (CBCL) and the CBCL for teachers: the Teacher Report Form (TRF) inquire about children's behaviors and categorize them as internalizing or externalizing.[15,16] The scales do not give specific information about anxiety disorders, but review of individual items may be helpful in directing the clinical interview. These scales are widely used and well normed.

The clinician may gain important information by observation. In the interview, the rate and volume of speech, verbal social skills, negative self-references, and automatic thoughts may give clues to anxiety. Overt anxious and oppositional behaviors, such as crying, tantrums, attempts to escape, refusal to come into the session or separate from the caregiver, and clinging are common. The interview may also be a forum for observation of parent behaviors, including coercion, collusion, conflict, and reinforcement as means of reinforcing or fighting anxiety behaviors. Researchers and clinicians may design a behavior avoidance task to assess severity and coping capacities around a specific symptom. In this task, a situation is engineered in a naturalistic setting to assess degree of approach.

9. Treatment

A Clinician's View: Case 2

Chris did not want to take medication. Feeling that it could really help Chris to be with other teenagers with OCD, the clinician suggested that he join the weekly adolescent OCD CBT group. He said that he would not talk, but he would go. It was recommended that his parents pick up books to help them learn more about the disorder (e.g. Brain Lock by Jeffrey Schwartz, Obsessive Compulsive Disorder in Children and Adolescents: A Cognitive Behavioral Treatment Manual by March and Mulle, Freeing Your Child from Obsessive Compulsive Disorder by Tamar Chansky, What to do When Your Child has Obsessive Compulsive Disorder by Aureen Pinto Wagner) and explore the OC Foundation website: ocfoundation.org.[17–20]

Chris started the group with five other teens, three of whom had already been through the group before. The first meeting, which included parents and siblings, was psychoeducational. It covered group rules, the neurological basis of OCD, information about epidemiology, and evidence for treatments. At the end, the teens met and talked about the symptoms and their interference. They were asked to get into the mindset of dueling OCD by naming it and by recalling another challenge they had successfully confronted. Chris thought about his initial stage fright and how, by practicing, he had become more comfortable and was well received. He decided to call OCD "OCD." For homework, he labeled obsessions and compulsions as OCD, without necessarily changing behavior.

Over 16 weeks, the group worked their way through the CBT protocol described in the March and Mulle book. At the end of each two hour meeting, parents came in to hear about what was worked on (without betraying confidentiality) and heard what homework goals the adolescents had set. The group learned about what a poor statistician OCD is ("If it could possibly happen, it will."), learned not to argue with it, but to acknowledge the thoughts as "spam" and to be attentive to other real-life goings-on. When the cognitive strategies were unsuccessful, Chris and his peers learned to do exposure therapy. For Chris, that meant addressing his showering and hand-washing rituals. To stop them all at once seemed impossible, because Chris believed that he would be dangerously contaminated and therefore unbearably anxious. So, he broke the rituals into pieces and tried to "mess with OCD" bit by bit. He tried washing his hands standing on one foot, and changing the order in which he dried them. He used a different shampoo. Eventually, he whittled down the rituals to nothing. To do so, he had to risk feeling uncomfortable and sustaining not doing the ritual until the anxiety had abated, often taking most of an hour.

The success was not instant. Chris's family continued to dog him to hurry up. They wondered why he could not just stop doing thing he admitted were irrational. When informed that a group was available for parents of kids with OCD, they were enthusiastic about joining. They arranged their schedules so that they could take turns coming. The parent group served as a good compliment to Chris's CBT group. It included continued psychoeducation, focusing on cognitive and behavioral strategies used to treat OCD. In this group, parents helped each other problem solve about solutions to the problems OCD caused. Research has demonstrated that OCD families are often not thinking-out-of-their-boxes, and problem-solving exercises proved fruitful. They stopped feeling alone in their frustration, and angry or helpless feelings began to diminish. They heard about others' progresses and pitfalls and learned by this.

OCD symptoms continue to impair Chris's school performance. Chris felt that OCD symptoms were distracting him enough that he could not get his homework done in a reasonable time and that, when taking tests, he did not have time to check his work because of having to write overly carefully (an OCD symptom). They ordered "OCD in the Classroom" from the OC Foundation, so as to have materials to inform the teachers of Chris's troubles in a credible way. Chris and his parents felt that Chris could benefit from having more time to complete his school work and tests. They requested a student study team meeting consisting of his teachers, the administration and counselor of his school. Because it was a private school, the parents needed to elicit the school's goodwill in order to get this accommodation. Had he been in a public school, the Individuals with Disabilities Education Act (IDEA) stipulates that the school and parents develop an Individual Educational Plan (IEP) to ensure that Chris could benefit from his educational opportunity.[21] *The school gave Chris extended time and copies of lecture notes.*

By the end of the group, Chris's symptoms, as measured by the CY-BOCS had improved from moderate-severe to mild. His family felt more comfortable when they could communicate with him using the "Fear Thermometer" — an estimation of the degree of anxiety a situation or an exposure would cause for Chris. When it was a 3, they pushed him, when it was a 10, they did not. Chris's mood improved and he wanted to continue the group for another round, glad to have found others with whom he could discuss this part of his life. It was too early to tell the impact the improvement and accommodations had. The family was vigilant for signs of illness or notices from school another student had strep. While they had not tried medication to treat Chris, they understood that this could be another help for him, if necessary in the future.

Before beginning treatment, the clinician must complete a diagnostic evaluation to adequately identify target symptoms and their baseline severity. When families permit, clinician's communication with school personnel gives important information to the assessment. The clinician should communicate the diagnosis clearly in language the patient and the family can understand and identify clear objectives for treatment. Then, the clinician may choose from treatments with adequate evidence to justify their use.

Currently, the treatments for which evidence exists include cognitive behavioral therapy (which has been rated as "well established" to "probably efficacious") and pharmacotherapy (probably efficacious status). For those with mild to moderate anxiety symptoms, treatment should begin with cognitive behavioral therapy. Those with moderate to severe anxiety may require medication to permit participation in cognitive behavioral therapy. Because more evidence supports cognitive behavioral therapy for childhood anxiety because it teaches enduring skills and does not risk adverse effects, it is the treatment of choice.

10. Psychotherapy for Anxiety

A Cochrane review of Cognitive behavioral therapy (CBT) for anxiety disorders in children and adolescents reviewed randomized controlled trials between the years 1970 and 2004. The 13 studies included over 800 outpatient subjects with mild to moderate anxiety symptoms. Fifty-six percent of treated versus 28% of control subjects responded with remission status. Three additional individuals were needed to treat (NNT) to observe an effect of treatment. The therapy in individual, group, and family formats was similarly helpful, as found in post-hoc analyses.[22] Aspects of CBT are described below.

Participant modeling qualifies as "well established" as an effective therapy for childhood phobias according to American Psychological Association criteria. In participant modeling, calm and successful contact with a feared stimulus is demonstrated by a "model," after which the patient contacts the stimulus. The model usually demonstrates *in vivo*, but filmed modeling exposures have also been used successfully. Initially, situations which are mildly anxiety provoking are chosen, then the patient and therapist advance to increasingly difficult ones.

Cognitive behavioral therapy (CBT) focuses on the interactions between what children think (cognitions), how children feel (affect), and what children do (behavior). Children and adolescents with anxiety disorders think negatively and fearfully and judge ambiguous situations as dangerous. When they experience such physical sensations as a pounding heart or a shortness of breath when anxious, they interpret these non-dangerous physiologic phenomena as dangerous and do not know how to calm or soothe themselves. They begin to avoid relatively innocuous stimuli to avoid these uncomfortable feelings. Cognitive behavioral therapy is a logical approach that has a growing body of supportive evidence. In fact, evidence for the effectiveness of cognitive behavioral therapy for anxiety disorders in children has the status of "probably efficacious": an advanced status in the field of child psychotherapy. Although the core cognitive skills required to effectively participate in a CBT program have not been standardized, a child must be able to consider and reflect on his/her own thoughts. The therapy is most effective if the participating child has an awareness of his/her own different emotions, an ability to connect thoughts, and feelings in a variety of situations, and have the ability to come up with different attributes about an event.

Multiple studies by various investigators have used manualized intervention in controlled studies of numbers of subjects and have demonstrated considerable benefit. Kendall, Silverman, and March have been leaders in this pursuit, designing and testing manualized treatment protocols to treat children and adolescents with anxiety disorders and OCD. Of these protocols, The Coping Cat by Kendall has undergone the most testing.[23] Manual-driven individual cognitive behavioral therapy, with and without parental involvement has lead to remission of symptoms to subclinical level in most children in multiple studies. Group therapies for separation anxiety, overanxious disorder, and social phobia using manualized cognitive behavior therapy have had similar successes in the clinical setting.

The cognitive behavior protocols include the basic interventions of psychoeducation, learning to identify dysfunctional thoughts and behaviors, and learning and applying more functional thinking and behavior. In the therapy, therapists act as coaches as children develop hierarchies of feared situations, expose themselves to feared stimuli, learn to control some anxiety symptoms through relaxation exercises and controlled breathing and receive rewards for adherence. In a large sample of children participating in manualized individual cognitive behavioral therapy, having comorbid anxiety or externalizing disorders did not influence outcome: approximately 70% in each group reached remission as defined by the ADIS-CP. Poor treatment response in a one-year follow-up study of children treated with cognitive behavioral therapy was related to pre-treatment teacher and maternal rated internalizing behavior severity, maternal depression, and older child age. Another group found that parental frustration and dysfunction perceived by children predicted poorer outcome to cognitive behavioral treatment.

Refinements to cognitive behavioral therapy have stemmed from addressing resistances. One group found that when parents are anxious, including a parental anxiety management component in the treatment plan doubled the treatment response.[24] When parents are not anxious, the family component did not add to short-term outcome. Parents of oppositional, anxious children require education about parenting strategies. A recent study found that parents can be successfully trained to be lay therapists for their anxiety-disordered children. Two-thirds of children whose parents learned to do CBT with them at home improved from clinical status to remission over a 12-week treatment. Post-hoc analysis suggested greatest improvement in children whose parents were anxious or depressed. Others have found that anxious offspring of anxious parents respond especially well to treatment when their parents were included. These findings suggest that children of anxious parents become less anxious when parents learn skills to address anxiety and that assessment of anxiety in the parent is indicated early in treatment, in order to gauge level of parent involvement needed.

Anxious parents may find anxiety-managing strategies useful both to themselves and children. Instead of running interference with the school systems in an overly protective way, checking-in too frequently in times of separation, and talking about dreaded outcomes of mildly risky situations, these parents reported using their new skills of cognitive reappraisal, mindfulness techniques, graded exposure, and analysis of their own parenting behaviors in a way that decreased anxiety for themselves and in an additive way, for their children.

11. Pharmacological Treatments for Anxiety Disorders

Pharmacotherapy for anxiety disorders in children and adolescents, as reviewed in 2009 by the Cochrane Library, can be effective.[25] Twenty-two randomized, controlled studies using selective serotonin-reuptake inhibiting antidepressants and venlafaxine, lasting less than or equal to 16 weeks were included in the analysis. Overall, including both OCD and other anxiety disorders, medication response (58%) was greater than placebo response (32%). For seeing an additional subject response, the number needed to treat with medication (NNT) was four. In these studies, medication was well tolerated, with 5% of participants withdrawing secondary to drug-related adverse responses.

More information exists on medication for children with OCD than for any other anxiety disorder. Double-blind placebo-controlled studies lasting from months to slightly more than one year demonstrate that the serotonin reuptake inhibitor class of anti-depressant medication is safe and effective in treating symptoms of OCD in children. Well-designed studies of clomipramine, fluoxetine, sertraline, and fluvoxamine have found medication superior to placebo and have found the medications tolerable for most. The most common side effects were headache, abdominal discomfort, behavioral activation, and sleep disturbance. Overall, approximately 60% of subjects were rated as improved.

In 2004, the Pediatric OCD Treatment Study (POTS) published the results of a randomized controlled trial comparing the efficacy of three treatments: CBT alone, medical management with the selective serotonin reuptake inhibitor sertraline alone, or CBT and sertraline combined as initial treatment for children and adolescents with OCD.[26] Combined CBT plus sertraline treatment proved superior to CBT alone and to sertraline alone which did not differ from each other. Remission rates were: for combined treatment 54%, for CBT alone 39%, for sertraline alone 21% (these two did not differ statistically) and for placebo 3.6%. The treatments proved acceptable and well tolerated.

A multicenter randomized trial compared fluvoxamine to placebo to treat anxious children.[27] Following a three-week psychoeducational lead-in phase, children aged 6–17 years and diagnosed with generalized, social, and separation anxiety disorders, and agoraphobia, underwent an eight-week trial of fluvoxamine. Subjects with histories of previous use of a serotonin reuptake inhibitor, OCD, post-traumatic stress disorder, mood disorders, Tourette's syndrome, pervasive developmental disorder, conduct disorder, suicidality, and stimulant medication use were excluded. Ratings on the Pediatric Anxiety Rating Scale (clinician administered) and Clinical Global Impressions-Improvement Scale (CGI) (clinician rated) demonstrated significant differences between fluvoxamine and placebo. Seventy-nine percent of those on fluvoxamine versus 29% of those on placebo were classified as responders (improved to symptom-free). The final dose of fluvoxamine was 5.9 ± 2.8 mg/kg (maximum 200 mg per day for children, 300 mg per day for adolescents). The most frequent adverse effects included abdominal discomfort: 49% on medication versus 28% on placebo and increased motor activity: 8% versus 1.4%. Only 8% discontinued fluvoxamine because of adverse effects.

A small, double-blind controlled study of another serotonin reuptake inhibitor, sertraline was published in 2002.[28] Boys and girls with generalized anxiety disorder underwent a two-week screen, then a nine-week trial of placebo or medication. Concurrent psychotherapy, with the exception of cognitive behavioral therapy, was allowed. Subjects receiving sertraline improved in anxiety symptoms significantly more than did those on placebo. Moreover, an analysis performed separating those low on depression ratings with those high in depression ratings suggested that improvement in anxiety was not merely secondary to an improvement in depressive symptoms. Those on placebo suffered 3 to 10 times more adverse effects seen in generalized anxiety disorder (dizziness, nausea, and stomach pain) than those on medication. For subjects taking medication, dry mouth (55% versus 27%), drowsiness (73% versus 45%), leg spasms (36% versus 9%), and restlessness (55% versus 27%) were the most common adverse effects.

A six-site, randomized placebo-controlled trial examined the relative efficacy of cognitive behavior therapy, sertraline, and their combination, against pill placebo (PBO) for the treatment of Separation anxiety disorder (SAD), Generalized anxiety disorder (GAD), and social phobia (SoP) in children and adolescents.[29] Children between the ages of 7 and 17 years who had a primary diagnosis of Separation anxiety disorder, Generalized anxiety disorder, or social phobia received 14 sessions of cognitive behavioral therapy, sertraline (at a dose of up to 200 mg per day), a combination of sertraline and cognitive behavioral therapy, or a placebo drug for 12 weeks in a 2:2:2:1 ratio. Percentages of children rated as very much or much improved on the Clinician Global Impression-Improvement were 81% for combination therapy, 60% for cognitive behavioral therapy, 55% for sertraline, and 23.7% for placebo. Adverse events, including suicidal and homicidal ideation, were no more frequent in the medication group than in the placebo group. Less insomnia, fatigue, sedation, and restlessness were associated with cognitive behavioral therapy than with sertraline.

A few, small studies of benzodiazepines have been conducted with children with anxiety disorders. Two double-blind placebo-controlled studies of alprazolam for anxiety had ambiguous outcomes. A double-blind cross-over study of clonazepam for children with separation anxiety showed no advantage for the medication. Clonazepam did show benefit in the treatment of adolescent panic in a small double-blind placebo-controlled study.

12. Course and Prognosis

In general, children recover from the initial episode of an anxiety disorder at a moderate to high rate. However, they remain at risk for development of additional psychiatric disorders. In 1996, Last reported the results of a prospective 3-to-4-year study including 217 anxiety-disordered subjects and comparison from previous treatment studies.[30] Eighty-two percent of initial anxiety disorders had remitted at follow-up. Relapse was rare. Thirty percent of subjects developed new psychiatric disorders, primarily anxiety disorders. Separation anxiety disorder showed greatest rate of recovery (96%). While 80% of subjects with overanxious disorder recovered, this subset had the greatest rate of developing a new anxiety disorder. Subjects involved in treatment did not differ from those receiving no treatment in recovery rates.

Sixty-eight anxious children were followed for three years. They reported, on the whole, that their anxiety decreased over time, with the exception of social concerns. Girls and younger children were found to be more anxious than boys.[31] The course of OCD is more persistent. Two-to-seven-year follow-up studies of children with obsessive-compulsive disorder revealed that 31 to 68% of children continued to suffer from OCD and the majority had developed additional psychiatric diagnoses.[32]

It has been reported that individuals with early-onset anxiety disorders are 40% less likely to finish high school. If they finish high school, they are 40% less likely to attend college.[33] If they attend college, they are 40% less likely to finish college. Those who have anxiety disorders are more likely to have children out of marriage, marry early, and to be divorced. An eight-year prospective outcome study compared 101 children with anxiety diagnoses to those with no psychiatric diagnosis. Anxious children were less likely to be living independently. Those with both anxiety and depression were less likely to be employed or in school, and more likely to be depressed and be in mental health treatment than those with only anxiety or no diagnosis. Young adults with the childhood or adolescent onset of OCD are more likely to be living at home, have been hospitalized, unemployed, and to have multiple diagnoses. Twenty-five to thirty-nine percent of those with school phobia show impairment in young adulthood.

13. Future Directions

The field of anxiety disorders leads others in the field of child psychiatry in its rigorous efforts to empirically validate psychotherapeutic interventions. Research continues to advance knowledge about psychotherapy, including settings (*e.g.* schools), individuals involved (families), formats (individual, group), as well as which components are necessary and sufficient for improvement. Future research regarding pharmacological treatments for anxiety disorders in children are required to determine long-term safety and efficacy, optimal dosages, and additional agents. Investigations into the risk factors of family interaction, physiologic reactivity, and genetic makeup are ongoing. At the basic-science level, mechanisms causing vulnerability and maintenance of anxiety symptoms are being explored using neuro-endocrine and neuro-imaging studies.

Two impulse control disorders deserve special mention and inclusion here in this chapter, because they very often are referred to anxiety clinics for evaluation because of the apparent obsessive/compulsive character of the symptoms. We include them here, although the most recent research suggests that their pathogenesis involves sensory-motor gating deficits. They are interesting from a theoretical point of view as they permit a glimpse of gene–environment interactions which is most likely relevant for many if not most child psychiatric syndromes.

14. Trichotillomania

14.1. *Introduction*

Fourteen-year-old Nora came to the Anxiety Disorders Clinic because she wanted to stop pulling out her hair. She was ashamed of being unable to control this behavior and ashamed of the way she looked without her eyelashes and eyebrows. Because of the repetitive nature of the symptoms of hair pulling, many children and adolescents who suffer from trichotillomania are referred for evaluation and therapy to an OCD or anxiety clinic.

Trichotillomania, an impulse disorder not otherwise specified in DSM-IV, overlaps phenomenologically with skin picking and nail biting and therefore fits best in the classification: body-focused repetitive behavior. These grooming behaviors, which are highly reinforced in the doing, continue relatively unchecked, despite the sufferer's intention to stop and distress at his/her actions. Of course, grooming has evolutionary value for health and mating. However, destructive, dysfunctional grooming is observed in humans and other animals (*e.g.* acral lick syndrome in dogs and feather plucking in birds). These repetitive behaviors likely represent grooming which increased in a time of stress and persisted due to powerful habit reinforcement. The reader is referred to a recent summary on trichotillomania by Michael Bloch[34] for further details.

14.2. *Diagnosis*

ICD and DSM-IV each classify trichotillomania as a disorder of impulse control. DSM-IV diagnostic criteria include: A. Recurrent pulling out of one's hair resulting in noticeable hair loss. B. An increasing sense of tension immediately before pulling out the hair or when attempting to resist the behavior. C. Pleasure, gratification, or relief when pulling out the hair. D. The disturbance is not better accounted for by another mental disorder and is not due to a general medical condition (*e.g.* a dermatological condition). E. The disturbance causes clinically significant distress or impairment in social, occupational, or other important areas of functioning. Proposed improvements in diagnostic criteria will account for the fact that hair loss may or may not be noticeable, and for the fact that criteria B and C are not always present in chronic hair pullers who differ from those with trichotillomania in no other way. Skin picking may be included in the same category as trichotillomania.

14.3. *Epidemiology*

The manifestations of trichotillomania may be obvious or invisible. Therefore, information about prevalence and incidence is difficult to determine. As mentioned above, determination of caseness is undergoing reevaluation as more data has become available from a survey study of respondents to the TLC Trichotillomania Impact Project.[35] Estimates place lifetime prevalence at 1 to 3% and age of onset as peripubertal.

14.4. *Differential diagnosis*

Pathological hair pulling may occur in such medical conditions as stimulant excess. "Baby-trich" may represent a different process, in which children up to age six twist, twirl, and tug at their hair, often while sucking their thumbs. (Interestingly, stopping the thumb sucking often leads to resolution of the hair loss.) Other causes of pathological hair loss without hair pulling include alopecia areata and tinea capitis, which may be established *via* dermatological consultation. The principal disorder involved in trichotillomania appears to be one of difficult to resist, repetitive impulses directed at a part of the body, which may include hair, nails, cuticles, and other parts of the skin.

Diagnosis is established by history and physical examination. A scale developed for adults, the Massachusetts General Hospital Hairpulling Scale (MGH-HPS) may be used to measure interference, distress, and severity of the trouble.[36] When patients with trichotillomania eat their hair, further examination is warranted to rule out the potentially dangerous condition of trichobezoar, or hair ball in the stomach.

14.5. *Pathogenesis*

Those with trichotillomania sometimes pinpoint the onset of symptoms to a specific stressful life event, such as having lice, a move, school transfer, or interpersonal loss. It is likely that biological factors are necessary for this type of repetitive behavior to become pathological. Genetic studies, a mouse model and brain imaging studies will help advance knowledge in this area. The hair pulling behavior may be reinforced by the thoughts and sensations associated, and influenced by behaviors of concerned family members and one's support system.

14.6. *Relevance for primary care*

When the primary care provider identifies trichotillomania, the practitioner must question the patient and his/her parent about whether the patient is eating his/her hair. If so, gastrointestinal complications require being ruled out.

14.7. *Interventions*

Behavioral analysis and targeted cognitive and behavioral intervention along with identification and treatment of comorbid stressors comprise the current cornerstone of treatment of trichotillomania. The authors, Vavrichek and Golumb have written an excellent workbook, *The Hair Pulling Habit and You*, which may be used with a psychotherapist or at home.[37] It leads the readers through a behavioral analysis of stimuli associated with pulling, suggestions for interventions, including habit reversal training, record-keeping materials, and a reinforcement plan. Habit reversal training is the only evidence-based treatment for trichotillomania.[38]

As the stress of comorbid conditions, including (but not limited to) unidentified learning disorders, attention deficit disorder, and family difficulties and transitions, may initiate and continue to drive the behaviors, the evaluator must consider and address these issues. Early research in adults with repetitive hair pulling disorder suggests a role for N-acetyl cysteine as the only medication with possible specific benefit for this type of repetitive body focused disorder.[39]

14.8. *Outcomes*

Trichotillomania and other body-focused repetitive behaviors are chronic and recurrent. The overwhelming majority of patients have reported that they have not experienced improvement in symptoms with treatment.[35] In addition to psychological and social troubles, chronic hair pulling may cause permanent damage to hair follicles.

14.9. *In practice*

Treating individuals with trichotillomania engages a large set of clinical skills, including creating therapeutic alliances with the patient and family about this often shame-producing condition, a thorough psychiatric evaluation to determine and treat comorbid stressors, a ruling-out of medical issues, psychoeducation, and a detailed behavioral analysis and treatment plan involving the patient and his family, if possible. The Trichotillomania Learning Center (TLC) (http://www.trich.org/) serves as a valuable source of information and support for individuals, families, and clinicians troubled by trichotillomania.

14.10. *Outcomes in your clinic*

Nora's trouble with hair pulling began as she entered middle school. Moving classroom to classroom taxed her organizational abilities. Writing assignments became more complex and she spent more time in front of her homework. She began plucking her eyebrows as part of her growing adolescent grooming routine, but found that in front of the mirror and at her desks at school and home she plucked not only her brows, but her eyelashes, too. Her mother and father entreated her to stop, but that embarrassed and agitated her and seemed to make her pull more.

Evaluation led to the diagnoses of trichotillomania, attention deficit disorder, inattentive type, and a learning disorder of written language. We catalogued the details of her pulling according to the mnemonic described in The Hair Pulling Habit and You: "Fiddle SHEEP." (Fiddle: need to be in motion, fiddling, Sensory triggers, Hands "automatically" pull without awareness, Environmental triggers, Emotional triggers, and Perfection — which references completeness, self-talk regarding symmetry, and type of hair pulled.) We reviewed a treatment plan which included stimulant medication for ADD, a meeting with school personnel to problem solve addressing Nora's learning disorder and executive functioning, referral to the TLC website for further education and support, and a behavioral plan. That plan included eliminating tweezers and the make-up mirror, administration of "fake" fingernails to make pulling less automatic and unconscious, and a reward system, not for not pulling, but for employing strategies to address pulling. Borrowing from acceptance and commitment therapy, we discussed the chronic nature of the impulses and Nora's need to be the one responsible for her success. In general, the quality of Nora's life improved as she, her parents and the school understood and intervened with obstacles to her school success. The fingernails worked well to interrupt the pulling until they came off. When symptoms recurred, she replaced them and resumed her efforts to coexist with the urges without complying with them.

14.11. *The next five years*

Over recent years, in part stimulated by the initiative of the TLC and its International Consortium for the Study of Trichotillomania and Related

Conditions, research projects are underway attempting to further characterize the phenomenology, genetic underpinnings, image-detected brain activity, and pharmacological, and sophisticated behavioral and psychotherapeutic interventions (derived from dialectical behavior therapy and acceptance and commitment therapy) for this disorder.

15. Tic Disorders

15.1. *Introduction*

Seven-year-old Julio came to the Anxiety Disorders and OCD Clinic because he was being teased at school about noises he made in the classroom and on the playground. He was unable to control this whooping behavior and ashamed of the way he looked when he ticked: shrugging his shoulders and turning his head. Because of the repetitive nature of the symptoms of tics and the frequent comorbidity of OCD and tic disorders, many children and adolescents who suffer from Tourette's disorder are referred for evaluation and therapy to an OCD Clinic.

The neuropsychiatric tic disorders described in DSM-IV and ICD-9 Tourette's disorder, chronic motor or vocal tic disorder, transient tic disorder and tic disorder not otherwise specified comprise a spectrum of movement problems that vary in duration and type. ICD 9 criteria refer to interference and distress, while DSM-IV criteria do not. The reader is referred to a recent summary on tic disorder not otherwise specified by Bloch and Leckman[40] for further details.

15.2. *Diagnosis*

According to DSM-IV, diagnostic criteria for Tourette's disorder include: A. Both multiple motor and one or more vocal tics have been present at some time during the illness, although not necessarily concurrently. (A tic is a sudden, rapid, recurrent, nonrhythmic, stereotyped motor movement or vocalization.) B. The tics occur many times a day (usually in bouts) nearly every day or intermittently throughout a period of more than one year, and during this period there was never a tic-free period of more than three consecutive months. C. The onset is before age 18 years. D. The disturbance is not due to the direct physiological effects of a substance (*e.g.* stimulants) or a general medical condition (*e.g.* Huntington's disease or post-viral encephalitis). Proposed changes to DSM-V include removing the words "stereotyped" and "usually in bouts," eliminating diagnostic constraint on tic-free intervals and eliminating mention of stimulant medication as an example of a substance-induced disorder[41] Chronic motor or vocal tic disorder describes a tic disorder that fails to meet diagnostic criteria for Tourette's disorder due to type of tics present, Transient tic disorder has lasted less than 1 year, and Tic disorder not otherwise specified captures other tic disorders, including those that begin after age 18. Diagnosis is established using history and physical examination.

15.3. *Epidemiology*

The onset of tic disorders peaks between the ages of three and eight years. Boys are affected twice as often as girls. Tics themselves occur in clusters or bouts, and typically wax and wane over the course of weeks to months. Transient tics may be seen in between 4 and 24% of children, while Tourette's disorder occurs in between 0.1 and 1%.

15.4. *Differential diagnosis*

Tics following infection may be seen in Sydenham's Chorea and Pediatric Autoimmune Neuropsychiatric Disorder Associated with Streptococcal Infection (PANDAS). Movement disorders may also be caused by general medical conditions (*e.g.* Huntington's disease, stroke, Lesch-Nyhan syndrome, Wilson's disease, multiple sclerosis, post-viral encephalitis, head injury) or side effects of a drug (*e.g.* akathisia and tardive dyskinesia associated with neuroleptic medication).[42] Individuals with stereotyped movement disorders or pervasive developmental disorder may demonstrate repetitive, purposeless movements which are not tics, but are stereotypes. Those with both OCD and tic disorders may have tic-like compulsions. Diagnosis is established by history and physical examination. Yale Global Tic Severity Scale[43] may be used to measure interference, distress, and severity of the disorder.

15.5. *Pathogenesis*

Tic disorders result from dysfunction in the basal ganglia and cortico-striatal thalamo-cortical systems and from abnormalities in dopaminergic function. Family studies demonstrate a strong genetic component. The average age of onset is between five and eight years of age. By age 10 years, most children with Tourette's disorder are aware of sensory urges that precede some of their tics. Known as premonitory urges, these sensations are often localized to a specific body region where the tic is about to occur and are frequently experienced as nearly irresistible. The urges themselves can be a major source of preoccupation and impairment. A fleeting feeling of relief often follows performance of a tic or series of tics. Tics increase during periods of stress, emotional excitement, and fatigue. Tics can be willfully suppressed for brief intervals and are highly suggestible.

Tics typically diminish during periods of goal-directed behavior, especially those that involve both focused attention and fine motor control, as occur in musical and athletic performances. Tics typically follow a waxing and waning pattern of severity, intensity, and frequency. Tic severity usually peaks between 8 and 12 years of age with many patients showing a marked reduction in severity by the end of adolescence.

15.6. *Relevance for primary care*

When the primary care provider identifies a tic disorder, the practitioner must rule out possible medical causes and begin a course of psycho education that may include helping the child and his/her parents understand the role that the premonitory urge plays in the emergence of the disorder. A psychiatric referral will help with determination of the nature of environmental psychoeducation and possible therapy indicated.

15.7. *Interventions*

Psychoeducation, pharmacotherapy, behavioral analysis and habit reversal therapy,[44] and identification and treatment of comorbid stressors comprise the current cornerstone of treatment of tic disorders. As the stress of comorbid conditions may initiate and continue to drive the tic disorders' severity, the evaluator must consider and address these issues. Important comorbidities include: unidentified learning disorders (commonly dysgraphia), attention deficit disorder, and OCD.

Social issues represent the most potential for suffering for those with tic disorders. Tics are often obvious visual and audible symptoms which can cause self-consciousness, and frighten and disturb others. Children with tics may be teased, mimicked, ostracized, and misunderstood. When family members, friends, and fellow students understand the relatively involuntary nature of the disorder and how calling attention to tics can precipitate bouts, the student with tics will have an improved experience. The Tourette's Syndrome Association (http://www.tsa-usa.org/) offers resources to help people and their families cope with the problems that occur with Tourette's disorder, including age-appropriate materials for children and adolescents with tic disorders and educational packets to be used in the classroom and with teachers.

Only when tics are painful, distressing, overly interfering, or causing social issues is pharmacological intervention indicated; for, medication does not cure tics and has potential side effects. Two classes of medications, the $alpha_2$-agonists and antipsychotics (formerly typical and more recently atypical) directly treat these movement disorders.[40] Recent expansion of research on CBT including habit reversal training for tic disorders shows that children and adolescents can benefit by performing behavioral analyses of their tics and performing a "competing response" motor movement incompatible with the tic (*e.g.* exhaling when they feel an urge to gasp). The first phase of this treatment is to help children become more aware of their premonitory urges so that they know when to initiate the competing response.

15.8. *Outcomes*

Tic disorders most typically begin in school age. Just 30% of those with tic disorders will continue into adulthood. A majority of children meeting criteria for Tourette's disorder in both general population studies as well as in clinic-based samples will have other neuropsychiatric disorders which can adversely impact their long-term outcome. In contrast, the rates of comorbidity are substantially lower for children with a chronic motor tic disorder or a transient tic disorder.

15.9. *In practice*

Treating individuals with tic disorders engages a large set of clinical skills, including creating therapeutic alliances with the patient and family, interfacing with the schools, thorough psychiatric evaluation to determine and treat comorbid stressors, a ruling-out of medical issues, psychoeducation, pharmacotherapy and a behavioral analysis and habit reversal treatment plan.

15.10. *Outcomes in your clinic*

Julio's trouble with tics began in second grade, beginning with occasional eye blinking. As time went by, different tics appeared as others left, becoming more complex and growing to include throat clearing and whooping sounds. When his teacher asked him to stop making noises in the classroom and he did not, a student study team meeting was called. At that time, his mother told the school that he was unable to control the sounds and asked for a psycho educational evaluation, as he was having trouble with penmanship as well.

Evaluation in the clinic and at school led to the diagnoses of Tourette's disorder and difficulties with fine motor tasks. We reviewed a treatment plan which included psychoeducational interventions separately with school personnel and peers and an occupational therapy evaluation for diagnosis and recommendations. As is typical, tics were most prominent in times of transition, excitement, and fatigue, so Julio's mother worked to maintain an adequate rest structure to his day. The family elected to try habit reversal training as a first step and perhaps a trial of guanfacine later, should the interference associated with his tics continue to be excessive.

15.11. *The next five years*

Basic science and clinical research projects are attempting to further characterize phenomenology, neurologic, and genetic underpinnings, and pharmacological interventions for tic disorders.

References

1. American Psychiatric Association. *Diagnostic and Statistical Manual of Mental Disorders,* 4th edition, Text Revision. Washington, DC: APA Press, 2000.
2. World Health Organization. *ICD-10: International Statistical Classification of Diseases and Related Health Problems.* 2nd edition. World Health Organization: Geneva, 2005.
3. Moretti G, Pasquini M, Mandarelli G, Tarsitani L, Biondi M. What every psychiatrist should know about PANDAS: A review, *Clin Pract Epidemol Ment Health* 2008; **21**: 4–13.
4. Newcorn JH, Halperin JM, Jensen PS, *et al.* Symptom profiles in children with ADHD: Effects of comorbidity and gender, *J Am Acad Child Adolesc Psychiatry* 2001; **40**(2): 137–146.
5. Bowlby J. *Attachment (Attachment and Loss Series, Vol 1)*, 2nd edition New York, NY: Basic Books, 1983.
6. Shaffer D, Fisher P, Lucas CP, Dulcan MK, Schwab-Stone ME. NIMH Diagnostic Interview Schedule for Children Version IV (NIMH DISC-IV): Description, differences from previous versions, and reliability of some common diagnoses, *J Am Acad Child Adolesc Psychiatry* 2000; **39**(1): 28–38.
7. Goodman W, Price L, Rasmussen S, *et al.* The Yale-Brown Obsessive-Compulsive Scale. I. Development, use and reliability, *Arch Gen Psychiatry* 1989; **46**: 1006–1011.
8. Silverman WK, Albano AM. *The Anxiety Disorders Interview Schedule for DSM-IV - Child and Parent Versions.* San Antonio, TX: Psychological Corporation, 1996.
9. Kovacs M. The Children's Depression Inventory (CDI), *Psychopharmacol Bull* 1985; **2**: 995–998.
10. Reynolds CR, Richmond BO. What I think and feel: A revised measure of children's manifest anxiety, *J Abnorm Child Psychol* 1978; **6**(2): 271–280.
11. Spielberger CD, Auerbach SM, Wadsworth AP, Dunn TM, Taulbee ES. Emotional reactions to surgery, *J Consult Clin Psychol* 1973; **40**(1): 33–38.
12. Ollendick TH. Reliability and validity of the Revised Fear Surgery Schedule for Children (FSSC-R), *Behav Res Ther* 1983; **21**(6): 685–692.

13. Muris P, Mayer B, Bartelds E, Tierney S, Bogie N. The revised version of the Screen for Child Anxiety Related Emotional Disorders (SCARED-R): Treatment sensitivity in an early intervention trial for childhood anxiety disorders, *Br J Clin Psychol* 2001; **40**(3): 323–336.
14. March JS, Parker JD, Sullivan K, Stallings P, Conners CK. The Multidimensional Anxiety Scale for Children (MASC): Factor structure, reliability, and validity, *J Am Acad Child Adolesc Psychiatry* 1997; **36**(4): 554–565.
15. Achenbach TM, Edelbrock CS. *Manual for the Child Behavior Checklist and Child Behavior Profile*. Burlington, VT: University of Vermont Department of Psychiatry, 1991.
16. Achenbach TM. *Manual of the Teacher's Report Form and 1991 profile*. Burlington, VT: University of Vermont, Department of Psychiatry, 1991.
17. Schwartz JM, Beyette B. *Brain lock — free yourself from Obsessive/Compulsive Behavior*. New York, NY: ReganBooks, 1996.
18. March JS, Mulle K. *Obsessive Compulsive Disorder in Children and Adolescents: A Cognitive Behavioral Treatment Manual*. New York, NY: Guilford Press, 2001.
19. Chansky T. *Freeing Your Child from Anxiety*. New York, NY: Random House, 2004.
20. Wagner AP. *What to do When Your Child has Obsessive-Compulsive Disorder: Strategies and Solutions*. Lighthouse Point, FL: Lighthouse Press, Inc, 2002.
21. The Individuals with Disabilities Education Act Amendments of 1997 Web site. http://www2.ed.gov/offices/OSERS/Policy/IDEA/index.html. Accessed on May, 2010.
22. James, AACJ, Soler A, Wetherall RRW. Cognitive behavioral therapy for anxiety disorders in children and adolescents (Review). *The Cochrane Library*. Issue 1. The Cochrane Collaboration. John Wiley & Sons, Ltd, 2009.
23. Kendall PC. *The Coping Cat Workbook*. Ardmore, PA: Workbook Publishing, Inc, 1992.
24. Thienemann M, Moore P, Tompkins K. A parent-only group intervention for children with anxiety disorders: Pilot study, *J Am Acad Child Adolesc Psychiatry* 2006; **45**(1): 37–46.
25. Ipser JC, Stein DJ, Hawkridge S, Hoppe L. Pharmacotherapy for anxiety disorders in children and adolescents (review). *The Cochrane Library*. Issue 3. The Cochrane Collaboration. John Wiley & Sons, Ltd, 2009.
26. Pediatric OCD Treatment Study (POTS) Team. Cognitive-behavior therapy, sertraline, and their combination for children and adolescents with obsessive-compulsive disorder: The Pediatric OCD Treatment Study (POTS) randomized controlled trial, *JAMA* 2004; **292**(16): 1969–1976.
27. Research Unit on Pediatric Psychopharmacology Anxiety Study Group for the treatment of anxiety disorders in children and adolescents, *N Engl J Med* 2001; **344**(17): 1279–1285.

28. Walkup JT, Albano AM, Piacentini J, *et al.* Cognitive behavioral therapy, sertraline, or a combination in childhood anxiety, *NEJM* 2008; **359**(26): 2753–2766.
29. Last CG, Perrin S, Hersen M, Kazdin AE. A prospective study of childhood anxiety disorders, *J Am Acad Child Adolesc Psychiatry* 1996; **35**(11): 1502–1510.
30. Last CG, Hansen C, Franco N. Anxious children in adulthood: A prospective study of adjustment, *J Am Acad Child Adolesc Psychiatry* 1997; **36**(5): 645–652.
31. Kessler RC, Berglund P, Demler O, Jun R, Merikangas KR, Walters EE. Lifetime prevalence and age-of-onset distributions of DSM-IV disorders in the National Comorbidity Survey Replication, *Arch Gen Psychiatry* 2005; **62**: 593–602.
32. Kessler RC, Foster CL, Saunders WB, Stang PE. Social consequences of psychiatric disorders, I: Educational attainment, *Am J Psychiatry* 1995; **152**(7): 1026–1032.
33. Kessler RC. The global burden of anxiety and mood disorders: Putting ESEMeD findings into perspective, *J Clin Psychiatry* 2007; **68**(Suppl 2): 10–19.
34. Bloch MH. Trichotillomania across the life span, *J Am Acad Child Adolesc Psychiatry* 2009; **48**(9): 879–883.
35. Woods DW, Flessner CA, Franklin, *et al.* The Trichotillomania Impact Project (TIP): Exploring phenomenology, functional impairment, and treatment utilization, *J Clin Psychiatry* 2006; **67**(12): 1877–1888.
36. Keuthen NJ, O'Sullivan RL, Ricciardi JN, *et al.* The Massachusetts General Hospital (MGH) hairpulling scale: I. Development and factor analyses. *Psychother Psychosom* 1995; **64**: 141–145.
37. Vavrichek SM, Golomb RG. *The Hair Pulling "Habit" and You: How to Solve the Trichotillomania Puzzle, Revised Edition.* Olney, MD: Writers' Cooperative of Greater Washington, 2000.
38. Bloch MH, Landeros-Weisenberger A, Dombrowski P, *et al.* Systematic review: Pharmacological and behavioral treatment for trichotillomania, *Biol Psychiatry* 2007; **62**(8): 839–846.
39. Grant JE, Odlaug BL, Kim SW. N-acetylcysteine, a glutamate modulator, in the treatment of trichotillomania: A double-blind, placebo-controlled study, *Arch Gen Psychiatry* 2009; **66**(7): 756–763.
40. Bloch MH, Leckman JF. Tourette disorder and obsessive–compulsive disorder in children and adolescents. In: Ebert MH, Loosen PT, Nurcombe B, Leckman JF. *Current Diagnosis & Treatment: Psychiatry,* 2nd edition. Columbus, OH: The McGraw-Hill Companies, Inc, 2008.
41. American Psychiatric Association DSM-5 Web site. Proposed Draft Revisions to DSM disorders and criteria. http://www.dsm5.org/Pages/Default.aspx. Accessed on May 23, 2010.
42. Bloch MH, Leckman JF. Tourette disorder and obsessive–compulsive disorder in children and adolescents, Tourette Syndrome and Tic Disorders: Essentials of Diagnosis 2008; **21**(8): 641–655.

43. Leckman JF, Riddle MA, Hardin MT, *et al.* The Yale Global Tic Severity Scale: Initial testing of a clinician-rated scale of tic severity, *J Am Acad Child Adolesc Psychiatry* 1989; **28**(4):566–573.
44. Piacentini J, Woods DW, Scahill L, *et al.* Behavior therapy for children with tourette disorder: A randomized controlled trial, *JAMA* 2010; **303**(19): 1929–1937.

Chapter 6

Depression and Related Mood Disorders

Kirti Saxena, Graham Emslie, Ryan Williams, and Kiki Chang

1. Introduction

Depression is a serious illness, the manifestations and treatment of which are well studied in adults. Over the past few decades, it has become increasingly recognized that depression does exist and is not uncommon in the pediatric population. Being able to diagnose and treat this illness in children and adolescents is of paramount importance, as it can cause significant morbidity and mortality.[1] Although the diagnostic criteria are the same for youth and adults, developmental differences often lead to different symptoms and presentations for children and adolescents. Hence, it can be difficult to recognize this disorder in this population, often leading to underdiagnosis and undertreatment.[1] There are now both well-studied psychopharmacological and psychotherapeutic treatment interventions for depressive disorders in youth to improve outcomes in this population.[2] This chapter discusses the epidemiology, symptomatology (including presentation and assessment), pathogenesis, and treatment of depressive disorders in the pediatric population.

1.1. *Evolutionary background*

In recent decades, researchers in numerous disciplines have theorized on the evidence of an evolutionary function in various phenomena. The behavioral sciences have been no exception, as evolutionary psychology is a thriving field. Is there a function in being sad? Nesse suggests that depression is an adaptation that functions to maintain or restore social order, allowing weaker individuals to coexist with the stronger, more dominant members of a particular population.[3] Watson and Andrews propose that depression offers an opportunity for an individual to gather new resources and change their current life strategies.[4] A hypothesis by Kinney and Tanaka predicts that depression can be elicited by various infections and environmental stressors which compromise immune function.[5]

2. Epidemiology

In children and adolescents, depression is a cause of substantial morbidity and mortality, and is associated with significant psychosocial impairment and impaired quality of life, which can persist into adulthood.[6] The prevalence of major depressive disorder (MDD) in children is approximately 2% (equal proportion in males and females), and in adolescents it is approximately 4–8% (male:female is 1:2). After puberty, particularly in females the risk for depression increases by a factor of two to four.[2] Dysthymia occurs in an estimated 4–5% of children.[7] In addition, about 5–10% of youth have subsyndromal symptoms of MDD which can cause significant psychosocial impairment and an increased risk for suicide and substance use in children and adolescents.[8,9] For each generation that has a depressive disorder, the next generation is at a greater risk for developing the disorder, with the onset of the disorder being at a younger age.[2]

3. Diagnosis

The Diagnostic and Statistical Manual of Psychiatric Disorders (DSM-IV-TR)[10] classifies depression into: Major Depressive Disorder (MDD), dysthymic disorder, and depressive disorder not otherwise specified (Depression NOS). Although the criteria for depressive disorders are similar across the lifespan, children and adolescents may present with irritable mood as the prominent mood symptom (with or without depressed mood).

Specifically, as per the DSM-IV-TR a child/adolescent meets diagnostic criteria for MDD when he/she has a minimum of five of the following nine symptoms present during the same two-week period: depressed mood or irritable mood or loss of interest or pleasure; markedly diminished interest or pleasure in activities; decrease or increase in appetite; insomnia or hypersomnia; psychomotor agitation or retardation; fatigue or loss of energy; feelings of worthlessness, diminished ability to concentrate; recurrent thoughts of death; recurrent suicidal ideation without a specific plan, or a suicide attempt or a specific plan for committing suicide. At least one of the symptoms has to be either depressed/irritable mood or loss of interest or pleasure. It is important that the symptoms represent a change from previous functioning and cause clinically significant distress or impairment in social, occupational, or other important areas of functioning.

The DSM-IV-TR criteria for dysthymia include a depressed or irritable mood for a duration of at least one year. While depressed or irritable, at least two of the following must be present: decreased or increased appetite, insomnia or hypersomnia, low energy or fatigue, low self-esteem, poor concentration, and feelings of hopelessness. Additionally, the child/adolescent has not been without the symptoms for more than two months at a time. For both MDD and dysthymia, the symptoms should not be due to substance abuse, use of medications, other psychiatric illness, bereavement, or medical illness.

DSM-IV-TR diagnosis of Depression NOS includes disorders with depressive features that do not meet the criteria for MDD or dysthymic disorder. This can include premenstrual dysphoric disorder, minor depressive disorder (episodes of at least two weeks of depressive symptoms but with less than five symptoms required for diagnosis of MDD), recurrent brief depressive episode (depressive episodes lasting from two days up to two weeks, occurring at least once a month for 12 months), or circumstances where the clinician concludes that a depressive disorder is present but is unable to determine whether it is primary, substance induced, or due to a general medical condition.

Major depressive disorder can further be broken down into subtypes, including atypical, psychotic, seasonal, catatonic, melancholic, and postpartum. Atypical features include an increase in appetite or significant weight gain, increased sleep, feelings of heaviness in arms or legs, and rejection sensitivity.[11] Psychotic depression, although rare before adolescence, represents a severe form of depression, with psychotic symptoms usually presenting as mood congruent. Children primarily have auditory hallucinations while adolescents usually have delusions. Adolescents with psychotic depression tend to do worse and some later develop bipolar disorder[2].

Youth whose symptoms of depression predominantly occur during winter or fall (the season when there is less daylight) are considered to have Seasonal Affective Disorder (SAD). Since school starts around the same time as the fall/winter months, it is important to distinguish depression triggered by school stress from SAD.[2]

Approximately 20% of youth with major depression experience manic episodes by adulthood.[12] Indeed, depression is usually the first symptom of bipolar disorder recognized in children and adolescents. Factors predicting development of mania in depressed youth include a family history of bipolar disorder, a depressive episode characterized by rapid onset, psychomotor retardation, and psychotic features.[2]

ICD-10

Similar to the DSM-IV-TR, the International Classification of Mental and Behavioral Disorders (ICD-10),[13] is used throughout Europe to classify psychiatric disorders.

Table 1: Common Symptom Presentations in Pediatric Depression

- Withdrawing from others
- Crying episodes
- Somatic complaints (headache/stomachache)
- Refusal to go to school
- Worsening school performance
- Social withdrawal or significant changes in peer relationships
- New behavioral problems
- Preoccupied with suicidal ideations
- Describe themselves in negative terms: "I am ugly," "I am stupid," "Nobody likes me."
- "I am bored" — is commonly indicative of loss of interest

The ICD-10 divides depression into mild to moderate to severe episodes. A duration of two weeks is usually required for diagnosis, but if the symptoms are particularly severe and of very rapid onset, the diagnosis of depression can be made earlier than two weeks. Diagnostic criteria are similar, although ICD-10 considers three core symptoms: depressed mood, anhedonia, and decreased energy to make the diagnosis of depression. This is in contrast to the DSM-IV-TR that requires the two symptoms of depressed/irritable mood or anhedonia to make the diagnosis of depression. Other symptoms included in the ICD-10 criteria for depression are: reduced concentration, reduced self-esteem/self-confidence, ideas of guilt and unworthiness, bleak and pessimistic views of the future, ideas or acts of self-harm or suicide, disturbed sleep, and diminished appetite. The number of symptoms defines depression severity. As noted, children and adolescents may not present with an overt depressed mood, which often leads to under recognition of the disorder.

The diagnosis of depressive disorders is made when the child/adolescent meets criteria based on DSM-IV-TR. However, the clinical presentation of depressive disorders in youth may be different than the classic presentation seen in adults due to the differences in physical, emotional, cognitive, and social developmental stage.[14,15] Although not specific diagnostic criteria, certain changes in behaviors may indicate the development of depression in youth. Table 1 details common symptoms leading to clinical referral for youth.

3.1. *Differential Diagnosis*

There are several psychiatric disorders whose symptoms overlap with the symptoms of MDD. They include bipolar depression, attention deficit hyperactivity disorder (ADHD), oppositional defiant disorder (ODD), pervasive developmental disorder (PDD), posttraumatic stress disorder (PTSD), adjustment disorder with depressed mood, bereavement, depression secondary to medical conditions (*e.g.* hypothyroidism, mononucleosis, anemia, autoimmune diseases, chronic fatigue syndrome) and substance-induced depression. Additionally, medications such as stimulants, corticosteroids, and contraceptives can cause symptoms similar to depression.[2,16]

When a child/adolescent presents with depressive symptoms, bipolar disorder must always be considered in the differential diagnosis as it is difficult to ascertain whether the youth is presenting with the depressive phase of bipolar disorder or a unipolar depression. Indicators for bipolar disorder include a family history of bipolar disorder, psychosis, and medication-induced mania. The clinician will need to follow the longitudinal course of the illness to assess if manic/hypomanic symptoms occur or not.[2] In the case of ADHD, inattentiveness and distractibility can be symptoms of depression so it is important to ascertain whether the youth met criteria for ADHD prior to the onset of the depressive episode. A depressed youth can be argumentative, disrespectful, and have behavioral problems that may lead the clinician to make a diagnosis of ODD and not depression. Youth with PDD lack social skills and can have poor peer relationships, thus leading one to think of depression as a primary diagnosis. Certain symptoms of PTSD overlap with depressive symptoms (*e.g.* difficulty falling or staying asleep, irritability, difficulty in concentrating, diminished interest in activities) and a depressive episode can follow a traumatic event; however, to make a diagnosis of PTSD there needs to be a exposure to a traumatic event. In adjustment disorder with depressed mood, symptoms of depressed mood, tearfulness, or feelings of hopelessness occur in response to an identifiable stressor occurring within three months of the onset of the stressor. After the death of a loved one, depressive symptoms can occur. If the depressive symptoms last for more than two months or are severe (*e.g.* psychosis, suicidality), then a diagnosis of MDD should be considered. To rule out depression secondary to a medical condition or depression secondary to medications or substance, a complete physical examination and pertinent laboratory investigations should be conducted. As always, a careful psychiatric evaluation is required to ascertain the primary diagnosis.

3.2. *Comorbidity*

As depressive disorders are usually accompanied by other psychiatric and medical conditions, it is important to have a complete physical examination and a medical work-up to ensure that there is no medical condition causing the depression (*e.g.* hypothyroidism, mononucleosis, anemia, certain cancers, autoimmune diseases, premenstrual dysphoric disorder, and chronic fatigue syndrome). Symptoms of medical conditions may overlap with the symptoms of depression (*e.g.* tiredness, poor concentration, and sleep and appetite disturbances), making the differential diagnosis complicated. Also, medications (*e.g.* stimulants, corticosteroids, and contraceptives) can induce depression-like symptomatology. The diagnosis of a depressive disorder can be made if depressive symptoms are not due solely to the illnesses or the medications and if the child fulfills the DSM-IV-TR criteria for a depressive disorder.[2]

In addition, comorbid psychiatric disorders are common in depression. In fact, it is estimated that 40–90% of youth with depressive disorders also have other psychiatric disorders, with up to 50% having two or more comorbid diagnoses.[2] The most frequent diagnoses comorbid with depressive disorders are anxiety disorders, followed by disruptive disorders, attention-deficit/hyperactivity disorder (ADHD), and, in adolescents, substance use disorders.[2] Being depressed also increases the risk for the development of non-mood psychiatric problems such as conduct and substance abuse disorders, although depressive disorders can manifest after the onset of substance use problems.[17]

4. Assessment

Although the criteria symptoms for depression are similar across the lifespan, the evaluation process of depression in youth is different from adults. The clinician utilizes multiple sources to obtain the history, including caregivers, teachers, and any other persons involved in the care of the child. Parents (caregivers) are often better able to provide information on the course of illness (*e.g.* timeline), including onset and duration of symptoms; this is particularly true with younger children, who may have difficulty remembering timelines. Adolescents should be interviewed alone as they may be more open to discussing symptoms privately with the clinician and also because this helps develop rapport with the clinician.

Rating scales are often helpful in eliciting symptoms, and are available for parents, youth, and clinicians. Several standardized structured and semistructured interviews are available for clinical evaluation of psychiatric symptoms in children older than seven years[15,18] and in younger children.[19] Currently, no biological or imaging tests are clinically available for the diagnosis of depression. Clearly, assessment of depression requires significant clinical acumen, as information from a variety of sources must be synthesized to develop an accurate picture of the illness and its course.

At the initial contact with the child/adolescent and the family, the clinician should discuss with the patient and parents the boundaries of the confidential relationship with the patient. The child/adolescent has a right to a confidential relationship that is determined by law and varies by state. In addition, each state has mandatory child abuse reporting requirements. The clinician must inform the parents about the child's treatment plan, the safety plan, and progress toward goals of treatment. The child should be informed that that suicide or violence risk issues will be communicated to the parents. The clinician should request the parents to sign a release of information form that enables the clinician to communicate with health care providers involved in the care of the patient and appropriate school personnel.[2] Obtaining a detailed biological family history is also very important in evaluating depressed youth, not only in determining biological predisposition to depression, but also in understanding any psychosocial stressors the family might be undergoing.

As a child's treatment outcome may be impacted by the presence of psychiatric disorders in the caregivers, an assessment and psychiatric referral for the caregiver may be warranted as part of the evaluation process for the child. Additionally, while performing a psychiatric evaluation of a child and his/her family the clinician should be cognizant of the family's ethnic, cultural, and religious characteristics as this may affect the presentation and treatment of the depression presentation. This assessment of the entire family as a unit is useful in developing a treatment plan that will be most beneficial to the family's needs.

In summary, the initial evaluation of a child or adolescent with depression includes a comprehensive psychiatric assessment with the child/adolescent and the parent (caregiver), a medical work-up, including a drug screen and collateral information from those involved in the youth's care.

5. Suicide and Depression

Suicide is the third leading cause of death in adolescents ages 15–19, leading to 2,000 deaths annually (NIMH, 2001) with 40–80% of adolescent attempters meeting diagnostic criteria for depression at the time of the attempt.[20,21] Hence, the evaluation of depressed youth must include assessment for the presence of harm to self or others. This evaluation is done by asking questions about suicidal and homicidal ideations as well as intent to carry out a suicidal or homicidal plan. Suicidal thoughts and behaviors must also be evaluated at subsequent visits. It is crucial to evaluate risk factors, such as stress and hopelessness, and protective factors, such as religion and family for suicidal behaviors. It is important to differentiate suicidal behavior from other types of self-harm behaviors, such as repetitive self-cutting, which are conducted to relieve anger and/or sadness rather than to end one's life. In evaluating and treating youth with suicidal thoughts, clinicians must assess the level of severity of the suicidal thoughts and the danger the patient may be to himself/herself.

6. Pathogenesis and Neuroscience Findings

Psychosocial, sleep, neuroimaging, and genetic research are underway to understand the development of depression in youth. Below are a few examples of the work that has been conducted in this field.

There is no one specific cause of depressive disorders, as evidenced by high-risk, adoption, and twin studies, which have shown that depression is a familial disorder likely caused by the interaction of genetic and environmental factors.[22–27] In fact, the single most predictive factor associated with the risk of developing MDD is high family loading for this disorder.[26,28] The onset of depressive disorders often appears associated with adverse or problematic environmental factors, in conjunction with genetic predisposition to the disorder.

Stressors such as losses, abuse, neglect, ongoing conflicts, and frustrations can moderate or mediate the onset and recurrence of MDD. The effects of these stressors also depend on the child's negative attributional styles for interpreting and coping with stress, support, and genetic factors. Other factors, such as the presence of comorbid disorders (*e.g.* anxiety, substance abuse, ADHD, eating disorders), medical illness (*e.g.* diabetes), use of medications, biological, and sociocultural factors have also been related to the development and maintenance of depressive symptomatology.[22,23,26,29–32]

Birmaher *et al.*[33] conducted a study to simultaneously and prospectively compare the clinical presentation, course, and parental psychiatric history between children and adolescents with MDD. This study followed 46 pre-pubertal children and 22 post-pubertal adolescents once every two years for approximately five years. It was found that both groups had similar depressive symptomatology, severity of the index episode, rates of recovery (85%), recurrence (40%), comorbid disorders, and parental psychiatric history. Factors associated with worse longitudinal course were female sex, increased guilt, prior episodes of depression, and parental psychopathology.

Research in adults has established that certain sleep polysomnographic abnormalities are commonly found in depressed patients, including sleep continuity disturbances, reduced slow-wave sleep, shortened rapid eye movement (REM) latency, and increased REM density. In a study conducted by Robert *et al.*[34] depressed adolescent boys had the greatest sleep disturbance with the highest amount of percentage of stage 1 sleep, the shortest REM latency, and the least percentage of slow-wave sleep and number of minutes of slow-wave sleep in the first non-REM period, as compared to controls. In a study conducted by Emslie *et al.*[35] baseline suicidal ideation and sleep dysregulation on sleep polysomnography predicted recurrence of depression in depressed children and adolescents.

Youth with MDD and controls participated in a comprehensive psychobiologic study including three nights of EEG sleep recording.[36] Depressed youth reported significantly worse sleep on subjective sleep quality, perceived number of awakenings, estimated minutes awake, and perceived ease of waking. However, objective EEG measures indicated no evidence of disturbed sleep in depressed youth compared to controls.[36] Wojnar *et al.*[37] studied the relationship between body mass index (BMI) and polysomnography in 72 children with major depressive disorder and 32 healthy controls aged 8–17. It was found that in depressed youth, higher BMI was significantly correlated with decreased sleep efficiency, decreased percentage of rapid eye movement sleep, and higher percentage of time spent awake and moving. In the healthy controls, higher BMI correlated with higher total sleep time. These findings suggest that youth with MDD and a high BMI have more fragmented sleep than healthy controls.

Depression and anxiety are associated with altered cortisol secretion around sleep onset, and these changes appear to be influenced by pubertal maturation, as evidenced in a study by Forbes *et al.*[38] where depressed adolescents had marginally higher perisleep-onset cortisol than control adolescents and significantly higher perisleep-onset cortisol than depressed children.

Feder *et al.*[39] found that anxious children seem to exhibit an altered pattern of night-time cortisol secretion, with an initially sluggish or delayed nocturnal rise before reaching similar peak levels of cortisol near the time of awakening.

With the development of Functional Magnetic Resonance Imaging (fMRI), there is increasing interest in functional imaging both in depressed and remitted individuals at different developmental stages. Preliminary data suggest similarities to adults, including neurobiological abnormalities in dorsolateral prefrontal cortex found with spectroscopy[40,41] and volumetric MRI.[42] Rao *et al.*[43] conducted longitudinal volumetric magnetic resonance imaging studies in 30 adolescents with MDD, 22 adolescents at high risk for depression, and 35 adolescent healthy controls. These adolescents were followed for up to five years to assess the onset and clinical course of depression. Results from the study showed that depressed adolescents and those at high risk for depression had significantly smaller left and right hippocampal volumes in comparison to the healthy controls. It was noted that smaller hippocampal volumes were associated with higher levels of early-life adversity.

An fMRI study conducted by Yang *et al.*[44] examined subgenual anterior cingulate activity in 26 depressed and normal 13–17-year olds during the performance of a stop-signal task. Relative to controls, significantly greater subgenual anterior cingulate activation was found in the depressed adolescents.

Proton magnetic resonance spectroscopy (MRS) allows for non-invasive measurement of brain chemistry and can measure choline compounds (Cho),

N-acetylaspartate (NAA), and creatine/phosphocreatine (Cr). Proton MRS Cho signal comprises of choline-containing compounds such as phosphorycholine, glycerolphosphocholine, and acetylcholine, and may play a role in signal transduction in MDD. Steingard *et al.*[41] conducted a study in depressed adolescents and found an increased Cho/Cr and Cho/NAA levels in left orbitofrontal cortex as compared to healthy adolescent controls. The dorsolateral prefrontal cortex (DLPFC) plays an essential role in mood regulation and integration of cognitive functions that are abnormal in major depressive disorder (MDD).

Caetano *et al.*[45] conducted magnetic resonance spectroscopy of the left DLPFC in depressed youth and healthy controls. Depressed subjects had significantly lower levels of glycerophosphocholine plus phosphocholine and higher myoinositol levels in the left DLPFC compared to healthy controls. In a study by Farchione *et al.*[40] choline compounds (Cho), N-acetylaspartate (NAA), and creatine/phosphocreatine (Cr) were measured in left and right DLPFC using magnetic resonance spectroscopic imaging in treatment-naïve MDD patients and case-matched controls. A significant increase in Cho was observed in left but not right DLPFC in MDD patients versus controls. Having increased left prefrontal Cho in depressed youth may reflect abnormalities in signal transduction in MDD and could possibly be associated with the pathogenesis of pediatric MDD. Gabbay *et al.*[46] conducted an MRS study in 14 adolescents with MDD and 10 healthy controls and found that the adolescents with MDD had significantly elevated concentrations of choline and creatine in the left caudate, in comparison to the controls.

While understanding affective disorders, researchers have emphasized not only clinical symptoms but also behaviors which reflect diminished positive affect. For instance, depressed persons may not have an increased motivation to obtain rewards, may have a reduced frequency of seeking rewarding behaviors and may not have as positive an experience with reward outcomes as someone who is not depressed.[47] To study this, Forbes *et al.*[48] examined behavioral and neural responses to reward in depressed youth using fMRI. A reward decision making task was used where depressed youth exhibited less neural response than controls in reward-related brain areas during both phases of the task. The authors concluded that depression involves altered reward processing.

Progress has also been made in the area of depression genetics research. It has been found that a common polymorphism in the 5-HTT gene promoter region (5-HTT LPR) is found to moderate the influence of stressful life events on depression. Individuals with one or two copies of the short allele polymorphism of the 5-HTT promoter exhibited more depressive symptoms, diagnoses of depression, and suicidality in relationship to stressful life events than individuals homozygote for the long allele.[22] Nobile *et al.*[49] also explored the possible association between childhood- and early-adolescent-onset depressive disorders and the serotonin transporter gene polymorphism. The case-control sample consisted of patients with depressive disorder (DD) and controls. An excess of the SS-genotype and of the S-allele was found among DD children. The family-based results suggested that the S-allele was preferentially transmitted to depressed children. Another study examined the association of 5-HTT LPR with suicidal behavior and related traits in Israeli suicidal adolescent inpatients. No significant allelic association of the 5-HTT LPR polymorphism with suicidal behavior was found. However, analysis of variance of the suicide-related trait measures for the three genotypes demonstrated a significant difference in violence measures between patients carrying the LL and LS genotypes, which suggests that the 5-HTT LPR polymorphism is unlikely to have major relevance to the pathogenesis of suicidal behavior in adolescence but may contribute to violent behavior in this population.[49] The 5-HT (2A) receptor gene polymorphism T102C is one of the candidate sites in the study of suicide and impulsive-aggressive traits. Hence Zalsman *et al.*[50] conducted a study of 30 families of inpatient adolescents from Jewish Ashkenazi origin, with a recent suicide attempt, and genotyped them. All subjects were interviewed for clinical diagnosis, depressive and impulsive-aggressive traits, and demographic data. The preliminary results suggested that the 5-HT (2A) T102C polymorphism is unlikely to be associated with suicidal behavior and related traits in adolescent suicide attempters. Hammen *et al.*[51] assessed 346 youth aged between 15 and 20 who had variations in polymorphisms of the 5HTT gene. The study attempted to distinguish between the effects of acute and chronic stress to predict depressive symptoms at age 20 in these youth. The authors assessed major acute life events in youth between the ages of 15 and 19. It was found that chronic family stress at age 15 predicted higher depression scores at age 20 among those with one or two S alleles. Only in females were the effects of genetic moderation significant. It was noted that with acute stress gene–environment interactions were non-significant.

7. Depression in Primary Care

Depressed youth usually present to their primary care physician initially. However, in the limited time available for pediatricians to see patients, it is unlikely that they can complete a thorough evaluation for making the diagnosis of depression. Apart from time constraints, factors limiting the diagnosis or management of pediatric depression by primary care physicians are training or knowledge of issues.[52] An important concern in depressed youth is understanding the difference between suicidal and self-injurious behaviors. There is often a lot of confusion surrounding this issue and not having the time or expertise to evaluate these behaviors can be detrimental to the safety of the child/adolescent. Hence, it can be helpful for the assessment of suicidality and depression to become a formal part of routine pediatric care. Toward this end, Zuckerbrot *et al.*[53] assessed the feasibility of depression screening among adolescents in primary care by implementing a pen-and-paper screen and a computerized assessment, into a busy pediatric practice. It was noted that patients and parents expressed more satisfaction with the screening procedures and this screening was well accepted by the providers. Given the recent warnings about the SSRIs, pediatricians have become hesitant to diagnose and treat depression in youth. This only delays the child getting into treatment for a depressive disorder. Another confounding factor in all this is even when pediatricians do decide to treat a depressed pediatric patient they are conservative in their dosing regimes. The decision of when and how primary care physicians decide to treat adolescent depression is strongly influenced by the physicians' perceptions of their role in treatment, availability of other treatment resources, and family and patient preferences and resources.[54]

8. Treatment

As noted above, psychosocial stressors, such as family and peer relationships, school performance, and other environmental factors can lead to depressive episodes. Equally important, however, is that depression may lead to substance abuse, suicide, and other long-term consequences. Treatment of depression must be individualized to address the specific consequences of depression being experienced by the child or adolescent. Non-specific interventions may include contact with school teachers and officials, referrals for family members to a psychiatrist or psychologist, or general problem-solving recommendations.

Determining the most efficacious treatment by understanding what is the evidence for effectiveness of specific interventions is important for both clinicians and patients. Evidence-based medicine is the integration of research evidence, clinical expertise, and patient preferences to determine the most effective treatment intervention. Currently, specific psychotherapies and selective serotonin reuptake inhibitors (SSRIs) are the most widely used treatments for pediatric depression (reviewed in detail below). In a metaanalysis of psychotherapy trials in pediatric depression, the effect size for depression studies was small (0.34 ± 0.4), but present.[55] A metaanalysis of antidepressants for pediatric depression also exhibited positive benefit for active medication over placebo.[56]

Information from clinical trials alone is usually insufficient to assist in developing treatment recommendations. This is best done utilizing guidelines (American Academy of Child and Adolescent Psychiatry) or algorithms.[57] Lack of sufficient evidence-based treatment options require clinicians to utilize other resources to evaluate treatment options. Therefore, it is important for clinicians to differentiate between clinical guidelines and clinical trials.[55,56,58,59] Clinical guidelines are developed from the research evidence, including randomized controlled trials (RCTs), open trials, clinical experience, epidemiological data, and (for children and adolescents) extrapolation from adult trials. There are many clinical situations in which there is only limited clinical information and no RCT data available. Guidelines can also address equally important issues, including adequacy of assessment, available treatment options, and staging of treatment. Clinical guidelines need to be developed from thoughtful examination of all available clinical information with input from clinicians and patients.

The treatment of depression in youth begins with a careful diagnostic evaluation as noted in Sec. 4. Once it is established that a depressive disorder exists, then the clinician should discuss the treatment recommendations with the child/adolescent and family. Treatment of the depressed youth includes developing a therapeutic alliance, psychoeducation, supportive management, and family and school involvement.

8.1. *Therapeutic alliance*

Developing a therapeutic alliance with the family and the child/adolescent is crucial during the treatment process. The clinician must meet individually with the child/adolescent and family at every visit. The boundaries of the therapeutic alliance must be carefully explained to both the patient and the family. Because it is the family that brings the child for treatment, it is imperative that the clinician keep the family closely involved in the treatment plan. The parents may see the depressive symptoms differently than the child does, or the child may not report all that is relevant for the clinician to know in order for treatment to be effective.

8.2. *Psychoeducation*

Psychoeducation involves educating family members and the patient about the causes, symptoms, course, and different treatments of depression, as well as the risks associated with various treatment interventions or lack of treatment. As noted above, the patient and family are involved in treatment decisions, so, providing clear information about all of the options helps to make the decision-making process easier for the family. It is important to emphasize that depression is an illness with both genetic and environmental contributions. Often parents blame themselves for their child's depression, so it is important to reduce these concerns for many parents. Parents can also be guided on methods of parenting a depressed child (*e.g.* when to be strict and when to be lenient in regards to the patient's functioning). It is also important for the family and patient to understand that the treatment of depression can be a slow process and that depression can become recurrent and chronic. Knowing this beforehand allows the family and patient to be aware of what to expect, to not get disappointed, and to remain in treatment. Giving all this information upfront can be beneficial in developing a strong therapeutic alliance.

8.3. *Supportive management*

At every stage of treatment, the patient and family require supportive psychotherapeutic management, which includes active listening and reflection, problem solving, coping skills, and strategies for continuing in treatment. Families who have depressed children/adolescents can benefit from problem-solving techniques and management of behavioral issues that can arise with their child. For the clinician to be supportive to the family, he/she needs to understand the individual concerns the family is presenting with and address the same. It is important to note that supportive therapy is not sufficient in the treatment of moderate or severe depression. However, a clinician who listens and is responsive to the family and youth can definitely help the treatment process move along. Indeed, supportive therapy alone may be sufficient in treating mild depression.

8.4. *Family and school involvement*

As noted above, the patient and family are involved in all treatment decisions. In addition, the clinician may provide intervention specific to the family. For example, depressed youth often have decreased school performance as a result of decreased concentration and/or decreased motivation. Parents with strict grade policies may be encouraged to slightly lower their scholastic expectations briefly while the child is depressed. Likewise, schools may be contacted to collaborate with the psychiatrist or therapist on minimizing school difficulties during the episode. The clinician can be of great help to the family by advocating for accommodations in the school setting. Depressed youth have difficulty getting schoolwork done, so if the workload can be accommodated until the child recovers from depression, this can be helpful for the child. Once the child has recovered from depression, if he/she has academic difficulties, then further testing for learning disabilities, other comorbid conditions, or environmental factors may be warranted to ascertain if there are additional nondepression causes for the child's persistent academic difficulties.

Thus, educating the family and patient about the causes, symptoms, course, and different treatments of depression and the risks associated with these treatments as well as no treatment at all is valuable. The current treatments for depression in youth include psychotherapy and pharmacotherapy. Always, the decision to treat with or without therapy and/or medications is made with the family and the child/adolescent. Factors that help in deciding how to proceed with treatment are: past episodes, severity of current episode, past responsiveness to medications and therapy, patient's and family's preference for treatment (*e.g.* medication or not; preference of medications), a detailed history of suicide attempts, and ideations and substance use history.

8.5. *Psychotherapy*

Effective treatments for depression are the specific psychotherapies, namely, Cognitive Behavioral Therapy (CBT) and Interpersonal Therapy (IPT), specifically in adolescents.[60,61] Weisz *et al.*[55] addressed the question of whether evidence based treatments (EBTs) produced better outcomes than the usual interventions employed in clinical care through a metaanalysis of 32 randomized trials that directly compared EBTs with usual care. The authors concluded that EBTs outperformed usual care. Although CBT and IPT are usually to be individual treatments, some modifications may include group treatments and family education sessions. Indeed, non-specific psychotherapy is not effective in moderate to severe depression.

8.5.1. *Cognitive behavioral therapy (CBT)*

Cognitive Behavioral Therapy (CBT) is the most commonly and widely used specific therapy for child and adolescent depression. The focus is on cognitive distortions, *i.e.* negative distortions of life experience, negative view of self, others, and the world. The goal is to alleviate depressive episodes, prevent recurrences by identifying and testing negative cognitions, and develop flexible, positive ways of thinking. CBT is time limited and focused on identifying thought and behavioral patterns which contribute to the child's depressed mood.[60]

Compton *et al.*[62] reviewed the literature on the cognitive-behavioral treatment of children and adolescents with anxiety and depressive disorders and concluded that from an evidence-based perspective, cognitive-behavioral therapy is currently the treatment of choice for anxiety and depressive disorders in children and adolescents.

8.5.2. *Interpersonal therapy*

IPT focuses on interpersonal problems — grief, interpersonal role disputes, role transitions, or interpersonal deficits or issues with single parent families (in adolescents) that occurred at the onset of depressive symptoms. The depression may be maintained because of these issues; hence, it is important to recognize these problems. In a 12-week open study of IPT for 25 moderately to severely depressed adolescents, 84% meet criteria for remission by the end of the treatment.[63] IPT is emerging as another efficacious psychotherapy for adolescent depression where it has been shown to be superior to twice a month supportive clinical management, with differences most prominent in those who were moderately or severely depressed and in older teens.[64] IPT appears to be relatively easy to disseminate as therapists in school-based health clinics with brief training and supervision were able to improve depression using IPT compared with treatment as usual.[65]

8.5.3. *Dialectical behavioral therapy*

DBT is an empirically supported psychotherapy that has been adapted for use particularly with those adolescents with suicidal ideation and/or borderline personality features.[66] DBT in adolescents focuses primarily on affect regulation, problem solving, improving communication, and maintaining a balance between acceptance and change. A pilot study of 12 adolescents was conducted by Fleischhaker *et al.*[67] to find out if DBT is an effective method of treatment for self-injurious behavior. During treatment, it was found that self-injurious behavior declined significantly with DBT.

8.5.4. *Family therapy*

There are studies pointing to the importance of family intervention in youth with mood disorders. A study conducted by Kolko *et al.*[68] found that those adolescents who had participated in family treatment had significantly improved parent–child relationships at a two-year follow-up. In a pilot study of nine children and adolescents, Fristad *et al.*[69] found that multi-family psychoeducational group therapy (a six-session treatment program) may improve the family climate in children with mood disorders immediately after the treatment and at four-month follow-up.

As a general rule, the clinician should evaluate the needs of the child/adolescent and family and make recommends for the appropriate form of therapy that can be beneficial for them.

8.6. *Pharmacotherapy*

Fluoxetine is the only antidepressant to show positive efficacy in more than one acute trial in pediatric depression, and is the only antidepressant with an FDA indication for the treatment of depression in both children and adolescents. Escitalopram has been approved by the Food and Drug Administration (FDA) for the treatment of MDD in adolescents. There is some evidence of efficacy of several selective serotonin reuptake inhibitors (SSRIs) in pediatric depression, including Fluoxetine,[70] sertraline,[71] citalopram,[72] and escitalopram.[73] Thus, the Children's Medication Algorithm Project (CMAP)[57] for MDD recommends that for the treatment of MDD in youth, an SSRI should be the first antidepressant to be started. The decision of which SSRI to start should be reviewed with the family and joint decisions made. All SSRIs have relative advantages and disadvantages, and adverse effects are not clearly different among SSRIs; therefore, prescribing clinicians should remain sensitive to family preferences.

Paroxetine has shown some efficacy on secondary outcomes in one adolescent trial[74]; however, two negative trials of paroxetine have also been reported.[75,76] Due to increased dropout rates due to adverse events in pre-pubertal children and potentially increase agitation/hostility than other SSRIs[58] paroxetine is not recommended for pre-pubertal children, but can be considered in adolescents as a second line treatment. All SSRIs are considered potential options as a second-line treatment following failure with an initial SSRI.[57] Following failure of two SSRIs, guidelines suggest switching to a different class of antidepressant, such as bupropion (wellbutrin), mirtazapine (remeron), or venlafaxine (effexor). Two trials each for mirtazapine and venlafaxine have failed to demonstrate positive efficacy of the medication over placebo in youth. Non-randomized, controlled trials in youth have been conducted to date with bupropion, although it has been shown to reduce depressive symptoms in youth with comorbid depression and ADHD.[77]

8.6.1. *Acute treatment*

Antidepressants should be started at low doses and monitored very carefully for the emergence of adverse effects and suicidal thoughts or behaviors. The dose of antidepressants in children and adolescents is titrated to those doses similarly used for adult patients.[78] Patients should be treated for four weeks with adequate and tolerable doses. Assess clinical response at four-week intervals, and if a complete response has not been obtained, the dosage may be increased, if the patient is tolerating the medication. If patients are started on one SSRI and are showing minimal or no response after eight weeks of treatment on an optimal dose, they can be switched to another SSRI. All antidepressants, except for fluoxetine, should be discontinued slowly. Because fluoxetine has a long half-life, it can be stopped at once. If antidepressants are discontinued abruptly, patients can experience withdrawal symptoms such as tiredness and somatic symptoms. If a partial response occurs with antidepressant monotherapy or when remission is not achieved despite significant clinical improvement, then the clinician can think of augmenting strategies. Randomized controlled trials have shown mirtazapine and sustained-release bupropion to be effective augmenting agents in adults who have experienced inadequate improvement with an SSRI, but this has not been studied in children.[79,80] The best augmenting agent in youth who are partial responders to an SSRI or fail to respond to an SSRI has yet to be determined.

After a child/adolescent has two failed trials of SSRIs, then he/she can be switched to an alternate antidepressant. However, before making the switch the clinician must reassess the accuracy of the diagnosis, comorbidity, and any other factors contributing to the depression. When MDD presents with psychotic features, the psychotic symptoms need to be treated in conjunction with the depressive symptoms. An antidepressant can be started in conjunction with an antipsychotic. Alternatively, an antipsychotic can be started initially and an antidepressant added if improvement is not seen.

8.6.2. *Continuation treatment*

The American Academy of Child and Adolescent Psychiatry recommends that until further research becomes available, continuation therapy for at least 6 to 12 months is recommended for all patients who have responded to the acute treatment. The duration of continuation treatment and need for maintenance treatment is based on severity of the index episode, ongoing residual symptoms, history of multiple episodes, patient and family preference, and side effects of continued treatment. When discontinuing the antidepressant, the dose should be tapered no more rapidly than 25% per week. Antidepressants should be tapered and discontinued over a 2- to 3-month period.[81] Patients and their families should be taught to monitor for recurrence of depressive symptoms. If depression recurs, then initiate treatment with the previously effective medication and follow the course of medication management previously followed to achieve remission of depressive symptoms. For patients with MDD with psychotic features, the antipsychotic medication should be continued for two to three months after remission of psychotic symptoms and then tapered off.[82]

Maintenance: Approximately, 70% of youths experiencing MDD will experience a recurrence.[83] Hence, all children and adolescents, experiencing recurrent depression and with risk factors (*e.g.* family history, severity of episode, suicidality during the episode) should be considered for maintenance treatment.[2] Maintenance medication should continue at full therapeutic doses. Although the optimal duration of maintenance medication has not been established in adults or youth, it is generally believed to be between three years and lifetime.

For further details on antidepressants, please refer to the *Handbook of Mental Health Interventions in Children and Adolescents: An Integrated Development Approach.*

8.6.3. *Warnings about antidepressants and increased suicidality*

The US Food and Drug Administration (FDA), after a metaanalysis of clinical trials assessing use of antidepressant medications among children and adolescents concluded that these medications pose an increased risk for "suicidal behavior or suicidal ideation." The FDA mandated that a boxed warning be put on the labels of all antidepressants indicating an increased risk of suicidal thoughts and behavior in youth taking these medications.[56] It is recommended that patients started on antidepressants should be closely monitored for suicidality or unusual changes in behavior, agitation, irritability during the initial few months of treatment and when there are changes in doses. The FDA recommends that treatment monitoring visits should be frequent when an antidepressant is initiated. Patients should be contacted weekly for the initial four week and biweekly through week 12. Further studies need to clarify if factors such as sex; patient's history of suicidality; family history of suicidality; time during treatment; withdrawal side effects; agitation, activation, or hypomania are related to increased risk for suicidality.[84–87]

Figure 1 shows how complex the situation is. The only way to handle this is to embed the patient in a carefully crafted integrated treatment network, thus allowing the clinician to decide whether emergent suicidality is indeed brought on by SSRI activation, insufficient response to treatment, injurious events, or other life stressors, *i.e.* loss of a boyfriend, etc.

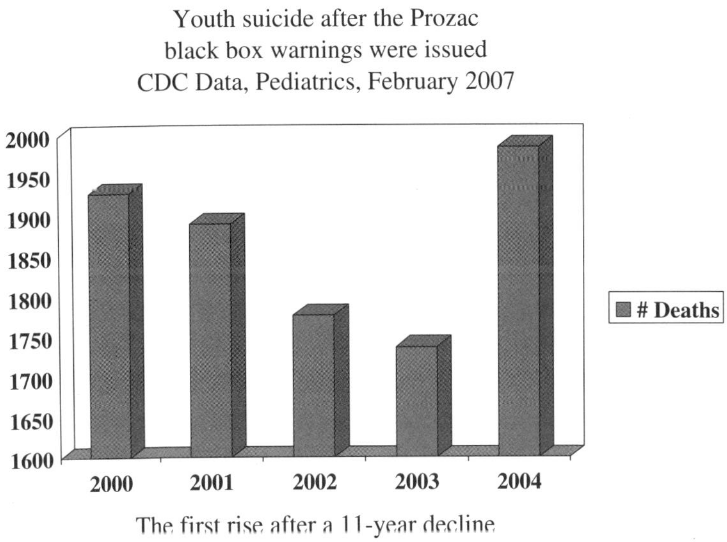

Fig. 1:

8.6.4. *Combination treatment*

The Treatment of Adolescent Depression Study (TADS)[88] was conducted at 13 centers in the United States. This was a randomized, 12-week clinical trial comparing the effectiveness of fluoxetine, CBT, and combination of fluoxetine and CBT to placebo in 439 adolescents (12–17 years) with major depression. The results of this study were as follows: of those who were on fluoxetine treatment 61% were responders, of those who were on placebo only, 35% were responders, of those who were on the combination of fluoxetine and CBT 71% were responders and of those receiving CBT only, 43% were responders to the treatment (Treatment of Adolescent Depression Study (TADS) Team). In the TADS study, combined treatment with fluoxetine and CBT was found to be effective in improving measures of overall functioning, global health, and quality of life.

The Treatment of SSRI-Resistant Depression in Adolescents (TORDIA) was a six site randomized controlled clinical trial of adolescents with MDD who had not responded to a two month initial trial with an SSRI. This study included 334 adolescents, aged 12–18 years. The study participants were randomized as follows: (1) to a different SSRI (paroxetine, citalopram or fluoxetine); (2) to a different SSRI with CBT; (3) to venlafaxine (effexor); or (4) to venlafaxine with CBT. The results showed that 54.8% of the participants responded to switching to a different SSRI with CBT, whereas 40.5% of the participants responded to switching to the different SSRI without CBT.[89]

In another study, Clarke *et al.*[90] compared SSRI treatment alone in 75 participants to a brief CBT intervention added to an SSRI in 77 participants. This study was conducted in primary care clinics. Results found no significant difference in decrease of depression symptoms between the two treatment groups.

Melvin *et al.*[91] in a study with 73 adolescents with MDD, dysthymia, or depression NOS found combination treatment to be no more effective than either medication alone or CBT alone.

9. Clinical Experience and Examples

Patients of all developmental ages are evaluated for depression and treated if appropriate. A comprehensive workup is conducted initially after which a treatment plan is put into place with the patient and family. Because fluoxetine is FDA approved for the treatment of depression in children/adolescents, this is the initial SSRI of choice unless the child/adolescent has been on fluoxetine before and has either not responded to an adequate dose with an adequate trial or has side effects with it, or unless the child is at high risk for developing bipolar disorder (see Chap. 7).

An SSRI is initiated at the lowest dose for depressed youth. If there is no improvement in clinical response after four weeks, then the dose of the medication should be increased. However, if patients are started on one SSRI and are showing minimal or no response after eight weeks of treatment they can be switched to another SSRI. It is only after two failed trials of an SSRI that we switch to another class of an antidepressant. If there is partial response to the maximum recommended dose of an SSRI, then we can add another class of an antidepressant to treat the depression. However, if at a low dose of an SSRI a patient is responding partially, but has side effects, then we add another class of an antidepressant to the SSRI. The common combination of antidepressants is an SSRI and bupropion. Individual and family therapy is individualized to address the patient's and family's needs.

Electroconvulsive Therapy (ECT) may be an effective treatment for adolescents with treatment-resistant depression and can be considered when there is a lack of response to two or more trials of pharmacotherapy or when the severity of symptoms prevents waiting for a response to pharmacological treatment.

More recently, a number of children and adolescents are presenting to clinicians with the primary complaint of daily verbal and/or physical aggression. Overt aggression can be a manifestation of depression, bipolar disorder, ADHD, anxiety disorder, substance use, and other psychiatric diagnoses. Thus, overt aggression is only a symptom, and determining the underlying diagnosis/diagnoses will lead to improved care and overall outcome. This is the scenario where the developmental timeline can help the clinician identify the primary diagnosis and true comorbidity.

To further illustrate, a 13-year-old boy presented to the psychiatrist's office with a history of oppositional, defiant behaviors, verbal and physical aggression both at home and in school. The patient himself denied any symptoms, and believed that all that was happening to him was everyone else's fault (an example of cognition distortions). Upon interviewing the mother, it was established that the patient had no prior psychiatric history and that for the year, he had been increasingly irritable, very defiant and aggressive with her, eating and sleeping more than usual and was failing most of his classes. He was suspended from school eight times in the current academic year. The patient's father moved out of state a year ago with much less frequent contact with the patient. A complete evaluation established the diagnosis of a major depressive disorder. The mother and patient gave their consent/assent for citalopram to be started. This was initiated at 10 mg per night. Family and individual therapy was initiated. Within six weeks, the patient's mood had improved, his aggression had reduced in intensity and frequency, and he started summer school. One year later, he showed full resolution of depressive symptoms and improvement in the quality of relationships with mother, peers, and teachers. He remains on citalopram 10 mg at night and continues weekly individual and family therapy.

10. Outcomes: Naturalistic, Clinical Trials

Thus far, outcomes of child and adolescent patients diagnosed with depression in either a naturalistic or clinical setting, have been shown to be better when therapy, specifically Cognitive Behavioral Therapy, is provided adjunctively with an antidepressant, typically fluoxetine[92,93]; however, when provided on its own, fluoxetine has been found to be quite effective in the treatment of depression in this cohort.[70,92] Data in the past few years has shown that 66% of those children or adolescents diagnosed with depression who are receiving some form of antidepressant, are being prescribed these medications by nonpsychiatrists (*i.e.* primary care physicians), and are not returning for the recommended number of follow-up visits.[94] In order to promote better future outcomes for these patients, it is imperative that more collaboration take place between psychiatrists or other mental health professionals treating these patients, and the primary care physicians who are also prescribing antidepressants.[94]

11. The Next Five Years

Future directions for the treatment of depression in children and adolescents should promote the tenet that remission is ultimately the desired endpoint for treatment.[95] To accomplish this, treatment should be personalized in studying patients' individual underlying biological factors (*e.g.* gross brain anatomy, genetic polymorphisms) and how they interact with environmental factors to either exacerbate or inhibit the development of depression in child and adolescent populations.[96] For example, Paddock and colleagues[97] found that genetic variations on a glutamate receptor plays a role on an antidepressant's efficacy, thereby helping to better predict which patients will respond better to that particular treatment for depression. By continuing to study these underlying biological factors, and how they interact with environmental factors, children and adolescents may have better outcomes as result of the greater breadth of knowledge about the disease state underlying depression, as well as the possible responses to varied kinds of treatment.[95]

12. Conclusion

Depression does exist in children and adolescents, although the presentation may be different from that in adults. Because it can be difficult to accurately diagnose depression in youth it remains underdiagnosed, and therefore undertreated in children and adolescents. This is a serious disorder causing significant morbidity and mortality; hence, research in psychosocial areas, sleep and hormonal areas, neuroimaging, and genetics is underway to find the pathogenesis causing this disorder. This will eventually help in maybe preventing and possibly finding the appropriate treatments for depressed youth. At present, only fluoxetine has received an indication from the FDA for treating pediatric depression. So far, the literature has clinical trials on the acute treatment of pediatric depression. Continuation and maintenance studies in psychopharmacological interventions are greatly needed. Certain psychotherapies, such as CBT and IPT are showing promise in the treatment of depression. However, long-term benefits of these treatments remain unknown, as limited research has been conducted in the continuation and maintenance treatment of children and adolescents with mood disorders.

References

1. Coyle JT, Pine DS, Charney DS, Lewis L, Nemeroff CB, Carlson GA, Joshi PT, Reiss D, Todd RD, Hellander M. Depression and bipolar support alliance consensus statement on the unmet needs in diagnosis and treatment of mood disorders in children and adolescents, *J Am Acad Child Adolesc Psychiatry* 2003; **42**: 1494–1503.
2. Birmaher B, Brent D, AACAP Work Group on Quality Issues, Bernet W, Bukstein O, Walter H, Benson RS, Chrisman A, Farchione T, Greenhill L, Hamilton J, Keable H, Kinlan J, Schoettle U, Stock S, Ptakowski KK, Medicus J. Practice parameter for the assessment and treatment of children and adolescents with depressive disorders, *J Am Acad Child Adolesc Psychiatry* 2007; **46**: 1503–1526.
3. Nesse RM. Is depression an adaptation? *Arch Gen Psychiatry* 2000; **57**: 14–20.
4. Watson PJ, Andrews PW. Toward a revised evolutionary adaptationist analysis of depression: The social navigation hypothesis, *J Affect Disord* 2002; **72**: 1–14.
5. Kinney DK, Tanaka M. An evolutionary hypothesis of depression and its adaptive symptoms, adaptive value, and risk factors, *J Nerv Ment Dis* 2009; **197**: 561–567.
6. Geller B, Zimerman B, Williams M, Bolhofner K, Craney JL. Adult psychosocial outcome of prepubertal major depressive disorder, *J Am Acad Child Adolesc Psychiatry* 2001; **40**: 673–677.
7. Goodman SH, Schwab-Stone M, Lahey BB, Shaffer D, Jensen PS. Major depression and dysthymia in children and adolescents: Discriminant validity and differential consequences in a community sample, *J Am Acad Child Adolesc Psychiatry* 2000; **39**: 61–70.
8. Fergusson DM, Horwood LJ, Ridder EM, Beautrais AL. Subthreshold depression in adolescence and mental health outcomes in adulthood, *Arch Gen Psychiatry* 2005; **62**: 66–72.
9. Lewinsohn PM, Solomon A, Seeley JR, Zeiss A. Clinical implications of "subthreshold" depressive symptoms, *J Abnorm Psychol* 2000; **109**: 345–351.

10. American Psychiatric Association. *Diagnostic and Statistical Manual of Mental Disorders*, 4th ed, Text Revision. Washington, DC: Americal Psychiatric Association, 2000.
11. Williamson DE, Birmaher B, Brent DA, Balach L, Dahl RE, Ryan ND. Atypical symptoms of depression in a sample of depressed child and adolescent outpatients, *J Am Acad Child Adolesc Psychiatry* 2000; **39**: 1253–1259.
12. Geller B, Zimerman B, Williams M, Bolhofner K, Craney JL. Bipolar disorder at prospective follow-up of adults who had prepubertal major depressive disorder, *Am J Psychiatry* 2001; **158**: 125–127.
13. World Health Organization. *International Classification of Diseases and Related Health Problems*-10th edition (ICD-10), Geneva: World Health Organization, 1992.
14. Fergusson DM, Woodward LJ. Mental health, educational, and social role outcomes of adolescents with depression, *Arch Gen Psychiatry* 2002; **59**: 225–231.
15. Klein DN, Dougherty LR, Olino TM. Toward guidelines for evidence-based assessment of depression in children and adolescents, *J Clin Child Adolesc Psychol* 2005; **34**: 412–432.
16. Carandang GC, Martin A. *Clinical Assessment of Children and Adoelscents with Depression. Treating Child and Adoelscent Depression.* Joseph RM, Boris B, Eds. 2009.
17. Fombonne E, Wostear G, Cooper V, Harrington R, Rutter M. The Maudsley long-term follow-up of child and adolescent depression. 2. Suicidality, criminality and social dysfunction in adulthood, *Br J Psychiatry* 2001; **179**: 218–223.
18. Myers K, Winters NC. Ten-year review of rating scales. II: Scales for internalizing disorders, *J Am Acad Child Adolesc Psychiatry* 2002; **41**: 634–659.
19. Luby JL, Mrakotsky C, Heffelfinger A, Brown K, Hessler M, Spitznagel E. Modification of DSM-IV criteria for depressed preschool children, *Am J Psychiatry* 2003; **160**: 1169–1172.
20. Beautrais AL. Risk factors for suicide and attempted suicide among young people, *Aust N Z J Psychiatry* 2000; **34**: 420–436.
21. Fergusson DM, Woodward LJ, Horwood LJ. Risk factors and life processes associated with the onset of suicidal behaviour during adolescence and early adulthood, *Psychol Med* 2000; **30**: 23–39.
22. Caspi A, Sugden K, Moffitt TE, Taylor A, Craig IW, Harrington H, McClay J, Mill J, Martin J, Braithwaite A, Poulton R. Influence of life stress on depression: Moderation by a polymorphism in the 5-HTT gene, *Science* 2003; **301**: 386–389.
23. Kendler KS, Gatz M, Gardner CO, Pedersen NL. Age at onset and familial risk for major depression in a Swedish national twin sample, *Psychol Med* 2005; **35**: 1573–1579.
24. Pilowsky DJ, Wickramaratne P, Nomura Y, Weissman MM. Family discord, parental depression, and psychopathology in offspring: 20-year follow-up, *J Am Acad Child Adolesc Psychiatry* 2006; **45**: 452–460.

25. Reinherz HZ, Paradis AD, Giaconia RM, Stashwick CK, Fitzmaurice G. Childhood and adolescent predictors of major depression in the transition to adulthood, *Am J Psychiatry* 2003; **160**: 2141–2147.
26. Weissman MM, Wickramaratne P, Nomura Y, Warner V, Verdeli H, Pilowsky DJ, Grillon C, Bruder G. Families at high and low risk for depression: A 3-generation study, *Arch Gen Psychiatry* 2005; **62**: 29–36.
27. Weissman MM, Wickramaratne P, Nomura Y, Warner V, Pilowsky D, Verdeli H. Offspring of depressed parents: 20 years later, *Am J Psychiatry* 2006; **163**: 1001–1008.
28. Nomura Y, Wickramaratne PJ, Warner V, Mufson L, Weissman MM. Family discord, parental depression, and psychopathology in offspring: Ten-year follow-up, *J Am Acad Child Adolesc Psychiatry* 2002; **41**: 402–409.
29. Costello EJ, Pine DS, Hammen C, March JS, Plotsky PM, Weissman MM, Biederman J, Goldsmith HH, Kaufman J, Lewinsohn PM, Hellander M, Hoagwood K, Koretz DS, Nelson CA, Leckman JF. Development and natural history of mood disorders, *Biol Psychiatry* 2002; **52**: 529–542.
30. Pine DS, Cohen P, Johnson JG, Brook JS. Adolescent life events as predictors of adult depression, *J Affect Disord* 2002; **68**: 49–57.
31. Pine DS, Lissek S, Klein RG, Mannuzza S, Moulton JL, 3rd, Guardino M, Woldehawariat G. Face-memory and emotion: Associations with major depression in children and adolescents, *J Child Psychol Psychiatry* 2004; **45**: 1199–1208.
32. Rey JM, Martin A, Krabman P. Is the party over? Cannabis and juvenile psychiatric disorder: The past 10 years, *J Am Acad Child Adolesc Psychiatry* 2004; **43**: 1194–1205.
33. Birmaher B, Williamson DE, Dahl RE, Axelson DA, Kaufman J, Dorn LD, Ryan ND. Clinical presentation and course of depression in youth: Does onset in childhood differ from onset in adolescence? *J Am Acad Child Adolesc Psychiatry* 2004; **43**: 63–67.
34. Robert JJ, Hoffmann RF, Emslie GJ, Hughes C, Rintelmann J, Moore J, Armitage R. Sex and age differences in sleep macroarchitecture in childhood and adolescent depression, *Sleep* 2006; **29**: 351–358.
35. Emslie GJ, Armitage R, Weinberg WA, Rush AJ, Mayes TL, Hoffmann RF. Sleep polysomnography as a predictor of recurrence in children and adolescents with major depressive disorder, *Int J Neuropsychopharmacol* 2001; **4**: 159–168.
36. Bertocci MA, Dahl RE, Williamson DE, Tosif AM, Birmaher B, Axelson D, Ryan ND. Subjective sleep complaints in pediatric depression: A controlled study and comparison with EEG measures of sleep and waking, *J Am Acad Child Adolesc Psychiatry* 2005; **44**: 1158–1166.
37. Wojnar J, Brower KJ, Dopp R, Wojnar M, Emslie G, Rintelmann J, Hoffmann RF, Armitage R. Sleep and body mass index in depressed children and healthy controls, *Sleep Med* 2010; **11**: 295–301.

38. Forbes EE, Williamson DE, Ryan ND, Birmaher B, Axelson DA, Dahl RE. Peri-sleep-onset cortisol levels in children and adolescents with affective disorders, *Biol Psychiatry* 2006; **59**: 24–30.
39. Feder A, Coplan JD, Goetz RR, Mathew SJ, Pine DS, Dahl RE, Ryan ND, Greenwald S, Weissman MM. Twenty-four-hour cortisol secretion patterns in prepubertal children with anxiety or depressive disorders, *Biol Psychiatry* 2004; **56**: 198–204.
40. Farchione TR, Moore GJ, Rosenberg DR. Proton magnetic resonance spectroscopic imaging in pediatric major depression, *Biol Psychiatry* 2002; **52**: 86–92.
41. Steingard RJ, Yurgelun-Todd DA, Hennen J, Moore JC, Moore CM, Vakili K, Young AD, Katic A, Beardslee WR, Renshaw PF. Increased orbitofrontal cortex levels of choline in depressed adolescents as detected by in vivo proton magnetic resonance spectroscopy, *Biol Psychiatry* 2000; **48**: 1053–1061.
42. Nolan CL, Moore GJ, Madden R, Farchione T, Bartoi M, Lorch E, Stewart CM, Rosenberg DR. Prefrontal cortical volume in childhood-onset major depression: Preliminary findings, *Arch Gen Psychiatry* 2002; **59**: 173–179.
43. Rao U, Hammen CL, Poland RE. Longitudinal course of adolescent depression: Neuroendocrine and psychosocial predictors, *J Am Acad Child Adolesc Psychiatry* 2010; **49**: 141–151.
44. Yang TT, Simmons AN, Matthews SC, Tapert SF, Frank GK, Bischoff-Grethe A, Lansing AE, Wu J, Brown GG, Paulus MP. Depressed adolescents demonstrate greater subgenual anterior cingulated activity, *Neuroreport* 2009; **20**: 440–444.
45. Caetano SC, Fonseca M, Olvera RL, Nicoletti M, Hatch JP, Stanley JA, Hunter K, Lafer B, Pliszka SR, Soares JC. Proton spectroscopy study of the left dorsolateral prefrontal cortex in pediatric depressed patients, *Neurosci Lett* 2005; **384**: 321–326.
46. Gabbay V, Hess DA, Liu S, Babb JS, Klein RG, Gonen O. Lateralized caudate metabolic abnormalities in adolescent major depressive disorder: A proton MR spectroscopy study, *Am J Psychiatry* 2007; **164**: 1881–1889.
47. Forbes EE, Dahl RE. Neural sytems of positive affect: relevance to understanding child and adolescent depression? *Dev Psychopathol* 2005; **17**: 827–825.
48. Forbes EE, Christopher May J, Siegle GJ, Ladouceur CD, Ryan ND, Carter CS, Birmaher B, Axelson DA, Dahl RE. Reward-related decision-making in pediatric major depressive disorder: an fMRI study, *J Child Psychol Psychiatry* 2006; **47**: 1031–1040.
49. Nobile M, Cataldo MG, Giorda R, Battaglia M, Baschirotto C, Bellina M, Marino C, Molteni M. A case-control and family-based association study of the 5-HTTLPR in pediatric-onset depressive disorders, *Biol Psychiatry* 2004; **56**: 292–295.
50. Zalsman G, Frisch A, Bromberg M, Gelernter J, Michaelovsky E, Campino A, Erlich Z, Tyano S, Apter A, Weizman A. Family-based association study of serotonin transporter promoter in suicidal adolescents: No association with suicidality but possible role in violence traits, *Am J Med Genet* 2001; **105**: 239–245.

51. Hammen C, Brennan PA, Keenan-Miller D, Hazel NA, Najman JM. Chronic and acute stress, gender, and serotonin transporter gene-environment interactions predicting depression symptoms in youth, *J Child Psychol Psychiatry* 2010; **51**: 180–187.
52. Olson AL, Kelleher KJ, Kemper KJ, Zuckerman BS, Hammond CS, Dietrich AJ. Primary care pediatricians' roles and perceived responsibilities in the identification and management of depression in children and adolescents, *Ambul Pediatr* 2001; **2**: 91–98.
53. Zuckerbrot RA, Maxon L, Pagar D, Davies M, Fisher PW, Shaffer D. Adolescent depression screening in primary care: Feasibility and acceptability, *Pediatrics* 2007; **19**: 101–108.
54. Richardson LP, Lewis CP, Casey-Goldstein M, McCauley E, Katon W. Pediatric primary care providers and adolescent depression: A qualitative study of barriers to treatment and the effect of the black box warning, *J Adolesc Health* 2007; **40**: 433–439.
55. Weisz JR, Jensen-Doss A, Hawley KM. Evidence-based youth psychotherapies versus usual clinical care: A meta-analysis of direct comparisons, *Am Psychol* 2006; **617**: 671–689.
56. Bridge JA, Iyengar S, Salary CB, Barbe RP, Birmaher B, Pincus HA, Ren L, Brent DA. Clinical response and risk for reported suicidal ideation and suicide attempts in pediatric antidepressant treatment: A meta-analysis of randomized controlled trials, *JAMA* 2007; **297**: 1683–1696.
57. Hughes C, Emslie G, Crismon ML, Posner K, Birmaher B, Ryan N, Jensen PS, Curry J, Vitiello B, Lopez M, Shon S, Pliszka SR, Trivedi M. Texas children's medication algorithm project: Update from the Texas consensus panel on medication treatment of childhood major depressive disorder, *J Am Acad Child Adolesc Psychiatry* 2007; **46**: 667–686.
58. Cheung AH, Emslie GJ, Mayes TL. Review of the efficacy and safety of antidepressants in youth depression, *J Child Psychol Psychiatry* 2005; **46**: 735–754.
59. Saxena K, Blasey C. Research methodology in clinical trials. *Handbook of Mental Health Interventions in Children and Adolescents: An Integrated Developmental Approach* 2004, pp. 222–244.
60. Curry JF. Specific psychotherapies for childhood and adolescent depression, *Biol Psychiatry* 2001; **49**: 1091–1100.
61. Weersing VR, Weisz JR. Community clinic treatment of depressed youth: Benchmarking usual care against CBT clinical trials, *J Consult Clin Psychol* 2002; **70**: 299–310.
62. Compton SN, March JS, Brent D, Albano AM 5th, Weersing R, Curry J. Cognitive-behavioral psychotherapy for anxiety and depressive disorders in children and adolescents: An evidence-based medicine review, *J Am Acad Child Adolesc Psychiatry* 2004; **43**: 930–959.

63. Santor DA, Kusumakar V. Open trial of interpersonal therapy in adolescents with moderate to severe major depression: Effectiveness of novice IPT therapists, *J Am Acad Child Adolesc Psychiatry* 2001; **40**: 236–240.
64. Mufson L, Dorta KP, Wickramaratne P, Nomura Y, Olfson M, Weissman MM. A randomized effectiveness trial of interpersonal psychotherapy for depressed adolescents, *Arch Gen Psychiatry* 2004b; **61**: 577–584.
65. Mufson LH, Dorta KP, Olfson M, Weissman MM, Hoagwood K. Effectiveness research: Transporting interpersonal psychotherapy for depressed adolescents (IPT-A) from the lab to school-based health clinics, *Clin Child Fam Psychol Rev* 2004b; **7**: 251–261.
66. Rathus JH, Miller AL. Dialectical behavior therapy adapted for suicidal adolescents, *Suicide Life Threat Behav* 2002; **32**: 146–157.
67. Fleischhaker C, Munz M, Bohme R, Sixt B, Schulz E. Dialectical behaviour therapy for adolescents (DBT-A) — a pilot study on the therapy of suicidal, parasuicidal, and self-injurious behaviour in female patients with a borderline disorder, *Z Kinder Jugendpsychiatr Psychother* 2006; **34**: 15–25.
68. Kolko DJ, Brent DA, Baugher M, Bridge J, Birmaher B. Cognitive and family therapies for adolescent depression: Treatment specificity, mediation, and moderation, *J Consult Clin Psychol* 2000; **68**: 603–614.
69. Fristad MA, Goldberg-Arnold JS, Gavazzi SM. Multifamily psychoeducation groups (MFPG) for families of children with bipolar disorder, *Bipolar Disord* 2002; **4**: 254–262.
70. Emslie GJ, Heiligenstein JH, Wagner KD, Hoog SL, Ernest DE, Brown E, Nilsson M, Jacobson JG. Fluoxetine for acute treatment of depression in children and adolescents: A placebo-controlled, randomized clinical trial, *J Am Acad Child Adolesc Psychiatry* 2002; **10**: 1205–1215.
71. Wagner KD, Ambrosini P, Rynn M, Wohlberg C, Yang R, Greenbaum MS, Childress A, Donnelly C, Deas D. Efficacy of sertraline in the treatment of children and adolescents with major depressive disorder: Two randomized controlled trials, *JAMA* 2003; **290**: 1033–1041.
72. Wagner KD, Robb AS, Findling RL, Jin J, Gutierrez MM, Heydorn WE. A randomized, placebo-controlled trial of citalopram for the treatment of major depression in children and adolescents, *Am J Psychiatry* 2004; **161**: 1079–1083.
73. Wagner KD, Jonas J, Findling RL, Ventura D, Saikali K. A double-blind, randomized, placebo-controlled trial of escitalopram in the treatment of pediatric depression, *J Am Acad Child Adolesc Psychiatry* 2006; **45**: 280–288.
74. Keller MB, Ryan ND, Strober M, Klein RG, Kutcher Sp, Birmaher B, Hagino OR, Koplewicz H, Carlson GA, Clarke GN, Emslie GJ, Feinberg D, Geller B, Kusumakar V, Papatheodorou G, Sack WH, Sweeney M, Wagner KD, Weller EB, Winters NC, Oakes R, McCafferty JP. Efficacy of parexetine in the treatment of adolescent major

depression: A randomized, controlled trial, *J Am Acad Child Adoelsc Psychiatry* 2001; **40**: 762–772.

75. Berard R, Fong R, Carpenter DJ, Thomason C, Wilkinson C. An international, multicenter, placebo-controlled trial of paroxetine in adolescents with major depressive disorder, *J Child Adolesc Psychopharmacol* 2006; **16**: 59–75.
76. Emslie GJ, Wagner KD, Kutcher S, Krulewicz S, Fong R, Carpenter DJ, Lipschitz A, Machin A, Wilkinson C. Paroxetine treatment in children and adolescents with major depressive disorder: A randomized, multicenter, double-blind, placebo-controlled trial, *J Am Acad Child Adolesc Psychiatry* 2006; **45**: 709–719.
77. Daviss WB, Bentivoglio P, Racusin R, Brown KM, Bostic JQ, Wiley L. Bupropion sustained release in adolescents with comorbid attention-deficit/hyperactivity disorder and depression, *J Am Acad Child Adolesc Psychiatry* 2001; **40**: 307–314.
78. Findling RL. The future of pharmacotherapy for paediatric anxiety, *Expert Opin Pharmacother* 2002; **3**: 573–574.
79. Carpenter LL, Yasmin S, Price LH. A double-blind, placebo-controlled study of antidepressant augmentation with mirtazapine, *Biol Psychiatry* 2002; **51**: 183–188.
80. Trivedi MH, Fava M, Wisniewski SR, Thase ME, Quitkin F, Warden D, Ritz L, Nierenberg AA, Lebowitz BD, Biggs MM, Luther JF, Shores-Wilson K, Rush AJ. Medication augmentation after the failure of SSRIs for depression, *N Engl J Med* 2006; **354**: 1243–1252.
81. Pine DS. Treating children and adolescents with selective serotonin reuptake inhibitors: How long is appropriate? *J Child Adolesc Psychopharmacol* 2002; **12**: 189–203.
82. Schur SB, Sikich L, Findling RL, Malone RP, Crismon ML, Derivan A, Macintyre Ii JC, Pappadopulos E, Greenhill L, Schooler N, Van Orden K, Jensen PS. Treatment recommendations for the use of antipsychotics for aggressive youth (TRAAY). Part I: A review, *J Am Acad Child Adolesc Psychiatry* 2003; **42**: 132–144.
83. Birmaher B, Arbelaez C, Brent D. Course and outcome of child and adolescent major depressive disorder, *Child Adolesc Psychiatr Clin N Am* 2002; **11**: 619–637.
84. Apter A, Lipschitz A, Fong R, Carpenter DJ, Krulewicz S, Davies JT, Wilkinson C, Perera P, Metz A. Evaluation of suicidal thoughts and behaviors in children and adolescents taking paroxetine, *J Child Adolesc Psychopharmacol* 2006; **16**: 77–90.
85. Brent DA. Antidepressants and pediatric depression — the risk of doing nothing. *N Engl J Med* 2004; **351**: 1598–1601.
86. Hammad TA, Laughren TP, Racoosin JA. Suicide rates in short-term randomized controlled trials of newer antidepressants, *J Clin Psychopharmacol* 2006; **26**: 203–207.
87. Safer DJ, Zito JM. Treatment-emergent adverse events from selective serotonin reuptake inhibitors by age group: Children versus adolescents, *J Child Adolesc Psychopharmacol* 2006; **16**: 159–169.
88. March J, Silva S, Petrycki S, Curry J, Wells K, Fairbank J, Burns B, Domino M, McNulty S, Vitiello B, Severe J, Treatment for adolescents with depression study

(TADS) Team. Fluoxetine, cognitive-behavioral therapy, and their combination for adolescents with depression: Treatment for adolescents with depression study (TADS) randomized controlled trial, *JAMA* 2004; **292**: 807–820.

89. Brent D, Emslie G, Clarke K, Wagner KD, Asarnow JR, Keller M, Vitiello B, Ritz L, Iyengar S, Abebe K, Birmaher B, Ryan N, Kennard B, Hughes C, DeBar L, McCracken J, Strober M, Suddath R, Spirito A, Leonard H, Melhem N, Porta G, Onorato M, Zelazny J. Switching to another SSRI or to venlafaxine with or without cognitive behavioral therapy for adolescents with SSRI-resistant depression: The TORDIA randomized controlled trial, *JAMA* 2008; **299**: 901–913.
90. Clarke G, Debar L, Lynch F, Powell J, Gale J, O'Connor E, Ludman E, Bush T, Lin EH, Von Korff M, Hertert S. A randomized effectiveness trial of brief cognitive-behavioral therapy for depressed adolescents receiving antidepressant medication, *J Am Acad Child Adolesc Psychiatry* 2005; **44**: 888–898.
91. Melvin GA, Tonge BJ, King NJ, Heyne D, Gordon MS, Klimkeit E. A comparison of cognitive-behavioral therapy, sertraline, and their combination for adolescent depression, *J Am Acad Child Adolesc Psychiatry* 2006; **45**: 1151–1161.
92. Pathak S, Kratochvil CJ, Silva S, Vitiello B, Weller EB, March JS. Comparative efficacy of cognitive behavior therapy, fluoxetine, and their combination in depressed adolescents: Initial lessons for the treatment of adolescents with depression study, *Current Psychiatry Reports* 2005; **7**: 429–434.
93. Kennard BD, Silva SG, Mayes TL, Rohde P, Hughes JL, Vitiello B, Kratochvil CJ, Curry JF, Emslie GJ, Reinecke MA, March JS. Assessment of safety and long-term outcomes of initial treatment with placebo in TADS, *Am J Psychiatry* 2009; **166**: 337–344.
94. Emslie GJ. Improving outcome in pediatric depression, *Am J Psychiatry* 2008; **161**: 1–3.
95. Keller MB. Past, present, and future directions for defining optimal treatment outcome in depression, *JAMA* 2003; **289**: 3152–3160.
96. Emslie GJ. Understanding placebo response in pediatric depression trials, *Am J Psychiatry* 2009; **166**: 1–3.
97. Paddock S, Laje G, Charney D, Rush AJ, Wilson AF, Sorant AJM, Lipsky R, Wisniewski SR, Manji H, McMahon FJ. Association of GRIK4 with outcome of antidepressant treatment in the STAR*D cohort, *Am J Psychiatry* 2007; **164**: 1181–1188.

Chapter 7

Bipolar Disorder in Children and Adolescents

Kiki D. Chang, Meghan Howe, Vishal Madaan, and Leena Khanzode

1. Introduction

Bipolar disorder (BD) is a common and potentially extremely debilitating disorder that affects people of all ages. BD in pediatric populations gained much more interest in the 1990s likely spurred by a combination of factors: a new understanding that there are childhood antecedents of many adult psychiatric disorders, inclusion of irritability as a primary mania mood symptom, realization of the high heritability of BD, and improved techniques of research in child development. Although there is no disagreement about whether pediatric BD exists, there is continued disagreement regarding the criteria experienced by a child to meet the diagnosis. Currently, realizations that children with chronic irritability might also suffer from manic symptoms and thus fulfill DSM-IV criteria for BD has led to inclusion of another whole category of children under the rubric of "bipolar disorder." Whether this inclusion is "correct," or that children should be subdivided into different categories based on the presence of elation and/or episodicity[1,2] is a source of argument within and outside the field. Some researchers feel that irritability is a sufficient mood symptom for childhood mania, and that euphoria or elation need not be present.[3] The requirement for duration criteria is another area of contention due to the difficulty in identifying a specified episode in the pediatric population. Indeed, Geller *et al.*[4] describe episodes lasting an average of 3.5 years in children with BD, so it may be difficult to identify episodes when one is expecting them to last weeks to months. This matter and our take on this controversy are addressed later in the chapter.

Suffice to say that for better or worse, the expansion of DSM criteria to include irritability as a primary manic symptom, the consideration of the bipolar spectrum in adults, and the lack of a well-validated method to uniformly apply adult-based DSM criteria to children has resulted in larger and larger numbers of children receiving the diagnosis of BD.[5,6] Multiple studies suggest that children with BD do indeed grow up to become adults with BD,[7] yet there is enough heterogeneity among adults with BD that this finding would not clarify the "true" phenotype of BD in humans.

Regardless, BD today is a $45 billion problem in the United States,[8] present in up to 4% of the population[9] and leading to suicide in 10–15% of patients.[10] Thus, copious research into BD has been conducted over the last few decades, leading to significant breakthroughs in understanding the genetics and neurobiology behind the disorder, advancements in psychotherapeutic and pharmacologic treatments, and finer understandings of the heterogenous presentations of the disorder, even within the same patient at different life stages. Here, we present the latest understanding of this disorder as it presents in pediatric populations.

2. Epidemiology

The prevalence of bipolar spectrum disorders in children and adolescents is unclear. A study in the Midwest has indicated rates of <2% in the general population.[11] One study of Oregon high school students found the incidence of bipolar spectrum disorders to be 0.99%. Of the 18 adolescents with BD, 2 had bipolar I disorder, 11 bipolar II disorder, and 5 cyclothymia.[12] Although a reliable semi-structured interview was used to interview adolescents, parents themselves were not interviewed. Furthermore, adolescents in alternate education programs (home school, special education schools, *etc.*) were not included, which may have significantly skewed the sample away from including the many children with BD that require alternate education placements.

Since 15 to 28% of adults with BD in the United States had their onset before age 13, and 50 to 66% before the age of 1,[13,14] and since up to 4% of the US adult population may have BD,[15] the prevalence in children before the age of 13 could be as high as 1% and in children under 19, 2–3%. Therefore, 420,000–2,072,000 US children alone could suffer from bipolar I or II disorder.[16]

The prevalence of BD NOS is even less clear, mostly owing to the lack of standard diagnostic criteria for BD NOS leading to a broad interpretation of this diagnosis. Therefore, it may not be useful to estimate this prevalence, although it has been noted that more children with this provisional diagnosis seek mental health treatment than those with full bipolar I or II disorder. Additionally, we are realizing that in many if not most cases there is a gradual progression toward BD leading to the first full manic episode. Thus, there are likely millions of children who are in the midst of a developing BD. For example, 1 in 5 children with ADHD,[17] and as many as 1 in 4 adolescents with unipolar depression[18] may develop BD.

Bipolar disorders account for a large percentage of psychiatry clinic visits and inpatient hospital stays.[19] For example, between 1995 and 2000 there was a 90% increase in likelihood of having a bipolar diagnosis among psychiatrically hospitalized children.[20] in the 2000s, it has been estimated that rates of BD diagnosis in children have risen 4000% in the community.[21]

It is important to note that the recent increase in diagnosis of BD in the United States has not necessarily been reflected in other countries. For example, while the six-month prevalence of BD in adolescents in Holland was 1.9%,[22] in Denmark, only 1.2% of psychiatrically hospitalized youth had a diagnosis of BD[23] and 1.7% in Finland.[24] The reasons for this discrepancy with US rates may be multifactorial, including researcher bias against or for the existence of BD in children, different interviews used, and lack of trained child psychiatrists internationally.[25] However, it is also possible that the prevalence of BD in children is indeed lower outside the US European countries, including the United Kingdom have reported a later age at onset of BD in adult patients (retrospectively reported) compared to adults with BD in the United States,[26] so there may be less youth with already fully developed BD. However, other studies suggest that Europe may be catching up to the United States.[27] It has been theorized that the relative less frequent use of stimulants and antidepressants in pediatric populations in Europe may account for less "creation" of BD in children,[28] but this phenomenon has not been well studied. More international research in pediatric BD is clearly needed to resolve this discrepancy.

3. Diagnosis

BD, is still a disorder that is diagnosed by the presence of a constellation of symptoms, qualifying it as a syndrome rather than a disease. Thus, adults, children, and adolescents are still diagnosed using DSM-IV criteria for BD. This convention might change in the upcoming DSM-V, similar to the changing of depression criteria for DSM-IV, in which children were allowed to have irritability as the main mood symptom. Allowing for developmentally relevant symptom presentations will help make diagnoses easier and more relevant across the age span.

Pediatric BD is defined as a mood disorder in which children experience significant period of irritability or euphoria, usually with periods of depression as well. These periods can be distinct or overlapping; frequently, they present together in mixed manic states similar to those reported in adults. During these mood disturbances, children with BD also must meet DSM-IV criteria.

3.1. *DSM IV*

The essential feature of bipolar I disorder is a clinical course that is characterized by the occurrence of one or more manic episodes or mixed episodes. Episodes of substance-induced mood disorder (due to the direct effects of a medication, or other somatic treatments for depression, a drug of abuse, or toxin exposure) or of mood disorder due to a general medical condition do not count toward a diagnosis of bipolar I disorder. In addition, the episodes are not better accounted for by schizoaffective disorder and are not superimposed on schizophrenia, schizophreniform disorder, delusional disorder, or psychotic disorder not otherwise specified.

Criteria for manic episode (DSM-IV, p. 332)

A. A distinct period of abnormally and persistently elevated, expansive, or irritable mood, lasting at least one week (or any duration if hospitalization is necessary).

B. During the period of mood disturbance, three (or more) of the following symptoms have persisted (four if the mood is only irritable) and have been present to a significant degree:

1. inflated self-esteem or grandiosity
2. decreased need for sleep (*e.g.* feels rested after only 3 h of sleep)
3. more talkative than usual or pressure to keep talking
4. flight of ideas or subjective experience that thoughts are racing
5. distractibility (*i.e.* attention too easily drawn to unimportant or irrelevant external stimuli)
6. increase in goal-directed activity (either socially, at work or school, or sexually) or psychomotor agitation
7. excessive involvement in pleasurable activities that have a high potential for painful consequences (*e.g.* engaging in unrestrained buying sprees, sexual indiscretions, or foolish business investments)

C. The symptoms do not meet criteria for a mixed episode.

D. The mood disturbance is sufficiently severe to cause marked impairment in occupational functioning or in usual social activities or relationships with others, or to necessitate hospitalization to prevent harm to self or others, or there are psychotic features.

E. The symptoms are not due to the direct physiological effects of a substance (*e.g.* a drug of abuse, a medication, or other treatments) or a general medical condition (*e.g.* hyperthyroidism).

Note: Manic-like episodes that are clearly caused by somatic antidepressant treatment (*e.g.* medication, electroconvulsive therapy, light therapy) should not count toward a diagnosis of bipolar I disorder.

3.2. *ICD-10*

The ICD-10 defines BD and a manic episode similarly to the DSM-IV. (World Health Organization. *The ICD-10 Classification of Mental and Behavioural Disorders: Diagnostic Criteria for Research.* WHO, Geneva, 1992). However, there are some notable differences. For example, the ICD-10 requires at least two episodes of mania for a diagnosis of BD, whereas the DSM-IV only requires one. This difference might be important specifically when diagnosing BD in children. One US study using the DSM-IV found the mean episode duration of mania in children with BD to be 79.2 weeks[4] Therefore, identification of multiple manic episodes in children may be difficult and lead to a lower rate of diagnosis by ICD-10 criteria. However, most international studies of BD in youth have so far used DSM-IV criteria.[25]

3.3. *Cardinal symptoms*

Children with BD appear to more often have irritability as a cardinal symptom of mania rather than euphoria.[3] Thus, there has been some discussion of whether BD in children should only be diagnosed with the presence of elation and/or grandiosity, which some groups have adopted.[29] Children with BD also have frequent mood shifts compared to adults, often throughout the day.[30] Thus, as children often present with ultrarapid or ultradian, cycling, discrete episodes of mania or depression are harder to discern.[31,32] Prepubertal children with BD commonly present with irritability that can often take on an explosive nature. Sleep is disrupted, more typically with significant initial insomnia rather than a decreased need for sleep. However, a true decreased need for sleep is required to count as a symptom of mania. Children with BD experience racing thoughts and pressured speech, which can be easier for parents and clinicians to identify, but often it is difficult to elicit these symptoms from the children themselves. Asking developmentally appropriate questions like "Does it ever feel that your mind is like a city with too many cars moving quickly around?" can help determine the presence of the symptom of racing thoughts. The presentation of grandiosity varies with the age — children with BD typically will be extremely bossy and profess to be able to do more than is possible, such as teach the math class or coach their own soccer team[31,33] while adolescents may be more boastful and display a more typical adult type of grandiosity. Hypersexuality may present in different forms: self-stimulation, graphic language too mature for their age, or an overt interest in sexual themes. Sustained heightened sexuality is an indicator and should not be confused with normal sexual exploration. Hypersexuality appears highly correlated with pediatric BD, when sexual abuse has been ruled out. Increased goal-directed activities may be present in the form of an over-focused interest in certain projects. For instance, an 8-year-old child may stay up late at night trying to make pancakes in his room, while a 14 year old may be engrossed in writing a film script or trying to compulsively copy movies onto tapes.

Poor judgment in younger children with BD may present as certain reckless behaviors, such as jumping from heights, climbing onto roofs, or performing dangerous bicycle tricks. In adolescents, this behavior presents as driving recklessly, experimenting with recreational drugs, or engaging in sex with multiple partners.

While only necessary for a diagnosis of BD II, depressive episodes are common in pediatric BD. Depressive symptoms in children and adolescents may appear as extreme irritability, frequent crying spells, periodic sadness or withdrawal socially, or frequent statements of wanting to be dead or wishing they were never born. These symptoms may be reflected in their artwork or play where they demonstrate morbid themes. As the age of the patient increases through adolescence, more typical depressive periods are seen, with bouts of anhedonia, depressed mood, decreased energy, apathy, falling school grades, poor concentration, and disrupted sleep and appetite. Passive suicidal ideation is common in younger children, yet, it becomes more frequent and is a serious symptom in adolescents because it often leads to lethal attempts.[34] Both children and adolescents often present with mixed states, where irritability and high energy may be interspersed with depression and suicidal ideation, which indeed puts them at higher risk for suicide attempts and completed suicide.

Taken alone, each of these symptoms may seem to be normal for a large percent of healthy children and adolescents. It is only after these symptoms present together, in the context of dysfunction, that a bipolar diagnosis should be considered.

3.4. *Episodicity*

It is often difficult to detect discrete episodes of mania or depression in children with BD. Even if they have enough manic symptoms to meet DSM-IV criteria for BD, they do not always meet the duration criteria of four days (hypomania) or seven days (mania). The natural course of children and adolescents with BD is manifested by frequent changes in symptom polarity with a fluctuating course showing a dimensional continuum of bipolar symptom severity from subsyndromal to full mood episodes.[30]

In the Course and Outcome of Bipolar Youth (COBY) study, 438 subjects, 7–17-years old, with BD were assessed. As much as 58% met criteria for BD I, 7% BD II, and 35% BD NOS, defined as needing one less symptom of mania and only 4 h duration of symptoms for a mania diagnosis.[35] The majority of NOS patients were diagnosed as such because they failed to meet the duration criteria for BD I, not because they did not have enough symptoms of mania. Notably, those with BD NOS did not differ from those with BD I in symptom severity, age at onset, rates of suicidal ideation, or degree of family history of BD. Faedda *et al.*[36] found that of 82 children who met DSM-IV criteria for BD, excluding episode-duration requirements, only 10% of patients had been diagnosed previously with BD. Thus, it may be difficult to detect BD in children due to their frequently changing mood state and difficulty in detecting an episode. Other researchers have considered "metaepisodes" since the daily cycling of mood is too confusing. When considering an overall change in mood consistent with mania, Geller *et al.*[4] reported mean manic episode duration to be children with BD to be 79.2 weeks! At Stanford, we prefer to use this "metaepisode" approach as we feel it better reflects the developmental differences in children from adults, in naturally having a more reactive mood within the day.

3.5. *BD NOS*

BD NOS encompasses a heterogenous group of children: those with not quite enough manic symptoms for a BD I diagnosis, those without a discernable episode that is at least four days long for a BD II diagnosis, and in the community, those with severe bouts of or chronic irritability with few other manic symptoms. In the COBY study, the investigators found that children with BD NOS (n = 153) were similar to those with BD I (n = 255) in age at onset, duration of illness, duration of comorbid disorders, suicidal ideation, family history, and types of manic symptoms.[35] Of note, elevated mood was present in 92% of children with BD I and 82% of children with BD NOS. However, children with BD I had more functional impairment, a greater number of hospitalizations, and a higher rate of psychosis. Over four years, 38.3% of children with BD NOS developed BD I or II.[37] Thus, BD NOS in certain children may represent a prodromal form of BD I. This finding argues children with BD NOS share similarity with BD I children, although if they are in a more prodromal phase, then perhaps they would still respond differently to treatment. It should be noted that may be another proportion of NOS children who are distinct and do not worsen, or even improve in symptomatology; future longitudinal studies should help better define these children.

Finally, it is likely that those youth without clear episodes and chronic irritability, such as those deemed by some researchers to have "severe mood dysregulation" are at higher risk for depression than true BD.[38] Further advances in genetic and neurobiological markers for BD will eventually help to determine which children with BD NOS fall squarely within the bipolar spectrum.

3.6. *Comorbidities*

Pediatric BD tends to have high rates of comorbid diagnosis such as: Attention-deficit/hyperactivity disorder (ADHD), oppositional defiant disorder (ODD), conduct disorder (CD), substance abuse, and anxiety disorders.[39] Additionally, encopresis and enuresis appear to be more common in pediatric bipolar compared to other pediatric psychiatric disorders.[40]

The high comorbidity rate for pediatric BD likely reflects the developmental nature of early-onset BD. That is, the earlier the onset, the more likely that multiple brain regions and circuits are involved, as development of these pathways are still occurring. Furthermore, mood episodes might cause further derailments to normal brain development in children with developing or full BD, leading to "comorbid" conditions. Thus, one could argue that some of these conditions are not truly comorbid, but rather varying presentations of one underlying brain disorder. For example, the comorbidity rates of ADHD and BD approach 100% in children under age 12.[41] This figure is too high to be coincidental — one can argue that similar brain circuitry must be involved. Indeed, brain regions such as dorsolateral prefrontal and anterior cingulate cortices have been implicated in the pathophysiology of both mood (BD) and attentional (ADHD) disorders.[42,43] Thus, prefrontal functional and/or structural abnormalities could lead to both bipolar mood episodes and inattentive/hyperactive symptoms consistent with ADHD.

Other comorbid conditions may reflect disruptions of normal psychosocial development (conduct disorder, substance abuse) or simply involvement of other brain circuitry abnormalities (anxiety, tics).

4. Etiology and Pathogenesis

The exact cause of BD in children or adults remains unknown. BD is most likely due to several genes creating a predisposition to affective instability. Then, when combined with psychosocial stress, the development of prodromal states and eventual full-blown BD occurs. This model follows the idea of kindling in affective disorders, as proposed by Post.[44] Thus, similar to other psychiatric disorders, it is likely that numerous psychosocial factors, including life stress and family environment, act together with an underlying genetic predisposition to create BD. Here, we concentrate on what is known about the etiology and pathogenesis of BD in children and adolescents.

4.1. *Genetics*

Numerous twin and family studies have supported the high heritability of BD, approaching 0.8,[45] similar to schizophrenia and ADHD.[46,47] However, as no single gene has emerged as causal, it is probable that BD results from the effects of multiple genes, perhaps greater than 20.[48] Significant efforts have been made to isolate these genes, but little progress has been made, likely due to the great numbers of subjects needed to detect the small effects of individual genes. Nonetheless, recent advances have included large sample size or resulted from metaanalysis of multiple studies of one gene region. The European Collaborative Study of Early Onset BPAD performed a genome-wide search with 384 microsatellite markers in 87 sib-pairs ascertained through an early-onset BD type I proband (AAO of 21 years or below) and found the region 3p14 on chromosome 3 to have the most significant linkage (by using non-parametric linkage analysis).[49] There are many other regions which have received attention, including 2p, 4p, 4q, 6q, 8q, 11p, 16p, 16q, 18p, 18q, 21q, and Xq.[50,51]

Another approach is to study candidate genes that have some relation to mood and brain function. While there are several such candidate genes that may be relevant, two promising ones are polymorphisms in genes that code for the serotonin transporter (5-HTT) and for brain-derived neurotrophic growth factor (BDNF). These polymorphisms have been associated with both depression and BD.[52–54] Other genes which are promising include catechol-o-methyl transferase (COMT), D-amino-acid oxidase activator (DAOA), and neuregulin (NRG1).[51]

4.2. *Neurobiology*

4.2.1. *Structural/morphometric studies*

The rapid explosion in brain imaging technological advances and applied research has begun to reveal the neurobiological underpinnings of BD. Structural MRI studies in adult patients with BD have reported varying results, with most indicating decreased frontal and prefrontal lobe volumes, increased ventricular size, or decreased thalamic, caudate and pituitary size compared to healthy controls.[55] Most of these regions have now also been studied in pediatric BD.[56] Decreased total cerebral volume (prefrontal cortex (ACC, orbitofrontal cortex, and left DLPFC) and temporal cortex) have been reported in bipolar children and adolescents compared to healthy youth. In contrast to studies in adults, most of the studies in children and adolescents (six out of seven) have shown decreased amygdala size.[57] Smaller hippocampal volumes have been reported in two studies[58,59] in children with BD, and in one study correlating to higher degree of anxiety.[60] No abnormalities were found in the thalamic volumes of the bipolar adolescents.[59,61,62] Putamen enlargement has been reported in adolescents with BD[62,63] but other studies[61,64] have reported no differences in the sizes of putamen or caudate.

Evidence from diffusion tensor imaging (DTI) points to white matter tract disturbances in internal capsule, fornix, corpus callosum, and prefrontal areas connecting prefrontal cortex to deeper subcortical structures.[65,66]

4.2.2. *Functional imaging*

Functional MRI (fMRI) studies have furthermore revealed differences in brain activation patterns in youth with BD. Notable findings have centered around amygdala hyperactivation when performing tasks that stimulate emotional centers, such as observing fearful faces, or watching negatively valenced pictures.[67] Prefrontal areas have also shown abnormal activation, including decreased and increased activation in DLPFC, orbitofrontal cortex, and ACC depending on the task used.[56] Thus, while specific and consistent functional differences have not yet been found in pediatric BD, it appears that children and adolescents with BD have abnormal activation patterns in prefrontal cortex, striatum, and amygdala, when performing tasks related to motor inhibition or affective stimulation.

These various findings all point toward the role of prefrontal cortex and limbic and paralimbic structures in the neuropathophysiology of BD. There are two interconnected pathways connecting these structures, the ventral-limbic pathway which includes ventromedial prefrontal and orbital cortex and amygdala (thought to regulate mood directly) and the dorsal subcortical pathway which includes dorsolateral prefrontal cortex, thalamus, and basal ganglia (thought to modulate mood through cognitive processes). It has been hypothesized that dysfunction within the two pathways, interconnected by the anterior cingulate, underlies the neuropathophysiology of BD.[68,69] As detailed above, abnormalities in these areas have been found in both children and adults with BD. One possibility is that limbic abnormalities (such as decreased amygdalar volume leading to limbic hyperactivity) may be inborn, or at least precede the onset of BD. Then, with repeated mood episodes after the onset of BD, neurodegeneration of PFC gradually occurs, which would lead to less mood control, and possibly rapid cycling and treatment-resistant states, consistent with the natural progression of BD and the kindling hypothesis.[70] Amygdalar volumes may be affected gradually by such variables as medication exposure,[61] number and severity of mood episodes, and substance use, leading to variable volumetric outcomes in adults with BD.[57]

5. Morbidity/Outcome

Pediatric BD is being increasingly diagnosed and recognized as a chronic mood disorder associated with a significant deterioration in quality of life and impairment of functioning of both the patient and the family. Recent research thus indicates that a younger age of onset, lower socioeconomic status and clinical features including the presence of mixed episodes, psychotic symptoms, cycling, comorbid substance use, and a strong family history may superimpose on trait-like neurocognitive deficits to contribute toward worse outcomes in pediatric BD.[37,71] Optimal clinical suspicion, an early diagnosis and adequate management of this chronic mood disorder, may help lessen the impact of pediatric BD on quality of life of the child and the family.

6. Importance in Primary Care

The primary care physicians' most important role in these cases is being able to refer these patients to child psychiatrists.

6.1. *Prevention — early identification*

Early identification of BD in youth is extremely important, as early and appropriate intervention may head off worse illness and a chronic and relapsing course. Identification of prodromal states of BD in children and adolescents is currently challenging, but pediatricians who detect early mood and behavioral problems in children with family histories of BD should consider referral to a specialist.

6.2. *Differential diagnosis and ADHD*

As pediatricians in the United States particularly are the front line for diagnosing and treating ADHD, they should be aware when a child presents with more than just ADHD, or when stimulants fail to elicit response or have adverse outcomes such as mood worsening. Similarly, when treating depression, family history of BD or adverse reactions to SSRI should prompt caution.

6.3. *Treatment and referral*

It is the rare pediatrician who feels comfortable, or really should, treat children with BD, due to the complexity of diagnosis and time needed to carefully decide on treatment. Therefore, currently we recommend that primary care physicians refer these children to child psychiatrists at the first hint of BD, to prevent delay in identification and intervention, and to prevent inappropriate treatments.

7. Interventions

Regarding interventions to treat youth with BD, there is beginning to be a preponderance of evidence to begin supporting treatment algorithms and recommendations. More formal discussion in the literature have emerged, including an expert consensus panel,[72] and treatment guidelines from the American Academy of Child and Adolescent Psychiatry.[73] These guidelines have been largely based on the large growth in research in this field over the past decade, which we summarize here.

7.1. *Psychopharmacologic interventions*

The use of psychotropic agents in children with BD has increased considerably over the past few years despite limited placebo-controlled trials involving the use of both mood stabilizers and atypical antipsychotics in the pediatric population. The data on safety and efficacy of these agents in the pediatric population were until recently largely based on case reports and small clinical trials. However, in the past four years, larger-scale placebo-controlled studies have been conducted, mostly using atypical antipsychotics. While most of these agents have only been studied for acute mania, recent studies are focusing on maintenance strategies and treatments for bipolar depression and comorbid conditions in pediatric BD.

7.1.1. *Lithium*

Lithium is approved by the United States Food and Drug Administration (FDA) for treatment of acute mania in children older than 12 years, largely based on extrapolation of adult data. Lithium exerts its effects by blocking the activity of inositol polyphosphate 1-phosphatase and inhibiting the adenylate cyclase system.[74]

Geller *et al.*[75] studied 25 adolescents in a prospective, placebo-controlled clinical trial of lithium in BD and reported that after six weeks of treatment, 6 of the 13 subjects on lithium had a significant decrease in positive urine toxicology screens as compared to 1 of 12 adolescents on placebo. This study also showed a significant improvement in global assessment of functioning in the lithium versus placebo group (46% versus 8%).[75] Regarding maintenance treatment, Strober *et al.*[76] conducted a study of 37 adolescents with BD and found that the 18-month relapse rate for non-compliant subjects was significantly higher (92%) compared to the rate for those who were compliant with treatment (37.5%). It has been suggested that lithium given as 30 mg/kg/day (three divided dosages) in prepubertal children (6–12 years) would result in therapeutic serum lithium concentration of 0.6–1.2 mmol/l,[77] the theoretical therapeutic range. However, it is not clear if children share the same such range as adults; in a magnetic resonance spectroscopy study, children were found to have lower brain-to-serum concentration ratios compared to adults and thus they might need higher serum concentrations to maintain therapeutic lithium levels in the brain.[78]

The common side effects associated with lithium use include nausea, gastrointenstinal upset, tremor, sedation, weight gain, polyuria, polydipsia, acne, hypothyroidism, and diarrhea. Long-term treatment with lithium may lead to nephrogenic diabetes insipidus resulting from its action on the distal tubules and antidiuretic hormone. Lithium also can cause cardiac conduction problems including atrioventricular blocks and irregular sinus rhythms. It can also cause seizures, coma, and death in toxic doses. Baseline labs including serum electrolytes, renal function tests, thyroid function tests, complete blood count along with an EKG, and a pregnancy test should be obtained before initiating treatment with lithium. Renal functions should be checked every 2–3 months in the first six months and thereafter every six months; thyroid function should be checked every six months.[79]

Lithium may be less effective in treating mixed mania episodes and rapid cycling, which are commonly seen in adolescents. Approximately 40 to 50% of children and adolescents with BD respond acutely to lithium alone[79] although discontinuation due to side effects and noncompliance are associated with a high relapse rate. Clinical factors that may predict a poor response to lithium include the presence of comorbid psychiatric disorders including ADHD, personality disorder, substance abuse and conduct disorder, and a prepubertal onset of the illness.[72] Despite the paucity of placebo-controlled data, lithium appears to be a fairly effective mood stabilizer in children and adolescents with "classic" mania and for children with more euphoric than irritable mania.

7.1.2. *Valproic acid (sodium divalproex)*

Valproic acid was initially introduced as an antiepileptic medication but has since been used as a mood stabilizer for management of BD as well. The exact mechanism as to how valproate works is not clear but it may potentiate GABAergic functions and also possibly provide neuroprotection against glutamatergic excitotoxicity.[80] While the therapeutic serum valproate concentrations for the pediatric population have not been established, those for adults have been reported to be 50–125 μg/ml.[81] Liver function tests, complete blood count including platelets, and a pregnancy test should be obtained initially at baseline and thereafter every six months.

The potential adverse effects from valproic acid include nausea, weight gain, sedation, low platelets, hair loss, tremor, hepatic toxicity, pancreatitis, neural tube defects, and blood dyscrasias. Valproic acid use has also been associated with the development of polycystic ovarian syndrome.[82]

In the United States, divalproex is the widely used form of valproic acid due to its greater tolerability. Divalproex (including the extended-release form) has been approved by the US FDA for the treatment of acute mania in adults with BD. While divalproex has been found efficacious in open-label trials of children and adolescents with BD,[83–85] the only large-scale placebo-controlled trial (of extended-release divalproex) was negative, finding both the placebo and active arms to have approximately 24% response rates.[86] Lack of efficacy may also have been due to relatively low serum levels (79.9 ug/ml), short study duration (four weeks), or use of the extended-release preparation. Valproate may prove to be more effective as a preventative intervention early in the course of BD development,[87] given early clinical data and *in vitro* neuroprotective qualities.[88] However, valproate was no better than placebo for acute amelioration of symptoms in a group of children at high risk for full bipolar I disorder,[89] so the evidence for long-term prevention is still pending.

7.1.3. *Carbamazepine*

Carbamazepine was launched as an antiepileptic medication and has since been FDA approved for trigeminal neuralgia and for generalized and partial seizures in adults and children over six years old. An extended release form is FDA approved for use in adults with bipolar mania. Its mechanism of action involves inhibition of c-AMP formation and also possibly, cell membrane stabilization.[90] Carbamazepine is readily absorbed from the gastrointestinal tract and thereafter undergoes hepatic metabolism by cytochrome P450 3A4 to carbamazepine 10, 11-epoxide, an active metabolite. It can also autoinduce its own metabolism using the same hepatic pathway, decreasing its own serum levels after 3–5 weeks of treatment. Therapeutic serum carbamazepine concentrations, extrapolated from the epilepsy and adult bipolar literature, are 4–12 μg/ml. When using carbamazepine in combination with other mood stabilizers, it is also important to note that carbamazepine can decrease the levels of lamotrigine and decrease lithium clearance while valproic acid can increase carbamazepine levels.[91,92]

The adverse effects from carbamazepine use include sedation, dizziness, ataxia, and blurred vision. Carbamazepine has also been associated with Stevens-Johnson syndrome, hyponatremia, aplastic anemia, and agranulocytosis. Apart from baseline complete blood counts, it is good clinical practice to educate the subject regarding the possibility of such a hematological event, and thus to carefully monitor for fever, sore throat, and easy bruising.

An open study of carbamazepine, extended release, found it only moderately effective for reducing manic symptoms in youth with bipolar spectrum disorders.[93] Carbamazepine is currently somewhat underutilized in child psychiatry due to adverse effects and P450 metabolism concerns. Further controlled studies in pediatric BD would help clinicians place this useful agent in the proper category for use.

7.1.4. *Newer anticonvulsants*

Newer antiepileptic medications including oxcarbazepine, lamotrigine, gabapentin, and topiramate have been used as adjunctive mood stabilizers for pediatric BD, with little evidence as of yet for monotherapy efficacy.

Oxcarbazepine is a 10-keto analog of carbamazepine that may have a somewhat reduced risk for leukopenia, rashes, interactions, and autoinduction when compared with carbamazepine. However, oxcarbazepine (mean dose = 1515 mg/day) was not more effective than placebo in reducing manic symptoms in a recent multicenter study involving 116 pediatric outpatients with bipolar I disorder, manic or mixed.[94] Furthermore, at least 5% of the patients in the oxcarbazepine group developed dizziness, nausea, somnolence, diplopia, fatigue, and rash with an incidence at least twice that of the placebo group. Thus, there is little evidence base that supports the use of oxcarbazepine in pediatric BD currently.

Lamotrigine has also been studied somewhat as an adjunctive treatment for pediatric BD, particularly bipolar depression. While lamotrigine holds promise especially for the depressed phase, there have been some concerns because of potentially lethal Stevens-Johnson syndrome and toxic epidermal necrolysis.[95] More recent data indicates a much lower rate of serious rash with slower dose titration.[96] An eight-week open trial prospectively studied the efficacy of lamotrigine as adjunctive or monotherapy in 20 adolescents with BD who were experiencing a depressive episode and found that 84% of these adolescents responded to the treatment while 58% achieved remission at week 8.[97] Thus, lamotrigine may emerge as an important agent in the management of bipolar depression in adolescents.

Gabapentin was initially used as an adjunct for treating BD in adults but later studies have not found it to be efficacious for mania.[98] Some case reports in adults, however, suggest a role for gabapentin in treating children with BD with comorbid anxiety disorders.[99,100]

Topiramate has been best studied as an adjunctive treatment for pediatric BD in open studies. DelBello *et al.*[101] reviewed the outpatient charts of 26 youth with pediatric BD-I or-II who were on topiramate and found that topiramate was effective as an adjunct in pediatric BD. In addition, topiramate's propensity to induce weight loss may help counter the weight gain associated with antipsychotic or mood stabilizer use. A double-blind, placebo-controlled study to assess the efficacy of topiramate monotherapy for acute mania in pediatric BD was negative, but also underpowered.[102] Further research is needed to determine whether topiramate is effective in reducing symptoms of pediatric BD.

7.2. *Atypical antipsychotics*

The atypical or second-generation antipsychotics have been better studied for pediatric mania, with recent large, placebo-controlled trials leading to FDA approvals for treating children and adolescents with bipolar mania for olanzapine (12–17 years old), risperidone (10–17), quetiapine (10–17), and aripiprazole (10–17).

7.2.1. *Olanzapine*

Olanzapine has been studied in monotherapy in a placebo-controlled, three-week study in children and adolescents with acute mania.[103] In this study involving 107 subjects randomized to olanzapine, versus 57 to placebo, it was found that olanzapine demonstrated greater reduction in mania symptoms and higher response rates (48% versus 22%) and remission rates (35% versus 11%) compared to placebo. The mean dose of olanzapine during the double blind period was 10.7 mg/day (SD = 4.5). Taking olanzapine was associated with greater mean weight gain (3.7 kg) compared with the placebo group (0.3 kg), with an incidence of clinically significant (at least 7%) weight gain of 42% in patients taking olanzapine and 2% in placebo. The olanzapine group also showed increases in prolactin relative to the placebo group, particularly among boys.[104] Thus, metabolic side effects may limit the utility of olanzapine as an acute and maintenance agent for youth with BD.

7.2.2. *Risperidone*

Risperidone was superior to placebo in a three-week study of 169 youth aged 10–17 years with manic or mixed episodes. Subjects received either risperidone 0.5–2.5 mg/day (mean dose = 1.9 mg/day) 3–6 mg/day (mean dose = 4.7 mg/day) or placebo. At endpoint, response rates were 59% in the low-dose risperidone group, 63% in the high-dose group, and 28% in the placebo group. Mean weight gain was about 2 kg with risperidone 0.5–2.5 mg/day, 1.5 kg with risperidone 3–6 mg/day, and 0.65 kg with placebo. The most common discontinuations due to adverse events included somnolence (5%), nausea (3%), abdominal pain

(2%), and vomiting (2%). In pediatric BD and schizophrenia trials, prolactin increases have been reported in 82–87% with risperidone compared to 3–7% with placebo.[105]

7.2.3. *Quetiapine*

Quetiapine was studied in a three-week double-blind, placebo-controlled trial of acute mania in youths 10–17 years of age (n = 277). The YMRS response rate was higher for those receiving quetiapine (n = 188) versus those receiving placebo (n = 89) (61% versus 37%). Common adverse effects with quetiapine were somnolence, sedation, and dizziness. Mean weight gain with placebo was 0.4 kg, and for both quetiapine groups was 1.7 kg.[106]

7.2.4 *Aripiprazole*

Aripiprazole, a partial dopamine agonist, has also received FDA approval as monotherapy for the treatment of acute manic and mixed episodes in children and adolescents (age 10–17 years), as well as for maintenance treatment of BD and adjunctive therapy for BD in children. Aripiprazole is also approved for the treatment of schizophrenia in adolescents aged 13–17 years. Aripiprazole was studied in a 4-week double-blind, placebo-controlled trial studied adolescents (age 10–17 years) with acute manic or mixed episodes.[107] The response rate in 197 subjects receiving either 10 or 30 mg/day of aripiprazole was higher (pooled rate, 54.2%) than in 99 subjects receiving placebo (26.1%). The 10 mg arm did not differ significantly in response rate from the 30 mg arm. Common adverse effects with aripiprazole were somnolence, extrapyramidal disorder, fatigue, nausea, akathisia, blurred vision, salivary hypersecretion, and dizziness. Mean weight gain was modest and statistically similar across groups (10 mg, 0.55 kg, 30 mg, 0.90 kg, and placebo 0.54 kg). The recommended dosing of aripiprazole in children and adolescents aged 10–17 years with acute manic or mixed episodes is to start with 2 mg/day, increase to 5 mg/day after two days, and increase to the target dose of 10 after two additional days once or divided twice daily. Subsequent dose increases should be administered in 5 mg/day increments up to a 30 mg/day target once or divided twice daily.

7.2.5. *Ziprasidone*

Ziprasidone was approved by the FDA for the treatment of acute manic episodes in adults in 2006, but it has not yet been approved for use in pediatric mania. In a four-week double-blind, placebo-controlled trial in children and adolescents (aged 10–17 years) with acute manic or mixed episodes, 149 subjects receiving ziprasidone

(80–160 mg/day) compared to 88 subjects receiving placebo had greater mean YMRS decreases (–13.8 versus –8.6, respectively).[108] Response rates were 62% for the ziprasidone group and 35% for the placebo group. The most common adverse effects with ziprasidone were sedation, somnolence, headache, nausea, fatigue, and dizziness. Mean weight change was –0.6 kg and –0.2 kg for the ziprasidone and placebo groups, respectively. There were no significant changes in mean BMI, lipids, liver enzymes, or glucose levels. One ziprasidone-treated subject had a QT prolongation to ≥460 msec. Thus, it is still recommended that prior to initiating treatment with ziprasidone, a careful personal history of congenital long QT syndrome be obtained, along with a family history of sudden cardiac death. It is recommended that an ECG be obtained at baseline and following attainment of ziprasidone target dosage.

7.2.6. *Clozapine*

Clozapine was found to show improvement in a series of five children and adolescents with mixed mania who had not previously shown any response with other antipsychotics. The side effects from clozapine include sedation, weight gain, increased salivation along with potentially lethal agranulocytosis, seizures, and myocarditis.[109,110] Clozapine is usually recommended only after inadequate response to at least two other antipsychotics at optimal dosages.

Recent research studying adverse events with atypical antipsychotics, especially olanzapine (and clozapine) have focused on significant metabolic problems resulting from a notable weight gain. These metabolic side effects have included excessive weight gain, type II diabetes mellitus, or hyperglycemia and hyperlipidemia.[111] Recent data suggests that children are particularly susceptible to weight gain, and thus potentially metabolic complications, when treated with all atypical antipsychotics.[112]

Thus, while olanzapine and quetiapine may be effective agents for pediatric mania, they can be associated with significant weight gain. Risperidone may be helpful especially with comorbid aggression, and aripiprazole and ziprasidone are promising given their more modest weight gain potential. Due to the potential for serious adverse effects, clozapine should be considered only for nonresponders to other agents.

7.3. *ADHD treatments*

Simulants have been under scrutiny for their potential role in "causing" or excerbating the course of BD in children.[113] However, recent data support that stimulants are generally likely to not be associated with an earlier AAO of mania.[114–116] In fact, a prospective study of children with ADHD found that children exposed to stimulants were less likely to develop BD than those without.[17] Certainly, on a case-by-case basis it is possible that some children may develop mania secondary to stimulant treatment, leading to spontaneous episodes of mania that occur earlier than otherwise would have occurred. However, overall it currently appears that stimulants do not have an adverse effect on the development of BD.

Therefore, there are two major concerns of treatment in this arena, (1) how do we treat children with ADHD who have a familial risk for BD?, and (2) how do we treat children who have both BD and ADHD? In the first case, currently we feel that if the child does not have significant symptoms of mania, the first line of treatment should include psychostimulants. They are first-line medication options for ADHD, with a long track record of safety and efficacy. Even long-acting stimulants are cleared fairly rapidly from the system, such that they could be stopped rapidly if the patient's mood worsens or manic symptoms appear. Efficacy is also quick, such that the clinician would know fairly soon whether the stimulant is effective in treating the target symptoms.

In the second case, the general consensus is to stabilize the mood as fully as possible. If residual ADHD symptoms are still present (such as inattention, hyperactivity, and impulsivity) even though the mood is euthymic, then a stimulant should be added to the mood stabilizer regimen.[72] This is still not a perfect solution though, as some children with BD may still have adverse reactions to stimulants. For example, 1/30 children with BD + ADHD taking divalproex experienced a subsequent manic episode after mixed-salts amphetamine was added, which quickly resolved after discontinuation of the stimulant.[117]

The alternative treatments for either case include atomoxetine, modafinil, an alpha-adrenergic agonist, buproprion, or a TCA. Atomoxetine was found useful in treating ADHD in children with BD who did not respond well to stimulants in an open prospective study.[118] None of the children had a fully manic reaction, but one such reaction was reported for an adult with BD.[119] Modafinil has positive data for treating uncomplicated ADHD,[120,121] but its utility in the BD + ADHD population is unknown. Buproprion may be problematic since antidepressants may also trigger mania (see below), although less so than SSRIs. TCAs are not recommended in children secondary to cardiac concerns.

7.4. *Antidepressants*

Another class of medications that appears more harmful to this population is the antidepressants, particularly SSRIs. Several case reports have confirmed clinical anectodal observances that SSRIs may trigger manic or mixed episodes in children and adolescents.[122,123] Larger retrospective studies report that this phenomenon may occur in 25–50% of adolescents with BD at some point in their treatment.[124]

Furthermore, new onset suicidal ideation may occur in up to 25%, a finding that may be related to the FDA warnings of increased suicidal behaviors now intrinsic to SSRIs.[124] However, in children with depression and no history of mania, it is unclear if SSRI exposure will hasten BD onset. One retrospective study found no evidence of this type of association.[116]

Similar to the issue with stimulants, the two relevant treatment issues here are (1) how do we treat pediatric depression with a family history of BD? and (2) how do we treat bipolar depression and comorbid anxiety in children and adolescents?

For the first case, such a child is clearly at increased risk for developing BD compared to the general population, perhaps 30% to above 50% depending on the degree of family history. Yet, if there are no symptoms of mania, it would be difficult to determine conclusively that this is a first episode of depression preceding an underlying, undeclared BD. Despite the relative lack of positive efficacy data of antidepressants in pediatric depression, an antidepressant could be started, at low dose, and the patient monitored carefully for any worsening or quick elevation of mood, increased agitation, or decreased sleep. If these symptoms appear, the antidepressant could be quickly stopped. Buproprion has been suggested as an antidepressant that may be less likely to cause a manic episode than SSRIs.[125] Fluoxetine, although having the most efficacy data in childhood depression, should be avoided due to its relatively long half-life. Starting a mood stabilizer or antipsychotic would require drawing labs and exposure to a higher possibility of more serious adverse effects. However, the risk of an SSRI triggering a manic episode may be even more problematic than these risks. Nevertheless, there is only mild evidence supporting the use of a mood stabilizer in this population.[87,89,126] Placebo-controlled studies of agents such as lithium, lamotrigine, and quetiapine are warranted in this population, due to suggestions that these agents are effective in adults with bipolar depression. Further, these agents are not known to trigger mania more often than placebo. Finally, if the patient does not have an acute adverse reaction to the antidepressant, it might be useful to continue the antidepressant as there is some data to suggest that long-term treatment with SSRIs may not hasten the development of BD[116] and in fact may guard against the development of mania in patients with psychotic unipolar depression.[127]

In the second case of clear bipolar depression or comorbid anxiety, we try to avoid using an antidepressant if at all possible. For bipolar depression, we first remove any antidepressants the child may be taking. We also strive to maximize the level of mood stabilizer or antipsychotic — this action alone may ameliorate depressive symptoms. However, data are lacking for these agents: the only placebo-controlled study in adolescent bipolar depression was a negative study for quetiapine.[128] In that study, 32 adolescents with bipolar depression were randomized to quetiapine or placebo over eight weeks, and response rates by CDRS-R were 67% and 71%, respectively.

Nonetheless, if depression persists, we consider adding lithium, lamotrigine, or quetiapine, due to positive open data and high response rates. Also, if TSH is high or high normal, we consider replacing with exogenous thyroid hormone (thyroxine) until the TSH is at 1.0 or below.[129] Only in cases of treatment-resistant bipolar depression do we add an antidepressant, and then we monitor carefully for any worsening of mood (mania or depression). For anxiety, we stress the use of CBT (see below) and if pharmacological treatment is needed, we consider the use of gabapentin, or benzodiazepines, such as clonazepam. Again, there is no controlled data on the treatment of comorbid anxiety in youth with BD.[72]

7.5. *Electroconvulsive therapy*

Electroconvulsive therapy (ECT) is an effective treatment for mania in adults. The research data regarding ECT in children and adolescents are very limited. The current practice involves considering ECT only for adolescents with well-characterized bipolar I disorder that have severe episodes of mania or depression that are unresponsive to standard psychotropic medications.[130] Given the current evidence base, ECT should not be considered for patients with BD NOS or atypical presentations of juvenile mania.

7.6. *Psychosocial interventions*

It is currently recommended that all patients with BD receive both medication and adjunct psychotherapy.[72] Similar to the literature in psychopathology and pharmacotherapy, psychotherapeutic interventions for adults with BD have been more extensively studied than for children with BD. Psychoeducation, bipolar-specified cognitive behavioral therapy, family therapy, and interpersonal and social rhythm therapy have all been demonstrated to significantly improve the overall well-being and functioning of adults with BD.[131] These psychotherapies have all shown a significant decrease in frequency of mood episodes, increase in medication compliance, and improvement in overall functioning. Although these approaches differ in theoretical approaches, they all include some type of educational component. For example, medication compliance, symptom recognition and management, problem solving, and improvement in communication skills[132] are all discussed in these different therapeutic modalities.

One of the most difficult challenges in modifying these interventions to fit child and adolescent populations is understanding the developing brain in conjunction with the environment of the child. Current recommendations for psychotherapeutic techniques for children with disorders such as BD suggest the need to include the family and to utilize a manualized intervention.[133] Additionally, two family-based treatment components appear to be overall beneficial in the psychosocial treatment of pediatric BD: psychoeducation and cognitive-behavioral techniques.[134] Psychoeducation is the process of teaching all family members about BD, its course, its prognosis, medication, and management. Cognitive behavioral therapy (CBT) is a psychotherapy based on modifying everyday thoughts and behaviors, with the aim of positively influencing emotions. Both psychoeducation and CBT can be used in individual and group therapy.

Recently researchers have begun to adapt and test the efficacy of adjunctive psychosocial interventions for children and adolescents with BD, largely including these modalities. Multi-Family Psychoeducation Groups (MFPG)[135] has been found to be effective for childhood mood disorders, including pediatric BD, adjunct to pharmacotherapy. MFPG includes an eight week, 90 min session format that covers psychoeducation of mood disorders, symptoms, medication, medication compliance, problem-solving skills, coping mechanisms, and self-preservation skills in a group format using cognitive-behavioral techniques. Additionally, the children's session includes a recreational activity implemented to foster social skills. The groups consist of children with BD and their parents initially. After a few minutes, the parents break away from the children and go to their own prospective sessions. After a six-week randomized controlled trial of 35 children with BD, 7-to-12-years old, parents reported an improved relationship with their children and increased knowledge in mood disorders and children reported perceived increase in social support.[136]

Similar to MFPG, Family Focused Therapy for Adolescents (FFT-A) uses a focused psychoeducational approach to working with children, includes family members, and is used in conjunction with pharmacotherapy.[137] FFT-A is a modification of the adult version of FFT, addressing developmental issues and unique clinical presentations of adolescents with BD. In adults with BD, FFT has been shown to reduce relapse rates, enhance stabilization of mood symptoms, improve medication compliance, and decrease stressful family interactions with adults with BD.[138] In a randomized, controlled trial involving 58 adolescents (mean = 14.5 years) with BD I, II, or NOS, patients receiving FFT along with standard medications had a more favorable and rapid recovery from index depressive symptoms than patients in a 3-session enhanced care (EC) condition, which consisted of psychoeducation treatment. Patients in FFT-A spent less time in states of depression during the two-year study and more time in remission than patients in EC.[137] In addition to an introductory session and a final wrap up session, the sessions were divided into 9 sessions of psychoeducation, 5 of enhancing communication skills, and 5 of learning problem-solving skills.

Finally, a modified cognitive behavioral therapy combined with family therapy (CFF-CBT) was developed specifically for children 8-to-12-years old with BD.[139] Similar to MFPG and FFT-A, CFF-CBT includes a psychoeducation approach, CBT techniques, and includes family members. The protocol itself consists of 12 individual parent and child sessions that also involve contact with school personnel. CFF-CBT has been shown to decrease the severity of symptoms of BD and increase over all well-being in an open study including 34 children with BD over a 12-week period.[139]

As noted previously, all three psychosocial interventions discussed here include a psychoeducational approach supplemented by techniques specific to the intervention. Additionally, family members are encouraged to participate and manuals have been developed for each intervention. More research is needed to provide direction on longitudinal effects of these modalities.

7.7. *Educational interventions*

A child suffering from BD usually requires special accommodations in school to be able to progress not only academically, but socially as well. Furthermore, proper educational settings can actually be part of the therapeutic plan for the child in that they can learn how to function within a certain behavioral framework (www.bpkids.org). Persistent mood swings as well as adverse effects from psychotropic medications used to treat BD can affect a child's school attendance, concentration, motivation, and energy levels. Furthermore, children with BD may suffer from baseline neurocognitive deficits even when euthymic. Twenty-eight subjects in each of unmedicated and medicated pediatric bipolar groups along with 28 healthy individuals were matched and compared using a computerized neurocognitive battery and standardized neuropsychological tests to assess attention, executive function, working memory, verbal memory, visual memory, visuospatial perception, and motor skills.[140,141] The study found that individuals with pediatric BD, regardless of medication and illness status, showed impairments in domains of attention, executive functioning, working memory, and verbal learning compared to healthy individuals. The absence of differences in the deficits of neurocognitive profiles between acutely ill unmedicated patients and euthymic medicated patients in this study suggested that these impairments may be a manifestation of trait-like characteristics of pediatric BD.

Parents should be first aware that they are the strongest advocate for their child receiving a proper education. Thus, they need to educate themselves on the state and federal laws and procedures that ensure that every child, regardless of disability, is entitled to a setting in which they can learn. After the proper school personnel have been contacted, or the child has been referred by their teacher to the special education program, the clinician then may interface with the school as well to help determine the proper educational plan for the child with BD. The clinician should first educate the family and school personnel that the child's functioning may vary greatly at different times throughout the academic year. Transitions to new teachers and new schools, return to school from vacations and absences, and changing to new medications are also common times of increased symptomatology for children with BD. The school personnel, parents, and mental health professionals should meet as a team to determine whether an individualized educational plan (IEP) is needed. If so, the input of the clinician on the IEP team can be very important to ensuring the development of a proper academic plan. The clinician should make the team aware of possible medication side effects that can be troublesome at school including increased thirst and urination, excessive sleepiness or agitation, and interference with concentration. Furthermore, weight gain, fatigue, and dehydration may impact a child's participation in gym and academic classes. Some of the accommodations that may help a child suffering from BD can be found at http://www.cabf.org.

8. Clinical Experience at Stanford: Practice-Based Evidence

It is becoming clear that due to the severe morbidity of pediatric BD and impact on normal development, youth suffering from BD require a multidisciplinary approach consisting of pharmacotherapy, psychotherapy, and educational interventions. We first perform a full clinical evaluation, often supported by a research-based diagnostic interview, and symptom severity scales (YMRS, CDRS, ADHD-RS, MASC) are completed. If additional neuropsychological or psychological testing is required, we obtain it. Ideally, a thorough educational evaluation would be next, but we are not equipped to provide this at Stanford. Based on these evaluations, a treatment plan is instituted, consisting of pharmacology, psychotherapy, and educational interventions.

Pharmacotherapeutic recommendations have been largely based on empirical evidence from the literature and expert clinical opinion. The overall recommended treatment strategy for children with acute mania is to use a traditional mood-stabilizer (lithium or valproate) or an atypical antipsychotic as the primary treatment, with other psychotropic medications to aid in mood stabilization and/or to treat comorbid conditions. Because of their strong efficacy data, we favor atypical antipsychotics first-line for acute mania. However, we strongly consider the use of lithium first or second line in patients in a clear cut manic episode. We agree with most experts in the field who feel that when treating pediatric BD, the initial goal is to stabilize the mood and then treat the associated comorbidities.[72] After stabilization, treatment largely consists of preventing relapse, minimizing side effects, eliminating medications where possible, and supporting healthy development psychotherapeutically and educationally.

The target goals of treatment should include a reduction in acute symptoms, prevention of relapse, reduction in long-term morbidity, and promotion of normal development. No single medication has been approved by the FDA for the treatment of all phases of BD; thus, the course of pharmacologic treatment usually involves a combination of psychotropic agents.

Here, we provide an illustrative case example:

CASE XR

XR is a 12-year-old boy with symptoms of depression (sad mood, anhedonia, decreased concentration, fatigue) who is starting to get Ds and Fs in school. He had been diagnosed with inattentive ADHD at age eight and treated for two years with methylphenidate with some success. However, MPH was stopped secondary to appetite suppression. XR has also had problems with irritability, anger attacks, and periods of giddiness at times. He has not had periods of decreased need for sleep, hypersexuality, increased goal-directed activity, or racing thoughts. XR has a mother with bipolar II disorder (undiagnosed, high functioning) and a 17-year-old brother with cyclothymia (undiagnosed). XR is now on divalproex 500 mg QHS, serum level = 58 ug/ml. He is also taking sertraline 50 mg QD.

XR is now 15-years old and was doing fairly well, but is starting to become depressed again. He is experiencing similar symptoms as previously, but with more severe depression, fatigue, and hypersomnia. Sertraline is raised to 100 mg QD. Within 10 days, XR has a two-week period of euphoria, racing thoughts, plans of wanting to trap animals in his backyard for their fur, buying trapping equipment online, sleeping 4 h/night, and pressured speech. His friends notice that he is "wackier" than usual. He ends up stealing a motorcycle and crashing it into a tree. He is hospitalized for acute mania. Sertraline is stopped, and divalproex is increased to 500 mg BID, achieving a serum level of 109 ug/ml. Olanzapine is added to the valproate, and titrated up to 15 mg QD. After one week, he continues to be mildly manic on the ward, so lithium is begun. Upon discharge another week later, he is stable, and lithium is now up to 450 mg BID, using extended release, with a serum level of 1.0 meq/l.

XR remains fairly stable over the next 12 months on this regimen. However, he has significant weight gain, acne, and tremors. He also now has an IEP instituted at school. This results in his being able to have a shortened school day, and extra time for tests. When he misses school days secondary to mood fluctuations or medication adverse effects, he is allowed to gradually make up the work with the assistance of an aide in a separate resource-type class. He is allowed to take frequent bathroom breaks secondary to the polyuria from lithium, and he has a laptop in class to type out assignments due to his tremor affecting his handwriting. His morning sedation is offset by a later start time of 9:30 am. Despite symptoms of ADHD, he chooses not to take additional medication at this time. He and his family participate in alternating weeks of family and individual therapy.

XR is now almost 17 and wants to stop all medications. After lengthy discussion, we realize he has already stopped his medications. Despite our recommendations, he chooses to not restart. Despite careful monitoring he experiences another manic episode, not triggered this time by medications or drugs. Aripiprazole is started at 2 mg QD and titrated to 10 mg over five days. Eventually, dose is titrated to 15 mg QD with good results. However, toward the end of his junior year, he notices problems concentrating in school, disorganization, and forgetfulness. Atomoxetine, at 1.0 mg/kg, is begun, titrating up to 1.2 mg/kg. He reports great success in his last year of high school, raising his GPA from a 2.3 to a 3.4. He does not have any recurrence of mania or depression.

XR is now 19-years old and in his freshman year at college. He has stopped taking the aripiprazole and atomoxetine four months prior. He is overwhelmed with school and isolating himself socially. He has begun drinking alcohol and using marijuana. He has significant insomnia and depressed mood, SI, decreased appetite, anhedonia, hopelessness. He is very resistant to taking medications, but comes to the office for help. Due to his low functioning, we recommend taking a semester off, and enrolling in a rehab program. At the same time, we prescribed lamotrigine, titrating up to 200 mg QD. With good response, but continuing anxiety and insomnia, we prescribed quetiapine 50 mg QHS, with good results.

XR completes the rehab program, and his mood and anxiety are much improved so that he is able to reenroll in college. He remains fairly euthymic and high functioning at 20-years old, and continues taking lamotrigine 200 mg QD and quetiapine 50 mg qhs.

Based on the factors mentioned above, Kowatch *et al.*[72] in their expert consensus guidelines on the subject, described two algorithms for acute treatment of pediatric BD, type I (manic or mixed type), depending on whether the child presents with or without features of psychosis. In patients without psychosis, they suggested initiating treatment with monotherapy involving traditional mood stabilizers (lithium, valproic acid, or carbamazepine) or atypical antipsychotics (olanzapine, quetiapine, or risperidone), with the majority of the consensus panel opting for lithium or valproic acid, as their first choice. Aripiprazole and ziprasidone were not yet recommended as first line due to their relative lack of efficacy data in this population at that time. But we would now add aripiprazole as first line, and ziprasidone among the second- or third-line alternatives. Furthermore, while we still use divalproex, usually this is not first line and it is adjunct to atypical antipsychotics. In children with BD with psychotic features, they recommend starting one of the traditional mood stabilizers concurrently with an atypical antipsychotic. An optimal trial with a pharmacological agent should last at least 6–8 weeks at optimal dosages of the medication before the clinician switches or augments the agent.

Maintenance therapy is often needed for youth with BD, with some youth requiring lifelong therapy. Although there is little research regarding the necessary duration of treatment in pediatric BD, most researchers and clinicians would agree that the treatment needed to stabilize acute mania should be maintained for 12–24 months. Clearly, if symptoms remain or there is a history of suicidality or dangerous behavior during mood episodes, children with BD may need to continue medications indefinitely.[72] This consensus panel led by Kowatch *et al.* noted that whereas lithium, divalproex, and carbamazepine have been the agents most commonly used to treat children and adolescents with BD, current research in adults supports the efficacy of lithium, lamotrigine, and olanzapine as maintenance treatments. We still believe this to be true, but more data are forthcoming for the other atypical antipsychotics and lamotrigine. Further, the recommendations include that medications be tapered and not abruptly discontinued with the taper occurring at a time associated with the lowest possible risk of dysfunction/poor outcomes, and with a stable environment and adequate monitoring systems in place. Thus, these expert consensus guidelines should be useful when added to the above discussed factors in choosing psychotropic agents for patients with pediatric BD.

9. Future Directions

The field of pediatric BDs has progressed dramatically in the past 10 years. According to Pubmed, there were approximately five papers published on this topic in 1996, compared to over 70 in 2006, not including papers published in non-English journals. It appears that increased funding has been allocated by the NIMH, private organizations, and pharmaceutical companies to study the presentation, genetics, neurobiology, and treatment of BD in children and adolescents. The field has several challenges before it: first, to address the controversy around the phenomenology of BD in children, including the discussed problems with episodicity and irritability. Next, additional longitudinal studies need to be done following children with BD through adulthood to establish or refute the continuity of pediatric and adult BD. Third, as children with BD are proving even more difficult to treat than adults, further treatment studies need to occur. Studies of combination treatments, treatment of mixed and depressed states, treatment of comorbidities, and maintenance treatment need to be established. The ultimate challenge may be in determining preventative interventions for children before they develop mood episodes and eventually full BD.

As children have vastly different neurobiological systems than adults and are still rapidly developing, there is no reason that BD in a child should exactly resemble BD in an adult. However, if one diagnoses BD based on symptoms only, which DSM-IV currently does, then the issue becomes, "what is BD?" Clearly, as there is a genetic and neurobiological basis to this disorder, it could be diagnosed partly using these measures. But ultimately, it is behavioral characteristics that come together in a repeatable fashion (between and within individuals) that makes this a consistent syndrome. Likely, there are many, many combinations of genes and many different brain make-ups that can lead to a bipolar spectrum disorder, the concept of "multifinality".[142]

Nonetheless, the most exciting and intriguing findings in the next decade will likely be related to the genetic and neurobiologic underpinnings of BD. By combining current symptomatology, family history, genetic profile, and neurobiological and other biomarkers, we will be able to determine the quantitative risk for BD development in at-risk children. Then, based on the likelihood of BD development, appropriate interventions can be instituted. At Stanford, we are studying both parts of this goal in parallel, in the hopes that we will be able to help the current generation of at-risk children, instead of waiting for definitive results from longitudinal studies to appear.[70] We anticipate that in the next 5–10 years, we will have such a quantitative screen, such that we can start to prevent the development of this chronic and debilitating disorder in millions of individuals in the United States and worldwide.

References

1. Carlson GA. Early onset bipolar disorder: Clinical and research considerations, *J Clin Child Adolesc Psychol* 2005; **34**(2): 333–343.
2. Geller B, Williams M, Zimerman B, Frazier J, Beringer L, Warner KL. Prepubertal and early adolescent bipolarity differentiate from ADHD by manic symptoms, grandiose delusions, ultra-rapid or ultradian cycling, *J Affect Disord* 1998; **51**(2): 81–91.
3. Wozniak J, Biederman J, Kwon A, *et al.* How cardinal are cardinal symptoms in pediatric bipolar disorder? An examination of clinical correlates, *Biol Psychiatry* 2005; **58**(7): 583–588.

4. Geller B, Tillman R, Craney JL, Bolhofner K. Four-year prospective outcome and natural history of mania in children with a prepubertal and early adolescent bipolar disorder phenotype, *Arch Gen Psychiatry* 2004; **61**(5): 459–467.
5. Blader JC, Carlson GA. Increased rates of bipolar disorder diagnoses among U.S. child, adolescent, and adult inpatients, 1996–2004, *Biol Psychiatry* 2007.
6. Healy D. The latest mania: Selling bipolar disorder, *PLoS Med* 2006; **3**(4): e185.
7. Chang K. Adult bipolar disorder is continuous with pediatric bipolar disorder, *Can J Psychiatry* 2007; **52**(7): 418–425.
8. Kleinman L, Lowin A, Flood E, Gandhi G, Edgell E, Revicki D. Costs of bipolar disorder, *Pharmacoeconomics* 2003; **21**(9): 601–622.
9. Kessler RC, Berglund P, Demler O, Jin R, Merikangas KR, Walters EE. Lifetime prevalence and age-of-onset distributions of DSM-IV disorders in the National Comorbidity Survey Replication, *Arch Gen Psychiatry* 2005; **62**(6): 593–602.
10. Baldessarini RJ, Pompili M, Tondo L. Suicide in bipolar disorder: Risks and management, *CNS Spectr* 2006; **11**(6): 465–471.
11. Carlson GA, Kashani JH. Manic symptoms in a non-referred adolescent population, *J Affect Disord* 1988; 15(3): 219–226.
12. Lewinsohn PM, Klein DN, Seeley JR. Bipolar disorders in a community sample of older adolescents: Prevalence, phenomenology, comorbidity, and course, *J Am Acad Child Adolesc Psychiatry* 1995; **34**(4): 454–463.
13. Leverich GS, McElroy SL, Suppes T, *et al.* Early physical and sexual abuse associated with an adverse course of bipolar illness, *Biol Psychiatry* 2002; **51**(4): 288–297.
14. Perlis RH, Miyahara S, Marangell LB, *et al.* Long-term implications of early onset in bipolar disorder: Data from the first 1000 participants in the systematic treatment enhancement program for bipolar disorder (STEP-BD), *Biol Psychiatry* 2004; **55**(9): 875–881.
15. Kessler RC, Chiu WT, Demler O, Merikangas KR, Walters EE. Prevalence, severity, and comorbidity of 12-month DSM-IV disorders in the National Comorbidity Survey Replication, *Arch Gen Psychiatry* 2005; **62**(6): 617–627.
16. Post RM, Kowatch RA. The health care crisis of childhood-onset bipolar illness: Some recommendations for its amelioration, *J Clin Psychiatry* 2006; **67**(1): 115–125.
17. Tillman R, Geller B. Controlled study of switching from attention-deficit/hyperactivity disorder to a prepubertal and early adolescent bipolar I disorder sphenotype during 6-year prospective follow-up: Rate, risk, and predictors, *Dev Psychopathol* Fall 2006; **18**(4): 1037–1053.
18. Geller B, Zimerman B, Williams M, Bolhofner K, Craney JL. Adult psychosocial outcome of prepubertal major depressive disorder, *J Am Acad Child Adolesc Psychiatry* 2001; **40**(6): 673–677.

19. Youngstrom EA, Duax J. Evidence-based assessment of pediatric bipolar disorder, part I: Base rate and family history, *J Am Acad Child Adolesc Psychiatry* 2005; **44**(7): 712–717.

20. Harpaz-Rotem I, Leslie DL, Martin A, Rosenheck RA. Changes in child and adolescent inpatient psychiatric admission diagnoses between 1995 and 2000, *Soc Psychiatry Psychiatr Epidemiol* 2005; **40**(8): 642–647.

21. Moreno C, Laje G, Blanco C, Jiang H, Schmidt AB, Olfson M. National trends in the outpatient diagnosis and treatment of bipolar disorder in youth, *Arch Gen Psychiatry* 2007; **64**(9): 1032–1039.

22. Verhulst FC, van der Ende J, Rietbergen A. Ten-year time trends of psychopathology in Dutch children and adolescents: No evidence for strong trends, *Acta Psychiatr Scand* 1997; **96**(1): 7–13.

23. Thomsen PH, Moller LL, Dehlholm B, Brask BH. Manic-depressive psychosis in children younger than 15 years: A register-based investigation of 39 cases in Denmark, *Acta Psychiatr Scand* 1992; **85**(5): 401–406.

24. Rasanen P, Tiihonen J, Hakko H. The incidence and onset-age of hospitalized bipolar affective disorder in Finland, *J Affect Disord* 1998; **48**(1): 63–68.

25. Soutullo CA, Chang KD, Diez-Suarez A, *et al.* Bipolar disorder in children and adolescents: International perspective on epidemiology and phenomenology, *Bipolar Disord* 2005; **7**(6): 497–506.

26. Post RM, Luckenbaugh DA, Leverich GS, *et al.* Incidence of childhood-onset bipolar illness in the USA and Europe, *Br J Psychiatry* 2008; **192**(2): 150–151.

27. Baldessarini RJ, Bolzani L, Cruz N, *et al.* Onset-age of bipolar disorders at six international sites, *J Affect Disord* 2010; **121**(1–2): 143–146.

28. Reichart CG, Nolen WA. Earlier onset of bipolar disorder in children by antidepressants or stimulants? An hypothesis, *J Affect Disord* 2004; **78**(1): 81–84.

29. Tillman R, Geller B. Diagnostic characteristics of child bipolar I disorder: Does the "Treatment of Early Age Mania (team)" sample generalize? *J Clin Psychiatry* 2007; **68**(2): 307–314.

30. Birmaher B, Axelson D, Strober M, *et al.* Clinical course of children and adolescents with bipolar spectrum disorders, *Arch Gen Psychiatry* 2006; **63**(2): 175–183.

31. Geller B, Zimerman B, Williams M, *et al.* Diagnostic characteristics of 93 cases of a prepubertal and early adolescent bipolar disorder phenotype by gender, puberty and comorbid attention deficit hyperactivity disorder, *J Child Adolesc Psychopharmacol* Fall 2000; **10**(3): 157–164.

32. Tillman R, Geller B. Definitions of rapid, ultrarapid, and ultradian cycling and of episode duration in pediatric and adult bipolar disorders: A proposal to distinguish episodes from cycles, *J Child Adolesc Psychopharmacol.* Fall 2003; **13**(3): 267–271.

33. Geller B, Luby J. Child and adolescent bipolar disorder: A review of the past 10 years [see comments] [published erratum appears in *J Am Child Adolesc Psychiatry* 1997; **36**(11): 1642]. *J Am Acad Child Adolesc Psychiatry* 1997; **36**(9): 1168–1176.
34. Goldstein TR, Birmaher B, Axelson D, *et al.* History of suicide attempts in pediatric bipolar disorder: Factors associated with increased risk, *Bipolar Disord* 2005; **7**(6): 525–535.
35. Axelson D, Birmaher B, Strober M, *et al.* Phenomenology of children and adolescents with bipolar spectrum disorders, *Arch Gen Psychiatry* 2006; **63**(10): 1139–1148.
36. Faedda GL, Baldessarini RJ, Glovinsky IP, Austin NB. Pediatric bipolar disorder: Phenomenology and course of illness, *Bipolar Disord* 2004; **6**(4): 305–313.
37. Birmaher B, Axelson D, Goldstein B, *et al.* Four-year longitudinal course of children and adolescents with bipolar spectrum disorders: The Course and Outcome of Bipolar Youth (COBY) study, *Am J Psychiatry* 2009; **166**(7): 795–804.
38. Leibenluft E. Severe mood dysregulation in children and adolescents. Paper presented at the 4th Annual Pediatric Bipolar Disorder Conference 2006; Chicago, IL, USA.
39. Pavuluri MN, Birmaher B, Naylor MW. Pediatric bipolar disorder: A review of the past 10 years, *J Am Acad Child Adolesc Psychiatry* 2005; **44**(9): 846–871.
40. Klages T, Geller B, Tillman R, Bolhofner K, Zimerman B. Controlled study of encopresis and enuresis in children with a prepubertal and early adolescent bipolar-I disorder phenotype, *J Am Acad Child Adolesc Psychiatry* 2005; **44**(10): 1050–1057.
41. Singh MK, DelBello MP, Kowatch RA, Strakowski SM. Co-occurrence of bipolar and attention-deficit hyperactivity disorders in children, *Bipolar Disord* 2006; **8**(6): 710–720.
42. Adler CM, Delbello MP, Mills NP, Schmithorst V, Holland S, Strakowski SM. Comorbid ADHD is associated with altered patterns of neuronal activation in adolescents with bipolar disorder performing a simple attention task, *Bipolar Disord* 2005; **7**(6): 577–588.
43. Bush G, Frazier JA, Rauch SL, *et al.* Anterior cingulate cortex dysfunction in attention-deficit/hyperactivity disorder revealed by fMRI and the Counting Stroop, *Biol Psychiatry* 1999; **45**(12): 1542–1552.
44. Post RM. Transduction of psychosocial stress into the neurobiology of recurrent affective disorder, *Am J Psychiatry* 1992; **149**(8): 999–1010.
45. Smoller JW, Finn CT. Family, twin, and adoption studies of bipolar disorder, *Am J Med Genet C Semin Med Genet* 2003; **123**(1): 48–58.
46. Cardno AG, Marshall EJ, Coid B, *et al.* Heritability estimates for psychotic disorders: The Maudsley twin psychosis series, *Arch Gen Psychiatry* 1999; **56**(2): 162–168.
47. Coolidge FL, Thede LL, Young SE. Heritability and the comorbidity of attention deficit hyperactivity disorder with behavioral disorders and executive function deficits: A preliminary investigation, *Dev Neuropsychol* 2000; **17**(3): 273–287.

48. Craddock N, Dave S, Greening J. Association studies of bipolar disorder, *Bipolar Disord* 2001; **3**(6): 284–298.
49. Etain B, Mathieu F, Rietschel M, *et al.* Genome-wide scan for genes involved in bipolar affective disorder in 70 European families ascertained through a bipolar type I early-onset proband: Supportive evidence for linkage at 3p14, *Mol Psychiatry* 2006; **11**(7): 685–694.
50. Hayden EP, Nurnberger JI, Jr. Molecular genetics of bipolar disorder, *Genes Brain Behav* 2006; **5**(1): 85–95.
51. Farmer A, Elkin A, McGuffin P. The genetics of bipolar affective disorder, *Curr Opin Psychiatry* 2007; **20**(1): 8–12.
52. Caspi A, Sugden K, Moffitt TE, *et al.* Influence of life stress on depression: Moderation by a polymorphism in the 5-HTT gene, *Science* 2003; **301**(5631): 386–389.
53. Geller B, Badner JA, Tillman R, Christian SL, Bolhofner K, Cook EH, Jr. Linkage disequilibrium of the brain-derived neurotrophic factor Val66Met polymorphism in children with a prepubertal and early adolescent bipolar disorder phenotype, *Am J Psychiatry* 2004; **161**(9): 1698–1700.
54. Neves-Pereira M, Mundo E, Muglia P, King N, Macciardi F, Kennedy JL. The brain-derived neurotrophic factor gene confers susceptibility to bipolar disorder: Evidence from a family-based association study, *Am J Hum Genet* 2002; **71**(3): 651–655.
55. Keener MT, Phillips ML. Neuroimaging in bipolar disorder: A critical review of current findings, *Curr Psychiatry Rep* 2007; **9**(6): 512–520.
56. Terry J, Lopez-Larson M, Frazier JA. Magnetic resonance imaging studies in early onset bipolar disorder: An updated review, *Child Adolesc Psychiatr Clin N Am* 2009; **18**(2): 421–439, ix–x.
57. Pfeifer JC, Welge J, Strakowski SM, Adler CM, DelBello MP. Meta-analysis of amygdala volumes in children and adolescents with bipolar disorder, *J Am Acad Child Adolesc Psychiatry* 2008; **47**(11): 1289–1298.
58. Blumberg HP, Kaufman J, Martin A, *et al.* Amygdala and hippocampal volumes in adolescents and adults with bipolar disorder, *Arch Gen Psychiatry* 2003; **60**(12): 1201–1208.
59. Frazier JA, Chiu S, Breeze JL, *et al.* Structural brain magnetic resonance imaging of limbic and thalamic volumes in pediatric bipolar disorder, *Am J Psychiatry* 2005; **162**(7): 1256–1265.
60. Simeonova DI, Jackson V, Attalla A, *et al.* Subcortical volumetric correlates of anxiety in familial pediatric bipolar disorder: A preliminary investigation, *Psychiatry Res* 2009; **173**(2): 113–120.
61. Chang K, Karchemskiy A, Barnea-Goraly N, Garrett A, Simeonova DI, Reiss A. Reduced amygdalar gray matter volume in familial pediatric bipolar disorder, *J Am Acad Child Adolesc Psychiatry* 2005; **44**(6): 565–573.

62. DelBello MP, Zimmerman ME, Mills NP, Getz GE, Strakowski SM. Magnetic resonance imaging analysis of amygdala and other subcortical brain regions in adolescents with bipolar disorder, *Bipolar Disord* 2004; **6**(1): 43–52.
63. Wilke M, Kowatch RA, DelBello MP, Mills NP, Holland SK. Voxel-based morphometry in adolescents with bipolar disorder: First results, *Psychiatry* 2004; **131**(1): 57–69.
64. Sanches M, Roberts RL, Sassi RB, *et al.* Developmental abnormalities in striatum in young bipolar patients: A preliminary study, *Bipolar Disord* 2005; **7**(2): 153–158.
65. Adler CM, Adams J, DelBello MP, *et al.* Evidence of white matter pathology in bipolar disorder adolescents experiencing their first episode of mania: A diffusion tensor imaging study, *Am J Psychiatry* 2006; **163**(2): 322–324.
66. Barnea-Goraly N, Chang KD, Karchemskiy A, Howe ME, Reiss AL. Limbic and corpus callosum aberrations in adolescents with bipolar disorder: A tract-based spatial statistics analysis, *Biol Psychiatry* 2009; **66**(3): 238–244.
67. Garrett A, Chang K. The role of the amygdala in bipolar disorder development, *Dev Psychopathol* Fall 2008; **20**(4): 1285–1296.
68. Chang K, Adleman NE, Dienes K, Simeonova DI, Menon V, Reiss A. Anomalous prefrontal-subcortical activation in familial pediatric bipolar disorder: A functional magnetic resonance imaging investigation, *Arch Gen Psychiatry* 2004; **61**(8): 781–792.
69. Strakowski SM, Delbello MP, Adler CM. The functional neuroanatomy of bipolar disorder: A review of neuroimaging findings, *Mol Psychiatry* 2005; **10**(1): 105–116.
70. Chang K, Howe M, Gallelli K, Miklowitz D. Prevention of pediatric bipolar disorder: Integration of neurobiological and psychosocial processes, *Ann N Y Acad Sci* 2006; **1094**: 235–247.
71. Geller B, Tillman R, Bolhofner K, Zimerman B. Child bipolar I disorder: Prospective continuity with adult bipolar I disorder; characteristics of second and third episodes; predictors of 8-year outcome, *Arch Gen Psychiatry* 2008; **65**(10): 1125–1133.
72. Kowatch RA, Fristad M, Birmaher B, Wagner KD, Findling RL, Hellander M. Treatment guidelines for children and adolescents with bipolar disorder, *J Am Acad Child Adolesc Psychiatry* 2005; **44**(3): 213–235.
73. McClellan J, Kowatch R, Findling RL. Practice parameter for the assessment and treatment of children and adolescents with bipolar disorder, *J Am Acad Child Adolesc Psychiatry* 2007; **46**(1): 107–125.
74. Belmaker RH, Bersudsky Y, Agam G. How does lithium work on manic depression? Clinical and psychological correlates of the inositol theory, *Annu Rev Med* 1996; **47**: 47–56.
75. Geller B, Cooper TB, Sun K, *et al.* Double-blind and placebo-controlled study of lithium for adolescent bipolar disorders with secondary substance dependency, *J Am Acad Child Adolesc Psychiatry* 1998; **37**(2): 171–178.

76. Strober M, Morrell W, Lampert C, Burroughs J. Relapse following discontinuation of lithium maintenance therapy in adolescents with bipolar I illness: A naturalistic study, *Am J Psychiatry* 1990; **147**(4): 457–461.
77. Weller EB, Weller RA, Fristad MA. Lithium dosage guide for prepubertal children: A preliminary report, *J Am Acad Child Psychiatry* 1986; **25**(1): 92–95.
78. Moore CM, Demopulos CM, Henry ME, *et al.* Brain-to-serum lithium ratio and age: An in vivo magnetic resonance spectroscopy study, *Am J Psychiatry* 2002; **159**(7): 1240–1242.
79. Chang K, Simeonova D. Mood stabilizers: Use in pediatric psychopharmacology. In: Steiner H, Chang K, Lock J, Wilson J, Eds. *Handbook of Mental Health Interventions in Children and Adolescents: An Integrated Developmental Approach.* New York: Jossey-Bass, 2004, pp. 363–412.
80. Chen G, Manji HK, Wright CB, *et al.* Effects of valproic acid on beta-adrenergic receptors, G-proteins, and adenylyl cyclase in rat C6 glioma cells, *Neuropsychopharmacology* 1996; **15**(3): 271–280.
81. Bowden CL, Janicak PG, Orsulak P, *et al.* Relation of serum valproate concentration to response in mania, *Am J Psychiatry* 1996; **153**(6): 765–770.
82. Isojarvi JI, Laatikainen TJ, Pakarinen AJ, Juntunen KT, Myllyla VV. Polycystic ovaries and hyperandrogenism in women taking valproate for epilepsy, *N Engl J Med* 1993; **329**(19): 1383–1388.
83. Henry CA, Zamvil LS, Lam C, Rosenquist KJ, Ghaemi SN. Long-term outcome with divalproex in children and adolescents with bipolar disorder, *J Child Adolesc Psychopharmacol* Winter 2003; **13**(4): 523–529.
84. Kowatch RA, Suppes T, Carmody TJ, *et al.* Effect size of lithium, divalproex sodium, and carbamazepine in children and adolescents with bipolar disorder [In Process Citation]. *J Am Acad Child Adolesc Psychiatry* 2000; **39**(6): 713–720.
85. Wagner KD, Weller EB, Carlson GA, *et al.* An open-label trial of divalproex in children and adolescents with bipolar disorder. *J Am Acad Child Adolesc Psychiatry.* 2002; **41**(10): 1224–1230.
86. Wagner KD, Redden L, Kowatch RA, *et al.* A double-blind, randomized, placebo-controlled trial of divalproex extended-release in the treatment of bipolar disorder, in children and adolescents, *J Am Acad Child Adolesc Psychiatry* 2009; **48**(5): 519–532.
87. Chang KD, Dienes K, Blasey C, Adleman N, Ketter T, Steiner H. Divalproex monotherapy in the treatment of bipolar offspring with mood and behavioral disorders and at least mild affective symptoms, *J Clin Psychiatry* 2003; **64**(8): 936–942.
88. Manji HK, Moore GJ, Chen G. Clinical and preclinical evidence for the neurotrophic effects of mood stabilizers: Implications for the pathophysiology and treatment of manic-depressive illness, *Biol Psychiatry* 2000; **48**(8): 740–754.

89. Findling RL, Frazier TW, Youngstrom EA, *et al.* Double-blind, placebo-controlled trial of divalproex monotherapy in the treatment of symptomatic youth at high risk for developing bipolar disorder, *J Clin Psychiatry* 2007; **68**(5): 781–788.
90. Manji HK, Chen G, Hsiao JK, *et al.* Regulation of signal transduction pathways by mood-stabilizing agents: Implications for the delayed onset of therapeutic efficacy, *J Clin Psychiatry* 1996; **57**(Suppl. 13): 34–46.
91. Bourgeois BF. Pharmacokinetic properties of current antiepileptic drugs: What improvements are needed? *Neurology* 2000; **55**(11 Suppl. 3): S11–16.
92. Reimers A, Skogvoll E, Sund JK, Spigset O. Drug interactions between lamotrigine and psychoactive drugs: Evidence from a therapeutic drug monitoring service, *J Clin Psychopharmacol* 2005; **25**(4): 342–348.
93. Joshi G, Wozniak J, Mick E, *et al.* A prospective open-label trial of extended-release carbamazepine monotherapy in children with bipolar disorder, *J Child Adolesc Psychopharmacol* 2010; **20**(1): 7–14.
94. Wagner KD, Kowatch RA, Emslie GJ, *et al.* A double-blind, randomized, placebo-controlled trial of oxcarbazepine in the treatment of bipolar disorder in children and adolescents, *Am J Psychiatry* 2006; **163**(7): 1179–1186.
95. Guberman AH, Besag FM, Brodie MJ, *et al.* Lamotrigine-associated rash: Risk/benefit considerations in adults and children, *Epilepsia* 1999; **40**(7): 985–991.
96. Messenheimer JA. The incidence of AED-related Stevens-Johnson syndrome in the German Registry of Serious Cutaneous Reactions: Pediatric vs adults rates. Paper presented at the American Academy of Neurology, 2002.
97. Chang K, Saxena K, Howe M. An open-label study of lamotrigine adjunct or monotherapy for the treatment of adolescents with bipolar depression, *J Am Acad Child Adolesc Psychiatry* 2006; **45**(3): 298–304.
98. Mcelroy SL, Keck PE, Jr Pharmacologic agents for the treatment of acute bipolar mania, *Biol Psychiatry* 2000; **48**(6): 539 557.
99. Pande AC, Davidson JR, Jefferson JW, *et al.* Treatment of social phobia with gabapentin: A placebo-controlled study, *J Clin Psychopharmacol* 1999; **19**: 341–348.
100. Pande AC, Pollack MH, Crockatt J, *et al.* Placebo-controlled study of gabapentin treatment of panic disorder, *J Clin Psychopharmacol* 2000; **20**: 467–471.
101. DelBello MP, Kowatch RA, Warner J, *et al.* Adjunctive topiramate treatment for pediatric bipolar disorder: A retrospective chart review. *J Child Adolesc Psychopharmacol* Winter 2002; **12**(4): 323–330.
102. Delbello MP, Findling RL, Kushner S, *et al.* A pilot controlled trial of topiramate for mania in children and adolescents with bipolar disorder, *J Am Acad Child Adolesc Psychiatry* 2005; **44**(6): 539–547.
103. Tohen M, Kryzhanovskaya L, Carlso G, *et al.* Olanzapine in the treatment of acute mania in adolescents with bipolar I disorder: A 3-week randomized double-blind

placebo-controlled study. Paper presented at the 44th Annual Meeting of the American College of Neuropsychopharmacology; December 13, 2006, 2005; Waikoloa, HI.

104. Tohen M, Kryzhanovskaya L, Carlson G, *et al.* Olanzapine versus placebo in the treatment of adolescents with bipolar mania, *Am J Psychiatry* 2007; **164**(10): 1547–1556.

105. Bishop JR, Pavuluri MN. Review of risperidone for the treatment of pediatric and adolescent bipolar disorder and schizophrenia, *Neuropsychiatr Dis Treat* 2008; **4**(1): 55–68.

106. DelBello MP, Findling RL, Early WR, *et al.* Efficacy of quetiapine in children and adolescents with bipolar mania: a 3-week, double-blind, randomized, placebo-controlled trail. 46th Annual Meeting of the American College of Neuropsychopharmacology; 2007 Dec 9–13; Boca Raton (FL).

107. Findling RL, Nyilas M, Forbes RA, *et al.* Acute treatment of pediatric bipolar I disorder, manic or mixed episode, with aripiprazole: A randomized, double-blind, placebo-controlled study, *J Clin Psychiatry* 2009; **70**(10): 1441–1451.

108. DelBello M, Findling RL, Wang PP, Gundapaneni B, Versavel M. Safety and efficacy of ziprasidone in pediatric bipolar disorder. Paper presented at the 55th Annual Convention and Scientific Program of the Society of Biological Psychiatry 2008; Washington, May 1–3.

109. Killian JG, Kerr K, Lawrence C, *et al.* Myocarditis and cardiomyopathy associated with clozapine, *Lancet* 1999; **354**(9193): 1841–1845.

110. Schulte PF. Risk of clozapine-associated agranulocytosis and mandatory white blood cell monitoring, *Ann Pharmacother* 2006; **40**(4): 683–688.

111. Yumru M, Savas HA, Kurt E *et al.* Atypical antipsychotics related metabolic syndrome in bipolar patients, *J Affect Disord* 2006; Sep 11; [Epub ahead of print].

112. Correll CU, Carlson HE. Endocrine and metabolic adverse effects of psychotropic medications in children and adolescents, *J Am Acad Child Adolesc Psychiatry* 2006; **45**(7): 771–791.

113. Chang K. Stimulant use in pediatric bipolar disorder with attention-deficit/hyperactivity disorder: Pro. *J Bipolar Disord: Rev Commentaries* 2003; **2**(3): 16–17.

114. Carlson GA, Loney J, Salisbury H, Kramer JR, Arthur C. Stimulant treatment in young boys with symptoms suggesting childhood mania: A report from a longitudinal study, *J Child Adolesc Psychopharmacol* Fall 2000; **10**(3): 175–184.

115. Galanter CA, Carlson GA, Jensen PS, *et al.* Response to methylphenidate in children with attention deficit hyperactivity disorder and manic symptoms in the multimodal treatment study of children with attention deficit hyperactivity disorder titration trial, *J Child Adolesc Psychopharmacol* Summer 2003; **13**(2): 123–136.

116. Chang KD, Saxena K, Howe M, Simeonova D. Psychotropic medication exposure and age at onset of bipolar disorder in offspring of parents with bipolar disorder, *J Child Adolesc Psychopharmacol* 2010; **20**(1): 25–32.

117. Scheffer RE, Kowatch RA, Carmody T, Rush AJ. Randomized, placebo-controlled trial of mixed amphetamine salts for symptoms of comorbid ADHD in pediatric bipolar disorder after mood stabilization with divalproex sodium, *Am J Psychiatry.* 2005; **162**(1): 58–64.
118. Chang K, Nayar D, Howe M, Rana M. Atomoxetine as an adjunct therapy in the treatment of co-morbid attention-deficit/hyperactivity disorder in children and adolescents with bipolar I or II disorder, *J Child Adolesc Psychopharmacol* 2009; **19**(5): 547–551.
119. Steinberg S, Chouinard G. A case of mania associated with tomoxetine. *Am J Psychiatry.* 1985; **142**(12): 1517–1518.
120. Biederman J, Swanson JM, Wigal SB, *et al.* Efficacy and safety of modafinil film-coated tablets in children and adolescents with attention-deficit/hyperactivity disorder: Results of a randomized, double-blind, placebo-controlled, flexible-dose study, *Pediatrics* 2005; **116**(6): e777–e784.
121. Greenhill LL, Biederman J, Boellner SW, *et al.* A randomized, double-blind, placebo-controlled study of modafinil film-coated tablets in children and adolescents with attention-deficit/hyperactivity disorder, *J Am Acad Child Adolesc Psychiatry* 2006; **45**(5): 503–511.
122. Cicero D, El-Mallakh RS, Holman J, Robertson J. Antidepressant exposure in bipolar children, *Psychiatry* Winter 2003; **66**(4): 317–322.
123. Faedda GL, Baldessarini RJ, Glovinsky IP, Austin NB. Treatment-emergent mania in pediatric bipolar disorder: A retrospective case review, *J Affect Disord* 2004; **82**(1): 149–158.
124. Baumer FM, Howe M, Gallelli K, Simeonova DI, Hallmayer J, Chang KD. A pilot study of antidepressant-induced mania in pediatric bipolar disorder: Characteristics, risk factors, and the serotonin transporter gene, *Biol Psychiatry* 2006; **60**(9): 1005–1012.
125. Leverich GS, Altshuler LL, Frye MA, *et al.* Risk of switch in mood polarity to hypomania or mania in patients with bipolar depression during acute and continuation trials of venlafaxine, sertraline, and bupropion as adjuncts to mood stabilizers, *Am J Psychiatry* 2006; **163**(2): 232–239.
126. DelBello MP, Adler CM, Whitsel RM, Stanford KE, Strakowski SM. A 12-week single-blind trial of quetiapine for the treatment of mood symptoms in adolescents at high risk for developing bipolar I disorder, *J Clin Psychiatry* 2007; **68**(5): 789–795.
127. DelBello MP, Carlson GA, Tohen M, Bromet EJ, Schwiers M, Strakowski SM. Rates and predictors of developing a manic or hypomanic episode 1 to 2 years following a first hospitalization for major depression with psychotic features, *J Child Adolesc Psychopharmacol* Summer 2003; **13**(2): 173–185.
128. DelBello MP, Chang K, Welge JA, *et al.* A double-blind, placebo-controlled pilot study of quetiapine for depressed adolescents with bipolar disorder, *Bipolar Disord* 2009; **11**(5): 483–493.

129. Chang KD, Ketter TA. Special issues in the treatment of paediatric bipolar disorder, *Expert Opin Pharmacother* 2001; **2**(4): 613–622.
130. Ghaziuddin N, Kutcher SP, Knapp P, *et al.* Practice parameter for use of electroconvulsive therapy with adolescents, *J Am Acad Child Adolesc Psychiatry* 2004; **43**(12): 1521–1539.
131. Miklowitz DJ, Scott J. Psychosocial treatments for bipolar disorder: Cost-effectiveness, mediating mechanisms, and future directions, *Bipolar Disord* 2009; **11**(Suppl. 2): 110–122.
132. Otto MW, Reilly-Harrington N, Sachs GS. Psychoeducational and cognitive-behavioral strategies in the management of bipolar disorder, *J Affect Disord* 2003; **73**(1–2): 171–181.
133. Burns BJ, Hoagwood K, Mrazek PJ. Effective treatment for mental disorders in children and adolescents, *Clin Child Fam Psychol Rev* 1999; **2**(4): 199–254.
134. Lofthouse N, Fristad MA. Psychosocial interventions for children with early-onset bipolar spectrum disorder, *Clin Child Fam Psychol Rev* 2004; **7**(2): 71–88.
135. Fristad MA, Verducci JS, Walters K, Young ME. Impact of multifamily psychoeducational psychotherapy in treating children aged 8 to 12 years with mood disorders, *Arch Gen Psychiatry* 2009; **66**(9): 1013–1021.
136. Fristad MA, Gavazzi SM, Mackinaw-Koons B. Family psychoeducation: An adjunctive intervention for children with bipolar disorder, *Biol Psychiatry* 2003; **53**(11): 1000–1008.
137. Miklowitz DJ, Axelson DA, Birmaher B, *et al.* Family-focused treatment for adolescents with bipolar disorder: Results of a 2-year randomized trial, *Arch Gen Psychiatry* 2008; **65**(9): 1053–1061.
138. Miklowitz DJ, Simoneau TL, George EL, *et al.* Family-focused treatment of bipolar disorder: 1-year effects of a psychoeducational program in conjunction with pharmacotherapy, *Biol Psychiatry* 2000; **48**(6): 582–592.
139. Pavuluri MN, Graczyk PA, Henry DB, Carbray JA, Heidenreich J, Miklowitz DJ. Child- and family-focused cognitive-behavioral therapy for pediatric bipolar disorder: Development and preliminary results, *J Am Acad Child Adolesc Psychiatry* 2004; **43**(5): 528–537.
140. Pavuluri MN, O'Connor MM, Harral EM, Moss M, Sweeney JA. Impact of neurocognitive function on academic difficulties in pediatric bipolar disorder: A clinical translation, *Biol Psychiatry* 2006; **60**(9): 951–956.
141. Pavuluri MN, Schenkel LS, Aryal S, *et al.* Neurocognitive function in unmedicated manic and medicated euthymic pediatric bipolar patients, *Am J Psychiatry* 2006; **163**(2): 286–293.
142. Cicchetti D, Rogosch FA. A developmental psychopathology perspective on adolescence, *J Consult Clin Psychol* 2002; **70**(1): 6–20.

Chapter 8

Traumatic Stress and Psychopathology

Victor G. Carrion, Sarah J. Erickson, Mary E. Bancroft, Julia Huemer, and Belinda Plattner

1. Introduction

When confronted with threat, individuals respond using the "fight or flight" response, a physiological and behavioral response that allows the individual to either confront or escape the danger. Despite its survival value, this system may become profoundly dysregulated in the presence of genetic vulnerability[1] or extreme accumulation of stress, referred to as allostatic load.[2] The permanent sequelae of such dysregulation we refer to as trauma-related psychopathology.

Behavioral theory posits that traumatic symptoms result from hyperactivation of the normal fear response. According to this theory, the initial exposure to a traumatic event activates a startle response that consists of physiological arousal and a behavioral response (such as fight or flight).[3] Through the process of fear conditioning, the elements of the trauma which directly cause the sensation of fear (the unconditioned stimuli) become paired with neutral elements present in the environment at the time of the trauma (the conditioned stimuli), leading to a sense of fear when presented with formerly neutral stimuli (conditioned response).[4] Thus, neutral stimuli come to serve as cues that trigger traumatic memories, reexperiencing, arousal, and avoidance. Trauma causes a normal fear reaction to be overactivated to such a degree that normal habituation and extinction fail to occur.[5] This fear response to traumatic stimuli may increase over time through sensitization and may even generalize to new stimuli. A survivor's attempts to avoid any stimuli associated with the trauma may backfire, causing memories to remain unprocessed and to resurface in the form of flashbacks and intrusive thoughts.[6] Normal exposure fails to take place because of attempts to avoid thinking about and coming into contact with traumatic reminders. Thus, the association between trauma cues and fear remains strong and cues are able to elicit posttraumatic symptoms long after the trauma.

Children who confront dangerous and threatening situations need to develop coping mechanisms with limited resources. Children who experience traumatic stress become angry and express this behaviorally (fight); or dissociate and deny the experience (flight). It is difficult for them, because of their dependent status, to consciously escape many situations. In this chapter, we discuss the behavioral and emotional repercussions of experiencing traumatic stress early in development and the treatment modalities we use in our practice to help these children.

1.1. *Traumatic stress*

Traumatic stress occurs when an individual is exposed to an event that is shocking, distressing, or emotionally painful and can result in negative mental and physical health effects.[7] Trauma exposure in childhood can result in a variety of psychological symptoms including posttraumatic stress disorder (PTSD), other anxiety disorders, depression, dissociation, and externalizing behavioral problems.[8,9] Trauma and its sequelae can also interfere with a child's cognitive,[10] social,[9,11] and emotional[12] development, and can negatively affect the individual's self-esteem[11] and self-control.[13] Due to its interference with normal developmental processes, trauma experienced during childhood may have an even more profound effect than trauma in adulthood.[14]

2. Epidemiology

Children may experience trauma that is acute (single-incident) or chronic (recurrent incidents or long-term exposure)[15] and may be exposed to trauma at an individual or community level.[16] Prevalence studies indicate that between 15 and 40% of adolescents in the general population have been exposed to trauma.[17] A community sample of 21 year olds found that 11% had experienced physical abuse or sexual abuse before the age of 18.[18] Another self-report study of late adolescents found that rape and child sexual abuse were the most commonly experienced traumas, followed by crime threats and witnessing crimes.[17]

The prevalence rate of PTSD in the general adolescent population is around 2%, with an estimated lifetime prevalence of roughly 3.5%.[19] Of those adolescents with trauma histories, the current prevalence of PTSD ranges from 12.4 to 14.5%, with a lifetime prevalence of between 51 and 67%.[19,20] If subsyndromal posttraumatic symptoms were taken into account, these prevalence rates might be even higher. Child survivors of interpersonal trauma may have even higher rates of PTSD, with approximately 36% of youth meeting full PTSD criteria after initial disclosure of the trauma,[21,22] and close to one-third still meeting full criteria two years later.[15] Higher PTSD prevalence rates have been documented in clinical and forensic samples. Among a sample of chemically dependent adolescents in residential treatment, PTSD was found to be the most common current and lifetime diagnosis, with 74.7% of participants reporting a history of trauma, and 19.2% meeting criteria for a current PTSD diagnosis.[23] Similarly, 22% of clinic-referred youth aged from 3 to 18 with a history of trauma met full PTSD criteria, while 32% exhibited some post-traumatic symptoms but did not meet full criteria.[24] Finally, between 51 and 82.7% of court-referred adolescents and juvenile delinquents report having experienced trauma, and many of these have symptoms of PTSD and dissociation.[25,26]

One consideration in identifying trauma prevalence rates across populations is the wide range of PTSD diagnostic interviews and self-report measures employed, often with different levels of sensitivity and specificity, thereby making comparisons difficult. Furthermore, as noted earlier, although PTSD is the most common syndromal sequelae following a traumatic experience,[27] other forms of psychopathology are also potential sequelae, including other anxiety disorders, depressive disorders, dissociative disorders , and behavioral disorders.

Beyond clinical and forensic populations, other child populations may be at heightened risk for experiencing trauma. Recent studies have examined the prevalence of post-traumatic symptoms and PTSD in children following exposure to a range of acute and chronic traumas, including medical conditions such as asthma[28] and cancer;[29–33] accidents and injuries;[34–37] natural disasters such as tsunamis[38] and earthquakes;[39] exposure to single acts of violence or terrorism;[40] exposure to war;[41,42] and exposure to domestic violence.[43,44] Further, technology has expanded the potential audiences for traumas from those proximal to the event to those who experience it distally from television.[45]

2.1. *Medical conditions*

In a study of children with posttraumatic stress symptoms (PTSS) in children following an accidental injury or recent diagnosis of cancer or diabetes, PTSS rates were found to vary significantly by diagnostic group and child's severity of PTSS was significantly correlated with their functional status.[32] Across groups, children who had experienced accidents evidenced the highest rate of moderate to severe PTSS (14.6%), followed by a cancer diagnosis (10%) and diabetes diagnosis (5.4%). PTSS rates were measured using the UCLA Posttraumatic Stress Disorder-Reaction Index (PTSD-RI)[46] at 5–6 weeks postaccident or diagnosis.

While this study examined rates of posttraumatic stress symptoms in children soon after a diagnosis, other studies have examined PTSD in children who have been coping with a diagnosis for a longer period of time and have experienced subsequent medical treatments, including studies with child survivors of cancer[31] and children with severe asthma.[28] A review of PTSD in pediatric cancer survivors found prevalence rates varying from 2 to 20% across studies, even after an average time lapse of 3–6 years since their last treatment.[33] More specifically, a recent study found moderate to severe levels of PTSS in 17.6% of adolescent cancer survivors after an average of 5.3 years of treatment using the PTSD-RI.[31] Prevalence rates of current PTSD were 4.7%, with 8% of adolescents having met diagnostic criteria for PTSD since their cancer diagnosis.[31] In addition to pediatric cancer, PTSD symptoms have been found in adolescents with severe asthma. As measured by the PTSD-RI, 20% of adolescents who had a life-threatening asthma episode met criteria for PTSD, compared with 11% in an asthma control group and 8% in a healthy control group.[28]

Across these studies, the impact of a child's illness on parents was also examined and rates of PTSD were found to be higher in parents than in the medically affected children. Kean *et al.*[28] found that 29% of parents (89% of respondents being mothers) of adolescents with severe asthma met criteria for PTSD. Landolt *et al.*[32] found that 16% of fathers and 23.9% of mothers met full DSM-IV-TR diagnostic criteria for PTSD following their child's accidental injury or recent diagnosis of cancer or diabetes. The highest levels of PTSD occurred in parents whose child had been recently diagnosed with cancer (44.4% mothers, 40% fathers). Interestingly, while mothers' and fathers' posttraumatic stress symptom scores were significantly correlated with each other, they were not related to children's levels of PTSS.[32] Kazak *et al.*[31] also reported higher rates of PTSS and PTSD in parents than in their child survivor of cancer. Moderate to severe levels of PTSS were found in 43.7% of the mothers and 35.3% of the fathers, with current PTSD prevalence rates of 13.7% and 9.6%, respectively. Furthermore, 29% of mothers met PTSD criteria at some point since their child's diagnosis. In partial contrast to the study of Landolt *et al.*[32] concordance rates of PTSD across family members were very low (0–5%), suggesting that while many families were affected by the trauma, typically one member was more affected than the others.[31] These findings point to the importance of evaluating posttraumatic stress symptoms in the family members of pediatric patients in addition to the pediatric patient themselves.[31]

2.2. *Accident/injury trauma*

In a review of studies examining psychological effects following traffic accidents in children, PTSD rates ranged from 6 to 34.5%.[36] Regarding prevalence rates in specific samples, a study of children admitted to a children's hospital trauma unit found PTSD rates of 7% at six-week follow-up, with significant PTSD symptomatology in an additional 17% of the sample.[35] By six-month follow-up, only 2% met criteria for PTSD and 4% for partial PTSD. Girls had significantly higher scores on the Clinician Administered PTSD Scale for Children and Adolescents (CAPS-CA)[47] than did boys.[35]

Another study using the CAPS-CA found a PTSD prevalence rate of 29.1% one-month postaccident in children who had been admitted to an ER following road traffic accidents.[36] Despite the wide age range included in this study, there were no significant differences by age in prevalence of PTSD. However, gender differences were significant, with girls being more likely than boys to evidence PTSD.[36] Delayed onset of PTSD following road traffic accidents in a small pediatric sample has been examined using the PTSD-RI.[34] PTSD symptoms were measured at 12–16 weeks postaccident and again at 18-months post-accident. An increase from 7 to 22% of children's moderate PTSD symptoms was found across the two time intervals, with severity of injury related to severity of PTSD symptomatology.[34]

Stress symptoms following injury have also been found in very young children. In a sample of young children (12–48 months old) admitted to a burn unit, 29% evidenced acute stress symptoms.[37] The Child Posttraumatic Stress Disorder Semi-Structured Interview (CPTSDSSI)[48] was used to assess child's stress symptoms via parental interview.

2.3. *Natural disasters*

Psychological effects of the December 2004 tsunami on children living in Southern Thailand were examined at two-months posttsunami. The prevalence of severe PTSD symptoms, as measured by the PTSD-RI, was significantly higher in children who had been displaced by the tsunami than those who lived in unaffected villages. In fact, the prevalence rate of severe PTSD symptoms for children who had lived in affected areas and were displaced from their homes was 13%, versus 6% among children living in unaffected areas. Prevalence rates for depression as measured by the Birleson Depression Inventory[49] were 11%, 5%, and 8% respectively. PTSD and depressive symptom rates did not change significantly when assessed again at nine months posttsunami.[38] In addition, a study of the effects of the 1999 Marmara earthquake in Turkey assessed for PTSD symptoms and found very high estimates of PTSD in children exposed to the earthquake (73%), as compared to rates in a control group not exposed to the earthquake (6%).[39]

2.4. *Acts of violence/war*

A large-scale study examined the psychological effects of children in New York City following the September 11th, 2001 attack on the World Trade Center.[40]

A sample of 8236 students in grades 4th through 12th were assessed using the Diagnostic Interview Schedule for Children (DISC) Predictive Scales (DPS)[50] which screens for probable mental disorders. Severity of exposure to the attack was also assessed in relation to levels of direct and family exposure. A high percentage of children evidenced one or more anxiety or depressive disorders (28.6%), with agoraphobia, separation anxiety, and PTSD being the most frequent probable diagnosis. Prevalence rates across anxiety and depressive disorders increased with increased severity of exposure (mild, 18.2%; moderate, 29.1%; and severe, 38.9%). Prevalence of probable PTSD in the total sample was 10%, and prevalence patterns also increased with increased severity of exposure (mild, 3.6%; moderate, 10%; and severe, 18.4%). Prevalence rates in girls were higher than in boys across anxiety and depressive disorders, with 34.7% of girls and 21.8% of boys meeting diagnostic criteria.[40]

A small sample of refugee children seen in a child specialty clinic in Oregon evidenced particularly high rates of PTSD (63%) as diagnosed by psychiatrists according to DSM-IV-TR criteria.[42] A majority of these children had experienced direct trauma from recent wars in Afghanistan and Bosnia. Furthermore, a recent review of the psychological effects on children exposed to war and children who are refugees found PTSD rates ranging from 25 to 75% across studies.[51]

2.5. *Domestic violence*

High rates of PTSD were found in an at-risk population of adolescents who had been referred to a center for severe behavior problems or youth correction facilities.[44] In addition to a history of witnessing domestic violence, these adolescents reported directly experiencing traumatic events such as serious physical assault, witnessing the death of another, and feared or actual abandonment. Gender differences emerged with sexual traumas, with girls being significantly more likely than boys to have experienced sexual assault (23% versus 6%). Using the Diagnostic Interview for Children and Adolescents — R (DICA-R),[52] 35% of the sample met full PTSD criteria. Girls displayed significantly higher rates of PTSD than boys, with 46% of girls versus 22% of boys meeting diagnostic criteria.[44]

Young children with a history of witnessing domestic violence and staying in a domestic violence emergency shelter with their mothers also evidenced high levels of PTSD symptoms.[43] Using the PTSD-RI, the entire sample evidenced moderate to severe PTSD symptomatology, with 40% classified as moderate, 50% severe, and 10% very severe. Severity of PTSD was related to both frequency and duration of witnessing interadult physical violence. No gender or age differences were found in rates of PTSD.[43]

2.6. *Ethnic variations*

Few studies have directly examined ethnic differences in rates of PTSD in young children. One study included an ethnically diverse sample (52% Caucasian, 34% African-American, 9.5% biracial, 1.4% Hispanic, 1.8% Native American, and 1.3% others) who had witnessed domestic violence.[53] The prevalence rate of PTSD was 25% as measured by maternal report using the Traumatic Stress Symptoms Child Scale (TSSC).[53] While the number of violent acts witnessed by the child (average of 31.3 incidents) did not vary by ethnicity, Caucasian children exhibited significantly higher rates of PTSD than did ethnic minority children, with 33% of Caucasian children and 17% of ethnic minority children meeting PTSD criteria. However, these findings must be interpreted cautiously as they are based on maternal report and the measure has not been widely used.[53]

In a large study of Northern Plains Native American adolescents, all of whom had experienced at least one traumatic event, 12% met criteria for lifetime PTSD as measured by the Composite International Diagnostic Interview (CIDI).[54,55] Prevalence rates of PTSD were higher for girls than for boys, with 16.7% of girls versus 6.0% of boys meeting diagnostic criteria.[55]

3. Diagnosis

Children's initial response to trauma is often characterized by physiological and behavioral hyperarousal and, when the trauma is ongoing, the response may become complicated by dissociation.[8] With evidence suggesting that children's response to trauma can be enduring and detrimental,[56,57] it is critical to ensure developmentally appropriate classification criteria.

3.1. *DSM-IV-TR*

Three symptom clusters form the basis for diagnosis: reexperiencing the traumatic event, avoidance or emotional numbing, and hyperarousal. This triad of symptoms following a traumatic experience has been termed posttraumatic stress PTSD according to the *Diagnostic and Statistical Manual of Mental Disorders-IV-TR*.[58] A traumatic experience is defined as an event in which: (1) the person experienced, witnessed, or was confronted with an event or events that involved actual or threatened death or serious injury, or a threat to the physical integrity of self or others; and (2) the person's response involved intense fear, helplessness, or horror.

The triad of symptoms include the following:

Reexperiencing (Cluster B; one symptom needed): Trauma persistently reexperienced in one or more of the following ways: (1) Recurrent and intrusive recollections of the event: images, thoughts, perceptions (in children, repetitive play); (2) Recurrent distressing dreams of the event (in children, frightening dreams); (3) Acting or feeling as if recurring (in children, trauma-specific reenactment may occur); (4) Intense distress upon cues; and (5) Intense physiological reactivity upon cues.

Avoidance (Cluster C; three symptoms needed): Avoidance of stimuli and numbing of general responsiveness: (1) Thoughts, feelings, or conversations; (2) Activities, places, or people; (3) Inability to recall important aspect of trauma; (4) Diminished interest; (5) Restricted range of affect; and (6) Sense of foreshortened future.

Hyper-arousal (Cluster D; two symptoms needed): Persistent symptoms of increased arousal: (1) Difficulty falling or staying asleep; (2) Irritability or outbursts of anger; (3) Difficulty concentrating; (4) Hypervigilance; and (5) Exaggerated startle response.

Criterion E: Symptoms persist for more than one month.

Criterion F: Clinically significant distress or impairment in, social, occupational, academic, or other important areas of functioning.

- acute or chronic (more or less than three months)
- with delayed onset (development six months or later after the traumatic event)

Research has demonstrated that the developmentally sensitive assessment of symptoms following trauma may be more valid than the DSM-IV-TR criteria in very young children, as symptoms of PTSD may differ substantially between children and adults.[48,59] In addition, youth experiencing subthreshold post-traumatic symptoms do not differ from youth who meet full PTSD criteria in terms of functional impairment.[60]

3.2. *Acute stress disorder, post-traumatic stress disorder and dissociation*

When analyzing "dissociation," one must differentiate between dissociation as a defense reaction in response to stress, an accompaniment of trauma-related psychopathology, such as acute stress disorder (ASD) and posttraumatic stress disorder (PTSD), and as a core feature of a set of disorders.[58]

Dissociation is defined by DSM as a defense that "deals with emotional conflict or external and internal stressors with a breakdown in the usually integrated functions of consciousness, memory perception of self or the environment, or sensory/motor behavior"[58] as opposed to splitting, a related defense, which is described as a process that deals with the same contingencies by "compartmentalizing opposite affective states and failing to integrate the positive and negative qualities of the self or others into cohesive images."[58]

In terms of Acute Stress Disorder (ASD), dissociative symptoms are core features of establishing a diagnosis. These symptoms are subsumed under five categories: derealization, emotional numbing, depersonalization, a lack of awareness for one's surroundings (*i.e.* stupor), and psychogenic amnesia.[58] The mentioned features were found in adults to be predictive of later PTSD symptoms, associated with other ASD symptoms and correlative with the severity of the exposure.[61–64] Both the emphasis of dissociative symptoms in the ASD diagnosis as well as the predictive and concurrent relationships of dissociative symptoms to PTSD remain controversial. This may lead to consideration for the DSM-V to include two redefined forms of PTSD, one that emphasizes dissociative symptoms and one that does not.

Furthermore, several diagnoses are present in the DSM-IV as dissociative disorders,[58] such as dissociative (psychogenic) amnesia, dissociative (psychogenic) fugue, depersonalization disorder, dissociative identity disorder (multiple personality disorder), and dissociative disorder not otherwise specified. Interpersonal childhood trauma is described as correlate with and most likely as antedate of the development of dissociative disorders, such as depersonalization.[26,65]

The persistence of traumatic events as "chronic trauma" in contrast to "acute trauma" precedes the development of dissociative disorders and is more strongly associated with comorbidity, self-injurious behaviors, suicidality, and treatment resistance.[66]

Butler *et al.*[67] described pathways from trauma to dissociative symptoms and disorders by postulating a diathesis-stress model, in which dissociative symptoms play an essential part in immediate and long-term stress responses to traumatic life events. The model, which still needs to be adapted to children and adolescents, postulates that pathologic dissociation develops in response to the combination of two factors: (1) the experience of one or more traumatic events and (2) the potential for a high innate hypnotizability, factors, which influence each other in a circular way.

This might be particularly relevant given the fact that children become increasingly hypnotizable from approximately five years of age until early adolescence and therefore presumably especially vulnerable to developing dissociative symptoms. Yet, the relationship between dissociation and hypnosis is still controversially discussed.[68]

Two further models of the effects of dissociative symptoms in psychopathology have been described by Terr and Putnam.[69,70] In Terr's model, the chronicity of dissociative and other traumatic stress symptoms is aggravated by the reappearance or persistence of traumatic life events, whereas Putnam's model emphasizes the states of consciousness that become more differentiated in people who live through dissociative disorders.

3.3. *ICD-10*

Similar to the DSM-IV-TR, the 10th revision of the *International Classification of Diseases (ICD-10)*[71] includes a categorical classification approach to disorders. While the ICD-10 clinical description includes the same triad of symptoms as the DSM-IV-TR, more emphasis is placed on intrusive memories and the reenactment of these memories, whereas symptoms of emotional numbing and avoidance may be experienced but are not required for a diagnosis. Given that symptoms of emotional numbing and avoidance are difficult to assess in young children,[51] the ICD-10 classification system may be particularly helpful to consider with young children.[27] The ICD-10 PTSD clinical diagnostic criteria include: evidence that symptoms arose within six months of a traumatic event of exceptional severity; a repetitive, intrusive recollection, or reenactment of the event in memories, daytime imagery, or dreams; and conspicuous emotional detachment, numbing of feeling, and avoidance of stimuli that may arouse trauma recollection are often present but are not essential for the diagnosis. The autonomic disturbances, mood disorder, and behavioral abnormalities all contribute to the diagnosis, but are not essential. Furthermore, the ICD-10 includes associated features: anxiety and depression, suicidal ideation, and excessive use of alcohol or drugs.

4. Differential Diagnosis and Comorbitidy

According to the DSM-IV-TR, associated features of PTSD may include guilt for the trauma, survival guilt and phobic avoidance of traumatic reminders, the latter often resulting in impaired interpersonal relations. In fact, we have found guilt to predict the development of posttraumatic stress symptoms in children affected by interpersonal violence.[72] Furthermore, in response to an interpersonal stressor (*e.g.* childhood abuse, domestic violence, war crimes), the following symptoms may occur more frequently: impaired affect modulation, self-destructive and impulsive behavior, dissociative symptoms, somatic complaints, shame and hopelessness, perceiving oneself to be irreparably damaged, loss of previously held beliefs about the nature of the world, hostility, social withdrawal, and impaired interpersonal relationships.

There is considerable symptom overlap between PTSD and other DSM-IV-TR diagnoses. Regarding differential diagnoses, adjustment disorders, other anxiety or mood disorders, acute stress disorder (ASD), obsessive compulsive disorder (OCD), and psychotic disorders warrant consideration. The high rates of comorbidity with other DSM-IV-TR diagnoses can present significant diagnostic challenges[73] and comorbidity among traumatized children has received limited empirical investigation. From the limited research, it appears that different comorbidity profiles may be characteristic of different traumatized groups. For example, Separation Anxiety Disorder was the most common comorbid diagnosis of sexually and physically abused 8–12-year-old children.[74] Attention Deficit Hyperactivity Disorder (ADHD) in relation to trauma has received some attention, with mixed results. In one study, 13% of all children and adolescents with PTSD also qualified for ADHD, with this rate jumping to 34% when the sample was limited to school-aged children (6–12 years old).[75] In contrast, Wozniak *et al.*[76] did not find an association between PTSD and ADHD. When they are present, it is unclear whether symptoms such as concentration difficulties, hyperactivity, and oppositionality are in response to a traumatic stressor or represent preexisting behavioral disorders. In the case of Conduct Disorder (CD), based on retrospective report, it appears that PTSD tends to develop subsequent to CD.[77] However, in our experience traumatic events precipitate many of the symptoms experienced by children in juvenile halls.[8] Finally, it is important to note that a traumatic event may be a catalyst for the development of any disorder an individual may be prone to develop, not only PTSD. Hence, it is not uncommon to clinically observe any of the conditions described above after the experience of a traumatic event.

5. Assessment

The assessment of traumatized children should consist of a face-to-face interview with both the child and his/her non-offending caretaker(s) during which they are asked directly and specifically about the traumatic event and its aftermath.[73,78,79] The inclusion of caretaker and child is important, as diagnosing post-traumatic symptoms may require the input of multiple reporters.[78] It should include both general questions about the child's psychological health and functioning and specific inquires about the trauma history and symptoms.[73,80] The use of standardized assessment instruments can provide a baseline by which to measure treatment gains and a standardization with which an individual child can be compared.[81,82] Children's functioning prior to trauma, during the trauma, and subsequent to trauma should be explored. The need to establish rapport is not unique to children with PTSD, but is especially crucial in the context of trauma and stress.

Diagnosis is strongly aided by the use of multiple informants, such as teachers, parents, and mental health and/or medical professionals. This allows for a multiperspective assessment and maximization of diagnostic validity. In particular, parents have a tendency to minimize PTSD-related symptoms in their children, and children themselves may experience considerable shame around discussing such issues. Multiple informants help to reduce the chance of minimization of symptoms and functional impairment. In addition to the need for multiple informants, there is a corresponding need for multiple forms of assessment. Such forms include behavioral observation, unstructured clinical interviews, semistructured interviews, and empirically validated pencil-and-paper instruments.[73,83]

5.1. *Behavioral observation/unstructured interview*

While a diagnosis of PTSD cannot be made solely on the basis of behavioral observation, this technique can provide valuable clinical information about the functioning of traumatized children. For example, informal observation of heightened startle reflex, reoccurring trauma themes in play, hypervigilance to the environment, and mood lability can inform the diagnosis of PTSD.

Important clinical data can also be garnered during an open-ended, unstructured interview. This approach is sometimes perceived as more child friendly than a structured interview, as it allows the opportunity for warm and empathic reactions. Significant drawbacks, however, exist with this method, which may not provide direct information about the child's experience, and children rarely spontaneously disclose trauma and resulting symptoms in unstructured situations.

5.2. *Semistructured interviews*

Several semistructured interviews and self- and parent-report instruments can be used to assess DSM-IV-TR in children and adolescents. Interviews can be PTSD-specific (such as the Clinician Administered PTSD Scale for Children and Adolescents (CAPS-CA)) or more broad-based and inclusive (such as the Anxiety Disorders Interview Schedule for DSM-IV: Child Version (ADIS-IV-C)).[84] Both types of interviews ensure standardization of question presentation and exploration of all diagnostic criteria. Clinicians can use their observations as well as responses of the child to modify the interview within specific parameters so as to maximize validity of the diagnosis. However, interviews about traumatic history and associated symptoms may be distressing, embarrassing, or even frightening for children. This format also gives clinicians some latitude to make the interview more therapeutic by way of using reflecting and rephrasing to foster therapeutic alliance and/or be of direct clinical benefit to the child. One major drawback, however, is the often lengthy administration time.

There are several semistructured interviews for determining current and lifetime diagnoses of PTSD that vary by inclusion of child, parent, or both child and parent informants in formulating diagnosis. The Clinician Administered PTSD

Scale for Children and Adolescents (CAPS-CA) is a semistructured, PTSD diagnostic clinical interview for use with children (ages 8–15). In addition to assessment of PTSD symptoms, it also includes assessment of child functioning across social, developmental, and academic domains. The CAPS-CA has been identified as one of the best tools for assessment of DSM-IV-TR PTSD in children[51] and has been employed in a variety of studies including children exposed to interpersonal traumas,[85] road traffic accidents,[36] and pediatric patients admitted to an ER after sustaining an Injury.[50]

The Diagnostic Interview for Children and Adolescents-Revised (DICA-R) is a comprehensive semistructured interview for use with children (ages 6–17) that assesses psychopathology and contains a PTSD module. While diagnosis can be based on either child or parent informant, it is recommended that both child and parent interviews are used for the most accurate assessment of child PTSD.[86] The DICA-R has been used in studies with at-risk adolescents exposed to longer-term abuse and violence,[44] and those with potential dual diagnoses,[77] and it has also been employed in studies with children following a single-incident trauma such as a road traffic accident.[87]

The Kiddie Schedule for Affective Disorders and Schizophrenia for School-age Children-Present and Lifetime version (K-SADS-PL),[88] is a semistructured interview that assesses general psychopathology in children (ages 7–17) and contains a PTSD module. Both child- and parental report are used in diagnosis. Other interview formats for diagnosing PTSD in children include the Childhood PTSD Interview-Childhood form;[89] the PTSD module of the Anxiety Disorders Interview Schedule for DSM-IV: Child Version (ADIS-IV-C) and the DSM-IV-TR version of the Children's Post-traumatic Stress Disorder Inventory.[90]

5.3. *Self-report measures of post-traumatic stress symptoms for diagnosis*

Valid and reliable paper-and-pencil instruments can be efficient, low-cost assessment tools to aid in reaching a diagnosis. They can be completed without the presence of a clinician, which may be of practical benefit, but cannot be substituted for a full clinical evaluation. Regardless of form, all assessment measures for pediatric PTSD must include developmentally appropriate language as well as take into account developmental differences in symptomatology.

Many self-report measures currently used in child populations are adaptations of adult self-report measures.[27,86] The UCLA Posttraumatic Stress Disorder-Reaction Index (PTSD-RI) has child, adolescent, and adult versions and can be used with children aged 5 and up. It assesses severity of post-trauma symptoms as well as providing a preliminary PTSD diagnosis based on DSM-IV-TR criteria.

The PTSD-RI is one of the most widely used measures across studies examining the effects of a variety of traumas in children, including medical conditions,[28,32,91] road traffic accidents,[34] natural disasters,[38] and domestic violence.[43] The Child PTSD Symptom Scale (CPSS)[92] is a child self-report measure for use with children that has been used to assess severity as well as diagnosis of PTSD according to DSM-IV-TR criteria[86] and has also been used to monitor child's progress.[51]

5.4. *Non-diagnostic self-report measures*

Although the Impact of Events Scale-Revised (IES-R)[93] was designed for use with adults, it has been used with children aged 12 and older. A shortened and adapted 13-item version has been used with children aged 8 and older.[94] This scale assesses intrusion, avoidance, and hyperarousal symptoms and, while not intended for use as a diagnostic tool[86] has been shown to be a reliable and valid measure of PTSD symptoms in children.[95] The Trauma Symptom Checklist for Children (TSCC)[96] is designed for use with children (aged 8–16) and measures exposure to trauma and more broadly defined posttraumatic stress symptoms. For example, the TSCC includes post-traumatic stress, anxiety, depression, anger, dissociation, and sexual concerns subscales. Other self-report measures have been designed for evaluating levels of PTSD symptoms in children following specific traumatic events such as the Children's Impact of Traumatic Events Scale-Revised (CITES-R)[97] designed to measure the traumatic impact of sexual abuse in children, and the war-trauma-questionnaire,[98] designed to measure war-related stressors.

5.5. *Self-report measures of associated symptoms*

Other scales may be employed to measure symptoms associated with, but not essential to, PTSD. These include the revised Fear Survey Schedule for Children (FSSC-R);[99] the Revised Children's Manifest Anxiety Scale (RCMAS);[100] the Children's Depression Inventory (CDI);[101] and the Birleson Depression Inventory. Additional supplemental information can be gathered from measures such as the Kidcope[102] that measures children's coping strategies and has been included in PTSD studies. The Posttraumatic Cognitions Inventory (PTCI),[103] measures beliefs about safety as well as cognitions around PTSD symptoms, has been predictive of the development and severity of PTSD, and is considered a valuable tool in treatment planning and evaluation of school-age children and adolescents.[27]

The Posttraumatic Growth Inventory for Children (PTGI-C) is an adaptation of the adult version of the PTGI[104] and includes "positive" sequelae of trauma, including factors of new possibilities, relating to others, personal strength, appreciation of life and spiritual change. There are few studies using the PTGI-C with children, although initial results with children following exposure to hurricane Floyd demonstrated variability among children's positive growth scores and a significant relationship between children's competency beliefs and positive life change following a traumatic event.[105] Continued research is needed on the potential for post-traumatic growth in children and adolescents. Such information regarding positive life change might help explain why some children do not develop PTSD following exposure to traumatic events, elucidate alternative pathways for children following traumatic events, and suggest ways that adults might intervene to support a child's posttraumatic beliefs.[105]

5.6. *Assessment of PTSD in young children*

The Post-traumatic Stress Disorder Semi-structured interview and Observational Record for Infants and Young Children[106] has been used to assess PTSD in very young children (up to 48 months old). This semistructured interview is based primarily on the DSM-IV-TR with developmental modifications made to 5 of the 17 criteria and is arguably more accurate and sensitive at detecting PTSD in very young children than traditional DSM-IV-TR assessment.[59,106] The Child Behavior Checklist (CBCL)[107] may be used to assess more general adjustment, including internalizing and externalizing behaviors, *via* parental report, in very young children (as young as two years old).[108] In addition, a proposed modified subscale of the CBCL, the Child Behavior Checklist -Post-traumatic Stress Disorder (CBCL-PTSD) Scale has shown promise more specifically as a parental-report screening tool of PTSD in preschool aged children.[109]

Although biological research utilizes new methodology to investigate biological correlates of stress and trauma, it is too early to use any of these methods (*i.e.*: MRI, cortisol measures, psychophysiology) diagnostically. Eventually these may be helpful in identifying currently behaviorally defined symptoms (*i.e.*: irritability, agitation, hyperarousal) that cut across diagnostic groups.

6. Pathogenesis

Not all traumatized populations develop PTSD or psychopathology. This underscores our need to understand environmental and genetic factors of stress vulnerability.

6.1. *Gender*

Female gender appears to be a risk factor for developing PTSD.[27,110] Across studies and trauma types, girls have evidenced significantly higher rates of PTSD than boys, including in response to road traffic accidents,[36] the attack on the World Trade Center,[40] and domestic violence trauma.[44] In pediatric populations, prevalence of sexual traumas is higher in girls than in boys, and girls are also significantly more likely to develop PTSD following a sexual trauma.[111] In addition, higher rates of sexual trauma and higher prevalence of PTSD in girls have also been found in Native American adolescents.[55] Girls tend to show more internalizing behaviors and boys more externalizing behaviors in response to physical violence and sexual abuse, which may in part explain the higher rates of PTSD in girls following sexual abuse.[75] However, it is largely unclear as to whether the gender differences observed in prevalence rates of PTSD have cultural or biological underpinnings.

6.2. *Physiological arousal*

Physiological arousal in children at the time of injury has been related to the development of PTSD. In a study of very young children (12–48 month olds) with burn injuries, higher pulse rate during hospitalization was a risk factor for developing acute stress symptoms.[37] Heart rate measurements of pediatric injury patients during emergency medical transport significantly predicted children's PTSD symptoms both at six-weeks and six-months posttrauma[35] and higher heart rate measured in the ER predicted higher levels of PTSD symptoms in injured adolescents.[112]

6.3. *Objective experience: Severity of trauma and exposure*

Proximity to the traumatic event and the objective severity of the trauma are highly correlated with the severity of a child's traumatic reaction.[40] Specifically, objective event severity has been related to higher PTSD symptoms in adolescents with a serious physical injury[112] and those witnessing the September 11th attacks[40]; functional impairment has been highly correlated with children's subsequent development of PTSD symptoms[32]; greater severity in injury has been associated with more severe PTSD following road traffic accidents in children;[34] and size of burn predicted higher levels of acute stress symptoms in very young children.[37] These studies suggest that children sustaining more severe injury are at higher risk for developing PTSD symptoms. In fact, several studies refer to a "dose–response effect" of trauma on the development of PTSD, whereby risk is increased with increased exposure and severity.[41] For example, exposure severity (measured by levels of personal and family impact) to the attack on the World Trade Center was related to higher rates of childhood anxiety and depressive disorders, including PTSD.[40] A review of studies on children exposed to war found that cumulative traumas as well as severity of trauma were associated with higher levels of psychological distress in children.[41] The same pattern holds with children exposed to domestic violence, whereby frequency and duration of witnessing interadult violence is related to more severe PTSD.[43] Prior trauma exposure and prior psychopathology also increase the likelihood of developing problems.[23,113,114]

6.4. *Subjective experience*

Subjective experience of trauma, including appraisals of the traumatic event, particularly those involving perceived life threat or potential future threat, have been linked to PTSD symptomatology in children as well. For example, significantly higher rates of PTSD were documented in children in response to a tsunami who reported having felt their own or a family member's life was in danger, determining that they were unable to escape, and experiencing extreme panic or fear at the time of the event.[38] In addition, a greater perceived risk of future threat partially explained why child survivors of parental bereavement reported significantly higher levels of PTSD symptoms than child survivors of cancer.[115] Furthermore, children's negative cognitive appraisals following a traumatic event accounted for 61–65% of the variance in PTSD symptoms following road traffic accidents. In short, children's subjective appraisal of the event appears to differentially challenge their sense of well-being.[116]

6.5. *Age/developmental considerations*

Age does not appear to be a risk factor for developing PTSD.[27] For example, across studies of PTSD following road-traffic accidents, children's age has not been related to their development of PTSD, even in samples including particularly wide age ranges. However, studies of PTSD following road-traffic accidents rarely include children under the age of 7.[36] Similarly, age has not been related with development of posttraumatic stress symptoms in children with medical conditions[35] or children witnessing domestic violence.[53] An exception is the finding that rates of probable PTSD, agoraphobia, and separation anxiety were higher in 4th and 5th grade students than in 6th–12th grade students in New York City following the attack on the World Trade Center. However, children in the 4th and 5th grade also had higher rates of direct and family exposure to the attack, and severity of exposure was highly associated with probable anxiety and depressive disorders.[40] While no consistent pattern has emerged suggesting that age may be a factor in developing PTSD following a traumatic event, researchers have noted the difficulty younger children have in responding to PTSD interview questions, potentially resulting in an underestimate of PTSD diagnoses among younger children.[36] Supporting this contention, parents tend to underestimate their child's PTSD symptomatology[117] and parental report is often used to assess PTSD in younger children.[37,53]

Furthermore, developmental status appears to affect the presentation of PTSD symptoms. Dyregrov and Yule[51] found that young children have particular difficulty reporting on symptoms of avoidance, perhaps due to an inability to understand and verbalize such covert behavior. Young children also tend to show less emotional numbing, more aggression, and more repetitive play in post-trauma responses. Between the ages of 8 and 10, children begin to present more like adults in response to trauma. They are more able to reflect on an event, and have a better understanding of their own behavior as well as the potential consequences of an event.

6.6. *Post-trauma parental support*

Parents' emotional distress and lack of child-perceived support following trauma have been correlated to depression, anxiety, post-traumatic symptoms, and externalizing behaviors in traumatized children.[114,118] Children's sense that their parents did not believe their account of the trauma has also been correlated with symptom severity.[118] Measures of overall family functioning such as conflict and adaptability have also been associated with both internalizing[118] and externalizing[119] behavior problems in child trauma survivors. Further, parental support has been shown to be a mediator of treatment outcome in abuse survivor.[120]

6.7. *Etiological factors*

Traumatic memories are stored in an associative network, or fear structure, containing information about the traumatic event and its sequelae, response patterns when presented with traumatic material, and interpretive information (appraisals) about the meaning behind the traumatic stimuli.[13] The memories contained in a trauma network are often qualitatively different than other memories: traumatic memories tend to be more sensory, less affected by subsequent learning, triggered by stimuli that are temporally rather than semantically linked to the original event, and experienced as occurring in the present.[6] Trauma memories are also less likely to be well elaborated and well integrated into autobiographical memory, context, and other knowledge.[6]

Pathological trauma reactions occur when excessive stress or avoidance results in a failure of the transfer of memories from sensory to verbal memory, leaving traumatic memories that are unprocessed, unintegrated, and easily triggered by situational cues.[121] Due to this pattern of sensory processing, trauma may cause widespread verbal memory deficits. For example, research has demonstrated lower verbal and full-scale IQ scores in children and youth who have experienced interpersonal trauma.[10,122] In fact, trauma severity and the degree of post-traumatic symptoms and impairment have a strong negative correlation to verbal and full-scale IQ scores.[10,122]

6.7.1. *Biology*

The process of fear conditioning, and the development of trauma symptoms that result, are accompanied by physiological processes. A normal stress response results in the activation of the sympathetic nervous system (SNS) and the central andrenergic mechanisms altering homeostasis.[3] In PTSD, these systems remain activated, even without external threat or exposure to cues. This pathological stress response is believed to be related to dyrsregulation of the hypothalamic-pituitary-adrenal (HPA) axis.[123] The HPA axis has been linked to the stress response (including hormone release, SNS activation, and behavioral responses) and to learning and memory (conditioning, habituation, extinction, and emotional valence to memories).[121] Because of these roles, and based upon experimental evidence regarding abnormalities in the HPA axis in children,[123–125] the HPA axis is believed to play a role in the pathophysiolgy of trauma, although its exact role is not yet understood.

The identification of biological markers of stress and PTSD could help guide the development of new treatment interventions and follow subsequent treatment response. In pediatric PTSD, this approach has concentrated in two arenas: brain structure and cortisol levels. In general, pediatric PTSD, has been associated with smaller total brain volumes[14,126] and an attenuation of frontal lobe asymmetry.[126] Regarding cortisol, elevated levels have been documented in children with PTSD, both by measures of salivary cortisol and by 24-h urinary collection.[123,125] Ongoing longitudinal studies are needed to identify the role of these factors in the pathogenesis of PTSD. Although cross-sectional studies have not replicated hippocampal abnormalities found in studies of adults with PTSD, our recent longitudinal study found that elevated cortisol levels and PTSD symptoms independently predicted hippocampal volume reduction in children with post-traumatic stress symptoms.[127] The hippocampus is of potential interest because of its limbic system location and its role in memory processing.

Regarding genetic studies, one study described how a functional polymorphism in the promoter region of the serotonin transporter (5-HTT) gene moderated the influence of stressful life events on depression.[1] In this study, depressed subjects with one or two copies of the short (S) allele of 5-HTT had increased severity of symptoms when compared to subjects that were homozygous for the long (L) allele. Kaufman and colleagues[128] continued this line of investigation by studying children with a history of maltreatment. Quality and availability of social support moderated the risk for depression associated with the presence of the SS allele.[128]

6.7.2. *Cognition*

Behavioral and physiological processes are accompanied by cognitive appraisals regarding why the traumatic event happened, its repercussions, and the survivor's perception of her/his own role in the event and others' responses upon learning about it.[6] These appraisals about the traumatic event and its aftermath help determine what emotions a child will experience, what will be remembered, and what behavioral and cognitive strategies will be used when exposed to traumatic reminders.[6] Post-traumatic symptoms develop as a result of processing the trauma such that the traumatic event continues to appear threatening even after it is over, leading to an ongoing sense of threat.[6] Negative cognitive attributions and attribution styles are associated with the development of depression, anxiety, dissociation, social problems, and post-traumatic symptoms subsequent to trauma.[118,119,129]

Cognitive distortions are conceptualized to arise as a result of trying to make sense of the traumatic experience and one's role in it,[130] and trying to accommodate this new information into preexisting cognitive schemas.[131] The new information received from the trauma must somehow fit into their prior worldview, or, alternately, the worldview must be altered to match the trauma information.[131] Due to their cognitive developmental level, children may be particularly likely to develop distorted thoughts following traumatic experiences.[130] These distortions may include survivor guilt, self-blame, a sense of responsibility for the trauma, omen formation, viewing oneself as different from others, a lack of trust, and the development of a view that the world is a dangerous place.[130,132]

According to cognitive theory, emotions and thoughts are intimately linked. Distorted cognitions can lead to negative emotional states and behaviors, such as depression, anxiety, and PTSD.[130,133] Following a traumatic event, thoughts and memories related to the trauma are accompanied by strong secondary emotions, such as guilt and anger, resulting in trauma memories being continually processed emotionally rather than logically and verbally.[134] Trauma, in addition to directly causing negative emotional states, can also result in a general pattern of emotional dysregulation.[12]

Emotions are stored within an integrated network of memory, thought, and behavioral responses.[12] Research has demonstrated that traumatized youth exhibit emotional deficits including emotional dysregulation and lability, increased negative emotionality and socially inappropriate emotional expression, and a lack of strategies for emotion coping.[135,136] These emotional problems are believed to be related to social and behavioral problems including aggression, withdrawal, and a lack of prosocial behaviors.[11,135]

There is growing evidence that cognitive difficulties may not only occur in the context of memory for the traumatic event, but also in other domains of executive function. Traumatized adults exhibit deficits in sustained attention,[137,138] mental manipulation,[139] and strategic and declarative memory abilities.[138,140] PTSD has been associated with symptom severity to IQ scores[141] with increased PTSD symptomatology in Vietnam combat veterans associated with lower scores on standardized IQ tests.[142]

Samet and colleagues[143] examined WISC-III scores in traumatized adolescents, and found no differences between those who met diagnostic criteria for PTSD and those who did not meet criteria.[143] In contrast, in a study comparing sexually abused children to controls, full scale and verbal IQ scores were similar, but traumatized children exhibited lower performance IQ than their peers.[144] Others have noted poorer performance on individual subtests of IQ measures, but not full scale, verbal, or performance IQ scores. Beers and De Bellis[145] reported that maltreated children performed worse than control subjects on the WISC-III similarities subtest, but performed similarly on the vocabulary, digit span, block design, object assembly, and coding subtests.

7. Naturalistic Course and Prognosis

Longitudinal research suggests that single-occurrence, non-abusive stressors result in trauma symptoms that peak within the first year after the trauma.[146,147] However, significant levels of symptomatology appear to persist in a subset of children years later.[19,148] In fact, although some investigators have found decreased rates of PTSD longitudinally, the course of pediatric PTSD is episodic in a substantial number of children. The limited longitudinal studies investigating the course of PTSD among children who have experienced repeated, multiple, or abusive stressors suggest that PTSD rates remain high regardless of the time elapsed since the cessation of traumatic exposure.[149,150]

The experience of traumatic stress and the development of post-traumatic stress symptoms have been linked to academic problems, school truancy and suspension, social withdrawal, aggressive and delinquent behavior, substance use and abuse, thought problems, emotional problems, poor physical health, suicidal ideation, and suicide attempts.[9,12,13,18,151] In addition, adults who experienced developmental trauma are at higher risk for anxiety, depression, and dissociative disorders.[152] Fifty-nine percent of adult psychiatric inpatients have experienced trauma before the age of 16.[153]

The experience of traumatic stress during development can have far-reaching public health consequences. Some adult health risk behaviors (such as smoking, obesity, numerous sexual partners, and a sedentary lifestyle) and associated medical diseases (such as sexually transmitted diseases, cancer, diabetes, cardiac disease, and chronic bronchitis and emphysema) have been shown to occur more often in adults abused as children.[151]

A large amount of variability has been found in the course and prognosis of childhood PTSD, with some children showing a delayed reaction, others showing early reaction and a gradual decrease over time, and still others demonstrating a high relapse rate after initial recovery.[20] Longitudinal research on the course of PTSD resulting from childhood trauma suggests that while some children may recover from PTSD relatively quickly, others may have symptoms that persist for 5 to 10 years or more.[19,20] If left untreated, childhood problems resulting from trauma may become chronic and persist into adolescence and adulthood. In fact, because traumamimetic triggers can cause relapse, it is recommended that intermittent therapeutic sessions follow the initial phase of treatment. Although there has been limited study of prognostic factors in children, a supportive environment, motivation, insight, and psychological mindedness help engagement in treatment.

8. Intervention

8.1. *Outcome studies*

The potential for chronicity[19,20] and relapse[20] of post-traumatic symptoms make early treatment imperative. Research suggests that cognitive-behavioral therapy (CBT) may be the treatment method of choice for traumatized youth. Several uncontrolled studies of cognitive behavioral treatment have demonstrated reductions in children's PTSD symptomatology, depression, anxiety, and anger following treatment.[154–156]

The few experimental studies that have been done with traumatized children show similar results. Studies comparing children treated with CBT to wait-list controls have shown positive therapeutic effects on PTSD, fear, anxiety, and depression.[157,158] A study comparing trauma-focused (TF-CBT) to supportive therapy found that TF-CBT had a significantly greater impact on traumatized preschool children's behavior problems posttreatment[159] and at 6 and 12-month follow-ups.[120,160]

Finally, a large randomized controlled study comparing TF-CBT and child-centered interventions for sexually abused youth and adolescents found that CBT resulted in significantly less PTSD, depression, behavior problems, shame, and abuse-related attributions in trauma survivors.[161] The parents involved in the CBT condition also had significantly less depression and distress and showed significantly more support and effective parenting toward their children post-treatment than did those parents in the child-centered condition.[161]

In addition to these cognitive behavioral components, several other methods have been successfully applied in treating young trauma survivors. Some studies have used a more expressive therapeutic approach and have shown success in treating post-traumatic symptoms.[162,163] Other studies have included parental training and/or treatment in addition to child CBT, resulting in positive effects in both the children and the parents.[154,159,79] Finally, many studies involve psychoeducation of both trauma survivors and their parents.[118,120,154,157–160,79]

8.2. *Exposure*

There are several key components of cognitive-behavioral treatment for children and adolescents. The behavioral technique of exposure to the trauma narrative and traumatic reminders has been applied in several studies.[154,156–159] Exposure helps to unpair ongoing feelings of fear from traumatic reminders.[164] Over time, exposure techniques can decrease trauma-related fear through the process of extinction.[130] The mental link between the trauma and the ongoing sense of fear and threat can be broken and the trauma can be placed in the past rather than the present.[164]

Child trauma studies have employed various forms of exposure, including imaginal flooding,[165] gradual exposure,[154] and systematic desensitization.[156] In gradual exposure, trauma cues and fear are unpaired through the process of habituation: the patient comes to tolerate symptoms of anxiety, and, eventually, no longer experiences the anxiety when presented with trauma reminders.[166] In contrast, systematic desensitization pairs exposure with relaxation techniques, leading a patient to feel the mutually exclusive sensations of anxiety and relaxation simultaneously.

Since trauma memories are often stored as sensations and feelings rather than as verbal narratives, it can be difficult for survivors to express their traumatic experiences verbally.[121] Verbalization may be particularly difficult for children.[167] Child therapy studies often allow for children to explore the trauma through imagery, play, and art, but generally have the ultimate goal of helping the patient to verbalize the trauma.[154]

Verbalization can be aided by a strong therapeutic alliance. One of the most important tasks of the early sessions of therapy with traumatized youth is building rapport.[154,155,168] Support from the therapist can help the patient manage the difficult therapeutic tasks that lay ahead.[80,163] The strength of the therapeutic alliance between the therapist and the patient has been found to be a predictor of PTSD symptom improvement in adult survivors of childhood abuse.[169]

Due to the trauma cue sensitivity experienced by survivors, many therapies include a cue exposure component in addition to narrative exposure. The trauma narrative has been used as a starting point to help identify cues.[157] The trauma narrative can also serve to expose the cognitive distortions and misattributions that survivors may develop subsequent to trauma.[164] Once cues are identified, they can be explored in relation to a patient's current distress, arousal, and avoidance,[157] with a particular focus on the cues that are of most concern to the child.[156] The cues can be approached gradually, beginning with imaginal exposure and role-plays within therapy, and progressing to *in vivo* at home assignments.

8.3. *Cognitive restructuring*

Repeated and graded exposure in therapy allows trauma survivors to begin to work through cognitive errors such as self-blame and guilt and work toward more positive attributions.[131] More direct cognitive restructuring techniques are also often included in addition to exposure,[154,156–159] often targeting such common post-traumatic beliefs as the sense that nowhere is safe, a short life is inevitable, the traumatized person is losing their mind, and others are untrustworthy. This process involves identifying the patient's current cognitions and the basis for them, and replacing them with more accurate ones.[130]

Cognitive processing therapy, a form of cognitive-behavioral therapy originally developed for adult sexual assault victims has also been modified for use with child trauma survivors.[156,159] This therapy attempts to help trauma survivors change the trauma's meaning and learn to assign appropriate meaning to both the trauma and their ongoing lives.[170] This is accomplished through cognitive reframing[159] and through providing corrective information on cognitive distortions and misattributions.[156] Other therapies use similar techniques, reprocessing the trauma to clarify distortions and misattributions,[157] and replacing negative cognitions with positive self-talk.[155] Other components of cognitive restructuring include assertiveness training,[159] self-efficacy development,[156] and redefining the patient as a survivor rather than a victim.[162]

The combination of exposure and cognitive restructuring techniques in trauma therapy enables the process of transforming traumatic memories from the sensory system to the verbal memory system. Through overcoming the pathological post-traumatic avoidance symptoms and processing the trauma consciously and verbally, intrusive emotional and physiological post-traumatic symptoms may also be overcome. According to this view, therapy is the process of creating detailed, controllable verbal memories, which inhibit the activation of sensory and emotional memories.[134] This process involves elaborating memories and integrating them into a coherent view of the self and the world.[6] The continual retelling of the trauma through narrative exposure leads to both symptom reduction and cognitive change.[164] Upon each retelling, the narrative should become less affective, less sensory, and more verbal.[164]

8.4. *Relaxation and coping skills*

Exposure can also be paired with relaxation and cognitive coping skills training.[79] Prior studies have used relaxation training components including cue-controlled and differential relaxation, [158] muscle relaxation, and diaphragmatic breathing,[156] as well as cognitive tools such as the fear thermometer,[164,156] and the traffic light. In their study of traumatized adolescents, Goenjian and colleagues[157] had patients develop their own relaxation strategies, such as listening to music or spending time with friends, in addition to those provided by the therapist. The identification and development of coping skills tailored to the individual patient has also been suggested by others as an effective tool when working with this population.[164]

The relaxation and cognitive coping tools gained during therapy can be helpful both within the therapy sessions and homework, and in a child's everyday life. Within therapy, they provide tools to help the patient manage the direct discussion of the traumatic event.[158] It is for this reason that these skills are often taught before the exposure aspect of the therapy. The skills learned within therapy can also generalize to the patient's everyday life, helping his/her feel in control of his/her feelings and providing him/her with skills to deal with the hyperarousal and reexperiencing symptoms that may result from trauma.[78,170] For instance, the child might be encouraged to use one of the techniques to help him/her fall asleep at night or to prevent intrusive thoughts during the school day.[157]

In addition to the role they play as relaxation tools, the patient-developed activities can serve as psychological rest and as a means to express trauma-related emotions. Art, play, and movement have been used as a means of rest and expression in several other child trauma therapies.[154,157,162,163] In addition to these benefits, it is suggested that aerobic exercise may help to facilitate cognitive acceptance of physiological arousal. Indeed, aerobic exercise shows promising early results as a treatment for adult post-traumatic stress disorder.[171] Moderate regular exercise was shown to decrease the amount and intensity of post-traumatic symptoms in adults with PTSD.[171]

8.5. *Targeting emotions*

Because of the link between cognitions and emotions,[133] exploration and expression of trauma-related emotions is another core aspect of trauma treatment. A few treatment studies have used interventions designed to allow for the expression of trauma-related grief, fear, and anger.[162,163] These studies have used art, play, discussion, and role-plays to facilitate emotional expression.[162,163] This direct targeting of emotions has been shown to have a positive impact on children's post-traumatic symptoms.[162,163]

8.6. *Parental involvement*

Because of the impact familial support and functioning can have on children's post-traumatic reactions and improvement in therapy, parental involvement in treatment is considered one of the integral components of child trauma treatment.[78] Parental distress and parental support have been found to be predictive of children's adjustment and outcome directly following treatment[159] and at 6 and 12-month post-treatment follow-ups.[120] Several studies have paired cognitive behavioral interventions with caretaker involvement and shown significant improvements in children's internalizing and externalizing behavior problems.[154,159] Such parent and child intervention studies have also found improvements in parents' appropriate parenting practices and emotional reactions to their children's trauma.[119,79]

Parents can play several important roles in child trauma treatment, helping to give their child a sense of safety and support[130] and manage the post-traumatic symptoms.[154,159] Prior interventions with children suffering from anxiety disorders have included a parental update session designed to allow parents to voice their ideas and give input on the child's problem areas, and to allow the therapist to reemphasize the treatment's focus and encourage parental support and compliance with treatment.[168] Therapies aimed specifically at traumatized youth have also emphasized the importance of parents in the treatment process.[154] Parental interventions have included training parents to communicate more effectively with their child, to discuss the traumatic experience in order to help with trauma processing, and to respond therapeutically to the child's post-traumatic fears, anxieties, and other symptom.[154,159,79]

8.7. *Psychoeducation*

Another important aspect of trauma intervention is providing patients with psychoeducation about their conditions and the treatment process. Parent and child education programs have been tested as a key component in several different efficacious treatment programs for traumatized children.[154,155,158,159,79] Prior studies have included educational components ranging from a discussion of treatment goals and the treatment framework[155] to providing a treatment rationale,[155,79] to educating about the general effects of trauma and the specific effects of different kinds of trauma, such as sexual abuse.[158,79] Psychoeducation allows the child and parent(s) to understand the rationale for elements of treatment, particularly exposure components, which may otherwise be avoided or declined because of their perceived aversive nature. Trauma intervention can also include educating survivors about the complex interaction of cognition, affect, and physiology in the etiology and symptoms of PTSD.[158] Relationships between thoughts, feelings, and behaviors can also be explored by asking patients to describe what they thought, felt, and did during stressful situations[155] and by exploring the relationship of negative cognitions to negative emotions and behaviors.[130]

8.8. *Emotion-regulation and social skills training*

Research on adult survivors of child abuse suggests that emotional regulation and social skills training is an important aspect of trauma intervention, allowing exposure to proceed more smoothly.[169,172] Child interventions have included education in identifying trauma-related emotions and understanding their links to thoughts, physiological responses, and behavior.[155,79] Several therapies also include training in adaptively managing and expressing trauma-related feelings such as anxiety, anger, and grief.[154,156,163]

8.9. *Psychopharmacology*

The psychopharmacology of trauma-related psychopathology in juveniles is in its infancy. Very few controlled studies are available to guide the clinician, and most treatment decisions are extrapolated from adult results (see Donnelly *et al.*[173] for a review on pediatric PTSD and Marmar *et al.*[174] for a review on adult PTSD psychopharmacology). In our practice, we utilize psychopharmacology in three different scenarios: (1) when the severity of the condition interferes with the child's ability to be an active participant of psychotherapy; (2) when needing to treat comorbidity; and (3) when one of the clusters of PTSD seems to predominate over others and it is severe in nature. The effect of trauma on several physiological systems can inform the choice of medication utilized. For example, alpha-2-agonists can help reduce sympathetic tone (hyperarousal, impulsivity). Because of the role of the dopaminergic system in frontal lobe activation, we reserve the use of atypical neuroleptics for treating psychosis, aggression, and self-injurious behaviors. Negative affect, such as anxiety, depression, and impulse control as well as agitation and hyperarousal symptoms in the presence of prolonged trauma may be reduced with antiepileptic medications,[175] supporting the conceptualization of chronic trauma as a kindled form of a psychopathological limbic system response.[66]

The first line for pharmacological treatment of anxiety and depression in children are the Selective Seratonin Reuptake Inhibitors (SSRIs). These medications are thought to delay disinhibition of 5-HT neurotransmission, resulting in more 5-HT being released from the axon terminal. Atypical antidepressants' mechanisms of action may involve receptors for the noradrenaline and dopamine systems as well as the serotonin system. Opioid antagonist can be utilized to decrease the potential increase in opioid release during self-injurious behaviors and substance abuse. Benzodiazepines can be used during the initial phase of treatment of severe comorbid anxiety. Future research on pharmacological treatment should include longitudinal outcome studies, treatment combination studies, and cross-over designs. New methods, such as functional magnetic resonance imaging, may be helpful in tracking improvement along with behavioral profiles.

8.10. *Termination phase of treatment*

Termination can be a difficult time for all children, but may be particularly difficult for traumatized kids who have prior experience with loss.[41] It is therefore important to begin to discuss termination issues early. Parents can also serve as helpers in the termination process.[24] The final sessions of exposure therapy should focus on summarizing, reviewing, reinforcing, and promoting generalization of the exposure and the coping and emotional control skills gained through therapy.[154,156] They might also emphasize the use of positive self-talk to counter PTSD intrusions and enforce a sense of personal efficacy.[156] Prior interventions have also included brainstorming future anxiety-provoking scenarios and how to apply coping skills to them.[24,155]

Other goals of the termination process include evaluating the progress made in treatment,[154] and emphasizing the child's achievements.[24] The potential for symptoms to return and the need for relapse prevention techniques such as therapy booster sessions should also be stressed.[156,157] The therapist must also address any preexisting comorbid disorders and their continued treatment.[78] Finally, the therapist should offer the patient and his/her parent(s) a list of referrals and resources to be used in the future if necessary.[24]

Although there is little consensus as to whether individual or group modalities are best suited to working with traumatized populations, some evidence does suggest that individual treatments are superior. A study comparing individual and group therapy for sexually abused girls found that, while the two conditions did not differ in general functioning following therapy, the individual condition showed more improvement in post-traumatic symptoms.[176] A metaanalysis of PTSD treatment studies of sexually victimized women found that individual therapeutic interventions had better outcomes overall than group interventions.[177]

Atypical intervention settings

In this chapter, we have given a conceptual framework for a multimodal approach to treatment of traumatized children. In addition to using this approach in our clinics, we have treated children at schools with the aid of a structured multimodal manual that is currently under development. School-based interventions have been applied with good outcomes, such as the Cognitive Behavioral Intervention for Trauma in Schools (CBITS).[178] Further, utilizing the consult liaison model, therapists can use these intervention components when treating children in hospital or primary care settings who have suffered trauma secondary to having severe medical conditions (see Chap. 13 of this handbook).

9. Experiences in Our Clinic

A hybrid approach — The case of Sammy

Sammy, an 11-year-old boy, was brought to our clinic because of increased aggression toward his siblings. His mom reported that this was very uncharacteristic of Sammy's previous demeanor. She also reported decreased academic performance. Feeling guilty and confused, she reported to the authorities that Sammy's father had regularly abused her and the children physically and emotionally for a number of years. Sammy had been hit numerous times with metal bars, wooden rods, and bamboo sticks. Sammy's mother felt the boy's behavior was directed at her for "breaking the family up"; mom and kids were now living in a new apartment after the father had been arrested and deported. Sammy had nightmares and difficulty sleeping. He scored 32 in his PTSD RI (moderate PTSD).

Sessions 1–5: Education into PTSD symptoms enabled mom to manage Sammy's nighttime episodes. Despite initial resistance, Sammy found relaxation exercises gave him a sense of control and a feeling of calmness. With support, guidance, and a structured mean to avoid suggestion, Sammy told his story (narrative). He now felt safe (his sense of security increased further as mom learned not to avoid him), but he also missed his father. During the aggressive episodes he felt confused, as in a daze and his heart rate would accelerate. After taking out his feelings on his siblings, he would feel guilty and ashamed.

Sessions 6–10: Sammy and his mother were introduced to the concept of traumatic cues. His father's violence was explored as a fearful event. Cues surrounding this event were most commonly neutral (not good or bad), but were reminders to his brain of the traumatic event. Sammy stated that when mom came home, the slamming of the car door reminded him of his father coming home. His brain associated these cues to aggression (classical conditioning). When exposed to the cue, an aggressive response would result. Sammy and his mother were taught how responses are characterized by four components: cognitive, physical, emotional and behavioral. We concentrated on changing any of these components as a means to develop appropriate responses (generalization).

Sessions 7–15: Although impossible to identify all pertinent cues, our ability to address some cues helped Sammy make a connection between history and behavior. The goal was not to get rid of the cues, but to be able to tolerate them as nonthreatening. Behavioral desensitization with gradual cue exposure (first; imagining, later; in-session and later; *in vivo*) helped Sammy develop new responses and strengthen his self-efficacy. He learned to process discordant emotions. By termination, Sammy was doing better at school, not arguing with his mother, not hitting his siblings and feeling better about his accomplishments. He scored 5 in his PTSD reaction score (subclinical).

9.1. *Outcomes in our clinic*

The case of Sammy illustrates a straightforward case. He was motivated, intelligent, and psychologically minded. When the trauma narrative is focused and there is a caring and consistent support system, we have found that individuals respond favorably to our cue-centered intervention. We have identified a second group of children that respond effectively to a second wave of intervention, basically repeating the sessions again. These children usually have difficulties focusing either secondary to physiological arousal or dissociative symptoms. These children need more time to engage in therapy and are prepared to be more active on the second round of intervention. For other kids, the protocol is part of an ongoing supportive and insight-oriented longer-term therapy. This group is characterized by increased severity, comorbidity, and chronic upheaval in their environment. No child has refused all components of the multimodal intervention. Children may refuse to talk about what happened to them, but they are usually open to address it in some fashion either through art work or play therapy. This manual continues to be under development and is being piloted in a school setting.

10. Upcoming Challenges

The field of developmental traumatology has advanced significantly during the past 15 years. Advancements have been made in the areas of epidemiology, phenomenology, biology, and treatment. However, the heterogeneity of children's experience of trauma and its sequelae will require a more specific and targeted approach. We need to continue to gather empirical data for treatment interventions and direct those interventions to specific populations. These subgroups will vary according to the type of trauma experienced, duration of the trauma, developmental age when the trauma occurred, current age, and other significant factors. New methodology, such as functional imaging, will help identify brain networks that have been impacted by chronic stress. This type of method will also aid in empirically validating different types of treatments. It is critical to note, however, that currently imaging has not reach this clinical utility and it is a research tool at this time. Other methods, such as psychophysiology and hormonal assessments will continue to give us insight into how trauma and stress affects biological systems during development. Neuropsychological testing will continue to increase our knowledge on cognitive function before and after trauma and before and after treatment.

References

1. Caspi A, Sugden K, Moffitt TE. Influence of life stress on depression: Moderation by a polymorphism in the 5-HTT gene, *Science* 2003; **301**(5631): 386–389.
2. McEwen BS. Allostasis and allostatic load: Implications for neuropsychopharmacology, *Neuropsychopharmacology*. 2003; **22**: 108–124.
3. Charney DS, Deutch AY, Krystal JH, Southwick SM, Davis M. Psychobiologic mechanisms of post-traumatic stress disorder, *Arch Gen Psychiatry* 1993; **50**(4): 294–305.
4. Mowrer OH. *Learning Theory and Behavior*. New York: Wiley, 1960.
5. Brewin CR, Holmes EA. Psychological theories of post-traumatic stress disorder, *Clin Psychol Rev* 2003; **23**(3): 339–376.
6. Ehlers A, Clark DM. A cognitive model of post-traumatic stress disorder, *Behav Res Ther* 2000; **38**(4): 319–345.
7. National Institute of Mental Health. *Helping Children and Adolescents Cope with Violence and Disasters*. (DHHS Publication No. 01–3518). Washington DC: U.S. Government Printing Office, 2001.
8. Carrion VG, Steiner H. Trauma and dissociation in delinquent adolescents, *J Am Acad Child Adolesc Psychiatry* 2000; **39**(3): 353–359.
9. Lansford JE, Dodge KA, Pettit GS, Bates JE, Crozier J, Kaplow J. A 12-year prospective study of the long-term effects of early child physical maltreatment on psychological, behavioral, and academic problems in adolescence, *Archiv Pediatr Adolesc Med* 2002; **156**(8): 824–830.
10. Carney NJ, Butter HJ, Persinger MA, Bialik RJ. Physiological and cognitive correlates of child abuse, *J Am Acad Child Adolesc Psychiatry* 1995; **34**: 1067–1075.
11. Kaufman J, Cicchetti D. Effects of maltreatment on school-age children's socioemotional development: Assessment in a day-camp setting, *Dev Psychol* 1989; **25**(4): 516–524.

12. Pollak S, Cicchetti D, Klorman R. Stress, memory, and emotion: Developmental considerations from the study of child maltreatment, *Dev Psychopathol* 1998; **10**(4): 811–828.
13. Rieder C, Cicchetti D. Organizational perspective on cognitive control functioning and cognitive-affective balance in maltreated children, *Dev Psychol* 1989; **25**(3): 382–393.
14. De Bellis MD, Keshavan MS, Clark DB, *et al.* Developmental traumatology: II. Brain development, *Biol Psychiatry* 1999; **45**(10): 1271–1284.
15. Vostanis P. The impact, psychological sequelae and management of trauma affecting children, *Curr Opin Psychiatry* 2004; **17**(4): 269–273.
16. Fullerton CS, Ursano RJ, Norwood AE, Holloway HH. Trauma, terrorism and disaster. In: Ursano RJ, Fullerton CS, Norwood AE, Eds. *Terrorism and Disaster: Individual and Community Mental Health Interventions.* New York, NY: Cambridge University Press, 2003, pp. 1–20.
17. Cuffe SP, Addy CL, Garrison CZ, Waller JL, *et al.* Prevalence of PTSD in a community sample of older adolescents, *J Am Acad Child Adolesc Psychiatry* 1998; **37**(2): 147–154.
18. Silverman AB, Reinherz HZ, Giaconia RM. The long-term sequelae of child and adolescent abuse: A longitudinal study, *Child Abuse Negl* 1996; **20**(8): 709–723.
19. Yule W, Bolton D, Udwin O, Boyle S, O'Ryan D, Nurrish J. The long-term psychological effects of a disaster experienced in adolescence: I: The incidence and course of PTSD, *J Child Psychol Psychiatry* 2000; **41**(4): 503–511.
20. Sack WH, Him C, Dickason D. Twelve-year follow-up study of Khmer youths who suffered massive war trauma as children, *J Acad Child Adolesc Psychiatry* 1999; **38**(9): 1173–1179.
21. Famularo R, Fenton T, Kinscherff R, Ayoub C. Maternal and child post-traumatic stress disorder in cases of maltreatment, *Child Abuse Negl* 1994; **18**(1): 27–36.
22. McLeer SV, Dixon JF, Henry D, *et al.* Psychopathology in non-clinically referred sexually abused children, *J Am Acad Child Adolesc Psychiatry* 1998; **37**(12): 1326–1333.
23. Deykin EY, Buka SL. Prevalence and risk factors for post-traumatic stress disorder among chemically dependent adolescents, *Am J Psychiatry* 1997; **154**(6): 752–757.
24. Silva RR, Alpert M, Munoz DM, Singh S, Matzner F, Dummit S. Stress and vulnerability to post-traumatic stress disorder in children and adolescents, *Am J Psychiatry* 2000; **157**(8): 1229–1235.
25. Brosky BA, Lally SJ. Prevalence of trauma, PTSD, and dissociation in court-referred adolescents, *J Interpers Violence* 2004; **19**(7): 801–814.
26. Plattner B, Silvermann MA, Redlich AD, *et al.* Pathways to dissociation: Intrafamilial versus extrafamilial trauma in juvenile delinquents, *J Nerv Ment Dis* 2003; **191**(12): 781–788.

27. Perrin S, Smith P, Yule W. Treatment of PTSD in children and adolescents. In: Barrett PM, Ollendick TH, Eds. *Handbook of Interventions that Work with Children and Adolescents: Prevention and Treatment*. Chichester: Wiley, 2004; pp. 217–242.
28. Kean EM, Kelsay K, Wamboldt F, Wamboldt MZ. Post-traumatic stress in adolescents with asthma and their parents, *J Am Acad Child Adolesc Psychiatry* 2006; **45**(1): 78–86.
29. Erickson SJ, Steiner H. Trauma spectrum adaptation: Somatic symptoms in long term pediatric cancer survivors, *Psychosomatics* 2000; **41**(4): 339–346.
30. Erickson SJ, Steiner, H. Trauma and personality correlates in long term pediatric cancer survivors, *Child Psychiatry Human Development* 2001; **31**(3): 195–213.
31. Kazak AE, Alderfer MA, Rourke MT, Simms S, Streisand R, Grossman JR. Post-traumatic stress disorder (PTSD) and post-traumatic stress symptoms (PTSS) in families of adolescent childhood cancer survivors, *J Pediatr Psychol* 2004; **29**(3): 211–219.
32. Landoldt MA, Vollrath M, Ribi K, Gnehm HE, Sennhauser FH. Incidence and associations of parental and child post-traumatic stress symptoms in pediatric patients, *J Child Psychol Psychiatry* 2003; **44**(8): 1199–1207.
33. Taieb O, Moro MR, Baubet T, Revah-Levy A, Flament MF. Post-traumatic stress symptoms after childhood cancer, *Eur Child Adolesc Psychiatry* 2003; **12**(6): 255–264.
34. Gillies ML, Barton J, DiGallo A. Follow-up of young road accident victims, *J Trauma Stress* 2003; **16**(5): 523–526.
35. Nugent NR, Christopher NC, Delahanty DL. Emergency medical service and in-hospital vital signs as predictors of subsequent PTSD symptom severity in pediatric injury patients, *J Child Psychol Psychiatry* 2006; **47**(9): 919–926.
36. Stallard P, Salter E, Velleman R. Posttraumatic stress disorder following road traffic accidents, *Eur Child Adolesc Psychiatry* 2004; **13**(3): 172–178.
37. Stoddard FJ, Saxe G, Ronfeldt H, *et al.* Acute stress symptoms in young children with burns, *J Am Acad Child Adolesc Psychiatry* 2006; **45**(1): 87–93.
38. Thienkrua W, Cardozo BL, Chakkraband MS, *et al.* Symptoms of post-traumatic stress disorder and depression among children in tsunami-affected areas of Southern Thailand, *J Am Med Assoc* 2006; **296**(5): 549–559.
39. Bulut S. Comparing the earthquake exposed and non-exposed Turkish children's post-traumatic stress reactions, *Anales de Psicologia* 2006; **22**(1): 29–36.
40. Hoven CW, Duarte CS, Lucas CP, *et al.* Psychopathology among New York City public school children 6 months after September 11, *Arch Gen Psychiatry* 2005; **62**(5): 545–552.
41. Ehntholt KA, Yule W. Practitioner review: Assessment and treatment of refugee children and adolescents who have experienced war-related trauma, *J Child Psychol Psychiatry* 2006; **47**(12): 1197–1210.

42. Kinzie JD, Cheng K, Tsai J, Riley C. Traumatized refugee children, *J Nerv Ment Dis* 2006; **194**(7): 534–537.
43. Jarvis KL, Gordon EE, Novaco RW. Psychological distress of children and mothers in domestic violence emergency shelters, *J Fam Violence* 2005; **20**(6): 389–402.
44. Moretti MM, Obsuth I, Odgers CL, Reebye P. Exposure to maternal vs. paternal partner violence, PTSD, and aggression in adolescent girls and boys, *Aggress Behav* 2006; **32**(4): 385–395.
45. Williams R. The psychosocial consequences for children and young people who are exposed to terrorism, war, conflict and natural disasters, *Curr Opin Psychiatry* 2006; **19**(3): 337–349.
46. Steinberg AM, Brymer MJ, Decker KB, Pynoos RS. The University of California at Los Angeles post-traumatic stress disorder reaction index (PTSD-RI), *Curr Psychiatry Rep* 2004; **6**: 96–100.
47. Newman E, Weathers FW, Nader K, *et al. Clinician Administered PTSD Scale for Children and Adolescents (CAPS-CA).* Los Angeles, CA: Western Psychological Services, 2004.
48. Scheeringa MS, Zeanah CH, Drell, MJ, Larrieu JA. Two approaches to the diagnosis of post-traumatic stress disorder in infancy and early childhood, *J Am Acad Child Adolesc Psychiatry* 1995; **34**(5): 191–200.
49. Birleson P. The validity of depressive disorder in childhood and the development of a self-rating scale: A research report, *J Child Psychol Psychiatry* 1981; **22**(1): 73–88.
50. Lucas CP, Zhang H, Fisher PW, *et al.* The DISC predictive scales (DPS), *J Am Acad Child Adolesc Psychiatry* 2001; **40**(4): 443–449.
51. Dyregrov A, Yule W. A review of PTSD in children, *Child Adolesc Ment Health* 2006; **11**(4): 176–184.
52. Reich W, Leacock N, Shanfield C. *Diagnostic Interview for Children and Adolescents – Revised (DICA-R).* St. Louis, MO: Washington University, 1994.
53. Graham-Bermann SA, DeVoe ER, Mattis JS, Lynch S, Thomas SA. Ecological predictors of traumatic stress symptoms in Caucasian and ethnic minority children exposed to intimate partner violence, *Violence Against Women* 2006; **12**(7): 663–692.
54. World Health Organization. *Composite International Diagnostic Interview (CIDI), Version 1.0.* Geneva, Switzerland: World Health Organization, 1990.
55. Gnanadesikan M, Kovins DK, Beals J. The relationship of gender and trauma characteristics to post traumatic stress disorder in a community sample of traumatized Northern Plains American Indian adolescents and young adults, *J Clin Psychiatry* 2005; **66**(9): 1176–1183.
56. Famularo R, Fenton T, Augustyn M, Zuckerman B. Persistence of pediatric post-traumatic stress after two years, *Child Abuse Negl* 1996; **20**(12): 1245–1248.

57. Terr LC. Childhood traumas: An outline and overview, *Am J Psychiatry* 1991; **148**(1): 10–20.
58. American Psychiatric Association. *Diagnostic and Statistical Manual of Mental Disorders*, 4th edition. Washington, DC: American Psychiatric Association, 1994.
59. Scheeringa MS, Peebles CD, Cook CA, Zeanah CH. Toward establishing procedural, criterion, and discriminant validity for PTSD in early childhood, *J Am Acad Child Adolesc Psychiatry* 2001; **40**(1): 52–60.
60. Carrion VG, Weems CF, Ray R, Reiss AL. Toward an empirical definition of pediatric PTSD: The phenomenology of PTSD symptoms in youth, *J Am Acad Child Adolesc Psychiatry* 2001; **41**(2): 166–173.
61. Classen C, Koopman C, Hales R, Spiegel D. Acute stress reactions as a predictor of post-traumatic stress symptoms following office building shootings, *Am J Psychiatry* 1998; **155**: 620–624.
62. Marmar CR, Weiss DS, Schlenger WE, Fairbank JA, Jordan BK, Kulka RA, *et al.* Peritraumatic dissociation and post-traumatic stress in male Vietnam theater veterans, *Am J Psychiatry* 1994; **151**: 902–907.
63. Shalev A, Peri T, Canetti L, Schreiber S. Predictors of PTSD in injured trauma survivors: A prospective study, *Am J Psychiatry* 1996; **153**: 219–225.
64. Spiegel D, Koopman C, Cardenã E, Classen C. Dissociative symptoms in the diagnosis of acute stress disorder. In: Michelson LK, Ray WJ, Eds. *Handbook of Dissociation*: *Theoretical, Empirical, and Clinical Perspectives*, New York: Plenum Press, 1996, pp. 367–380.
65. Simeon D, Guralnik O, Schmeidler J, *et al.* The role of childhood interpersonal trauma in depersonalization disorder, *Am J Psychiatry* 2001; **158**: 1027–1033.
66. Steiner H, Carrion V, Plattner B, Koopman C. Dissociative symptoms in post-traumatic stress disorder: Diagnosis and treatment. In: Laor N, Ed. *Child Adolesc Psychiatric Clinics North America* 2003; **122**(2): 231–249.
67. Butler LD, Duran REF, Jasiukaitis P, *et al.* Hypnotizability and traumatic experience: A diathesisstress model of dissociative symptomatology, *Am J Psychiatry* 1996; **153**(Suppl): 42–63.
68. Spiegel D. Dissociation and hypnosis in post-traumatic stress disorders, *J Traumatic Stress* 1988; **1**: 17–33.
69. Putnam FW. Dissociation in children and adolescents: A developmental perspective, New York: Guilford Press, 1997.
70. Terr L. Childhood traumas: An outline and overview, *Am J Psychiatry* 1991; **148**: 10–20.
71. World Health Organization. *The ICD-10 Classification of Mental and Behavioural Disorders, Clinical Descriptions and Diagnostic Guidelines*, Geneva: World Health Organization, 1992.

72. Kletter H, Weems CF, Carrion VG. Guilt and post-traumatic stress symptoms in child victims of interpersonal violence, *Clin Child Psychol Psychiatry* 2009; **14**(1): 71–83.
73. Perrin S, Smith P, Yule W. Practitioner review: The assessment and treatment of posttraumatic stress disorder in children and adolescents, *J Child Psychol Psychiatry* 2000; **41**(3): 277–289.
74. Dykma, RA, Ackerman, PT, Newton JE, Joseph EO. Post-traumatic stress disorder: A sensitization reaction, *Integrative Physiol Beh Sci* 1997; **32**(1): 75–83.
75. Fletcher K. The childhood PTSD interview-child form. In: Carlson E, Ed. *Trauma Assessments: A Clinician's Guide*. New York, NY: Guilford Press, 1997, pp. 248–250.
76. Wozniak J, Crawford MH, Biederman J, *et al.* Antecedents and complications of trauma in boys with ADHD: Findings from a longitudinal study, *J Am Acad Child Adolesc Psychiatry* 1999; **38**(1): 48–55.
77. Reebye P, Moretti MM, Wiebe VJ. Symptoms of posttraumatic stress disorder in adolescents with conduct disorder: Sex differences and onset patterns, *Can J Psychiatry* 2000; **45**(8): 746–751.
78. American Academy of Child and Adolescent Psychiatry. Practice parameters for the assessment and treatment of children and adolescents with post-traumatic stress disorder, *J Am Acad Child Adolesc Psychiatry* 1998; **37**(Suppl): 4S–26S.
79. Deblinger E, Stauffer LB, Steer RA. Comparative efficacies of supportive and cognitive behavioral group therapies for young children who have been sexually abused and their nonoffending mothers, *Child Maltreat* 2001; **6**(4): 332–343.
80. American Psychiatric Association. Acute stress disorder and post-traumatic stress disorder part A: Treatment recommendations, *Am J Psychiatry* 2004; **161**(Suppl. 11): 4–31.
81. Ruggiero KJ, Morris TL, Scotti JR. Treatment for children with post-traumatic stress disorder: Current status and future directions, *Clin Psychol Sci Prac* 2001; **8**(2): 210–227.
82. American Psychiatric Association. *Diagnostic and Statistical Manual of the Mental Disorders,* 4th edition rev. Washington, DC: American Psychiatric Association, 2000.
83. March, JS. Assessment of pediatric post-traumatic stress disorder. In: Saigh PA, Bremner JD, Eds. *Post-traumatic Stress Disorder: A Comprehensive Text.* Needham Heights, MA: Allyn and Bacon, 1998: pp. 199–218.
84. Silverman WK, Albano AM. *ADIS: Anxiety Disorders Interview Schedule for DSM-IV: Child version*. San Antontio, TX: Psychological Corporation, 1996.
85. Cortes AM, Saltzman KM, Weems, CF, Regnault HP, Reiss AL, Carrion VG. Development of anxiety disorders in traumatized pediatric population: A preliminary longitudinal evaluation, *Child Abuse Neglect* 2005; **29**(8): 905–914.

86. Hawkins SS, Radcliffe, J. Current measures of PTSD for children and adolescents, *J Pediatr Psychol* 2006; **31**(4): 420–430.
87. Keppel-Benson JM, Ollendick TH, Benson MJ. Post-traumatic stress in children following motor vehicle accidents, *J Child Psychol Psychiatry* 2002; **43**(2): 203–212.
88. Kaufman J, Birmaher, B, Brent D, *et al*. Schedule for affective disorder and schizophrenia for school-age children-present and lifetime version (K-SADS-PL): Initial reliability and validity, *J Am Acad Child Adolesc Psychiatry* 1997; **36**(7): 980–988.
89. Fletcher K. Childhood post-traumatic stress disorder. In: Mash, EJ, Barkley RA, Eds. *Child Psychopathology, 2nd edition* New York, NY: Guilford Press, 2003; pp. 330–371.
90. Saigh PA, Yasik AE, Oberfield R, Indamar S, Rubinstein H, Nester J. *The development and validation of the DSM-IV version of the Children's Post-traumatic Stress Disorder Inventory.* Unpublished.
91. Kazak AE, Kassam-Adams N, Schneider S, Zelikovsky N, Alderfer MA, Rourke M. An integrative model of pediatric medical traumatic stress, *J Pediatr Psychol* 2006; **31**(4): 343–355.
92. Foa EB, Johnson KM, Feeny NC, Treadwell KH. The child PTSD symptom scale: A preliminary examination of its psychometric properties, *J Clin Child Psychol* 2001; **30**(3): 376–384.
93. Weiss DS, Marmar CR. The impact of events scale-revised. In: Wilson JP, Keane TM, Eds. *Assessing Psychological Trauma and PTSD*. New York, NY: Guilford Press, 1997, pp. 399–411.
94. Yule W, Udwin O, Murdock K. The "Jupiter" sinking: Effects on children's fears, depression and anxiety, *J Child Psychol Psychiatry* 1990; **31**(7): 1051–1061.
95. Smith P, Perrin S, Yule W, Rabe-Hesketh S. War-exposure and maternal reactions in the psychological adjustment of children from Bosnia-Hercegovina, *J Child Psychol Psychiatry* 2001; **42**(3): 395–404.
96. Briere J. *Trauma Symptoms Checklist for Children*. Odessa, FL: Psychological Assessment Resources, 1996.
97. Wolfe VV, Gentile C, Sas L, Wolfe DA. Children's impact of traumatic events scale: A measure of post-sexual abuse PTSD symptoms, *Behav Assess* 1991; **13**(4): 359–338.
98. Macksound M. Assessing war trauma in children: A case study of Lebanese children, *J Refug Stud* 1992; **5**: 1–15.
99. Ollendick TH. Reliability and validity of the revised fear survey schedule for children (FSSC-R), *Behav Res Ther* 1983; **21**(6): 685–692.
100. Reynolds C, Richmond B. *Revised Children's Manifest Anxiety Scale Manual (RMCAS)*. Los Angeles, CA: Western Psychological Services, 1985.
101. Kovacs M. *Children's Depression Inventory (CDI)Manual*. North Tonawanda, NY: Multi-Health Systems, 1992.

102. Spirito A, Stark J, Williams C. Development of a brief coping checklist for use with pediatric populations, *J Pediatr Psychol* 1998; **13**: 555–574.

103. Foa EB, Ehlers A, Clark DM, Tolin D, Orsillo SM. The post-traumatic cognitions inventory (PTCI): Development and validation, *Psychol Assess* 1999; **11**(3): 303–314.

104. Tedeschi RG, Calhoun LG. The posttraumatic growth inventory: Measuring the positive legacy of trauma, *J Trauma Stress* 1996; **9**(3): 455–471.

105. Cryder CH, Kilmer RP, Tedeschi RG. An exploratory study of post-traumatic growth in children following a natural disaster, *Am J Orthopsychiatry* 2006; **76**: 65–69.

106. Scheeringa MS, Zeanah CH, Myers L, Putnam FW. New findings on alternative criteria for PTSD in preschool children, *J Am Acad Child Adolesc Psychiatry* 2003; **42**(5): 561–570.

107. Achenbach T. *Achenbach System of Empirically Based Assessment.* Burlington, VT: ASEBA Publications, 2000.

108. Carr A. Interventions for post-traumatic stress disorder in children and adolescents, *Pediatr Rehabil* 2004; **7**(4): 231–244.

109. Dehon C, Scheeringa MS. Screening for preschool posttraumatic stress disorder with the child behavior checklist, *J Pediatr Psychol* 2006; **31**(4): 431–435.

110. Caffo E, Forresi B, Lievers LS. Impact, psychological sequelae and management of trauma affecting children and adolescents, *Curr Opin Psychiatry* 2005; **18**(4): 422–428.

111. Walker JL, Carey PD, Mohr N, Stein DJ, Seedat S. Gender differences in the prevalence of childhood sexual abuse and in the development of pediatric PTSD, *Arch Womens Ment Health* 2004; **7**(2): 111–121.

112. Zatzick DF, Grossman DC, Russo J, *et al.* Predicting post-traumatic stress symptoms longitudinally in a representative sample of hospitalized injured adolescents, *J Am Acad Child Adolesc Psychiatry* 2006; **45**(10): 1188–1195.

113. Breslau N, Chilcoat HD, Kessler RC, Davis GC. Previous exposure to trauma and PTSD effects of subsequent trauma: Results from the Detroit area survey of trauma, *Am J Psychiatry* 1999; **156**(6): 902–907.

114. Daviss WB, Mooney D, Racusin R, Ford JD, Fleischer A, McHugo GJ. Predicting post-traumatic stress after hospitalization for pediatric injury, *J Am Acad Child Adolesc Psychiatry* 2000; **39**(5): 576–583.

115. Stoppelbein LA, Greening L, Elkin D. Risk of post-traumatic stress symptoms: A comparison of child survivors of pediatric cancer and parental bereavement, *J Pediatr Psychol* 2006; **31**(4): 367–376.

116. Stallard P, Smith E. Appraisals and cognitive coping styles associated with chronic post-traumatic symptoms in child road traffic accident survivors, *J Child Psychol Psychiatry* 2007; **48**(2): 194–201.

117. Dyb G, Holen A, Braenne K, Indredavik M, Aarseth J. Parent-child discrepancy in reporting children's post-traumatic stress reactions after a traffic accident, *Nordic J Psychiatry* 2003; **57**(5): 339–344.
118. Cohen JA, Mannarino AP. Predictors of treatment outcome in sexually abused children, *Child Abuse Negl* 2000; **24**(7): 983–994.
119. Brown EJ, Kolko DJ. Child victims' attributions about being physically abused: An examination of factors associated with symptom severity, *J Abnorm Child Psychol* 1999; **27**(4): 311–322.
120. Cohen JA, Mannarino AP. Factors that mediate treatment outcome of sexually abused preschool children: Six- and 12-month follow-up, *J Am Acad Child Adolesc Psychiatry* 1998; **37**(1): 44–51.
121. Brewin CR. A cognitive neuroscience account of post-traumatic stress disorder and its treatment, *Behav Res Ther* 2001; **39**(4): 373–393.
122. Saltzman KM, Weems CF, Carrion VG. IQ and post-traumatic stress symptoms in children exposed to interpersonal violence, *Child Psychiatry Hum Dev* 2006; **36**(3): 261–272.
123. Carrion VG, Weems CF, Ray RD, Glaser B, Hessl D, Reiss AL. Diurnal salivary cortisol in pediatric post-traumatic stress disorder, *Biol Psychiatry* 2002; **51**(7): 575–582.
124. Cicchetti D, Rogosch FA. The impact of child maltreatment and psychopathology on neuroendocrine functioning, *Dev Psychopathol* 2001; **13**(4): 783–804.
125. De Bellis MD, Baum AS, Birmaher B, *et al.* Developmental traumatology: I. Biological stress systems, *Biol Psychiatry* 1999; **45**(10): 539–564.
126. Carrion VG, Weems CF, Eliez S, Reiss AL. Attenuation of frontal asymmetry in pediatric post-traumatic stress disorder, *Biol Psychiatry* 2001; **50**(12): 943–951.
127. Carrion VG, Weems CF, Reiss AL. Stress predicts brain changes in children: A pilot longitudinal study on youth stress, post-traumatic stress disorder, and the hippocampus, *Pediatrics* 2007; **119**(3): 509–516.
128. Kaufman J, Bao-Zhu Y, Douglas-Palumberi H, *et. al.* Social supports and serotonin transporter gene moderate depression in maltreated children, *Proc Natl Acad Sci* 2004; **101**(49): 17316–17321.
129. Ehlers A, Mayou RA, Bryant B. Cognitive predictors of post-traumatic stress disorder in children: Results of a prospective longitudinal study, *Behav Res Ther* 2003; **41**: 1–10.
130. Cohen JA, Mannarino AP, Berliner L, Deblinger E. Trauma-focused cognitive behavioral therapy for children and adolescents: An empirical update, *J Interpers Violence* 2000; **15**(11): 1202–1223.
131. Bower GH, Sivers H. Cognitive impact of traumatic events, *Dev Psychopathol* 1998; **10**(4): 625–653.

132. Mannarino AP, Cohen JA. Abuse-related attributions and perceptions, general attributions, and locus of control in sexually abused girls, *J Interpers Violence* 1996; **11**(2): 162–180.
133. Beck, AT. *Cognitive Therapy and the Emotional Disorders.* Oxford: International Universities Press, 1976.
134. Brewin CR, Dalgleish T, Joseph S. A dual representation theory of post-traumatic stress disorder, *Psychol Rev* 1996; **103**(4): 670–686.
135. Shields A, Cicchetti D. Reactive aggression among maltreated children: The contributions of attention and emotion dysregulation, *J Clin Child Psychol* 1998; **27**(4): 381–395.
136. Shipman KL, Zeman J. Socialization of children's emotion regulation in mother-child dyads: A developmental psychopathology perspective, *Dev Psychopathol* 2001; **13**(2): 317–336.
137. Sachinvala N, von Scotti H, McGuire M, *et al.* Memory, attention, function, and mood among patients with chronic post-traumatic stress disorder, *J Nerv Ment Dis* 2000; **188**(12): 818–823.
138. Vasterling JJ, Duke LM, Brailey K, Constans JI, Allain AN, Sutker PB. Attention, learning, and memory performance and intellectual resources in Vietnam veterans: PTSD and no disorder comparisons, *Neuropsychology* 2002; **16**(1): 5–14.
139. Vasterling JJ, Brailey K, Constans JI, Sutker PB. Attention and memory dysfunction in post-traumatic stress disorder, *Neuropsychology* 1998; **12**(1): 125–133.
140. Gilbertson MW, Gurvits TV, Lasko NB, Orr SP, Pitman RK. Multivariate assessment of explicit memory function in combat veterans with post-traumatic stress disorder, *J Trauma Stress* 2001; **14**(2): 413–432.
141. Gurvits T, Gilbertson MW, Lasko NB, *et al.* Neurologic soft signs in chronic post-traumatic stress disorder, *Arch Gen Psychiatry* 2000; **57**(2): 181–186.
142. McNally RJ, Shin LM. Association of intelligence with severity of post-traumatic stress disorder symptoms in Vietnam combat veterans, *Am J Psychiatry* 1995; **152**(6): 936–938.
143. Samet MJ. A comparative analysis of WISC-III performance of traumatized and non-traumatized children, *Diss Abstr Int: Sect A: Hum Soc Sciences* 1998; **58**(9-A): 3419.
144. Sadeh A, Hayden RM, McGuire JP, Sachs H, Civita R. Somatic, cognitive and emotional characteristics of abused children in a psychiatric hospital, *Child Psychiatry Hum Dev* 1994; **24**(3): 191–200.
145. Beers SR, De Bellis MD. Neuropsychological function in children with maltreatment-related post-traumatic stress disorder, *Am J Psychiatry* 2002; **159**(3): 483–486.
146. Becker DE, Weine SM, Vojdoda D, McGlashan, TH. Case series: PTSD symptoms in adolescent survivors of "ethnic cleansing." Results from a 1-year follow-up study, *J Am Acad Child Adolesc Psychiatry* 1999; **38**(6): 775–781.

147. Pfefferbaum B, Seale TW, McDonald NB, *et al.* Post-traumatic stress two years after the Oklahoma City bombing in youths geographically distant from the explosion, *Psychiatry* 2000; **63**(4): 358–370.
148. Tyano S, Iancu I, Solomon Z, *et al.* Seven-year follow-up of child survivors of a bus-train collision, *J Am Acad Child Adolesc Psychiatry* 1996; **35**(3): 365–373.
149. Mannarino AP, Cohen JA, Smith JA, Moore-Motily S. Six- and twelve-month follow-up of sexually abused girls, *J Interpers Violence* 1991; **6**(4): 494–511.
150. Stuber ML, Nader K, Yasuda P, Pynoos RS, Cohen S. Stress response after pediatric bone marrow transplantation: Preliminary results of a prospective longitudinal study, *J Am Acad Child Adolesc Psychiatry* 1991; **30**(6): 952–957.
151. Felitti VJ, Anda RF, Nordenberg D, *et al.* Relationship of childhood abuse and household dysfunction to many of the leading causes of death in adults: The adverse childhood experiences (ACE) study, *Am J Prev Med* 1998; **14**(4): 245–258.
152. Roesler TA, McKenzie RN. Effects of childhood trauma on psychological functioning in adults sexually abused as children, *J Nerv Ment Dis* 1994; **182**(3): 145–150.
153. Bryer JB, Nelson BA, Miller JB, Krol PA. Childhood sexual and physical abuse as factors in adult psychiatric illness, *Am J Psychiatry* 1987; **144**(11): 1426–1430.
154. Deblinger E, McLeer SV, Henry D. Cognitive behavioral treatment for sexually abused children suffering post-traumatic stress: Preliminary findings, *J Am Acad Child Adolesc Psychiatry* 1990; **29**: 747–752.
155. Farrell SP, Hains AA, Davies WH. Cognitive behavioral interventions for sexually abused children exhibiting PTSD symptomatology, *Behav Ther* 1998; **29**(2): 241–255.
156. March JS, Amaya-Jackson L, Murray MC, Schulte A. Cognitive-behavioral psychotherapy for children and adolescents with post-traumatic stress disorder after a single-incident stressor, *J Am Acad Child Adolesc Psychiatry* 1998; **37**(6): 585–593.
157. Goenjian AK, Karayan I, Pynoos RS *et al.* Outcome of psychotherapy among early adolescents after trauma, *Am J Psychiatry* 1997; **154**(4): 536–542.
158. King NJ, Tonge BJ, Mullen P *et al.* Treating sexually abused children with posttraumatic stress symptoms: A randomized clinical trial, *J Am Acad Child Adolesc Psychiatry* 2000; **39**(11): 1347–1355.
159. Cohen JA, Mannarino AP. A treatment outcome study for sexually abused preschool children: Initial Findings, *J Am Acad Child Adolesc Psychiatry* 1996; **35**(6): 42–50.
160. Cohen JA, Mannarino AP. Factors that mediate treatment outcome of sexually abused preschool children, *J Am Acad Child Adolesc Psychiatry* 1996; **35**(1): 1402–1410.
161. Cohen JA, Deblinger E, Mannarino AP, Steer RA. A multisite, randomized controlled trial for children with sexual abuse-related PTSD symptoms, *J Am Acad Child Adolesc Psychiatry* 2004; **43**(4): 393–493.

162. Galante R, Foa D. An epidemiological study of psychic trauma and treatment effectiveness for children after a natural disaster, *J Am Acad Child Adolesc Psychiatry* 1986; **25**(3): 357–363.
163. Chemtob CM, Nakashima JP, Hamada RS. Psychosocial intervention for post disaster trauma symptoms in elementary school children: A controlled community field study, *Arch Pediatr Adolesc Med* 2002; **156**: 211–216.
164. Silva RP, Cloitre M, Davis L. Early intervention with traumatized children, *Psychiatric Quarterly* 2003; **74**(4): 333–347.
165. Saigh PA. In vitro flooding of an adolescent's post-traumatic stress disorder, *J Clin Child Psychol* 1987; **16**(2): 147–150.
166. Jaycox LH, Foa AB, Morral AR. Influence of emotional engagement and habituation on exposure therapy for PTSD, *J Consult Clin Psychol* 1998; **66**(1): 185–192.
167. Albano AM, Miller PP, Côté G, Barlow DH. Behavioral assessment and treatment of PTSD in prepubertal children: Attention to developmental factors and innovative strategies in the case study of a family, *Cogn Behav Pract* 1997; **4**(2): 245–262.
168. Kendall PC. Treating anxiety disorders in children: Results of a randomized clinical trial, *J Consul Clin Psychol* 1994; **62**(1): 100–110.
169. Cloitre M, Stovall-McClough KC, Miranda R, Chemtob CM. Therapeutic alliance, negative mood regulation, and treatment outcome in child abuse-related post-traumatic stress disorder, *J Consult Clin Psychol* 2004; **72**(3): 411–416.
170. Cohen JA, Perel JM, DeBellis MD, Friedman MJ, Putnam FW. Treating traumatized children: Clinical implications of the psychobiology of post-traumatic stress disorder, *Trauma Violence Abuse* 2002; **3**(2): 91–108.
171. Manger TA. The effects of a community-based aerobic exercise program on post-traumatic stress disorder-related symptoms and concomitant anxiety and depression, *Diss Abstr Int: Sect B: Sci Eng* 2000; **61**(3-B): 1643.
172. Cloitre M, Koenen KC, Cohen LR, Han H. Skills training in affective and interpersonal regulation followed by exposure: A phase-based treatment for PTSD related to childhood abuse, *J Consult Clin Psychol* 2002; **70**(5): 1067–1074.
173. Donnelly CL, Amaya-Jackson L. Post-traumatic stress disorder in children and adolescents: Epidemiology, diagnosis and treatment options, *Paediatric Drugs* 2002; **4**(3): 159–170.
174. Marmar CR, Neylan TC, Schoenfeld FB. New directions in the pharmacotherapy of post-traumatic stress disorder, *Psychiatric Quarterly* 2002; **73**(4): 259–270.
175. Steiner H, Saxena K, Carrion V, Khanzode L, Silverman M, Chang K. Divalproex sodium for the treatment of PTSD and conduct disordered youth: A pilot randomized controlled clinical trial, *Child Psychiatry Hum Dev* 2007; **38**(3); 183–193.
176. Trowell J, Kolvin I, Weermanthri T, *et al.* Psychotherapy for sexually abused girls: Psychopathological outcome findings and patterns of change, *Br J Psychiatry* 2002; **180**(3): 234–247.

177. Chard KM. A meta-analysis of post-traumatic stress disorder treatment outcome studies of sexually victimized women, *Diss Abstr Int: Sect B: Sci Eng* 1995; **55**(10-B): 4589.
178. Stein BD, Jaycox LH, Kataoka SH, Wong M, Tu W, Elliott MN, Fink A. A mental health intervention for schoolchildren exposed to violence: A randomized controlled trial, *JAMA* 2003; **290**(5): 603–611.

Chapter 9

Learning Disorders

Richard D. Abbey

1. Introduction

Learning disorders can have a detrimental affect on the people in whom they occur. Often identified years after they began, learning disorders may cause children, adolescents, and adults to feel defeated, frustrated, and "stupid." It is therefore vital to identify learning disorders as early as possible while the student is still motivated to achieve and perform at a high level. The "wait-to-fail" model often results in underachievement, low self-esteem, and associated emotional problems. Early intervention provides the most favorable prognosis. This chapter focuses on the identification, assessment, and neurobiology of the most common learning disorders.

Learning disorders were first recognized by Pringle-Morton in 1896 and Kerr in 1897.[1] However, the last 25 years of neuroscience research has provided significant advances in our understanding of their neurocognitive phenotypes, which has been made possible by momentous developments in psychological assessment and neuroimaging. Although our knowledge has increased, there remains considerable controversy regarding the diagnosis and treatment of learning disorders.

2. Epidemiology

The prevalence of learning disorders ranges from 2 to 10%.[2,3] However, prevalence rates of learning disorders reported in the literature vary and depend on several factors, including sex, socioeconomic status, medical conditions, language development, the method used to identify them, and the developmental stage in which they are identified. Prevalence rates also vary depending on the type of learning disorder.

Gender ratios of learning disorders vary widely depending on the method of data collection. Clinical studies have found male to female ratios to be as high as 2:1 to 5:1[4]; however, research-identified samples have been closer to 1:1,[5] and experts generally agree that learning disorders occur in both genders at about the same rate. However, boys tend to be identified more often than girls because they tend to be more disruptive with various comorbid conditions (*e.g.* ADHD), and are therefore assessed more frequently.

The prevalence of reading disorders, the most commonly diagnosed learning disorder, ranges from 4%[2] to as high as 20%.[6,7] Although most studies of dyslexia have been conducted with primarily English-speaking populations, cross-language studies are beginning to emerge. Research has found that the prevalence of poor reading skills in French speaking second graders was highly influenced by socioeconomic status (SES), ranging from 3.3% in neighborhoods with high SES to 20.5% in neighborhoods with low SES.[8] Poor readers were identified by deficits in phonological awareness and rapid naming skills while controlling for verbal and non-verbal intelligence. Other research investigating the incidence of dyslexia among young offenders in Kuwait found that more than 20% of them were dyslexic compared to a national average of approximately 6%.[6] Dyslexia is also found in logographic-based languages. For example, out of a sample of 690 Cantonese-speaking Chinese children, 99 (12.6%) of them were dyslexic. [9]

Most research suggests that developmental dyscalculia occurs in about 5–7% of children.[10, 11] A much larger portion of children and adults have less severe difficulties with mathematics which may nevertheless cause problems in academic and occupational functioning.

3. Diagnosis and Assessment

Although a child with symptoms of learning disorders may first present to a pediatrician, psychiatrist, or other professional, psychoeducational and/or neuropsychological assessments are necessary to clinically assess and diagnose a specific learning disability. In addition, assessments vary in depth and breadth, so a failure to diagnose a learning disability may merely reflect a false negative. Evaluations by school "psychologists" are generally completed by Master's level evaluators who may be limited by the resources available to the school. District budgets may restrict the time and scope of testing batteries that the school evaluator is able to administer. Psychologists who have earned their Ph.D. have more extensive training in psychoeducational evaluations, and typically provide a more in-depth assessment. In addition to providing comprehensive psychoeducational evaluations, neuropsychologists also assess neurocognitive functioning that may be underlying the learning disorder. Choosing the appropriate clinician to complete the diagnosis is crucial for identifying learning disorders. Thus, if an evaluation has not uncovered a specific weakness, and you and/or the parent feels that one does exist, a more comprehensive evaluation done by a clinician independent of the school district may be warranted.

Assessment of learning disorders often begins in the school setting. Unfortunately, it is common for children with learning disorders to go unidentified for years before the problem is detected. The current system tends to be based on a "wait-to-fail" model, in which a child does not qualify unless there is a significant impairment and is functioning below the level of same-age peers. Although this model captures a portion of the children in need of specialized instruction and accommodations, there is a significant portion who are functioning lower than expected based on their own neurocognitive strengths and weaknesses. Student's giftedness, as measured by a superior intellect on cognitive abilities tests, may be masked by average, yet relatively weak, academic achievement.[12] These children tend to get overlooked because their performance was not "failure" enough. It is important to identify why the child may be struggling in school. Some children are labeled as "lazy" with "poor motivation." Although this may be true and may be the cause of poor academic performance, there may be underlying reasons that either resulted in this condition or that may better explain why the child appears to be poorly motivated.

Describing two very different cases may be helpful in illustrating various etiologies of poor academic performance. In the first case, a child may be functioning at a high level despite having average intellectual abilities. Through extra effort and motivation, the child is able to achieve at a high level. In the second case, a child with superior intellect may be putting forth extra effort to compensate for his or her learning disabilities. That is, relative to superior intellect, reading skills may be only average, and so the child must spend extra time to compensate for this disorder and to achieve at a high level commensurate with intelligence. In each case, when the academic demands are raised to a high enough level, both children struggle to meet the demands, but for very different reasons. For the child with average abilities, performing at a high level presents a challenge that is easily understood. However, in the latter case, the child is struggling academically for very different reasons, which, most importantly, could be remediated, at least in part, through interventions. Unfortunately, many of these children go unidentified and go on to perform below their potential, leading to lost opportunities and associated frustration, loss of motivation, and potential emotional problems.

Thus, early detection of learning disorders is the key to providing the greatest opportunity for favorable outcomes. For example, early phonological and language processing deficits at 3.5 years of age have shown to predict reading accuracy at

5.5 years.[13] These researchers used structural equation modeling to form a highly stable factor of early phonological and language processing (EPLP) comprised of core dyslexic predictors (*i.e.* phonological awareness, rapid naming, pseudoword repetition, vocabulary, and short-term memory). A strong association was identified between EPLP and reading and spelling accuracy. The importance of interventions and their potential effect on the brain is discussed later in this chapter. Let us now focus on the importance of comprehensive evaluations that help uncover the cause of the academic failures and guide interventions and academic planning.

Assessment of learning disorders varies depending on the age and specific problem of the child. Assessments of children in early childhood should focus on the core aspects of the neurocognitive functions that are important in learning basic academic skills, whereas assessments in school-aged children, adolescents, and young adults should hone in on higher level academic skills and associated executive functions.

With regard to IQ, caution should be taken when interpreting the overall or full scale IQ. Significant intersubtest scatter requires the clinician to provide a more sophisticated analysis. It is common for assumptions to be made about significant discrepancies in the data. However, a one-to-one relationship between the data and its implications should not be assumed. For some children, the overall IQ score is not an accurate indicator of their neurocognitive abilities. For example, in the case of gifted and talented students, it is not uncommon for IQ testing to reveal a discrepancy between either verbal or non-verbal reasoning abilities, and working memory and processing speed, resulting in a much lower full scale IQ. In this case, the general abilities index (GAI) would more accurately reflect the child's true neurocognitive abilities because it factors out processing speed and working memory. Thus, it would be more appropriate to use the GAI to detect academic achievement discrepancies.[12,14]

Another case in which caution should be taken when interpreting IQ scores is in the case of a significant discrepancy between verbal and non-verbal reasoning skills. For example, a significant weakness in non-verbal reasoning skills is often assumed to indicate a non-verbal learning disorder. However, more extensive testing is necessary to determine if this diagnosis is appropriate. The interested reader is referred to books and articles by Byron Rourke (also see his website: http://www.nld-bprourke.ca/BPRCV.html) for a review on this topic. Although a non-verbal learning disorder may exist, the weakness in this area could be due to a number of other factors, such as impulsive responding to visual stimuli.

Gifted and talented students who have a specific learning disability (SLD) are referred to as "twice exceptional" and are among the most challenging groups to identify. Thus, these students tend to be among the most underserved in our schools.[12] They are often perplexing to parents and teachers because they simultaneously demonstrate significant academic strengths and specific relative weaknesses. For example, gifted students are often observed to be highly verbal and can discuss complex abstract concepts at a conceptually high level. However, they may fall short when writing or completing assignments on these very topics. This often presents a confusing picture to parents, teachers, and the students, as the resulting classroom performance is unpredictable.

Contemporary trends in the field of learning disabilities has made diagnosing gifted children with learning disabilities even more challenging.[12] Historically, the ability-achievement model has been used since it was first introduced by federal special education regulations in 1977 to determine whether a significant discrepancy existed between a child's cognitive ability and academic achievement. For example, a student with an average cognitive ability would be expected to perform in the average range academically. This model assumes adequate exposure to academic instruction and is not otherwise explained by a lack of motivation. Further complicating the picture is the widely held belief by many educators that gifted students cannot have a diagnosable learning disability. That is, in the case of the gifted student, a significant discrepancy would occur when the child demonstrates superior cognitive abilities with average academic skills. However, because this child is performing at an "average" level when compared to same-age/grade peers, many educators would assert that a learning disability does not exist because it is not impacting the student's performance relative to peers. The tragedy in the case of gifted students with an undiagnosed SLD is that they are not only waiting to fail, but they are also failing to flourish.[12]

Response to intervention (RTI) is a relatively new approach in the U.S. educational system designed to provide early detection and support for students with SLDs at the first sign of difficulty. It was originally intended as an alternative to the comprehensive assessment approach to identifying learning disabilities.[15] RTI best serves children who are experiencing academic difficulties due to a variety of factors, including learning disabilities, limited English proficiency, and socioeconomic disadvantage. However, there is a fundamental difference in the way in which RTI identifies SLDs when compared to the ability-achievement discrepancy model. Whereas diagnosing learning disabilities was typically done by psychologists through assessment of cognitive abilities and achievement, the RTI model relies more on the classroom teacher to identify early learning problems. This fundamental shift makes it even more challenging to identify gifted children with SLDs.

3.1. *Reading disorders*

According to the National Institute of Mental Health, approximately 80% of individuals diagnosed with a learning disorder have dyslexia. The International Dyslexia Association (IDA) defines dyslexia as "difficulties with accurate and/or fluent word recognition and by poor spelling and decoding abilities. These difficulties typically result from a deficit in the phonological component of language that is often unexpected in relation to other cognitive abilities and the provision of effective classroom instruction."[16] There has been a fundamental shift in the scientific understanding of learning disabilities over the past 25 years, from general descriptions to specific types of reading problems.[17] Reading problems can be broken down into three specific categories: (1) Dyslexia — problems decoding single words, (2) Fluency — difficulties reading words and text automatically without a word reading problem, and (3) Comprehension problems in the absence of decoding and fluency problems. Children with dyslexia tend to have problems with all three of these categories. However, a smaller subset of children have difficulties with fluency and/or comprehension. This distinction allows reading problems to be identified at a more precise level, making it possible for the practitioner to pinpoint specific reading interventions and accommodations.

Assessing reading disorders in early childhood should focus on the core aspects of reading. The standard of care begins with an assessment of intellectual functioning, to establish ability level that is used to compare the level of academic achievement. Although IQ tests are no longer required to establish learning disorders, they are useful for comparing weaknesses that are relative to the child's own functioning. Assessments that only compare the child's academic performance against same-age and same-grade peers may fall short of identifying these weaknesses, and may result in a missed opportunity to uncover a problem specific to the child.

The assessment of reading disorders should be comprehensive and tailored to the individual. That is, a false negative may be the result of an assessment that falls short of administering all of the necessary tests required to detect a reading disorder if in fact one exists. The specific tests to be used should be determined by the individual case. Unfortunately, school evaluations often fall short of a comprehensive evaluation. It is common for a school evaluation to consist of an IQ test accompanied by a measure of academic functioning such as the Woodcock-Johnson-III. Although this approach would likely capture some children with learning disorders, it may result in false negatives due to inadequate measurement of the cognitive and academic skills. For example, in the case of a child who is just learning to read, it would be important to include additional measures of phonological awareness, rapid naming, and working memory abilities. These core aspects of reading can be found in the Comprehensive Test of Phonological Awareness (CTOPP) and Phonemic Awareness Test-2, the latter of which is more sensitive to core reading problems at younger ages (five and six years of age). Virginia Berninger has made it possible to assess the core processes of reading at a more precise level (*Process Assessment of the Learner* — 2nd Edition; PAL-II), allowing the clinician to identify the specific weaknesses that are contributing to the child's reading problems. The more specific information obtained from an evaluation, the more likely the clinician will obtain an accurate diagnosis, allowing detailed recommendations for early interventions to be made.

When children reach third grade, the focus tends to shift from learning to read to reading to learn. Moreover, children are required to read longer lengths of text and are expected to comprehend what they read. To adequately evaluate a child at this stage, a measure of oral reading of paragraph-length passages should be administered and analyzed to aid in diagnosis (*e.g. Gray Oral Reading Test* – 4th Edition; GORT-4). Providing measures of single word reading may result in a false negative, as many children begin to memorize words to which they have been exposed. Timed measures of irregular words and pseudowords (*e.g. Test of Word Reading Efficiency*) add important information in determining the child's true decoding abilities.

As the child progresses into high school and beyond, they are expected to read, comprehend, and make inferences from more sophisticated text. At this stage, it is often necessary to add measures that reflect this demand, such as a timed measure that includes several paragraphs of text (*e.g.* Nelson Denny). The Nelson Denny also allows extended time so that the clinician can determine to what degree the student would benefit from such an accommodation. Even with significant improvements through the course of interventions, adolescents and young adults with dyslexia are inefficient readers. Attentional resources are taxed,[18] making reading fluency and comprehension challenging. They often continue to need extended time to demonstrate their true abilities and to be placed in a level-playing field with their peers. For example, Undheim[19] found dyslexics continued to show impairment through adulthood. These students were diagnosed at 10 years of age, and reassessed at 16 years and 23 years. Although nearly all of the participants showed weaknesses in decoding ability, they had only slightly lower educational attainment levels compared to controls.

The interested reader is directed to additional resources to learn more about psychoeducational and neuropsychological evaluations, including books by Pennington,[1] Baron,[20] and Lezak.[15]

3.2. *Mathematics disorder*

Developmental dyscalculia is defined as severe difficulties learning and doing arithmetic that cannot be explained by a lack of educational opportunity or intellectual impairment.[21] Despite the high prevalence of this disorder, the current knowledge about the neurocognitive characteristics of this learning disability is limited.[21] However, new research is emerging.

Number sense develops in early childhood and is felt to be an important contributing factor to mathematics disorders. Mathematics skills represent a combination of neurocognitive systems including knowledge built on the language system, visuospatial system, and central executive functioning that both inhibits irrelevant information and sustains attention.[22] Difficulties in mathematics may result in deficits in one or a combination of these systems. Mathematics involves the retrieval of facts and the application of procedural knowledge.[5] Problem solving, especially as it applies to word problems, may involve a combination of reading skills, verbal reasoning, computation, and visuospatial skills. Additional neurocognitive systems also important in mathematics include ability to shift set, plan, organize, and utilize working memory. Solving math facts quickly is critical in order to avoid overloading working memory stores that are important for needed on-line access of various kinds of information.[5] Given the number of neurocognitive systems involved in mathematics disorders, a comprehensive evaluation is usually necessary to detect them.

3.3. *Disorders of written expression*

Developmental disorders of written expression include impairments in handwriting, spelling, and/or composition. Written expression can been broken down into "transcription" and "generational" components.[23] Transcription involves translating ideas into a written component and is represented by the production of letters and spelling. The generational component requires translating ideas into language, which then must be organized and retrieved from memory.[5]

Handwriting

Handwriting can be assessed through speeded retrieval and reproduction of alphabetic letters, rapid coding of orthographic information, and fine motor coordination. It is important to note that handwriting is more than merely a motor act, it also involves planning and knowledge of orthography.

Spelling

Spelling involves several neurocognitive mechanisms, including access to the meaning of the word, access to its orthographic representation, the conversion of abstract representations into specific shapes, and execution of fine motor skills. Assessments of spelling involve dictation of single words presented in sentences. Spelling can also be assessed in the context of a written composition.

Composition

Composition not only consists of the transcription and generation components of writing, but it also calls upon language skills and executive functions. Several aspects of executive functioning are involved in writing.[24] Analysis requires the student to size up the demands of the situation. Many students with executive functioning deficits become overwhelmed when determining the best approach to writing assignments. Idea generation may complicate the planning process by being overwhelmed by the number of ideas generated. Moreover, the relationship among the ideas may not be clear, and planning a strategy to express them may be difficult. Attentional control is also important in the writing process. The student must focus and maintain attention in addition to inhibiting interfering behaviors. Finally, cognitive flexibility allows the student to adjust plans and goals to meet changing situations. All or a portion of these executive functions may impede the writing process and may contribute to writing difficulties.

3.4. *DSM-IV criteria*

A learning disorder is present when standardized testing in reading, math, or writing reveals an impairment that is substantially below expectations based on age, academic instruction, and intellectual functioning.[2] The learning problem must also significantly interfere with academic achievement or daily living skills. The discrepancy between academic achievement and IQ must be between 1 and 2 standard deviations to meet criteria for the diagnosis of the learning disorder according to the DSM-IV. In the case of a comorbid sensory disorder, the learning disorder must be in excess of what would normally be expected. Learning disorders are indicated on Axis II of the DSM-IV multiaxial system.

3.5. *ICD-10 criteria*

The general criteria for learning disorders in the ICD-10 are similar to those in the DSM-IV although they are not identical. The ICD-10 identifies learning disorders as a disturbance in the normal patterns of academic skill acquisition that are not better explained by a lack of opportunity to learn, impaired intellectual functioning, or is not due to an acquired brain injury or disease.[25] Although the ICD-10 uses different terms to describe similar disorders, their criteria are nearly identical. For example, the ICD-10 terms learning disorders as specific developmental disorders of scholastic skills, which include a specific reading disorder, specific spelling disorder, and a specific disorder of arithmetical skills. The term "other developmental disorders of scholastic skills" is reserved for developmental expressive writing disorder. If more than one learning disorder is present, then the diagnosis is a mixed disorder of scholastic skills.

In contrast to the DSM-IV, the ICD-10 does not provide discrepancy guidelines for diagnosing learning disorders. The clinician must determine what constitutes a "significant impairment" in the development of the specific disorder. Moreover, standardized testing is not required. The lack of specific guidelines makes it challenging to reliably diagnose a specific disorder, which could explain the differences in prevalence rates found in the United States and Europe. We prefer the guidelines provided in the DSM-IV, because they allow for differential diagnoses leading to a principal diagnosis whenever possible. As interventions become more precise, this precision will become increasingly more important.

4. Differential Diagnosis and Comorbidity

4.1. *Differential diagnosis*

It is important to distinguish the case of a child with a learning disorder from academic difficulties due to an impoverished environment, resulting in a lack of opportunity or poor teaching. Cultural factors are also important to consider. Children whose primary language is something other than English or whose cultural background is significantly different than the school culture may perform poorly on academic achievement tests. Thus, the clinician must consider the whole person when considering a diagnosis of a specific learning disorder.

Psychiatric functioning is another important factor to consider when determining if a child has a learning disorder. For example, a child with schizophrenia who is experiencing positive and/or negative symptoms will likely show a very different neurocognitive profile once the symptoms have reduced or the child is symptom free. For complicated cases in which treating the symptoms completely is not possible, an evaluation can help establish the current level of functioning, which can be extremely useful in determining academic needs and placement. Upon significant changes in psychiatric functioning, the child should be re-evaluated to determine the new level of academic functioning and the child's Individualized Education Plan (IEP) should be updated to reflect these changes.

Although academic functioning in children with intellectual disabilities (*i.e.* formerly known as mental retardation) is generally commensurate with the level of intellectual functioning (defined by an IQ 2 standard deviations below the mean, ≤ 70), in some cases, the level of achievement in reading, writing, and math is significantly below expectations. In these cases, an additional diagnosis of the specific learning disorder should be made.[2] In addition, children with intellectual disabilities may demonstrate neurocognitive strengths and weaknesses depending on their etiology. For example, children with Fragile X tend to have relative strengths in vocabulary, verbal comprehension, reading, and spelling, but relative weaknesses in intellectual abilities, pragmatics, arithmetic, attention, and executive functioning skills.[1] Thus, a comprehensive evaluation will help determine the individual strengths and weaknesses and whether a specific learning disability exists. This information is crucial for effective academic planning.

4.2. *Comorbidity*

A child with one learning disorder is more likely to have another diagnosed learning disorder, making the prognosis less favorable.[26] Children experiencing deficits in one academic domain are four to five times more likely to have deficits in another compared to their non-impaired peers.[27] Thus, psychoeducational evaluations should assess all aspects of academic functioning to determine if comorbid learning disorders exists.

Children with learning disabilities are also at increased risk for psychosocial problems, and those with a learning disorder and comorbid ADHD are at greater risk for developing associated mood disorders.[28] Having a learning disorder often results in high levels of frustration and low self-esteem, and these symptoms are exacerbated by comorbid conditions. Moreover, although the primary symptoms of ADHD are inattention and hyperactivity, associated problems often co-occur, including academic underachievement, conduct problems, interpersonal difficulties, anxiety, and depression. Thus, psychosocial functioning should be considered when working with a child with learning disabilities. For more information on comorbid internalizing disorders, please see Chaps. 5–8.

Children with learning disorders are also at increased risk for having comorbid externalizing disorders (Chaps. 9–11), pervasive developmental disorders (Chap. 14), and sleep disorders (Chap. 16). These conditions make interventions more challenging and the prognosis for these patients tends to be less favorable.

5. Neuroscience

Multiple studies have found a number of interrelated neural systems that are activated when reading. These studies have identified two neural systems in the posterior brain regions and distinct and associated systems in the anterior regions of the brain.[39]

Fig. 1 illustrates the neural systems activated in proficient readers. According to Shaywitz,[18] the parietotemporal system is involved in word analysis and decoding of phonemes (*i.e.* individual units of words). Once the phonemes are analyzed, they are further processed in the visual word form area (VWFA) located in the left

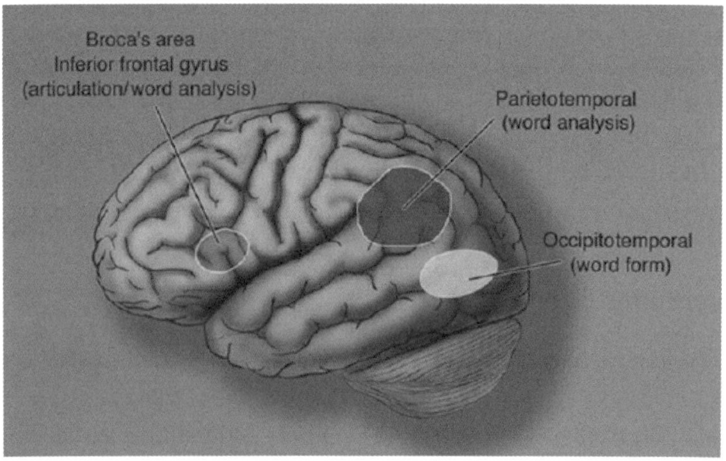

Fig. 1: Neural systems for reading. From: *Overcoming Dyslexia* (S. Shaywitz, 2003).

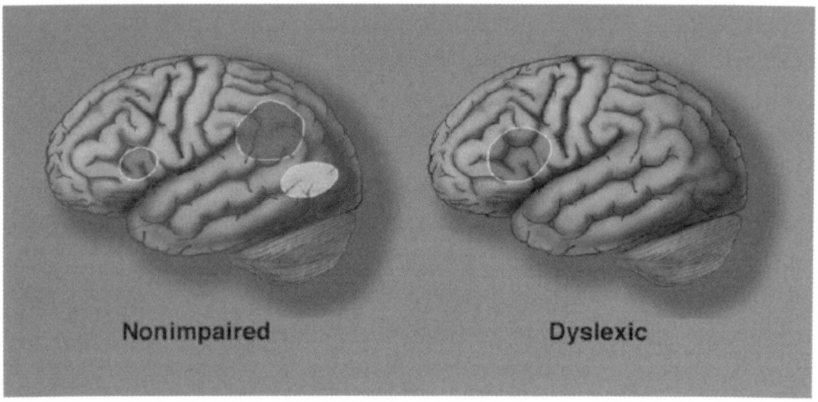

Fig. 2: From *Overcoming Dyslexia: A New and Complete Science-Based Program for Reading Problems at any Level*, by S. Shaywitz, 2003. New York: Alfred A. Knopf. Copyright 2003 by Shaywitz. Reprinted with permission.

occipito-temporal sulcus.[29] The VWFA then projects to the frontal lobes to process phonological or lexico-semantic information.[30]

Research has demonstrated that dyslexic children and adults activate different neural systems than their non-impaired counterparts when reading. This neural system has been coined the "neural signature for dyslexia."[18] Shaywitz and colleagues[31] used functional magnetic resonance imaging (fMRI) to assess 144 dyslexic and nonimpaired children during pseudoword and real-word reading tasks. As illustrated in Fig. 2, dyslexic readers showed a disruption of posterior reading systems and a compensatory over-activation in the anterior reading systems. Non-impaired readers showed greater brain activation than dyslexics, primarily in the left hemisphere neural systems, specifically in the parietotemporal and the occipitotemporal systems.

5.1. *Biopsychosocial factors*

Fletcher[5] provides a framework for understanding the contributing biopsychosocial factors that influence outcomes of children with learning disorders (see Figure 3). This framework can be used for the major types of learning disorders, including reading, mathematics, and written expression. At the primary level of analysis are the specific academic skills deficits (*e.g.* reading fluency, math problem solving, and written expression). The second level of analysis involves the core cognitive processing of the child. For example, a child's phonological awareness deficits are directly contributing to the academic skill deficits (*e.g.* reading fluency). The third level of analysis illustrates the effects of neurobiological and environmental factors. Note that the bidirectional arrow linking neurobiological and environmental factors represents the interaction between these two domains. Research has demonstrated that learning disorders are highly heritable and are found within families and across generations. For example, children of parents with a reading disorder or math disorder are 8 to 10 times more likely to have the same disorder than the general population.[32,33] Although there is a strong genetic component to

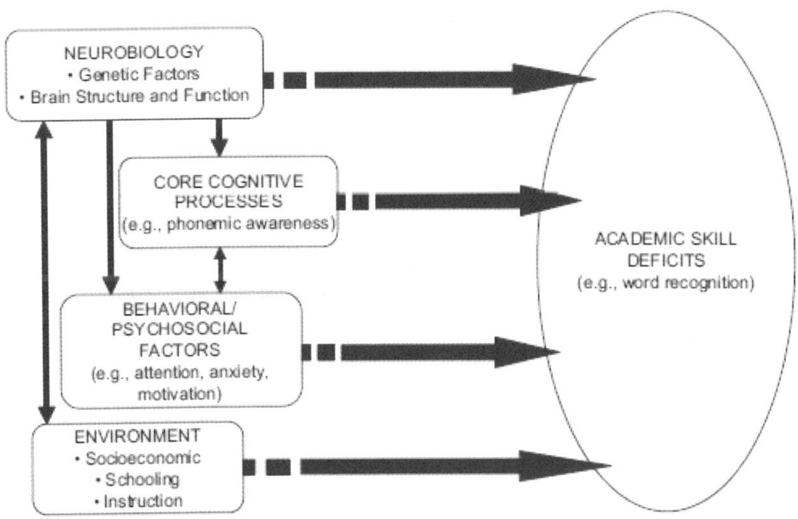

Fig. 3: Framework representing different sources of variability that influence academic outcomes in children with learning disorders. From Fletcher *et al.* (2007, p. 3). Reprinted with permission.

learning disorders, whether or not they will develop is a complex question. As Fig. 3 illustrates, there are several biopsychosocial factors influencing a child's academic skills set. Moreover, environmental factors, such as interventions, can change important structures in the brain associated with the specific learning disorder. Unfortunately, socioeconomic status may determine whether adequate interventions are available.

6. Learning Disorders in Primary Care

Pediatricians are well positioned to enhance the well-being of children with learning disabilities and contribute to their academic success.[34] As summarized in Chap. 10, pediatricians have provided diagnostic and therapeutic services to children with ADHD. Because learning disorders are highly comorbid with ADHD, the pediatrician may be the first to recognize this problem. Parents reporting that their children avoid homework, spend too much time on homework, require extensive assistance to complete it, or describe a significant discrepancy between their intellectual functioning and specific academic skills may present the first opportunity for the pediatrician to intervene. Once a learning disorder is suspected, pediatricians can guide parents to obtaining an appropriate assessment, including differentiating between competing and/or comorbid diagnoses, such as ADHD, anxiety, and depression. They could also help parents consider the multidimensional aspects of learning disorders. That is, those providing any level of care should acknowledge and address the whole child, including medical, behavioral, social, and emotional needs, as well as the specific instructional interventions and accomodations.[34]

7. Interventions

Interventions for learning disorders are largely delivered in schools in the mainstream classroom and/or in the special education classroom. The Individuals with Disability Education Act (IDEA) was originally passed in 1997 and updated and reauthorized in 2004. IDEA reflects the Congressional purpose to ensure that all children with disabilities have a free and appropriate public education (FAPE) "designed to meet their unique needs and prepare them for further education, employment, and independent living."[35] Thus, children who qualify for special education services are required by law to receive them in the public school setting. IDEA requires schools to identify children with disabilities and to determine their eligibility through non-discriminatory assessments.[36] Once identified, these children have the right to the least restrictive environment to the extent that it is appropriate. Thus, some children will receive services in the mainstream classroom while others will receive them in the special education classroom depending on the unique needs of the child. When there is a disagreement between the parents and the school, children with disabilities and their parents are afforded the right to a due process hearing to resolve them. In addition, every child in special education is required to have an Individualized Education Program (IEP), which documents the special education services that will be provided and specific goals to be achieved throughout the year.

Head Start is one example of an early intervention program that was established in 1965 to promote school readiness by enhancing the social and cognitive development of children. Its focus is to help low-income children from ages three to five years. Associated programs are also available, including early Head Start for infants and toddlers. Migrant and seasonal Head Start is available for children of migrant and seasonal farm workers. In addition, American Indian and Alaska Native Head Start programs promotes school readiness for disadvantaged infants, toddlers, and preschool children. Eligibility for head start services is primarily based on income being below the federal poverty level. Moreover, all programs are required to provide full services to children with disabilities. Long-term research studies have demonstrated that Head Start programs are associated with higher academic achievement and lower rates of school suspension and grade repetition.[37,38]

Interventions provided within the school setting are often a good start; however, school resources are often limited and the interventions may not be sufficient in remediating the problem. The clinician should evaluate the services being provided by the school through a review of the student's IEP. Regardless of the specific program that is being used, it should include the important elements based on the latest scientific research. Reading interventions is one area that has been extensively researched, and guidelines for interventions are outlined in the next section. Many private learning centers across the country are now available (*e.g.* Lindamood-Bell). There are also excellent home-based programs that provide parents with the latest interventions for their children (*e.g.* Barton Reading and Spelling System; see http://www.bartonreading.com/). These programs are especially helpful in rural areas and for families who could not otherwise afford private tutoring.

Most children will also require accommodations as a part of their IEP. Depending on the students needs, extended time to complete homework and tests may be necessary. Students may also need reduced homework assignments due to poor efficiency or slow processing speed. For students with executive dysfunction, it may be helpful for teachers to break down complex, abstract material into its component parts so that the student can better understand what is expected of them and complete tasks without becoming overwhelmed. For more information about interventions and accommodations, the interested reader should consult additional texts.[5,39]

7.1. *Results from the national reading panel*

In 1997, Congress requested that the Secretary of Education as well as the Director of the National Institute of Child Health and Human Development convene a national panel of experts to assess the research-based knowledge of the effectiveness of various approaches to teaching children to read.[40] As a result, the National Reading Panel (the NRP or the Panel) was assembled and consisted of 36 experts in reading research who reviewed the extant reading literature.

The national reading panel found that phonological awareness was critical in teaching children to read. Specifically, they found that programs that taught children to manipulate phonemes into words were highly effective across a range of grade and age levels. Moreover, programs that included teaching phonemic awareness directly were superior to those that lacked this type of instruction. The review of the experimental studies led the Panel to conclude that phonemic awareness training caused improvements in phonemic awareness, spelling, and reading skills.

The Panel also found instruction in phonics to be important in teaching children to read. Phonics instruction is a way of teaching how letters are linked to sounds (phonemes) so the reader can form letter-sound correspondences. A meta-analysis indicated that systematic phonics instruction improved reading skills for students in kindergarten through sixth grade. Children taught phonics at an early age (first grade) showed improvements in decoding skills, spelling, and reading comprehension. Although older children receiving phonics instruction improved in decoding and spelling, their comprehension did not improve significantly.

Fluency refers to reading speed, accuracy, and proper expression. Children who have impairments in reading fluency read in a laborious and inefficient manner. For these children, reading is not an automatic effortless process, making it difficult to comprehend the text and relate the information to his or her background knowledge. Unfortunately, reading fluency is often neglected in classroom instruction. The NRP found that guided repeated oral reading, which involves students reading passages orally with explicit guidance and feedback from the instructor, had a significant positive impact on reading fluency, word recognition, and comprehension across a range of grade levels. In contrast, the Panel was unable to find a positive relationship between independent silent reading with minimal guidance or feedback and reading achievement. It is important to note that although independent silent reading may improve reading skills, the National Reading Panel found that there was insufficient data from well-designed studies capable of testing a causal link between silent reading and reading achievement.

Reading comprehension is critical to the development of reading skills and obtaining an education. The studies reviewed by the NRP indicated that vocabulary instruction improves reading comprehension. In addition, teaching a combination of reading comprehension techniques, including comprehension monitoring, use of graphic organizers, question generation (readers ask themselves questions about the text), and summarization (readers are taught to generalize new information and integrate ideas), tended to have the best outcomes.

7.2. *The effects of intervention on brain function*

Several studies have used Functional Magnetic Resonance Imaging (fMRI) to demonstrate the impact of intensive remedial instruction on brain functioning. For example, Meyler and colleagues[41] used fMRI to longitudinally assess whether intensive remedial reading instruction would correspond with changes in cortical activity (Fig. 2). Fifth grade students' reading comprehension was assessed prior to remediation, after 100 hours of intensive instruction, and at one-year follow-up. A control group of fifth grade non-impaired readers were also assessed during these time points for comparison. Prior to instruction, children that comprised the poor reading group had significantly less activation bilaterally in the parietal cortex compared to good readers. However, after intensive instruction, poor readers not only made significant gains in reading ability, they also demonstrated changes in brain activation. Specifically, poor readers demonstrated increased activation in the left angular gyrus and left superior lobule. At one-year follow-up, poor readers continued to increase their reading skills and brain activation in the respective areas. However, poor readers had increased activation across the medial frontal cortex as compared to good readers, which was felt to reflect a more effortful and intentionally based reading strategy.

7.3. *Pharmacotherapy for the treatment of dyslexia*

Recent research has suggested that medication may help improve reading in children with ADHD and dyslexia.[42,43] Sumner and colleages[43] provided open-label atomoxetine to 47 children aged 10–16 years with ADHD and ADHD with comorbid dyslexia. Results of this study suggested that children taking atomoxetine over 16 weeks not only demonstrated substantial improvements in attention and hyperactivity, they also showed improvements in reading skills. Specifically, patients with ADHD and patients with ADHD plus comorbid dyslexia demonstrated statistically significant improvements in mean standard scores and age equivalencies on measures of reading comprehension. Notably, patients with ADHD plus comorbid dyslexia also showed improvements in reading decoding. This study also included measures of working memory (*i.e.* the ability to hold information in mind and mentally manipulate it), which has found to be an important component to reading.[44,45] Patients with ADHD and comorbid dyslexia made significant improvements on a measure assessing the phonological loop, and both the ADHD and ADHD plus dyslexia groups made overall improvements in working memory. Although this study provides preliminary support for the treatment of atomoxetine in children with ADHD and comorbid dyslexia, it did not include a control group. Thus, further research is warranted to investigate the potential benefits of atomoxetine in children with this comorbid condition.

Methylphenidate (MPH) has also shown some potential in the treatment of ADHD and comorbid dyslexia.[46] In an unblinded study evaluating the effect of methylphenidate in children with ADHD and comorbid dyslexia, Keulers and colleagues[42] found that children made significant improvements on reading raw scores. However, these effects were not found for standard scores, which was felt to be a result of floor effects not detecting the small reading improvements. Future research is necessary to study the potential effects of MPH on reading in children with ADHD.

8. Outcomes (evidence-based follow-up studies)

Long-term outcome studies of individuals with diagnosed learning disorders indicate that they continue to experience a number of problems across the entire lifespan.[47] In a longitudinal study, Undheim[19] followed students who were diagnosed at 10 years of age and reassessed at 16- and 23 years. Although nearly all of the participants showed weaknesses in decoding ability, they had only slightly lower educational attainments levels compared to controls. In another study, 73% of university graduates indicated that their learning disorder affected their job in some way.[48] However, only 55% reported disclosing their learning disability, and only 12% requested accommodations in their work setting. The most common areas that the respondents indicated experiencing problems included writing (51%), processing speed (43%), reading comprehension (36%), and organizational skills (29%). In order to compensate, these individuals reported working extra hours and implementing organization strategies. An international study revealed that individuals with learning disorders had higher unemployment rates (21%) compared to those who did not report having a learning disorder (9%).[49] Moreover, individuals with learning disorders were twice as likely to be employed in blue collar jobs (68%) as opposed to white collar jobs (32%). In contrast, the proportions were nearly equal for the non-impaired group (50% white collar, 49% blue collar).[49]

With regard to long-term outcomes of interventions, the most is known about interventions for reading disorders. Although dyslexics show significant improvement in accuracy, reading continues to be slow and effortful, not fluid and effortless.[39] In a long-term study, Shaywitz and colleages[50] followed children into adulthood to examine the differences between poor readers and non-impaired readers. Three groups were identified. The first group was comprised of compensated readers who became more accurate in their reading but did not show significant improvement in fluency. These patients continued to show an underactivation in the word form area. A second group, comprised of persistently poor readers who did not show improvements in accuracy or fluency, appeared to rely on memory-based reading strategies rather than analytic word identification strategies. Thus, this study provides evidence that reading problems identified in childhood persists into adulthood, even for those who showed improvements in accuracy through reading interventions.

9. Clinical Experiences: Practice-Based Evidence

During my tenure at Stanford and now in our private clinic, patients have represented the entire age spectrum. While the modal age is eight years, clients range in age from three years to the mid-50s. Patients in the older age groups typically represent returning college students with unidentified learning disorders, ADHD, those who find themselves having difficulty in the workplace, and autism spectrum disorders. Due to recent advances, these patients tend to be more aware of their own deficits and the potential impact they may be having on their academic performance.

The assessment begins with a clinical interview to gather current and historical information that have contributed to the patient's difficulties. Medical records, school records, previous assessments, and any additional information is collected and reviewed. We routinely work with schools to obtain academic and behavioral information from teachers and staff to contribute to the assessment.

Approximately 30% of our cases are completely new referrals who are either being seen to assess early learning problems/concerns or adolescents and young adults who have undetected learning disorders and ADHD. A majority of the children have been evaluated by the school (40%) whose parents are either seeking a second opinion or have been referred for a more comprehensive evaluation by a child psychiatrist or pediatrician. We also see complex cases referred to us by the school for independent evaluations. The remaining cases tend to come from the community as self-referrals or reevaluations for more complex cases with comorbid executive functioning problems and/or severe emotional problems.

Case A

This case illustrates missed diagnoses and the importance of a comprehensive evaluation. All identifying information has been changed to protect the confidentiality in these case examples.

This patient is a 13-year-old adolescent boy with a history of academic difficulties. Birth and development were within normal limits with the exception of poor articulation for which he received speech therapy. He had never demonstrated significant behavior problems or difficulties with attention. Parental concerns of reading and writing problems resulted in a school evaluation at the age of nine years. Although "relative weaknesses" were identified in reading and spelling, they did not meet criteria for a specific learning disorder so he did not qualify for interventions at school. However, the patient received extra help from his parents and a private tutor for his reading problems. He maintained strengths in mathematics, science, and history through 8th grade. Despite receiving As in all of his subjects, his parents were concerned due to the amount of time required to complete his homework. They expected the demands would increase as he transitioned into high school the following year. There were no present concerns of emotional problems, but the family feared that they may develop if he continued on the current course.

The patient found grammar and verb agreement confusing. He reported that although he enjoyed reading, he did not feel comfortable reading aloud in class because he "often stumbled when reading aloud."

Results

Given significant discrepancies in scores between verbal comprehension (very superior) and perceptual reasoning (superior) as compared to working memory (average) and processing speed (low average), the general ability index (GAI; a composite score that is based on verbal comprehension and perceptual reasoning subtests) was felt to be a more accurate estimate of the patient's true intellectual abilities (superior) Table 1.

On measures of reading, the patient's performance was variable. Although his ability to read single words was average relative to same-age peers (standard score = 90), it was greater than 2 standard deviations below his intellectual abilities. His reading difficulties were more pronounced for timed tasks of reading pseudowords (standard score = 80), which exploited his impairments in decoding unfamiliar words. The patient was also administered an oral reading task of paragraph-length passages (*i.e.* GORT-4). On this measure, his fluency score was impaired (standard score = 70), and his reading was characterized by slow, choppy reading in addition to frequent errors of substitution and repetition. The

Table 1: Intellectual Functioning: Composite Scores Summary

Scale	Sum of scaled scores	Composite score	Percentile rank	95% confidence interval	Qualitative description
Verbal comprehension (VCI)	46	132	98	123–137	Very superior
Perceptual reasoning (PRI)	40	121	92	112–127	Superior
Working memory (WMI)	21	102	55	94–109	Average
Processing speed (PSI)	16	88	21	80–98	Low average
Full scale (FSIQ)	123	118	88	113–122	High average

patient also completed a silent reading measure consisting of passages of several paragraphs in length that included reading comprehension questions (*i.e.* Nelson Denny). After the allotted 20 minutes, the patient's performance (standard score = 80) was below expectations relative to his IQ but was low average relative to same-age peers. The patient performed within normal limits on additional measures of neurocognitive functioning, including attention, learning, memory, and executive functioning.

Based on his profile, the patient received a diagnosis of dyslexia and met criteria for receiving accommodations at school. In this case, the additional reading measures were important for providing an accurate diagnosis. The patient received reading interventions at school and was referred to a private learning center that followed the guidelines set forth by the National Reading Panel. The patient was seen for a follow-up assessment two years later. Although he made substantial gains in his reading accuracy, his reading speed was slow. At four-year follow-up, the patient received extended time on his college entrance exams and was admitted to a prestigious college. Based on our recommendations, he planned to seek accommodations through the university's learning resource center, which included extended time on tests and preferred registration so he could enroll in the courses that would best fit his academic needs.

Case B

This is an eight-year-old boy who was referred for a comprehensive evaluation by a child psychiatrist in the community to clarify whether the patient had specific learning disabilities and/or ADHD. Birth and early development was within normal limits. Vision and auditory exams were normal. His mother indicated a childhood history of difficulties with focus, concentration, and sustained attention since early childhood. In the school setting, he was described as being "highly distractible" with no concerns of excessive activity levels. His mother was primarily concerned about his difficulties with reading and the impact his academic challenges may be having on his emotional functioning. His performance on measures of intellectual functioning was quite variable, with very superior non-verbal reasoning abilities (standard score = 130) in the context of average verbal reasoning abilities (standard score = 100), low average processing speed (standard score = 85), and impaired working memory (standard score = 74).

The patient demonstrated weaknesses across reading skills relative to his intellectual abilities, and in some cases, relative to same-age peers. Single word reading was relatively weak (standard score = 86), as was reading of pseudowords (standard score = 82). Moreover, his performance on measures of phonological awareness was impaired (standard scores ranged from 71 to 79). Reading impairments were more pronounced for reading paragraph-length passages, as his reading rate and accuracy was in the 2nd percentile. Comprehension skills were relatively better (16th percentile). We typically see this pattern of results in which the child's comprehension abilities are better than reading accuracy and rate. Thus, unless the child receives an oral reading test, silent reading measures of comprehension will result in a false negative.

In addition to significant weaknesses in working memory noted above, this patient demonstrated significant weaknesses in sustained attention. On the Test of Variables of Attention (TOVA), a 21-min measure of sustained attention, the patient failed to respond to the target stimuli at an age-appropriate level, resulting in a significant number of errors of omission (See Chart 1). The patient also demonstrated significant reaction time variability on the TOVA, reflecting substantial problems with sustaining attention (Chart 2).

Parent and teacher ratings of the patient's attention were significantly elevated, indicating impairments in his attention span and in his level of distractibility.

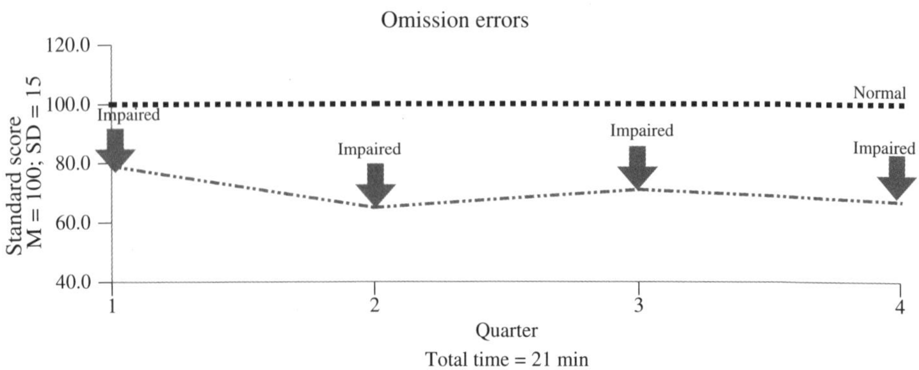

Chart 1: Number of omission errors across a 21-min measure of sustained attention.

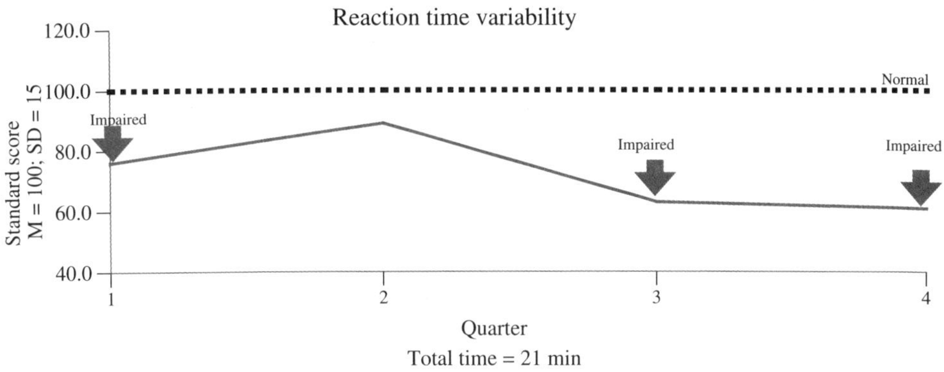

Chart 2: Reaction time variability over a 21-min interval.

Parent and teacher ratings also reflected significant concerns of anxious, depressive, and somatic symptoms, and they noted that the patient frequently worried about his academic performance. He was described as being easily upset, persistently negative, and tearful. The patient endorsed these symptoms during the clinical interview and reported feeling sad because he felt "stupid."

The child was diagnosed with dyslexia and comorbid ADHD-inattentive type. He was referred back to his psychiatrist for a medication evaluation for his attention problems and depressive symptoms. The psychiatrist provided psychotherapy for his emotional problems and he responded well to atomoxetine for inattention. He was also enrolled in a specialty school for children with dyslexia. His mood improved considerably as a result of engaging in therapy, receiving reading interventions, and attending school with peers who had similar difficulties. After this evaluation, the patient's mother requested a second evaluation for her 6 year-old son. Because we were able to detect several early risk factors for dyslexia, this patient began receiving early reading interventions and had a favorable prognosis.

10. Outcomes in Our Clinic

We receive the majority of our referrals for diagnostic clarification for complex cases. We closely follow the practice parameters put forth by the American Academy of Child and Adolescent Psychiatry to provide differential diagnoses and specific recommendations.[51] We are constantly updating our testing instruments to provide state-of-the-art neurocognitive and psychoeducational assessments. Moreover, we integrate the biopsychosocial model in our assessments to consider all of the important factors that may be contributing to the client's difficulties.

The findings from our assessments generate specific recommendations that are integrated into the comprehensive report. Our recommendations are realistic and are based on the needs of the child. The majority of our reports provide the guidance necessary for the school to design IEPs to meet the child's needs. However, we often attend IEP meetings at the request of the parents. The IEP meeting is an opportunity to educate school officials on the specific needs of the child and the evidenced-based interventions that will be needed to treat their difficulties. Although most schools provide useful interventions, they often cannot provide the intensity of interventions that is supported by scientific research. However, we strongly advocate for the child to get the interventions they so desperately need.

The appropriate school placement is crucial for children with learning disabilities and associated comorbid conditions. Some of their needs can be met in the regular classroom with appropriate accommodations, such as extended time on testing or help from a teacher's aide. For children who require specialized instruction to remediate their learning disorder, pull-out services in a resource room is often necessary. In these cases, it is usually best to vary the days and times the child receives these services so they do not miss out on instruction in the same subjects. Alternatively, the child could attend the resource room during an elective activity (*i.e.* art). Parents should be allowed to help make these decisions with school officials and they should be integrated into the student's IEP.

Some parents opt for additional instruction by private learning centers or enroll their child in a school that specializes in remediating specific learning disabilities. Private learning centers should provide more than merely tutoring; they should provide interventions based on scientific research. Lindamood-Bell learning centers are found in various parts of the country and are a good example of a learning center that provides scientifically based interventions. Unfortunately, many areas throughout the country do not have such resources. Careful consideration should be given when determining effective options. Home-study programs can be extremely effective if they are based on scientific research. The Barton Reading and Spelling System (http://www.bartonreading.com/) is just one example of an effective program that can be used by parents in their home. However, when there are existing problems with the parent–child relationship, interventions from outside resources should be considered until these problems are resolved.

We work closely with psychiatrists at Stanford and the community for our patients who need medication consultations. Results from our assessments are communicated directly with the psychiatrists in writing and through a phone consultation. We also provide brief, serial evaluations for our psychiatrists to provide objective data for response to medication.

Our decision to treat the child in our clinic depends upon the referral. When the referral comes to us from the treating psychiatrists for diagnostic clarification and treatment recommendations, we provide consultation and refer the patient back to the referral source. For cases in which we are the primary care provider, we provide psychotherapy services to children and their families in our clinic and consult with psychiatrists for medication related issues. Our goal is to provide patients with comprehensive care for the best outcomes.

11. Future Directions in the Diagnosis and Treatment of Learning Disorders

Although considerable advances have been made over the past decade in the identification and treatment of learning disorders, recent technologies and conceptual advances have the potential to provide an understanding of the learning process that could not have been imagined 10 to 20 years ago. These advances will guide assessment and treatments in new ways, providing hope for the future of children with learning disabilities. Functional imaging will continue to advance the identification of specific brain structures involved in learning disorders, resulting in unequivocal evidence that these once "hidden disabilities" are real.[18] Although diagnosing learning disorders will not be made by neuroimaging alone, combining imaging and neuropsychological testing may allow us to be more precise in our diagnoses, so we can target specific interventions. Recent research that has identified the role of attention in reading may lead to a better understanding of the neurochemical mechanisms of reading and dyslexia and how they are related to the neural circuits in ADHD.[18]

There is strong evidence that executive functioning has a significant impact on learning and academic skills. For example, extensive research has demonstrated the importance of working memory on reading[44,45,52] and math.[53,54] There is now growing evidence that Cogmed working memory training — an intervention designed to improve working memory — has an associated positive effect on academic achievement.[55,56] Moreover, the gains in working memory have generalized to other areas as well, including sustained attention, impulsive responding, and executive functioning abilities.[57] These treatments may be increasingly used to supplement existing therapies for learning disorders and comorbid ADHD. Although this ground breaking research and associated interventions are just beginning to emerge, continued advancements will develop over the next five years and beyond to treat underlying neurocognitive functions important in successful academic progress.

References

1. Pennington BF. *Diagnosing Learning Disorders: A Neuropsychological Framework* (2nd edition). New York, NY US: Guilford Press, 2009.

2. Association. AP, Ed *Diagnostic and Statistical Manual of Mental Disorders.* 4th edition, *Text Rev.* American Psychiatric Association, 2000.
3. Lagae L. Learning disabilities: Definitions, epidemiology, diagnosis, and intervention strategies, *Pediatr Clin North Am* 2008; **55**(6): 1259–1268.
4. Liederman J, Kantrowitz L, Flannery K. Male vulnerability to reading disability is not likely to be a myth: A call for new data, *J Learning Disabilities* 2005; **38**(2): 109–129.
5. Fletcher JM, Lyon GR, Fuchs LS, Barnes MA. *Learning Disabilities: From Identification to Intervention.* New York: Guilford Press, 2007.
6. Elbeheri G, Everatt J, Al Malki M. The incidence of dyslexia among young offenders in Kuwait, *Dyslexia* 2009; **15**(2): 86–104.
7. Shaywitz SE, Shaywitz BA. Dyslexia (specific reading disability), *Pediatr Rev* 2003; **24**(5): 147–153.
8. Billard C, Fluss J, Ducot B, *et al.* Deficits in reading acquisition in primary school: Cognitive, social and behavioral factors studied in a sample of 1062 children, *Rev Epidemiol Sante Publique* 2009; **57**(3): 191–203.
9. Chan DW, Ho CS-H, Tsang S-M, Lee S-H, Chung KKH. Prevalence, gender ratio and gender differences in reading-related cognitive abilities among Chinese children with dyslexia in Hong Kong, *Educational Studies* 2007; **33**(2): 249–265.
10. von Aster M, Schweiter M, Zulauf MW. Rechenstörungen bei kindern: Vorläufer, prävalenz und psychische symptome, *Zeitschrift für Entwicklungspsychologie und Pädagogische Psychologie* 2007; **39**(2): 85–96.
11. Shalev RS, Manor O, Gross-Tsur V. Developmental dyscalculia: A prospective six-year follow-up, *Developmental Med Child Neurol* 2005; **47**(2): 121–125.
12. Assouline SG, Nicpon MF, Whiteman C. Cognitive and psychosocial characteristics of gifted students with written language disability, *Gifted Child Quarterly* 2010; **54**(2): 102–115.
13. Puolakanaho A, Ahonen T, Aro M, *et al.* Developmental links of very early phonological and language skills to second grade reading outcomes: Strong to accuracy but only minor to fluency, *J Learn Disabil* 2008; **41**(4): 353–370.
14. Harrison AG, DeLisle MM, Parker KCH. An investigation of the general abilities index in a group of diagnostically mixed patients, *J Psychoeducational Assessment* 2008; **26**(3): 247–259.
15. Coyne MD, Harn BA. Promoting beginning reading success through meaningful assessment of early literacy skills, *Psychol Schools* 2006; **43**(1): 33–43.
16. Lyon GR, Shaywitz SE, Shaywitz BA. A definition of dyslexia, *Annals Dyslexia* 2003; **53**: 1–14.
17. Fletcher JM. Dyslexia: The evolution of a scientific concept, *J Int Neuropsychol Soc* 2009; **15**(4): 501–508.
18. Shaywitz SE, Shaywitz BA. Paying attention to reading: The neurobiology of reading and dyslexia, *Dev Psychopathol* Fall 2008; **20**(4): 1329–1349.

19. Undheim AM. A thirteen-year follow-up study of young Norwegian adults with dyslexia in childhood: Reading development and educational levels, *Dyslexia* 2009; **15**(4): 291–303.
20. Baron IS. *Neuropsychological Evaluation of the Child.* New York, NY US: Oxford University Press, 2004.
21. Dowker A, Kaufmann L. Atypical development of numerical cognition: Characteristics of developmental dyscalculia, *Cognitive Development* 2009; **24**(4): 339–342.
22. Geary DC. Mathematical disabilities: Reflections on cognitive, neuropsychological, and genetic components, *Learning Individual Differences* 2010; **20**(2): 130–133.
23. Berninger VW. Understanding the "Graphia" in developmental dysgraphia: A developmental neuropsychological perspective for disorders in producing written language. In: Dewey D, Tupper DE, Eds. *Developmental Motor Disorders: A Neuropsychological Perspective.* New York, NY US: Guilford Press, 2004, pp. 328–350.
24. Graham S, Harris KR, Olinghouse N. Addressing executive function problems in writing: An example from the self-regulated strategy development model. In: Meltzer L, Ed. *Executive Function in Education: From Theory to Practice.* New York, NY US: Guilford Press, 2007, pp. 216–236.
25. *International Classification of Diseases.* 10th Revision edition. World Health Organization, 1992.
26. Dirks E, Spyer G, van Lieshout EC, de Sonneville L. Prevalence of combined reading and arithmetic disabilities, *J Learn Disabil* 2008; **41**(5): 460–473.
27. Landerl K, Moll K. Comorbidity of learning disorders: Prevalence and familial transmission, *J Child Psychol Psychiatry* 2010; **51**(3): 287–294.
28. McNamara JK, Willoughby T, Chalmers H. Psychosocial status of adolescents with learning disabilities with and without comorbid attention deficit hyperactivity disorder, *Learning Disabilities Res Practice* 2005; **20**(4): 234–244.
29. Cohen L, Martinaud O, Lemer C, *et al.* Visual word recognition in the left and right hemispheres: Anatomical and functional correlates of peripheral alexias, *Cerebral Cortex* 2003; **13**(12): 1313–1333.
30. Bolger DJ, Hornickel J, Cone NE, Burman DD, Booth JR. Neural correlates of orthographic and phonological consistency effects in children, *Human Brain Mapping* 2008; **29**(12): 1416–1429.
31. Shaywitz BA, Shaywitz SE, Pugh KR, *et al.* Disruption of posterior brain systems for reading in children with developmental dyslexia, *Biological Psychiatry* 2002; **52**(2): 101–110.
32. Pennington BF, Olson RK. Genetics of dyslexia. In: Snowling MJ, Hulme C, Eds. *The Science of Reading: A Handbook.* Malden: Blackwell Publishing, 2005, pp. 453–472.
33. Shalev RS, Manor O, Kerem B, *et al.* Developmental dyscalculia is a familial learning disability, *J Learning Disabilities* 2001; **34**(1): 59–65.
34. Horowitz SH. From research to policy to practice: Prescription for success for students with learning disabilities, *J Child Neurology* 2004; **19**(10): 836–839.

35. Blau AF, Allbright AL. 50-State roundup: Ensuring children with disabilities a free appropriate public education, *Mental Phy Disability Law Reporter* 2006; **30**(1): 11–19.
36. Smith TEC. IDEA 2004: Another round in the reauthorization process, *Remedial Special Education* 2005; **26**(6): 314–319.
37. Joo M. Long-term effects of head start on academic and school outcomes of children in persistent poverty: Girls vs. boys. *Children Youth Services Rev* 2010; **32**(6): 807–814.
38. Barnett WS. Long-term cognitive and academic effects of early childhood education of children in poverty, *Preventive Med: Int J Devoted Practice Theory* 1998; **27**(2): 204–207.
39. Shaywitz S. *Overcoming Dyslexia: A New and Complete Science-Based Program for Reading Problems at any Level.* New York, NY US: Alfred A. Knopf, 2003.
40. Panel NR. *Report of the National Reading Panel: Reports of the subgroups*, 2000.
41. Meyler A, Keller TA, Cherkassky VL, Gabrieli JDE, Just MA. Modifying the brain activation of poor readers during sentence comprehension with extended remedial instruction: A longitudinal study of neuroplasticity, *Neuropsychologia* 2008; **46**(10): 2580–2592.
42. Keulers EH, Hendriksen JG, Feron FJ, *et al.* Methylphenidate improves reading performance in children with attention deficit hyperactivity disorder and comorbid dyslexia: An unblinded clinical trial, *Eur J Paediatr Neurol* 2007; **11**(1): 21–28.
43. Sumner CR, Gathercole S, Greenbaum M, *et al.* Atomoxetine for the treatment of attention-deficit/hyperactivity disorder (ADHD) in children with ADHD and dyslexia, *Child Adolesc Psychiatry Ment Health* 2009; **3**: 40.
44. Sesma HW, Mahone EM, Levine T, Eason SH, Cutting LE. The contribution of executive skills to reading comprehension, *Child Neuropsychol* 2009; **15**(3): 232–246.
45. Swanson HL, Xinhua Z, Jerman O. Working memory, short-term memory, and reading disabilities: A selective meta-analysis of the literature, *J Learn Disabil* 2009; **42**(3): 260–287.
46. Grizenko N, Bhat M, Schwartz G, Ter-Stepanian M, Joober R. Efficacy of methylphenidate in children with attention-deficit hyperactivity disorder and learning disabilities: A randomized crossover trial, *J Psychiatry Neurosci* 2006; **31**(1): 46–51.
47. Goldberg RJ, Higgins EL, Raskind MH, Herman KL. Predictors of success in individuals with learning disabilities: A qualitative analysis of a 20-year longitudinal study, *Learning Disabilities Res Practice* 2003; **18**(4): 222–236.
48. Madaus JW. Employment self-disclosure rates and rationales of university graduates with learning disabilities, *J Learning Disabilities* 2008; **41**(4): 291–299.
49. Vogel SA, Holt JK. A comparative study of adults with and without self-reported learning disabilities in six English-Speaking populations: What have we learned? *Dyslexia: Int J Res Practice* 2003; **9**(4): 193–228.

50. Shaywitz SE, Shaywitz BA, Fulbright RK, *et al.* Neural systems for compensation and persistence: Young adult outcome of childhood reading disability, *Biol Psychiatry* 2003; **54**(1): 25–33.
51. Beitchman JH, Cantwell DP, Forness SR, Kavale KA, Kauffman JM. Practice parameters for the assessment and treatment of children and adolescents with language and learning disorders, *J Am Acad Child Adolesc Psychiatry* 1998; **37**(Suppl. 10): 46S–62S.
52. Swanson HL, O'Connor R. The role of working memory and fluency practice on the reading comprehension of students who are dysfluent readers, *J Learn Disabil* 2009; **42**(6): 548–575.
53. Schuchardt K, Maehler C, Hasselhorn M. Working memory deficits in children with specific learning disorders, *J Learn Disabil* 2008; **41**(6): 514–523.
54. Rotzer S, Loenneker T, Kucian K, Martin E, Klaver P, von Aster M. Dysfunctional neural network of spatial working memory contributes to developmental dyscalculia, *Neuropsychologia* 2009; **47**(13): 2859–2865.
55. Holmes J, Gathercole SE, Dunning DL. Adaptive training leads to sustained enhancement of poor working memory in children, *Dev Sci* 2009; **12**(4): F9–15.
56. Holmes J, Gathercole SE, Dunning DL. Adaptive training leads to sustained enhancement of poor working memory in children, *Dev Sci* 2009; **12**(4): F9–F15.
57. Klingberg T, Fernell E, Olesen PJ, *et al.* Computerized training of working memory in children with ADHD — A randomized, controlled trial, *J Am Acad Child Adolesc Psychiatry* 2005; **44**(2): 177–186.

Chapter 10

ADHD and Other Disorders of Attention Regulation

Hans Steiner, Pascale G. Stemmle, Rebecca E. Hall, Shashank V. Joshi, and Paresh D. Patel

"If I had to start my career as a neuroscientist today, I would pick the problem of attention and its regulation to study."

Eric Kandel, M.D, Nobel Laureate winner in Physiology or Medicine, 2000, on the occasion of his talk at Stanford University, May 11, 2006.

1. Introduction

Attention regulation is a core piece of human mental functioning. As only approximately 5% of all mentation is conscious,[1] human beings have developed a system that reliably and flexibly selects the most salient inputs across a broad range of situations, helps us attend to novel external and internal stimuli, and prepares an appropriate executive response. The system also allows for the tracking of multiple inputs in specific situations. Thus, the attention regulation system can become dysregulated in several different ways. It may fail to track multiple inputs; it may fail to identify the most salient ones for response; and it may not issue forth the most appropriate response.

Attention regulation is especially important when learning new information. Learning proceeds in systematic fashion and inputs need to be properly sequenced as well as effectively stored. As our academic and professional lives become increasingly complex, refined processing of sophisticated inputs becomes central; malfunction in a system that facilitates our acquisition of knowledge becomes increasingly deleterious. Perhaps, it is this intersection of increased demands on children, adolescents, and adults that helps explain why disorders of attention have become a prominent focal point of our computer and web-based societies. The attention regulation system is an exceedingly complex one.[2–4] Complex systems leave much room for developmental deviations, the impact of environmental influences in addition to genetic underpinnings, and the possibility that there are multiple pathogenetic pathways leading to the final common outcome of an attention deficit disorder.

The pathologization of problems with attention has not been uniformly accepted. There are some very vocal critics of the concept of ADHD.[5–7] Some arrive at their position from a high level of tolerance of normative variation of attentional processes,[6] and some from a position of concern that the condition is overdiagnosed and too commonly treated with potentially harmful medications.[7,8] Our view, that this condition is truly a maladaptive extension of normative processes, is informed by the tenets of developmental psychopathology.[9] Importantly, the "maladaptiveness" of symptoms is somewhat context dependent; *e.g.* "inattention to extraneous stimuli" might be adaptive in a chaotic environment in which the extraneous stimulus is a capricious and abusive caregiver. After a certain point, however, a syndrome becomes so potent that it results in disordered functioning in multiple domains and a failure of developmental progression. By this point, we have traversed the distance from isolated symptoms to a syndromal disorder in need of treatment. The symptoms constituting the syndrome may not be qualitatively different from the normative processes of attention, but the magnitude of their dysfunction and the associated negative outcomes signals the need for intervention.

Some of the tendency to overdiagnose ADHD in the United States compared to other countries is most likely generated by the absence of reliable and valid diagnostic methods other than historical/clinical ones. In the absence of such methods, errors in both directions are possible (*i.e.* both the under- and overdiagnosing of ADHD). Currently, we must rely on the convergence of historical data from at least two domains of functioning to generate a reliable diagnosis with some degree of certainty, and such a standard is surely minimal compared to what will certainly be the more highly specific and sensitive instrumentation of the future.

Problems with attention have received a great deal of focus in the child psychiatric literature for several decades. The literature supporting current practices is voluminous and generally speaking, of high quality, as far as evidence-based medicine standards are concerned. Still, several deficiencies are also apparent and need to be discussed. This chapter relies heavily on the practice parameters of the American Academy of Child and Adolescent Psychiatry,[10] the American Academy of Pediatrics,[11] and Europeans clinical guidelines,[12] to develop an appropriately summarized database.

2. Epidemiology

The current consensus among experts is that ADHD is estimated to occur in 3% to 7% of school-age children,[13,14] with a wide range reported in the literature; some figures reported are as low as 1% and some are as high as 20%. The variation in these estimates can be explained as a consequence of key methodological differences between studies. (For a detailed discussion, see Barkley[15]). Further, although DSM nosology has consistently required that mental illness must be defined by both symptom criteria and clinically significant distress or impairment, clinicians often disregard this requirement when operationalizing "caseness".[16] Bird *et al.* (2000) has suggested the use of a global impairment scale, such as the Children's Global Assessment Scale (CGAS).[17] Bird *et al.* (2000) found that when utilizing this type of measure in addition to disorder-specific measures, the prevalence rates of many childhood disorders decrease; ADHD prevalence estimates dropped from 7.8% using symptom criteria only, to 3.9% when combining symptom criteria and a CGAS score less than or equal to 68.[16] Finally, it is significant that ADHD is diagnosed two to three times more frequently in boys than in girls.

3. Symptoms and Diagnosis

3.1. *DSM-IV criteria*

ADHD has an onset in early childhood, with evidence of impairment often evident as early as age three in a small subset of children. Symptoms of hyperactivity and impulsivity are the first to arise, usually in the pre-school years. Symptoms of inattention come later, increasing as school demands increase; typically they are evident by late childhood. Factor analysis studies[18] have demonstrated that there are two separate but significantly correlated constructs underlying the behavioral problems that are characteristic of ADHD: inattention and hyperactivity-impulsivity. Latent class analysis suggested that ADHD symptomatology could be broken into three problem domains: predominantly inattentive, (ADHD-PI) predominantly hyperactive/impulsive (ADHD-PHI), and combined type (ADHD-C).[18] Criteria for each subtype require six or more of nine symptoms in each category. Additional criteria require onset of symptoms by age seven, pervasive and clinically significant impairment of functioning, and exclusion of other psychiatric conditions. Of note, several changes to the ADHD criteria are being considered by the DSM-5 Task Force. One of the most substantial changes would entail eliminating the three subtypes, possibly making two separate diagnoses (ADHD, which would be what is currently called ADHD-C), and ADD, which would include inattentive symptoms but no hyperactive symptoms would be required. One of the most substantial changes would entail eliminating the three subtypes, possibly making two separate diagnoses: ADHD (which would be what is currently called ADHD-C), and ADD (which would include inattentive symptoms but no hyperactive symptoms would be required) These proposed changes are being reviewed by the task force because of several criticisms of the current diagnosis.[19]

3.1.1. *Inattention*

Attentional deficits in ADHD are characterized primarily by an inability to sustain attention, particularly when performing repetitive, structured, and less enjoyable tasks. This inability to sustain attention results in distractibility, disorganization and forgetfulness, failure to finish assignments or chores, frequent changing of activities, and difficulty persisting in an activity even when the child is engaged with said activity. Children with ADHD may also exhibit impairments in attentional capacity and selective attention.

Recent research suggests that a subgroup of children (30–50%) with ADHD-PI may, in fact, represent an entirely different disorder. These children are hypoactive rather than hyperactive, are prone to daydreaming, and exhibit fewer externalizing symptoms (ODD, CD), and greater internalizing symptoms (depression, anxiety) than children with ADHD-C. This subset of symptoms has been described as Sluggish Cognitive Tempo or SCT.[20] Barkley suggests that because this subgroup appears to evidence problems with selective/focused attention rather than sustained attention and lacks the behavioral disinhibition characteristic of other types of ADHD, it may require different modes of intervention.

3.1.2. *Hyperactivity/impulsivity*

Hyperactive-impulsive behavior is excessively energetic, intense, inappropriate, and not goal directed. Children with ADHD are often described as being "driven by a motor," and they tend to show more motor activity than children without ADHD. This has been demonstrated in several studies with the use of an actigraph.[21] Hyperactive children are fidgety, excessively talkative, and have trouble staying seated when they are required to do so. Impulsivity can manifest itself as cognitive impulsivity, behavioral impulsivity, or both. These children have difficulty resisting immediate gratification, are likely to resist stopping a behavior when asked to do so, and have trouble waiting their turn. They frequently interrupt others and may speak or act without regard to consequences.

3.1.3. *Limitations of DSM-IV criteria*

DSM-IV criteria for ADHD were rigorously empirically derived, but are not without limitations (for a review see Barkley[19,20]). First, the symptom checklists for both the inattention and hyperactivity-impulsivity domains are behaviorally oriented and situation specific. Thus, these criteria may apply to 4–16 year olds, but may be of limited usefulness when evaluating older teenagers or adults. This would not be problematic if ADHD was a static disorder that did not change over time. However, substantial research has shown that particular behaviors, such as the items included in the hyperactivity-impulsivity symptom list, tend to dissipate with age. Stability of subtypes over time is also questionable. This suggests that individuals may outgrow certain symptoms without necessarily outgrowing the disorder itself.[20] Further, the essence of the diagnosis of ADHD is that the behaviors must be developmentally inappropriate, which suggests that different sets of criteria are needed for the different developmental stages of life. These issues are currently being addressed by the DSM-5 Task Force.[19]

Other criteria utilized by DSM-IV to describe ADHD may also be problematic. There is a lack of empirical support for the requirement that symptoms must be present prior to age seven, and indeed, many cases are reported with a later age of onset.[19] Earlier onset of symptoms may be indicative of poorer prognosis, but there is no evidence to suggest any qualitative differences between children with ADHD-onset prior to age seven and those children whose symptoms began later.

As discussed above, there may be a need to develop different ADHD criteria for boys and girls. Boys typically display more of the behaviors characteristic of ADHD than girls do, and in a more observable manner. In the absence of gender-specific criteria, girls must meet a higher threshold of impairment compared to peers in order to meet criteria for a diagnosis of ADHD. Developing different sets of criteria for males and females may narrow the current gap in diagnosis of ADHD between boys and girls.

3.2. *ICD-10 criteria*

ICD-10 criteria[22] for Hyperkinetic Disorder (HKD) are similar, although not identical, to the DSM-IV criteria for ADHD. The ICD-10 and DSM-IV work groups adopted the same list of symptoms for HKD and ADHD, and both ICD-10 and DSM-IV require functional impairment in home and school settings, and onset prior to age seven. However, ICD-10 differs from DSM-IV in that it requires the presence of both hyperactivity-impulsivity and inattention in order to make a diagnosis of HKD; it does not distinguish the subtypes that DSM-IV does. Another important difference is that the diagnosis of HKD cannot be made when the child concurrently meets criteria for an anxiety disorder, depression, or any other significant psychiatric disorder. DSM-IV allows for comorbid diagnoses (with the exception of autism spectrum or pervasive developmental disorders), provided that the symptoms in question do not occur exclusively within episodes of such other disorders. The ultimate result of these criterion differences would be to make the diagnosis of HKD more exclusionary, and therefore more stringent, in ICD-10. This, in part, could explain the differences in prevalence rates found in the United States and Europe. Therefore, the clinician has to make a choice as to how he/she prefers to practice. As outlined throughout this book, we prefer the differential diagnostic approach leading to a principal diagnosis, if at all possible, as treatments become increasingly specific and diagnostic differences begin to matter.

In a longitudinal study,[23] all children who met full criteria for HKD also met full DSM-IV criteria for ADHD, but only 26% of ADHD children met criteria for HKD. Children were followed over a period of six years, and all children (those who met criteria for HKD and those who met criteria for ADHD) exhibited more symptoms of ADHD, lower adaptive functioning on the Children's Global Assessment Scale (CGAS), more problems in peer relations, and more difficulties in the classroom over time than non-referred comparison children. This suggests that both the ICD-10 and DSM-IV criteria are predictively valid across different impairment constructs. Moreover, the ADHD group continued to exhibit symptoms and functional impairment over time, in some cases more severely so than those in the HKD group, leading Lahey *et al.*[23] to suggest that the more stringent ICD-10 criteria may underidentify children with significant problems related to inattention and hyperactivity-impulsivity.

4. ADHD Across the Lifespan

It was originally believed that ADHD was a disorder that only affected young children, and that most would "outgrow" the disorder by the time they reached their teen years. However, as more longitudinal research is conducted, there are indications that ADHD continues to be a problem throughout the lifespan for many individuals. The range of persistent problems is large (from 2 to 80%), depending on whether full syndromal criteria are required for adult diagnosis, and depending on which instruments are employed. Barkley recently discussed these difficulties.[24,25] The National Comorbidity Survey[26] estimated the prevalence of adult ADHD to be 4.4%; however, many of these adults continue to exhibit significant impairments in functioning due to ADHD-related symptoms. Adults with ADHD are often found to have marked inattention, distractibility, organization difficulties, poor efficiency, and as a result report a history of academic and occupational failures. Adults who report a childhood history of ADHD have higher rates of employment and martial difficulties, health problems, injuries, accidents, and antisocial and criminal behavior.[27] They also commonly report teen pregnancies[28] and bearing children out of wedlock.[29] Although this chapter is concerned with the diagnosis and treatment of

ADHD in children and adolescents, it is important to note that for some, ADHD can be a chronic condition that requires treatment across the lifespan.

Several studies of underage populations have shown that 80–90% of teenagers diagnosed with ADHD in childhood will continue to exhibit significant symptoms of the disorder in adolescence and early adulthood,[20,25] with the core symptoms affecting almost all domains of functioning.

A sample of clinic-referred children aged 4–12 at the outset of the study who were "rigorously diagnosed as hyperactive," were followed into adulthood.[25] Participants were evaluated again at ages 19–25 (mean age 21) and finally in their early thirties (2008). There was a high persistence of both diagnosis and dysfunction in academic, vocational, interpersonal, and other health domains when compared to age-matched controls. Based upon the results of this longitudinal study, ADHD seems to be a highly persistent disorder, and while symptoms of hyperactivity and impulsivity decline over time, problems with attention persist and put ADHD patients at a marked disadvantage compared to same-age peers.

4.1. *Predictors of adolescent and adult outcomes*

No single predictor of outcome has emerged in determining the adolescent and adult outcomes of childhood ADHD. Most recently, the results of the 36-month follow-up of the NIMH MTA study[30,31] did not find any predictors of treatment response (including initial symptom severity, sex (male), comorbidity (either internalizing or externalizing disorders), public assistance, and/or parental psychopathology). However, there are several factors which, operating alone or in tandem, may have prognostic power.[20] Family SES is associated with outcome, as is the overall intelligence of the child. The extent of peer relationship problems in childhood is associated with future interpersonal difficulties; conduct disorder and aggression in children is associated with poorer outcomes in adolescence. Familial psychopathology, in particular a family history of ADHD, is also associated with emotional and psychiatric problems in adolescence; this risk is increased when family members also have comorbid conduct problems.

5. Comorbid Disorders

A diagnosis of ADHD carries with it a significant risk for the cooccurrence of other disorders. In a study of clinic-referred children with ADHD, 80% had at least one other disorder besides ADHD.[32] The incidence of true comorbidity is important, as it intensifies impairment among the child. It has also been shown that the presence of certain key comorbidities, including depression, delinquency, and learning disorders, do not respond optimally to ADHD treatments.

The most commonly comorbid disorders with ADHD are Oppositional Defiant Disorder (ODD) and Conduct Disorder (CD) (see Chap. 9 of this volume for discussion). Studies have suggested that between 54 and 84% of children and adolescents with ADHD may meet criteria for an additional diagnosis of ODD; a significant portion of these will develop CD.[33] Children with comorbid ADHD and ODD/CD appear to have more severe impairment than children with ADHD alone. They exhibit more impulsivity than children with ADHD alone, and are more impulsive than they are hyperactive.[34] Evidence is mounting to suggest that the combination of ADHD and CD is likely a unique disorder. These children have an earlier onset of symptoms, particularly conduct problems, than children with either disorder alone. They also show more aggression, more peer/social rejection and more callous/unemotional traits.

Children with ADHD show impaired performance on standardized measures of intelligence and achievement compared to controls. They also have more problems with school performance; various studies have found that children with ADHD are more likely to repeat grades, more likely to require placement in special classrooms, more likely to need tutoring, and more likely to earn lower grades in academic subjects. However, studies have shown that not all children with ADHD have lower IQs than controls; rather, they seem to span the spectrum of intellectual ability, from highly gifted to mild mental retardation. Regardless, it is currently estimated that 25–35% will have a coexisting language or learning problem.[25,35]

Anxiety disorders are estimated to occur in approximately one-third of patients with ADHD.[36] In addition, a longitudinal study[25] found that the prevalence rates of comorbid mood and anxiety disorders among children with ADHD increased significantly at the four-year follow-up, suggesting that children with ADHD are at substantial risk for developing further impairment across multiple domains. A detailed discussion of the issue of comorbidity of ADHD and bipolar disorder can be found in this volume (Chap. 7).

ADHD and substance abuse are known to cooccur. This association seems particularly prevalent in those patients with coexisting disruptive behavior disorders, such as CD and (to a lesser degree) ODD. These diagnoses may serve as a marker for the potential for drug abuse, both within treatment and outside of treatment. There is evidence that successful treatment reduces the risk for and presence of substance and alcohol abuse. The most recent MTA follow-up study[37] found that although MTA children had higher rates of delinquency and substance use than a normative sample, there were no effects of initial treatment assignment (*e.g.* medication, community care or behavioral treatment) on delinquency or substance use. However, as the children in this sample were only 11–13 years old, further follow-up is needed as these children enter their mid-late teens and early adulthood (when rates of substance use peak).

As we are entering a new phase in ADHD treatment with several compounds being available which have no abuse or diversion potential, it is important to understand the possible relationship between type of ADHD treatment and future delinquent behavior, as such an association creates risk scenarios which have only recently come under increased scrutiny. Some patients, while being treated for ADHD, will abuse their stimulant medications for non-medical purposes. This issue was somewhat academic when only stimulants were available for treatment. However, over the past 5–7 years, multiple other treatments have emerged that suggest alternate interventions first when abuse is a prominent problem.[38]

New information gathered in studies from NIDA and SAMHSA examine hitherto ignored risks. The Drug Abuse Warning Network (DAWN) report[39] found that the most frequent reason for ADHD-related emergency room visits was non-medical use of stimulant medications (48%). Rates of emergency room visits for amphetamine or methylphenidate-related conditions were higher among 12–17 year olds than among patients aged 18 or older. Finally, approximately 68% of emergency visits involving non-medical use of amphetamines or methylphenidate also involved another substance (alcohol, an illicit drug, or other prescription medicines).

A recent edition of the *Harvard Newsletter*[40] summarizes the abuse profile within a treated ADHD population. Of the ADHD patients in grades 7–12 surveyed, 30% have been asked to divert their medication: 7–15% have done so, and 11% have sold their medication. They have also abused stimulant medications themselves: 22% had taken more of the medication than prescribed, and 10% had used their medication to get high. Most of those who reported abuse of ADHD medications also had a comorbid CD diagnosis.

Thus, a substantial fraction of treated ADHD patients may divert and/or abuse their medications. The mechanisms of stimulant abuse have been described.[41] The stimulant-abusing patient will seek to rapidly reach maximal efficacy of the medication prescribed. This results in a very short time to 50% dopamine transporter (DAT) occupancy, and a "high" is reported when there is a steep rise to this level. Rapid bioavailability is achieved by several possible methods: (1) alteration of route of administration (snorting, intravenous); or (2) the ingestion of large amounts of the compound over a short period. Methylphenidate is twice as potent as cocaine at blocking the DAT. The dose of methylphenidate needed to achieve 50% DAT occupancy (ED50) is 0.075 mg/kg. This means that an intranasal dose of 20–50 mg is likely to be well above the ED50 and equivalent to about 100 mg cocaine IV. This can easily be achieved with currently prescribed doses of stimulants. Dextroamphetamine is more potent still, but has yet to be studied. The therapeutic effects of stimulants seem to be tied to its slow and constant delivery at steady and low doses; rapid administration and high doses activate appetitive and reinforce "rush" responses.

Other variables also influence these factors, namely age, social context, and other intraindividual variables. However, the potential for abuse of treatment medications by patients cannot be ignored. As the data suggest, adolescents seem especially vulnerable.

Most interestingly, a recent study reported that children with concentration problems seem to have increased risk for trauma later in life.[42,43] This is hardly surprising, as impulsivity and lack of consideration of possible consequences will often expose individuals to dangerous situations.

6. Neuroscience

From the viewpoint of neuroscience, ADHD is a heterogeneous disorder for which the neurobiology is just beginning to be understood. Studies in animal models, cognitive neurosciences, and genetics are uncovering a clearer picture that may soon permit us to go beyond mere phenomenology to address specific deficits in functioning. However, in the past 10 years, great strides have been made in identifying the neuroscientific underpinnings of human attention regulation. Convergent evidence from neuropsychological studies, imaging studies, especially fMRIs, evoked potentials in humans and monkeys, as well as lesion studies and other anatomical studies support the model depicted in Fig. 1. Pessoa *et al.*[44]

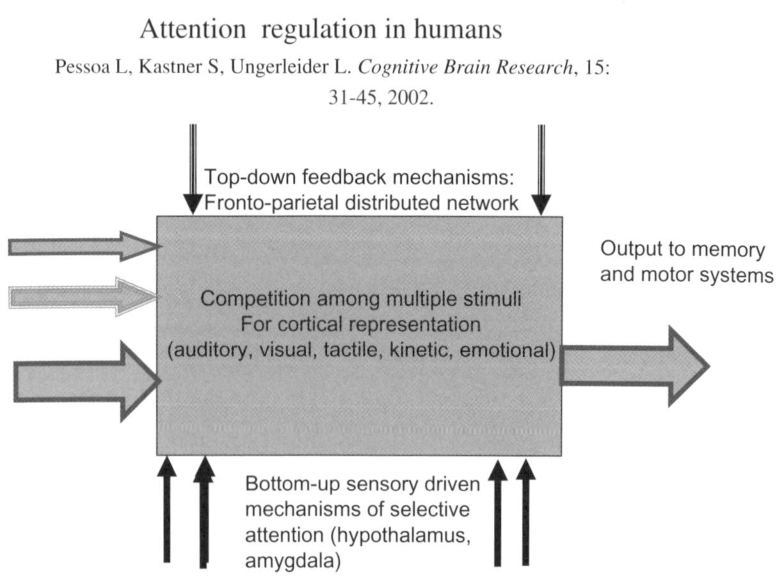

Fig. 1: Attention regulation in humans (modified from Pessoa 2002)[44].

summarizes work that is based on the study of visual stimuli. The model described is therefore only strictly applicable to this sensory input, but it is very likely that similar regulatory influences will be found for other sensory modalities, such as auditory and tactile.

At any given time humans are immersed in complex visual space from which they must select certain inputs for particular salience, assess their relevance to what they are doing at that moment, and help them prepare an appropriate executive response. The selection of these stimuli can occur in two basic formats: by bottom-up driven mechanisms which originate in the emotion circuits of the amygdala and the hippocampus; or via the top-down control of a parallel distributed network in the frontoparietal regions. These two systems are in competition for the selection of stimulus response. Imaging, neuropsychological, and anatomical evidence supports the existence of the top-down regulation circuits. The support from imaging studies is especially strong, as is demonstrated by metaanalytic evidence from 10 independent studies indicating similar patterns of activation.[44]

These two systems have important characteristics which set them apart. The bottom-up driven system is closer to hardwired, reflects more emotionally salient inputs, and thus selects stimuli with relative rigidity and disregard for the demands of a particular situation. A good example would be the type of inattention created by overactive an amygdala, which can be found in patients suffering from PTSD and bipolar illness. In such cases inattention is part of the disorder, but that does not necessarily mean that the top-down regulation system is disordered. More likely, the amount of bottom-up hyperselectivity simply overwhelms the capacity of a normally functioning top-down regulation system. The competition between various stimuli is ultimately resolved in the visual cortex, but the top-down biasing signals come from the frontoparietal network.

Additionally, there is evidence from fMRIs and experimental work in humans that these frontoparietal systems are compromised[45] in ADHD. In an interference suppression paradigm, there was evidence that the frontal–striatal–temporal–-parietal network was not as active as in healthy controls. ADHD subjects also relied on a different region than controls to inhibit responses (right superior region in those with ADHD versus fronto–striatal regions in controls).

There is sufficient evidence to outline the neural network of directed attention.[44] Four cerebral regions appear to provide an integrated network for the modulation of directed attention; each region has a unique functional role. The posterior parietal cortex provides an internal sensory map; a limbic component in the cingulate gyrus regulates the spatial distribution of motivational valence; the frontal cortex coordinates the motor programs, and the reticular component provides the underlying level of arousal and vigilance. Single lesions to any of these four areas will yield partial unilateral neglect syndromes in the contralateral extrapersonal space. Lesions encompassing more than one region will result in more profound attentional deficits.

Additionally, we have convergent evidence regarding the neurotransmitters that enable the top-down system to function properly: norepinephrine, dopamine, and most recently 5-hydroxytryptamine (serotonin) are all implicated. This is important, as new psychopharmacological advances have made possible the more specific targeting of these systems and thus make possible more specific treatments. Dopamine is of great interest,[46] but other monoamines may play a larger role than previously appreciated. It is increasingly apparent that norepinephrine (NE) is important, gleaned from the observation that stimulants are also potent inhibitors of the norepinephrine transporter (NET)[47] and the effectiveness in ADHD of non-stimulant NET inhibitors such as desipramine and atomoxetine.[48] Clinically heterogeneous responses to medications may be evidence for distinct imbalances in DA versus NE signaling compounded by the specific pharmacology of each agent. The classic stimulants, amphetamine (AMPH) and methylphenidate (MPH), differentially modulate synaptic reuptake versus vesicular accumulation of DA and NE, resulting in differential augmentation.[49] Regional differences may also underlie response heterogeneity or side effects, *e.g.* atomoxetine and MPH increase extracellular NE and DA in prefrontal cortex, but only the latter increases extracellular DA in striatum and nucleus accumbens.[50] These findings speak to the integral crosstalk between DA and NE systems, since atomoxetine is almost 300-fold less potent at the DAT,[50] yet, robustly modulates prefrontal DA levels. One model integrating these two systems proposes a bipartite attention network. A posterior system, mediated by ascending noradrenergic fibers from the locus coeruleus, biases behavioral orientation between external and internal stimuli.[51] NE seems to support disengagement from stimuli, shifting attention to novel stimuli, and engaging the new stimuli. Meanwhile, an anterior executive system, mediated by DA and NE, subsequently prepares the organism for response.[52] DA seems to govern the analysis of new inputs and preparation for an appropriate response. Dysregulation in either of these systems may result in an ADHD phenotype, but effective treatment may depend on the relative balance of the impairment.

The "dopamine hypothesis"[53] was initially supported by a report of increased DATs in the striatum of a small group of adult ADHD patients,[54] but replications have been inconsistent and a recent study of unmedicated ADHD subjects found lower DAT binding in caudate and nucleus accumbens.[55] Interestingly, attention impairment scores correlated with increased DAT binding, but for a given DAT level, ADHD subjects exhibited greater attention problems, suggesting that impairments in other systems interact with dopamine signaling to regulate attention.

Consonant with clinical experience, these data emphasizes that a monotonic model centered on dopamine is not likely to yield the total picture.

Most recently, data have emerged regarding a possible role for serotonin (5-HT) in ADHD. Impulsivity is a cardinal feature of most individuals with ADHD, and one of the strongest associations in psychiatry is that between impulsivity and low CSF concentrations of the serotonin metabolite 5-hydroxyindoleacetic acid.[56] Rodent models implicate serotonin in the pharmacologic effects of MPH and AMPH.[47,57] Depletion of serotonergic projections to prefrontal cortex in primates results in impairments in prepulse inhibition[58] and 5-HT depletion dampens the ability of amphetamine to decrease impulsive choice.[59] A growing number of studies implicate serotonin signaling pathway genes in the phenotype of ADHD.[60,61] Polymorphisms in TPH2, the rate-limiting enzyme in brain serotonin biosynthesis, are associated w/measures of response inhibition[62] and conflict-related executive processing.[63] Conflict is thought to be monitored by the dorsal anterior cingulate cortex (ACC).[64] Error-related negativity, an event-related potential that maps to the ACC and peaks shortly after an incorrect response is decreased in ADHD,[65] suggesting these individuals fail to adequately monitor negative responses. Output from ACC is proposed to modulate decision centers in dorsolateral frontal cortex that coordinate behavioral output.[66] Interestingly, the executive processing differences associated with the TPH2 promoter polymorphism[63] map to ACC.[67]

It is tempting to speculate that in ADHD, raphe serotonin governs activity of conflict monitoring regions in the frontal cortex that interact with salience signals regulated by the dopaminergic system and alerting functions of the noradrenergic system. The concerted actions of these neurotransmitters may be responsible for normal functioning in the attention network. Disruptions in individual pathways may give rise to different degrees of impairment in attention, impulse control, hyperactivity, and/or comorbid symptoms. This conclusion is supported by the high comorbidity in ADHD[13] and results from the MTA study supporting distinction of ADHD with internalizing versus externalizing symptoms.[68] The model should not, however, be viewed as an invitation to injudicious polypharmacy, but rather a clarion call for more detailed study of the biology, genetics, and phenomenology of ADHD.

The progress in the neuroscientific underpinnings of attention regulation and its pathology is exciting. It has opened up new windows on diagnosis, treatment, and possibly etiological pathways. We, however, would like to add a cautionary note at this point: all these findings have been produced in tightly-controlled experiments, with highly selected subject groups. The apparatuses used to produce these findings are usually of the highest quality and complexity, and barely comparable to those available on a routine clinical basis. There are some claims that relatively simple programs can assess these deficits, a claim that is not supported by high-level evidence. It is quite clear that ultimately we will be able to use neuroscience to our advantage in the clinical setting. At this time, however, we are simply not in a position to do so for ADHD.

7. Etiologies

Although there may be multiple etiologies all leading to the development of ADHD, consensus is emerging that developmental, neurological, and genetic factors are the most contributory. Scientists have frequently noted the similarities between patients with ADHD and those with frontal lobe lesions or injuries. While the majority of children with ADHD do not suffer from a traumatic brain injury, research has continued to examine possible structural, functional, and/or neurochemical bases for ADHD.

Although neuroimaging is not currently useful as a diagnostic tool for ADHD, we are beginning to define some neurobiological differences between children with ADHD and controls. Structural differences in the brain have been found in children with ADHD, including smaller cerebellar volume,[69,70] smaller right hemisphere plana temporale, smaller corpus callosum, smaller anterior right frontal regions, smaller size of the caudate nucleus, and smaller globus pallidus regions.[69] The reduced volume of the cerebellum in children with ADHD is consistent with what is known about the function of this region of the brain, which is that it performs many tasks related to executive functioning. Reduced volumes in key frontal–striatal regions is also consistent with the role of these structures in governing executive functioning, including attention, cognition, and behavioral modification.

Functional imaging of ADHD is still in its infancy, but some preliminary studies have found that children with ADHD show differences in brain activation compared to controls. As described by Bush *et al.*,[71] children were asked to perform tasks requiring inhibitory control (*e.g.* Go-No-Go task) while in an fMRI machine. Healthy volunteers activated their dorsal anterior cingulated cortex (dACC), whereas children with ADHD did not. The dACC has been shown to play important roles in attention, cognition, motor control, and reward-based decision making.[72,73]

Other neurobiological (non-genetic) causes of ADHD have been reported,[74] consisting of such factors as perinatal stress and low birth weight,[75] maternal smoking during pregnancy[76] and very severe early deprivation (this must be extreme deprivation, not simply a lack of adequate parenting).[77]

Pathways in the brain that govern attentional processes are surely implicated in the development of ADHD. Executive inhibition,[78] or poor inhibition of behavioral responses to external stimuli, has been implicated in ADHD. Deficits or dysfunctions in neurotransmitters (as discussed in detail above) may also play a role.

8. Genetics

Research suggests that ADHD is a highly heritable disorder. Evidence in support of this theory comes from family and adoption studies, twin studies, and molecular genetic studies. A recent study found a threefold increase in ADHD among biological parents of children with ADHD, as compared to adoptive parents of adopted children with ADHD.[79] More recent studies have attempted to determine the percent of variance between twins that can be accounted for by genetic, as opposed to environmental, factors. The results of these studies suggest that the heritability of ADHD is nearly 0.80, making it one of the most highly heritable psychiatric disorders.[80] Finally, molecular genetics is being applied to the search for a gene or a combination of genes that might account for the development of ADHD. This can be done in one of two ways: a genome-wide scan, which looks for any and all genes that might be involved in a disorder, or a candidate gene analysis, which targets specific genes hypothesized to play a role in the disorder.[81] ADHD candidate genes for which genetic associations have been reported include the dopamine 4 and 5 receptors, the dopamine transporter, the enzyme dopamine beta hydroxylase, the serotonin transporter gene, the serotonin 1B receptor, and the synaptosomal-associated protein-25 gene (DRD4, DRD5, DAT, DBH, 5-HTT, HTR1B, and SNAP-25).[82] More recently, three groups have reported on an association for polymorphisms in TPH2.[83–85] While the rapid progress in molecular genetics is exciting and encouraging, it should be noted that no confirmed polymorphism explains enough variance to warrant genetic testing as a predictive tool.

9. Interventions

The psychopharmacologic treatment of ADHD rests on an impressive amount of high-quality empirical data. In general, studies show that a variety of medications are effective in powerfully ameliorating the target symptoms of ADHD. Psychotherapeutic interventions, although effortful and costly, can be a useful adjunct to medication for some patients. Nonetheless, as best as we can tell at the present time, none of our interventions are curative. All are palliative, having their beneficial effects only while administered, without lasting residual effects after treatment is stopped. It is generally thought that if the disorder ceases to cause problems, this is due to maturation or a learning effect, whereby a person learns to willfully control their symptoms.

For those interested in familiarizing themselves with the entire range of interventions in ADHD, we suggest consulting the latest update by Barkley.[33] Those interested in more details of the specific interventions listed in this section are referred to our previous publication on *Developmental Approaches to Psychopathology*.[9]

9.1. *Pharmacotherapy for the treatment of ADHD*

Many of these compounds have been in use for many decades and are well known and studied. While the side-effect profiles are not ideal, they are known quantities and can be monitored carefully. There is also a steady accumulation of information on the treatment of the disorder across the lifespan. The best and most rigorously designed studies, funded by NIMH, employ stimulants and related compounds[86–89] without special delivery systems.

However, because of the side-effect profiles and abuse potential these are not necessarily the interventions of automatic first choice, now that we have available to us compounds which essentially bypass these issues altogether. There are two clinical scenarios where the use of stimulants as the medications of choice should be carefully considered: (1) the presence of externalizing comorbid disorders in the patient, such as ODD, CD, and/or substance abuse/dependence; or the presence of substance abuse/dependence in the child's social context (family, peer or otherwise); (2) the presence of anxiety and mood problems which might be negatively impacted by the use of stimulants. These considerations must be weighed against the fact that non-stimulant treatments of ADHD have a relatively limited database, compared to stimulants, and therefore, many of the truly long-term effects are not understood.

Still, although atomoxetine (strattera) has a relatively short life as a researched agent (about seven years), and thus potential cumulative side effects are not known, its complete lack of abuse potential and mild side effect profile recommends it for serious first-line consideration. The American Academy of Child and Adolescent Psychiatry (AACAP) has endorsed it as one of the three agents for initial drug treatment trial, along with methylphenidates and amphetamines.[90] This will hopefully be true for the new extended-release preparation of guanfacine (intuniv).[91]

An additional caution with respect to stimulants is their well-documented psychotropic effect on unaffected individuals. The German Luftwaffe used stimulants frequently among its pilots to enhance performance in World War II,[7,92] as did the United States Air Force up until fairly recently; college students and academics have recently begun receiving attention in the media for their use of these compounds to "get ahead" in our competitive, career-driven society.[93] Stimulants have profound effects on normal populations. In two landmark studies, normal prepubescent adolescents and adults were given methylphenidate and exhibited similar effects on motor activity and vigilance[94,95] as would be expected from patients with ADHD. As discussed in a thoughtful and complete review,[92] many studies have shown that stimulants have performance-enhancing effects in athletes. The issue of generating a response when there is no disorder is a serious one to be taken into account in evaluating treatment effects and risk.

The other classes of compounds used in the treatment of ADHD (bupropion, modafanil, desipramine, atypical antipsychotics, alpha-adrenergic agents, pemoline) are best thought of as second line, for special circumstances and judicious combination treatment. This chapter details mostly first-line treatments (atomoxetine and stimulants) and will not include a detailed discussion of second- and third-line treatments mentioned above. Discussion of these agents, their efficacy, side effects, dosing, and pharmacokinetics, can be found in Joshi[96] or psychopharmacology textbooks.

9.1.1. *Clinical indications*

Atomoxetine is indicated for the treatment of adult, adolescent, and childhood ADHD. Most recently it has been reported that it may also have some mild anxiolytic properties, or at least, it does not worsen anxiety symptoms in the context of ADHD.[97] There are a large number of independent studies of atomoxetine, reported as posters at national meetings, currently in various stages of review, promising to round out the clinical profile of this interesting compound.

In cases of more complicated ADHD (comorbid with externalizing disorders and anxiety), we suggest seriously considering drugs without abuse and diversion potential as well as mood neutral side effects as first agents of intervention. We tend to draw a parallel in the treatment of ADHD with the treatment of anxiety disorders: we aim to employ a relatively safe up-regulator of the attention system and are willing to accept less than perfect efficacy in order to avoid addiction and abuse potential. We then add, if necessary, a rescue medication (a stimulant in ADHD), which is employed in small amounts and targeted for times of known allostatic overload (*e.g.* final exams, job interviews, standardized tests).

Guanfacine extended-release (intuniv), a selective alpha-2A-receptor agonist, recently became the second non-stimulant medication approved by the FDA for the treatment of ADHD.[93] Alpha-2A-receptor agonists enhance neurological activity in the prefrontal cortex, which may improve impulse control as well as planning and organizational skills. One study compared the efficacy of guanfacine extended release (GXR) with placebo in children and adolescents in a double-blind, nine-week, dose-ranging, parallel-design, multicenter trial. six-to-seventeen-year olds were randomly treated by either once-daily oral GXR in 1-, 2-, 3-, and 4-mg doses or placebo. Primary outcome was change in total ADHD Rating Scale-IV score from baseline to endpoint. Statistically significant reductions in ADHD scores were observed from baseline to endpoint at all doses of GXR, with effect sizes ranging from 0.43 to 0.62. Mean heart rate and systolic and diastolic blood pressure decreased as the dose of GXR increased. Once the dose was maintained or tapered, the side effects subsided. Other frequent side effects were somnolence, headache, fatigue, sedation, dizziness, irritability, upper abdominal pain, and nausea, emerging usually in the first two weeks of treatment.[91]

Stimulant medications continue to be the most commonly prescribed agents in child and adolescent psychiatry. There is a vast body of literature to support their use, and recently, there has been a marked increase in the types of stimulant compounds available.[98] Amphetamines are the prototypical agent. Psychostimulants are thought to exert their mechanisms of action on the catecholamines dopamine (DA) and/or norepinephrine (NE) by reuptake inhibition, enhanced release, or a combination of these.[50,99] Bupropion (wellbutrin) is also thought to act by this mechanism, although its clinical effects on ADHD symptoms are not as robust.[100,101] Amphetamines (AMPH) seem to affect many aspects of release, uptake, and storage, while methylphenidates (MPH) act primarily presynaptically to prevent reuptake of dopamine and norepinephrine though the inhibition of the DA transporter protein.

The MTA study was the first to systematically compare treatment with medication to other forms of treatment. Almost 600 children between the ages of seven and nine years old who had been diagnosed with ADHD, combined-type, were divided into four groups. Over 14 months, one group received medication alone, overseen by the study operators who monitored the dosage and performed monthly visits. A second group received intensive behavioral therapy over the same period. A third received medication combined with behavioral therapy, and the fourth was given standard community treatment, which may have included treatment with medication. The study found unequivocally that medication, when given under a "carefully crafted" treatment program, was significantly more effective at treating the ADHD symptoms than treatments that did not include medication. Although all four groups showed substantial improvement, those in the supervised medication group and the combined treatment group showed substantially more improvements than those who received behavioral therapy alone, or community care.

Although medication alone proved very effective, the study also found that children in the combined group, which received behavioral therapy in addition to medication management, showed similar levels of improvement on lower doses of medication. It is also important to note that the medication management program administered through the study did significantly better than routine community care. Since routine care often involves medication, the implication is that not all courses of medication treatment will have similar outcomes. According to the NIMH FAQ (http://www.nimh.nih.gov/events/mtaqa.cfm), "During the first month of treatment, special care was taken to find an optimal dose of medication for each child receiving the MTA medication treatment. After this period, these children were seen monthly for one-half hour at each visit. During the treatment visits, the MTA prescribing therapist spoke with the parent, met with the child, and sought to determine any concerns that the family might have regarding the medication or the child's ADHD-related difficulties. If the child was experiencing any difficulties, the MTA physician was encouraged to consider adjustments in the child's medication (rather than taking a "wait and see" approach)."

More recent reports of the three-year follow-up[30] indicate another interesting fact, which may further support psychosocial interventions. Although the 14- and 24-month follow-up studies found an advantage for the medication management and combination treatment (medication management and behavior therapy) groups compared to behavior therapy only and community care groups, after three years, outcomes between the four groups did not differ (with all groups showing symptom improvement since baseline). Thus, it may be possible that latent (or sleeper) effects of psychosocial interventions leveled the playing field. Rates of improvement may also be related to intensity of treatment; this might explain the gains that the community care group showed over time, where contact may have been less frequent or the intervention less intense and so improvement occurred more slowly. In any case, these results suggest the need to discontinue medication treatment after a couple of years, when substantial improvement has been observed, to ascertain whether treatment with these agents is still warranted (*e.g.* over the summer months).

A special issue concerning stimulant and related compound treatment emerged after Canada decided to ban its use following post-marketing reports of 12 unexplained cases of pediatric cardiac arrest. This led to a stringent review by two panels of the FDA in 2006 (http://www.fda.gov/medwatch/safety/2006/safety06.htm#Dexedrine) which recommended ultimately that practitioners need to give stronger warnings to parents and patients taking stimulants. This is in addition to the included cardiac-related risk warnings in the package inserts.

On closer examination, at least five of the cases that prompted the review and ban had undiagnosed structural cardiac deficits. The remainder had combinations of metabolic, hydration, and toxicity problems. These are the only cases reported in the 0–18 year age range over seven million patient years of treatment. Additionally, the absolute number of cases is lower than in the general population.[102]

Still, the clinician must exercise special caution when prescribing activating compounds such as stimulants. We ask that a recent pediatric physical examination be on file that speaks directly to the issue, in addition to routinely taking vital signs ourselves, along with a detailed cardiac history of the patient and the family. In the presence of documented cardiac problems we tend not to prescribe the stimulants.[40]

Contraindications to the use of stimulants include a previous sensitivity to these agents, a history of glaucoma, symptomatic cardiovascular disease, clinically important hypertension, or hyperthyroidism, and repeated occurrence of metabolic problems, dehydration, and diversion as well as noncompliance with our prescription. Stimulants cannot to be taken concomitantly with monoamine oxidase inhibitors (MAOI), or with a history of active psychosis. The presence of tics or Tourette syndrome per se is not a sufficient reason to withhold stimulants, but we tend not to use them in the presence of tics now that alternative treatments are available. Atomoxetine, in principle, should be used as the alternate agent of choice, because it does not seem to be active in the striatum. Other alternate agents, such as alpha-agonists (guanfacine, clonidine) or D2 antagonists (risperidone, ziprasidone, haloperidol, pimozide) may be considered as additions to treat tics. Other strategies include lowering of the stimulant dose, which may become more possible with a second medication in the regimen, or switch to monotherapy with a nonstimulant such as atomoxetine, an atypical antidepressant (bupropion, venlafaxine), or a tricyclic antidepressant. MPH is not approved for use in children under six, but there are at least eight published studies documenting their efficacy in preschoolers. D-amphetamine and pemoline can be used down to age three, despite the lack of published controlled studies in children this young.[99]

9.2. *Alternative treatments in ADHD*

As in many other parts of medicine, interest has been stimulated in finding homeopathic alternatives to allopathic treatments. Rojas and Chan[103] published an excellent review of some of the main complementary and alternative medicine (CAM) treatment approaches to ADHD. They reviewed elimination of artificial food additives, colors, and/or preservatives, the effect of simple sugar on behavior in children, and the use of EEG biofeedback. The authors note that they have been well studied, but lack support as effective sole treatments for ADHD.[104] The authors advise, however, that more rigorously designed studies are needed to evaluate their effectiveness as monotherapy for ADHD. Finally, a recent review on the use of omega-3 fatty acids by Richardson[105] presents interesting findings culled from the world literature on this frequently utilized CAM treatment. Although the evidence for this as a single intervention is still emerging, it seems potentially promising for a subset of patients and families who may be unwilling to try more well-known allopathic pharmacologic interventions.

9.3. *Future directions in psychopharmacology*

Several newer agents for ADHD are currently under development. This area of developmental psychopathology is one of the most active in terms of search for effective established and novel compounds. Prince[106] has summarized some of the most important studies done thus far with emerging compounds. The following is a summary from that work and reviews of other authors.

Modafinil (provigil), approved for the treatment of narcolepsy, continues to be studied for use in ADHD. It is a schedule IV substance, which seems to work through activation of the hypocretin–orexin system in the hypothalamus, an area thought to be involved in the mediation of wakefulness and vigilance. It also appears to have a direct effect on the dopamine transporter.[107] Results from double-blind placebo controlled studies in adults with ADHD have been mixed.[108–111] Turner and colleagues conducted a randomized placebo-controlled trial of 20 adults with ADHD, and found that the modafinil-treated group had improved short-term and visual memory, spatial planning, vigilance, and accuracy.[112] In a pooled analysis of 3 studies in children and teens, Wigal *et al.*[113] showed that modafinil was well tolerated among 623 school-aged children. Doses were "fixed" and based on weight, with those <30 kg receiving 300 mg, and those >30 kg receiving 425 mg QD. However, despite the large database of positive responders to this compound (including both children and adults), safety issues remain. For example, among the original group of patient data submitted during the course of FDA approval (n = 1236), three pediatric patients developed a serious drug rash, and one of these was a seven-year-old boy with presumed Stevens-Johnson syndrome. In addition, four adults developed serious erythema multiforme rashes in post-marketing surveillance studies. Thus, the FDA ruled in 2006 that, although there was consensus among panel members that modafinil was efficacious, the drug was not without potential serious safety issues. More information can be found at http://www.fda.gov/ohrms/dockets/ac/06/slides/2006-4212S1-01-02-FDAAndreason.ppt.

Reboxetine (edronax) has already been used in Europe for the treatment of depression. This SNRI (selective norepinephrine reuptake inhibitor) has been studied by Ratner *et al.*[114,115] and others. Results of both studies indicated a general reduction in ADHD symptom severity, with the most common side effects being drowsiness and gastrointestinal complaints. In this manner, its side effect profile and receptor selectivity is not unlike its better-known SNRI relative, atomoxetine. The dose ranges in these two open-label studies were 4–8 mg/day.

The H3 receptor antagonist GT-2331 (perceptin) may also have some DA-, NE-, and ACh(acetylcholine)-enhancing properties, and the histaminergic system is known to be involved in vigilance, attention, and cognition.[116,117] Gliatech, the drug's maker, reports that it is safe and well tolerated as a once-daily medication in Phase I trials. Phase II trials are currently underway with adult subjects.[118,119]

The compound GW 320659, a norepinephrine (NE) and dopamine (DA) reuptake inhibitor, was studied in prospective open-label fashion over a 11-week period.[120] As many as 51 patients were enrolled in this multisite trial, and 46 completed the study. By the end of the treatment phase, 76% of patients reported an improvement in symptoms. Side effects with the greatest frequency included headaches (31%), GI discomfort/pain (25%), emotional lability (20%), anorexia (18%), insomnia (14%), and nausea/ vomiting (12%).

A (R)-sibutramine (meridia) metabolite, marketed by sepracor, is currently being evaluated as both a potential ADHD treatment and useful medication for depression.[119] It has reuptake properties for DA, NE, and 5-HT. Recent data suggest effectiveness in targeting the attentional problems of ADHD and improving attention on a vigilance task. It also showed improvements in postural control, which may have special significance in ADHD, given recent findings regarding cerebellar abnormalities in children and adults with ADHD.[118,119,121] Research done so far indicates that sibutramine has little-to-no abuse potential, and may have utility in reducing attentional problems that are alcohol induced.

Selegiline (deprenyl), an irreversible MAO-B inhibitor, has shown promise as a potentially effective and well-tolerated medication for treating ADHD in both children and adults across several studies.[122,123] Among stimulant alternatives, these medicines may be particularly useful for inattentive symptoms. Recent comparisons versus MPH have been favorable in terms of tolerability and symptom improvement.[122,123] Doses across these studies for selegiline, used in children as young as 4-years old in one study,[122] were 5 mg/d in children <5 years old, and 10 mg/day if >5 years old. The most common side effects in these studies were mild, and included headache, labile mood, and GI upset, although the studies were relatively short term (between 4 and 10 weeks). The often-touted risk for adverse interaction with tyramine-rich foods appears less common with the use of a patch, if doses remain below 9 mg/day in adults,[124] and deserves formal study in children.

Anti-Alzheimer drugs such as donepezil (aricept) have shown promise in some small open series[125] and not others.[126] Further study is needed to better understand what role cognitive enhancers such as galantamine, revastigmine, and memantine may play in youth with ADHD. Two reports by Wilens[127–129] have shown evidence for the use of donepezil as a cognitive enhancer for patients with ADHD, especially for executive function deficits. An open series was conducted with five youths, aged 8–17 years, all of whom demonstrated improvement.[125]

Nicotine has shown evidence of cognitive enhancing effects.[130] Potter and Newhouse[131] compared the effects of a nicotine patch (7 mg) and MPH (10–20 mg, 0.15–0.21 mg/kg) in eight non-smoking teens with ADHD. While both the nicotine and MPH-treated patients showed improvements in stop-signal reaction times, nicotine beat MPH in measures of distractibility (Stroop test: interference by irrelevant stimuli), compared to placebo. The authors recommended that nicotine and the nicotinic system should remain an active area of study for novel treatment development.

Theophylline, a bronchodilator and adenosine receptor antagonist, appears to have effects on central norepinephrine and dopaminergic transmission, and as such, may have utility in ADHD. Mohammadi and colleagues[132] compared this treatment against MPH in 32 newly diagnosed boys (aged 6–14 years) with ADHD-CT (combined type). Random assignment was either to theophylline at 3–4 mg/kg/day (<12 year olds received the lower dose, 12 years or older received the higher), or MPH at 1 mg/kg/day). Both groups responded in similar fashion with regard to core symptoms of ADHD, as measured by parent and teacher ratings. Decreased appetite, sleep disturbances, and heart palpitations were the most commonly reported side effects, and were comparable among the groups. Of interest, all side effects were nearly equal between the two medications, with headache slightly more common in the MPH group ($p < .03$).

9.4. *Psychosocial interventions for the treatment of ADHD*

Psychosocial treatments for ADHD are important for a variety of reasons. First, there are several limitations to the use of pharmacological treatments.[133] Studies have suggested that approximately 20–30% of children and adolescents do not show a clinically significant response to medication, and may even show an adverse response. The addition of psychosocial treatment may provide the boost needed to produce an excellent treatment response. Finally, while there is abundant literature supporting the short-term efficacy of stimulant medications, research that supports the effectiveness of medications over the long-term is still in development.[134] Medication adherence may be an issue, either on the part of the child or the parent, but more likely, residual symptoms remain that are not addressed by medications.[135] Many parents express a preference for behavioral treatments in lieu of pharmacological treatment, or at the very least, in addition to it.[96] Concerns over medication use, or fear that stimulant medications might lead to later drug abuse or addiction may prompt some parents to refuse pharmacological treatment.

In addition, more complex presentations of ADHD may require psychosocial treatments that target symptoms that cannot be managed by medication alone. For example, it should not be expected that medication alone is sufficient for ADHD children whose families are dysfunctional in multiple domains, or for children who may have certain comorbid disorders. The findings of the MTA study at the 14-month assessment period suggested that combined medication and behavioral management therapies may be preferable for subgroups of ADHD children with anxiety disorders or high levels of socio-economic and/or family stressors.[136] Further, combined medication and psychotherapy may be more effective in producing certain related outcomes, which are not necessarily part of the core symptoms of the disorder, namely reducing parent–child conflict, improving social skills, oppositional/aggressive symptoms, academic difficulties, and anxiety symptoms.[136] It is also possible, as has been found in several studies of psychosocial interventions[137] that psychosocial interventions produce many "sleeper" effects, which only become apparent after the passage of months to years.

For these reasons, it is important to consider psychosocial interventions, when appropriate, in the treatment of ADHD. There is a vast array of psychosocial interventions which have been tried in the context of ADHD. A thorough review is beyond the scope of this chapter and available elsewhere,[33] we discuss here those that have received most empirical support and are readily available to practitioners. The most reasonable targets for these interventions vary by age and setting.

9.4.1. *Cognitive-behavioral therapy*

This array of interventions is probably most appropriate to consider in older patients (older children, adolescents, and adults) and those whose families for a variety of reasons are not available for treatment. Cognitive-behavioral therapy (CBT) for the treatment of ADHD targets impulse control and deficits in self-control and self-regulation (for a review of cognitive behavioral therapy in children and adolescents, see Erickson and Achilles).[138] CBT, because it focuses on individual self-management, is more appropriate for older children and adolescents because they are more likely to have the cognitive abilities necessary to understand the treatment. In fact, much research is currently being conducted on CBT in the treatment of ADHD in adults, with successful results in randomized controlled trials.[135] However, it has been difficult to establish the efficacy of CBT treatment in children. Hinshaw and his colleagues have found support for CBT in treating various types of interpersonal difficulties faced by youths with disruptive behavior disorders (including ADHD). Changing problem behaviors through self-monitoring and self-evaluation seems to be most effective with respect to reducing anger, aggression, and other negative social interactions.[139] Although the effect sizes are relatively small compared to medication trials, CBT can yield incremental effects and target areas of function that are not necessarily targeted by medication. These treatments can be useful in enhancing problem-solving skills, identifying and correcting cognitive distortions, and increasing emotional awareness.[138]

9.4.2. *Social skills training*

Social skills training programs are increasingly popular because of the significant peer relationship problems among those with ADHD. Children with ADHD have been found to be often rejected by their peers after only brief interactions; they also have fewer friends than their non-ADHD peers.[139] As mentioned previously, poor peer relationships are predictive of negative long-term outcomes for children with disruptive behavior disorders (*e.g.* ADHD, ODD, CD). Social skills training has demonstrated efficacy in improving skill knowledge, *e.g.* teaching children how to make friends, handle teasing, solve problems, be a good sport, and accept others.[140] Some studies have found social skills training to be effective in improving symptoms of ADHD, but a combined intervention of social skills training and parent training to be more so. This suggests that social skills training may function best as part of an overall treatment package (discussed later in this chapter). Of note, consideration must be given to grouping children within social skills training programs. There is concern that deviant behaviors among all participants may increase when aggressive and non-aggressive children are grouped together in these programs.[141]

Finally, there are some promising new social skills-based interventions on the horizon, notably friendship training[142] and student-mediated conflict resolution programs.[143] These are reviewed in detail by Barkley.[33] Friendship training focuses on helping the child build dyadic friendships that are mutually satisfying, which in turn improves for the overall well-being of the child. Student-mediated conflict resolution programs utilize student mediators on the playground, who are trained to intervene when conflict occurs, offer students the opportunity to resolve disputes, and if necessary, assist in the negotiation of a resolution.[143] Although this type of work may be frequently done by an adult, such as a teacher or parent volunteer, having a peer fill this role may provide a unique learning opportunity for the child. There can be many important benefits from this type of treatment, when it is implemented properly and given the appropriate oversight, as discussed by Cunningham.[144]

9.4.3. *Parent management training*

Families with ADHD children experience high levels of stress. Parents often feel incompetent and helpless to deal with their child's behavioral problems, and burdened by the increased caretaking demands. These families exhibit higher rates of maternal depression[145] and other kinds of psychopathology. Increased rates of marital conflict may lead to separation or divorce.[25] Finally, conflict between parents and children is common, and there is evidence that this conflict often originates or is perpetuated by the parents, who may have adopted counterproductive or maladaptive parenting strategies to cope with a child's behavioral difficulties.

PMT is one of the best-studied and supported set of psychosocial interventions in behavioral medicine, with many studies meeting the strictest criteria for evidence-based rigor.[140] PMT provides parents with skills to help manage their child's behavior, reduce parent–child conflict, and cope with difficulties of raising a child with ADHD. The main goal of PMT is to make parents more effective in identifying social and antisocial behaviors, rewarding prosocial behaviors (*e.g.* through point systems) and consistently implementing consequences for antisocial behaviors (e.g. time-outs or response costs). In addition, PMT teaches specific skills, such as how to utilize positive communication styles, and how to effectively set rules and boundaries.[140] For a thorough review of the theory and approach to parent training in developmental psychiatry, see Forgatch.[146]

PMT for ADHD can be administered in group or individual settings, and is typically brief (8–12 sessions). In studies of efficacy of PMT, researchers found improvement in ADHD symptoms, reduced aggression, and improvements in parental functioning, including reduced stress and enhanced parenting self-esteem and confidence.[140,147] The mechanisms of change in PMT are not understood, and there is an issue of whether or not the gains can be maintained over the long term.[140] However, family-based approaches can be extremely helpful, especially for families with younger children (school age and younger).

9.4.4. *School-based interventions*

One of the most common challenges faced by children with ADHD is functioning in educational settings. Children spend much of their time in classrooms and as such, school personnel can be in a unique position to positively impact functioning. Further, because of the increasing number of children receiving services for ADHD in schools nationwide, school-based interventions have become increasingly popular. One of the first steps in establishing successful school-based interventions is providing psychoeducation for teachers and administrators about the nature, causes, and course of the ADHD.[33] The next step is to establish effective communication and collaboration between parents and educators, so that a consistent treatment plan can be implemented. Behavioral interventions for ADHD in the classroom can include a range of modifications to the classroom environment, including accommodations to assist the student in completing assigned academic tasks, in-class consequences and rewards, and self-management strategies. Most of these interventions are concerned with creating predictable structure, reasonable and clear consequences for undesirable behaviors, and positive reinforcements for desired behaviors.[141] Studies have supported positive outcomes with the use of daily report cards or school-home contracts, peer tutoring, accommodations to tasks, changes in classroom structure, curricula changes,[148] and teacher consultation programs.[149] Useful tools for clinicians consulting in school settings can be found at http://schoolpsychiatry.org and http://schwablearning.org.

9.4.5. *Community education programs*

The Community Parent Education (COPE) program, is an extension of the PMT model discussed above, implemented at a community level. These workshops are designed to be more accessible to parents than clinic-based parent training programs, and are conducted at schools in the evenings and on weekends. This type of workshop may reduce some of the stigma associated with seeking mental health assistance, which is particularly evident crossculturally.[33] The content of the program focuses on many of the same social learning concepts employed in other parent training programs, and incorporates behavioral techniques, including modeling, role playing, homework goal setting, and self-monitoring to build skills.

10. ADHD and Related Disorders in Primary Care

For several decades now, developmental/behavioral pediatricians have provided diagnostic and therapeutic services to children and adolescents with ADHD.[102] Thus, unlike in many other domains of developmental psychopathology, primary care physicians are usually attuned to the symptoms and signs of this spectrum of disorders. Existing pediatric practice parameters address the standard of care for this spectrum of disorder.[11] In comparison to the practice parameters of child and adolescent psychiatry, these may appear somewhat conservative. The main issue in terms of the appropriate handling of cases of ADHD is the limited amount of time permitted for each practitioner to diagnose, treat, and follow-up these patients. Thus, we find, issues of true comorbidity are not appropriately addressed in these settings. Primary care providers also relatively overuse short acting, immediate-onset treatments, which typically have significant abuse and diversion potential.

11. Our Clinical Experiences: Practice-Based Evidence

In our program at Stanford, we see the entire age spectrum of disruptive behavior disorders. While our modal age range is around 12, patients range in age from 3.5 to their early 40. Genders are split at a rate of approximately 6:1 in favor of males, but as age increases genders tend to be more evenly represented.

We strictly adhere to the practice of obtaining data on attention/impulsive problems from school/work, family, and the clinical setting and strive to have concordance between these different domains of functioning before we diagnose and start treatment. We follow the recommendations of the AACAP practice guidelines in establishing diagnosis and following treatment systematically to assess progress and continued need for intervention.

Sometimes, the principal diagnosis is not clear from a single diagnostic interview. In such cases, we will provide serial follow-up and tracking in order to obtain longitudinal data from home and school. At times, such practice is not supported by the insurance; however, we will still insist on proceeding in this manner and request the parents' financial support to do so. Usually parents appreciate the caution that we exercise in diagnosis and determination of treatment. From the very first contact we make it clear that we are practicing in accordance with what we deem to be the highest consensual and evidence-based standards of care. Insurances may or may not support this, but we will not practice medicine dictated by insurance. In order to achieve this with minimal interference in the child's life, we closely mold our intervention schedule to the school year, as much as is possible.

Only about 15% of our patients are completely new referrals. Usually we are asked to reevaluate treatment of cases seen in other pediatric or psychiatric clinics (30%) or are formally approached regarding a second opinion (25%), at times with forensic implications. The remaining cases usually come from the community as either direct self-referrals or requests for reevaluation of a very complex case. We usually see complicated cases with externalizing and internalizing comorbidity. We suspect that individuals with relatively pure ADHD, roughly 30% of cases, are treated primarily in primary care practices, although occasionally, we encounter such a case, as we illustrate in our first example. The presence of comorbid conditions is an important aspect of how we approach cases, as they are a factor in determining our specific treatment of a case.

Case A

This case highlights problems associated with potential diversion and non-medical use of properly prescribed treatment.

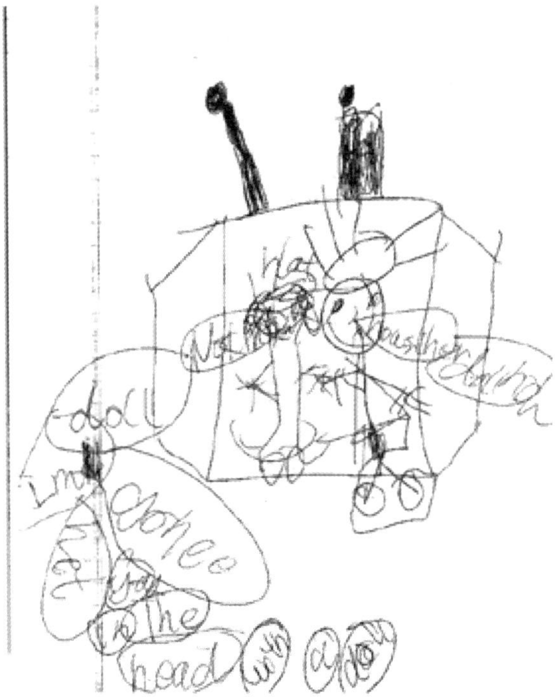

Fig. 2: Drawing produced by an eight-year-old girl before initiation of treatment for ADHD symptoms.

This is an eight-year-old girl (35 kg) brought in by her parents for complaints of inattention at school and poor organizational skills, just before summer vacation started. As part of our workup, we asked her to draw her house and her family. She did so and with much effort produced the first drawing (Fig. 2).

Reports from school confirmed very poor organizational skills, despite will ingness and effort. There were no reports of hyperkinesis or aggression. The patient was mildly inattentive yet cooperative in our tranquil exam setting. As testing demands increased, more disorganization and orientation to extraneous stimuli became apparent. There was little doubt in our minds that this patient could be helped by ADHD treatment.

However, our suspicions were aroused when her father insisted that his daughter would only respond to methamphetamine preparations. He claimed a history of ADHD and LD, and received treatment as a child and an adult. After some discussion, and with his permission, we retrieved his medical record to find that he had a lengthy alcohol and drug abuse history but was reportedly sober now. This was a multicultural family with many transcultural issues and significant marital discord.

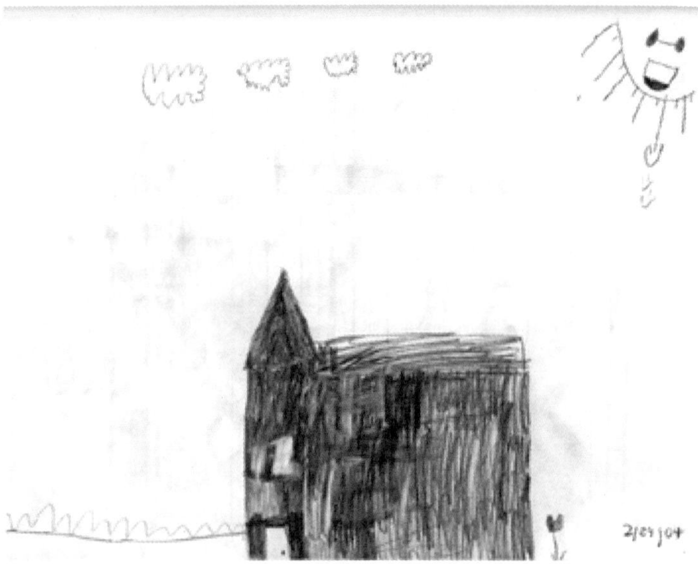

Fig. 3: Second drawing produced by an eight-year-old patient after treatment with atomoxetine.

These issues repeatedly disrupted our PMT efforts. During the summer months, we titrated the patient onto atomoxetine, much to the father's disappointment. School was not informed regarding this intervention and independently confirmed that the patient was doing well on 60 mg (1.71 mg/kg/d). At this point the patient repeated the initial drawing exercise and produced the second drawing (Fig. 3).

At 2-year follow-up, we ascertained that she continued to do well on 60 mg of atomoxetine, until the current attending went off service. The father then kept insisting that the medication was not effective any more, a report that was at odds with the excellent school reports. The new attending and resident then switched the patient to adderall, which was not effective except at very high doses. As soon as the previous attending became aware of this change, the patient was immediately switched back to atomoxetine with excellent efficacy (2.0 mg/kg/d). Mother confirmed that father was always in charge of giving the medicine and seemed to divert it for his own personal use. Child protective services were involved and offered helpful consultation and follow-up.

Approximately 35–40% of our cases do not respond to atomoxetine, even at the best titrated and optimized doses. Given the complexities of the neurotransmitters underpinning the attention system, this should not come as a surprise because of the relatively specific actions of atomoxetine and its relatively weak and downstream effects on DA. The following case illustrates this type of scenario.

Case B

This is a very thin five-year-old Asian-American girl (barely third percentile for weight and between fifth and tenth percentile for height), with ADHD-C and severe temper tantrums, which used to occur several times per week. After an initial trial of atomoxetine, which was ineffective, she was brought in for consultation. Her parents were appropriately involved in her treatment. She had some biological risks in that her older sister and several second-degree relatives were also diagnosed with ADHD. Psychosocially, she appeared to have a secure attachment with both parents, and was highly intelligent and fairly well adjusted in terms of self-esteem, although she had few regular friends. She was considered "too bossy" by most of her peers, and as a result she had a rich fantasy life which she was all-too-happy to be immersed in, playing mostly by herself and with her sister. She was originally referred to our clinic because of severe, recurrent temper tantrums at home, especially around homework assigned by the kindergarten teacher (often requiring up to 1 h of dedicated work in the evenings).

After one year of treatment, she responded well to a combination of monthly pharmacotherapy, therapeutic play during these monthly sessions as a means of alliance formation and maintenance, psychoeducational school-based interventions through a 504 plan to reduce the daily homework load, and parent training for ADHD. Her current medications consist of an MPH chewable tablet, 5 mg, and guanfacine, 1 mg bid.

In about 60% of other consult cases, our job is to simplify diagnoses, perform interventions, and restore health and growth. Many patients have received prior treatment, which strictly adhered to the simple additive model of comorbidity. Unfortunately, this treatment regimen was not useful for these patients, and little improvement was noted (in some cases, a worsening of symptoms may even have occurred). In our clinics, the psychiatrist provides psychotherapy, pharmacotherapy, and family consultation in all of these cases, illustrating the emphasis on integrated, biopsychosocial, and culturally informed treatment for these patients and families affected by ADHD. These vignettes underline the central role of the family in treatment, and of utilizing evidence-based interventions whenever possible (all patients first started with monotherapy, and subsequent dose adjustments and medication augmentation strategies were required due to side effects). Most importantly, it illustrates the central role of the therapeutic alliance in both pharmacotherapies and psychotherapies, as it took several months of work before sustainable symptom improvement was achieved, requiring that the children and families maintain their patience and trust with their doctor and treatment team on a sometimes bumpy road to symptom remission.

11.1. *Outcomes in our clinic*

The modal length of treatment in our program is 18 months, but there are approximately 50% of individuals who remain with us through their young adult years. We have followed these individuals an average of about 15 years. As there are no curative interventions for these disorders at the present time, we think it is wise to assume a lifetime perspective of practice in treating patients within this syndrome cluster. Our patients are clearly very grateful for the "institutionalized" knowledge base of their developmental trajectories. Most of our young adults do not come in for active treatment more frequently than one or twice a year for a check up. They will come sooner when crossing major developmental nodal points, in the context of unexpected crises, increased allostatic load, and emergencies. Subsequent interventions are then easily tailored to extant need and symptom control and developmental progress is rapidly restored.

Our intervention packages are usually specifically tailored to complicating target symptoms or comorbid conditions. Broadly, these can be divided along the following lines. About 20% of our patients present with uncomplicated ADHD. Another 50–60% of our patients present with comorbid externalizing symptoms (specifically aggressive and disruptive behavior, substance and/or alcohol abuse/dependency). The remainder have predominantly internalizing symptoms and comorbidities, typically an anxiety and/or mood problem. This type of profile maps roughly on the recent findings of the National Comorbidity Survey,[26] with perhaps a lower percentage of our patients having uncomplicated ADHD. We would expect such a profile from a tertiary care clinic in an academic research center. The high percentage of overlap of our patients with disorders of aggression most likely reflects one of the author's special expertise and research in this specific area, as well as this author's forensic practice.

Most typically, we treat these subgroups as follows:

Uncomplicated ADHD in the absence of any crisis (school, family, or juvenile justice system) is prepared for a 6–12-week trial of a stimulant or an SNRI (atomoxetine) with weekly follow-up medication management visits as the medication is being titrated to efficacy. We require a pediatric exam to be on file within the previous six months that speaks directly to the issue of any potential cardiac structural deficit issues and/or and hypertension. We require a screening panel of lead, LTFs, TSH, and a CBC to be on file as well. Once the patient is cleared for ADHD treatment, we begin pharmacotherapy. The dosing schedule is as follows: in the case of atomoxetine, patients receive a 0.5 mg/kg/day trial dose of approximately 1–2 weeks (single hs dosing). In weeks 3 to 12, we aim for the first therapeutic window, which is usually around 1.4–1.6 mg/kg/d, depending on side effects. If efficacy is transient or not optimal, then we push the dosing to a final 1.8 to 2.0 mg/kg/d. We do not usually go beyond this last threshold, as there is evidence that one only incurs more serious and frequent side effects without substantial gain in efficacy.[150] If stimulants are selected, we begin with a recommended starting dose, depending on which particular medicine is being used.[9] If bipolar symptoms are also present, they should be stabilized first, as stimulants may potentially cause or exacerbate mania.[151] Both MPH and AMPH preparations appear to be equally effective, although adderall may have a slight edge in head-to-head studies over standard release MPH.[152] For methylphenidates, the recommended starting dose is 5 mg, once or twice daily, or 0.3 mg/kg/day divided bid with subsequent increases to target doses in the range of 0.3–2 mg/kg/day. Weight-based dosing may be useful for smaller children in order to minimize side effects. We use lower doses for children <25 kg, in the range of 0.3–1 mg/kg/day. The maximum recommended dose for MPH preparations is 60 mg or 54 mg for concerta (OROS-MPH). The methylphenidate patch (daytrana) is an interesting alternative because it cannot be extracted or snorted. It may offer a solution to MPH abuse and may also be helpful in the treatment of young children who are unwilling or unable to swallow tablets.

AMPH preparations are thought of as 1.5–2 times as potent as MPH preparations. Accordingly, the corresponding dose works out to roughly 0.15–1 mg/kg/day, with the maximum daily dose being 40 mg. We recommend giving no more than single doses of 15 mg MPH or 10 mg AMP/DEX for children under 25 kg. There are some teens and adults who will tolerate and require higher doses, such as 40 mg of adderall-XR in the morning. The physician should aim for a consistent and regular dose titration schedule. A fixed dose schedule may also be used, such that the child gets exposure to his/her "best dose," which can be deduced at the end of such a trial (typically one month or so, as in the MTA study). Parents must also be informed regarding the method of evaluating drug response, and, importantly, strategies for managing treatment-emergent side effects.

On follow-up visits, we examine the following routinely: weight, height, blood pressure, pulse, appetite, sleep, side effects (most notably somnolence and gastrointestinal upset). We routinely ask about compliance and mnemonic devices to remember taking the medicine and we ascertain whether there have been any attempts at misuse or diversion. We are alert to the signs and symptoms of liver toxicity and potential interactions with other routinely taken medications.

In cases of true comorbidities, we will select our first-line intervention in keeping with risks posed by the interventions we propose. Thus, in the 40–60% of ADHD comorbid with externalizing disorders, which are very susceptible to problems with diversion and abuse, atomoxetine becomes the logical first choice. Atomoxetine also is a strong consideration when problems of anxiety and mood are present. If there is any suspicion of bipolar disorder, we aim to stabilize mood first, then treat residual problems with either stimulants or atomoxetine while carefully tracking activation and worsening of anxiety and mood symptoms (see also Chap. 7 of this volume).

In our clinics, we usually manage to restore symptom control in 4–12 weeks, depending on the exact details of the case. We usually then employ a mix of interventions, most typically ordered as described in the figure below. As symptoms are in improved control, our sociotherapeutic interventions recede; our family contacts become more supportive and the main basis of our interventions are an integration of supportive therapy and psychopharmacology. We remain alert to the possible recurrence of symptoms during times of stress (marital discord, separations), great allostatic load (finals), and other intercurrent events. We are always ready to review the current treatment package and examine its efficacy and continued need for the specific modalities.

We use individual sessions and tailored pharmacotherapy as the basis for long-term treatment. Both these modalities tend to achieve maximum efficacy only after a period of time. We consider the individual contact to be essential to establish a working alliance with the patient, which then allows us to gradually build a tailored integrated intervention package which has a very high chance of being followed to the best of the patient's ability. Controlling structured environments and working with the family are most important as we are trying to stabilize symptoms and alleviate crises and emergencies. Sociotherapy may take the form of simple consultation with teachers and tutors, or it may become as complex as helping design behavioral programs for the management of impulsive, disruptive, and/or aggressive behavior. At the minimum, family therapy is centered on creating a sophisticated understanding of ADHD and impulsivity, while reinforcing the need for parenting consistency and rescue systems in times of high allostatic load. At other times, family intervention can become as specific as parent management training (PMT), or structural family therapy.

12. Future Directions in the Diagnosis and Treatment of ADHD and Related Disorders

The knowledge base in ADHD and related disorders is extensive and arguably of the best quality in developmental psychiatry. There are several exciting leads which should be tracked in the next five years or so, as they most likely will profoundly affect our diagnostic and therapeutic practices and make treatment more efficacious. Imaging is clearly an important part of future assessment and differential diagnosis. Our knowledge of different brain structures that drive phenomenologically identical behavior will increase and help us determine with greater precision the most appropriate targets for intervention. The identification of such targets will be increasingly important, as we are beginning to map with some accuracy the neural circuits supporting the varying functions of the brain/mind system and as we map the neurotransmitters involved in this process. The latter provide the most tangible targets for our interventions. We are much better poised to understand the facilitatory and inhibitory roles neurotransmitters have proximally and distally, and continued exploration will result in more precise response profiles of medications and other interventions, increasing specificity of treatment. Sorely needed are studies of combination treatments with more modern compounds, building on our knowledge base created by the MTA study. Genetics will begin to exert an influence: the hope is that pharmacogenetic studies will increase in number and provide us with the results needed to optimize intervention agent selection. The application of genetics to identify risk for disorder seems to be more distant, as our understanding of the complexities of polygenetic inheritances of highest level mental functions (such as attention regulation) is only in its infancy.

References

1. Bargh J. *Social Psychology & the Unconscious: The Automaticity of Higher Mental Processes*. New York, NY: Psychology Press, 2007.
2. Kastner S, Ungerleider L. Mechanisms of visual attention in the human cortex, *Annu Rev Neurosci* 2000; **23**: 315–341.
3. Russell VA. Neurobiology of animal models of attention-deficit hyperactivity disorder, *J Neurosci Methods* 2007; **161**: 185–98.
4. Sarter M, Gehring WJ, Kozak R. More attention must be paid: The neurobiology of attentional effort, *Brain Res Rev* 2006; **51**: 145–60.
5. Biederman J, Spencer T, Wilens T, Prince J, Faraone S. Treatment of ADHD with stimulant medications: Response to Nissen perspective in The New England Journal of Medicine, *J Am Acad Child Adolesc Psychiatry* 2006; **45**(10): 1147–1150.
6. MacNeil J. Reject psychiatric view of attention disorders, *Pediatric News* 2006; **40**: 28–29.
7. Nissen S. ADHD drugs and cardiovascular risk, *N Engl J Med* 2006; **354**: 1445–1448.
8. Rothenberger AB. Informing the ADHD debate, *Sci Am Mind* 2004; **14**: 50–55.
9. Steiner H. *Handbook of Mental Health Interventions for Child and Adolescents: An Integrated Developmental Approach.* San Francisco, CA: Jossey-Bass, 2004.
10. American Academy of Child and Adolescent Psychiatry. *Practice Parameter for the Assessment and Treatment of Children and Adolescents with Attention-Deficit/Hyperactivity Disorder* (in press).
11. American Academy of Pediatrics. Clinical practice guideline: Treatment of the school-aged child with attention-deficit/hyperactivity disorder, *Pediatrics* 2001; **108**(4): 1033–1044.

12. Taylor E, Dopfner M, Sergeant J *et al.* European clinical guidelines for hyperkinetic disorder–first upgrade, *Eur Child Adolesc Psychiatry* 2004; **13**(Suppl. 1): 7–30.
13. Kessler RC, Berglund P, Demler O, Jin R, Merikangas KR, Walters EE. Lifetime prevalence and age-of-onset distributions of DSM-IV disorders in the national comorbidity survey replication, *Arch Gen Psychiatry* 2005; **62**: 593–768.
14. Faraone S, Sergeant J, Gillberg C, Biederman J. The worldwide prevalence of ADHD: Is it an American condition? *World Psychiatry* 2003; **2**: 104–112.
15. Barkley R. Attention-deficit/hyperactivity disorder. In: Mash E, Barkley R, Eds. *Child Psychopathology.* New York, NY: Guilford Press, 2003; pp. 75–143.
16. Bird H, Davies M, Fisher P *et al.* How specific is specific impairment? *J Am Acad Child Adolesc Psychiatry* 2000; **39**(9): 1182–1189.
17. Shaffer D, Gould M, Brasic J, Ambrosini P. A children's global assessment scale (CGAS), *Arch Gen Psychiatry* 1983; **40**: 1228–1231.
18. Rohde L, Barbosa G, Polanczyk G, *et al.* Factor and latent class analysis of DSM-IV ADHD symptoms in a school sample of Brazilian adolescents, *J Am Acad Child Adolesc Psychiatry* 2001; **40**(6): 711–718.
19. Barkley, R. Against the status quo: Revising the diagnostic criteria for ADHD, *J Am Acad Child Adolesc Psychiatry* 2010; **49**(3): 205–207.
20. Barkley R. *Attention-Deficit Hyperactivity Disorder: A Handbook for Diagnosis and Treatment*, 3rd edition. New York, NY: Guilford Press, 2006.
21. Wood AC, Asherson P, Rijsdijk F, Kuntsi J. Is overactivity a core feature in ADHD? Familial and receiver operating characteristic curve analysis of mechanically assessed activity level, *J Am Acad Child Adolesc Psychiatry* 2009 Aug 18 [Epub ahead of print].
22. World Health Organization. *International Classification of Diseases*, 10th Revision. 1992.
23. Lahey B, Pelham W, Chronis A, *et al.* Predictive validity of ICD-10 hyperkinetic disorder elative to DSM-IV attention-deficit hyperactivity disorder among younger children, *J Child Psychol Psychiatry* 2006; **47**(5): 472–479.
24. Barkley R, Fischer M, Smallish L, Fletcher K. The persistence of attention-deficit/hyperactivity disorder into young adulthood as a function of reporting source and definition of disorder, *J Abnorm Psychol* 2002; **111**: 279–289.
25. Barkley RA, Murphy KR, Fischer M. *ADHD in Adults: What the Science says*. New York, NY: Guilford, 2008.
26. Kessler R, Adler L, Barkley R. The prevalence and correlates of adult ADHD in the United States: Results from the national comorbidity survey replication, *Am J Psychiatry* 2006; **163**(4): 716–723.
27. Barkley R, Fischer M, Smallish L, Fletcher K. Young adult follow-up of hyperactive children: Antisocial activities and drug use, *J Child Psychol Psychiatry* 2004; **45**: 195–211.

28. Barkley R, Fischer M, Smallish L, Fletcher K. Young adult outcome of hyperactive children: Adaptive functioning in major life activities, *J Am Acad Child Adolesc Psychiatry* 2006; **45**: 192–202.
29. Johnston C. The impact of attention deficit hyperactivity disorder on social and vocational functioning in adults. In: Jensen P, Cooper J, Eds. .*Attention Deficit Hyperactivity Disorder; State of the Science, Best Practices*. Kingston, NJ: Civic Research Institute, 2002.
30. Jensen PS, Arnold LE, Swanson JM, *et al.* 3-year follow-up of the NIMH MTA study, *J Am Acad Child Adolesc Psychiatry* 2007; **46**: 989–1002.
31. Swanson JM, Hinshaw SP, Arnold LE, *et al.* Secondary evaluations of MTA 36-month outcomes: Propensity score and growth mixture model analyses, *J Am Acad Child Adolesc Psychiatry* 2007; **46**: 1003–1014.
32. Wilens T, Biederman J, Brown S, Tanguay S, Monuteaux M, Blake C. Psychiatric comorbidity and functioning in clinically-referred preschool children and school-age youth with ADHD, *J Am Acad Child Adolesc Psychiatry* 2002; **41**: 262–268.
33. Barkley R. *Attention-Deficit Hyperactivity Disorder: A Handbook for Diagnosis and Treatment*, 3rd edition. New York, NY: Guilford Press, 2006.
34. Newcorn J, Halperin J, Jensen P. Symptom profiles in children with ADHD: Effects of comorbidity and gender, *J Am Acad Child Adolesc Psychiatry* 2001; **40**(2): 137–146.
35. Pliszka SR. *ADHD with Comorbid Disorders: Clinical Assessment and Management.* New York, NY: Guilford Press, 1999.
36. Tannock R. Attention deficit disorders with anxiety disorders. In: Brown T, Ed. .*Attention-Deficit Disorders and Comorbidities in Children, Adolescents and Adults*. New York, NY: American Psychiatric Press, 2000: pp. 125–175.
37. Molina BSG, Flory K, Hinshaw SP, *et al.* Delinquent behavior and emerging substance use in the MTA at 36 months: Prevalence, course, and treatment effects, *J Am Acad Child Adolesc Psychiatry* 2007; **46**: 1028–1040.
38. Wolraich M, McGuinn L, Doffing M. Treatment of attention deficit hyperactivity disorder in children and adolescents: Safety considerations, *Drug Safety* 2007; **30**: 17–26.
39. US Department of Health and Human Services SAMHSA, Office of Applied Studies, and Drug Abuse Warning Network (2006), Drug Abuse Warning Network, 2004. National estimates of drug-related emergency department visits. In: *DAWN Series D-28, DHHS Publication No. (SMA) 06-4143.* Rockville, MD, 2006.
40. Harvard Mental Health Letter. ADHD update: New data on the risks of medication, *Harvard Ment Health Lett* 2006: 3–5.
41. Volkow N, Swanson J. Variables that affect the clinical use and abuse of methylphenidate in the treatment of ADHD, *Am J Psychiatry* 2003; **160**: 1909–1918.
42. Breslau N, Lucia V, Alvarado G. Intelligence and other predisposing factors in exposure to trauma and posttraumatic stress disorder, *Arch Gen Psychiatry* 2006; **63**(11): 1238–1245.

43. Storr C, Ialongo N, Anthony J, Breslau N. Childhood antecedents of exposure to traumatic events and posttraumatic stress disorder, *Am J Psychiatry* 2007; **164**: 119–125.
44. Pessoa L. Neural correlates of visual working memory fMRI amplitude predicts task performance, *Neuron* 2002; **35**: 975.
45. Gabrieli J. Altered neural substrates of cognitive control in childhood ADHD: Evidence from functional magnetic resonance imaging, *Am J Psychiatry* 2005; **162**: 1605.
46. Russell VA. Neurobiology of animal models of attention-deficit hyperactivity disorder, *J Neurosci Methods* 2007; **161**: 185–98.
47. Davids E, Zhang K, Kula NS, Tarazi FI, Baldessarini RJ. Effects of norepinephrine and serotonin transporter inhibitors on hyperactivity induced by neonatal 6-hydroxydopamine lesioning in rats, *J Pharmacol Exp Ther* 2002; **301**: 1097–1102.
48. Maidment ID. The use of antidepressants to treat attention deficit hyperactivity disorder in adults, *J Psychopharmacol* 2003; **17**: 332–336.
49. Easton N, Steward C, Marshall F, Fone K, Marsden C. Effects of amphetamine isomers, methylphenidate and atomoxetine on synaptosomal and synaptic vesicle accumulation and release of dopamine and noradrenaline in vitro in the rat brain, *Neuropharmacology* 2007; **52**: 405–414.
50. Bymaster FP, Katner JS, Nelson DL, *et al.* Atomoxetine increases extracellular levels of norepinephrine and dopamine in prefrontal cortex of rat: a potential mechanism for efficacy in attention deficit/hyperactivity disorder, *Neuropsychopharmacology* 2002; **27**(5): 699–711.
51. Aston-Jones G, Bloom FE. Activity of norepinephrine-containing locus coeruleus neurons in behaving rats anticipates fluctuations in the sleep-waking cycle, *J Neurosci* 1981; **1**: 876–886.
52. Pliszka SR, McCracken JT, Maas JW. Catecholamines in attention-deficit hyperactivity disorder: Current perspectives, *J Am Acad Child Adolesc Psychiatry* 1996; **35**: 264–272.
53. Levy F. The dopamine theory of attention deficit hyperactivity disorder (ADHD), *Aust N Z J Psychiatry* 1991; **25**: 277–283.
54. Dougherty DD, Bonab AA, Spencer TJ, Rauch SL, Madras BK, Fischman AJ. Dopamine transporter density in patients with attention deficit hyperactivity disorder, *Lancet* 1999; **354**: 2132–2133.
55. Volkow ND, Wang GJ, Newcorn J, *et al.* Brain dopamine transporter levels in treatment and drug naive adults with ADHD, *Neuroimage* 2007; **34**: 1182–1190.
56. Linnoila M, Virkkunen M, Scheinin M, Nuutila A, Rimon R, Goodwin FK. Low cerebrospinal fluid 5-hydroxyindoleacetic acid concentration differentiates impulsive from nonimpulsive violent behavior, *Life Sci* 1983; **33**: 2609–2614.
57. Gainetdinov RR, Wetsel WC, Jones SR, Levin ED, Jaber M, Caron MG. Role of serotonin in the paradoxical calming effect of psychostimulants on hyperactivity, *Science* 1999; **283**: 397–401.

58. Walker SC, Mikheenko YP, Argyle LD, Robbins TW, Roberts AC. Selective prefrontal serotonin depletion impairs acquisition of a detour-reaching task, *Eur J Neurosci* 2006; **23**: 3119–3123.
59. Winstanley CA, Dalley JW, Theobald DE, Robbins TW. Global 5-HT depletion attenuates the ability of amphetamine to decrease impulsive choice on a delay-discounting task in rats, *Psychopharmacology (Berl)* 2003; **170**: 320–331.
60. Oades RD, Lasky-Su J, Christiansen H, *et al.* The influence of serotonin- and other genes on impulsive behavioral aggression and cognitive impulsivity in children with attention-deficit/hyperactivity disorder (ADHD): Findings from a family-based association test (FBAT) analysis, *Behav Brain Funct* 2008; **4**: 48.
61. Banaschewski T, Becker K, Scherag S, Franke B, Coghill D. Molecular genetics of attention-deficit/hyperactivity disorder: An overview, *Eur Child Adolesc Psychiatry* 2010; **19**(3): 237–257.
62. Stoltenberg SF, Glass JM, Chermack ST, *et al.* Possible association between response inhibition and a variant in the brain-expressed tryptophan hydroxylase-2 gene, *Psychiatr Genet* 2006; **16**: 35–38.
63. Reuter M, Ott U, Vaitl D, Hennig J. Impaired executive control is associated with a variation in the promoter region of the tryptophan hydroxylase 2 gene, *J Cogn Neurosci* 2007; **19**: 401–408.
64. Botvinick M, Nystrom LE, Fissell K, Carter CS, Cohen JD. Conflict monitoring versus selection-for-action in anterior cingulate cortex, *Nature* 1999; **402**: 179–181.
65. van Meel CS, Heslenfeld DJ, Oosterlaan J, Sergeant JA. Adaptive control deficits in attention-deficit/hyperactivity disorder (ADHD): The role of error processing, *Psychiatry Res* 2007; **151**(3): 211–220.
66. Heekeren HR, Marrett S, Bandettini PA, Ungerleider LG. A general mechanism for perceptual decision-making in the human brain, *Nature* 2004; **431**: 859–862.
67. Fan J, McCandliss BD, Fossella J, Flombaum JI, Posner MI. The activation of attentional networks, *Neuroimage* 2005; **26**: 471–479.
68. Jensen P, Hinshaw S, Kraemer H, *et al.* ADHD comorbidity findings from the MTA study: Comparing comorbid subgroups, *J Am Acad Child Adolesc Psychiatry* 2001; **40**: 147–158.
69. Castellanos F, Lee P, Sharp W. Developmental trajectories of brain volume abnormalities in children and adolescents with attention-deficit/hyperactivity disorder, *JAMA* 2002; **288**: 1740–1748.
70. Durston S, Hulshoff H, Schnack H, Buitelaar J, Steenhuis M, Minderaa R. Magnetic resonance imaging of boys with attention-deficit/hyperactivity disorder and their unaffected siblings, *J Am Acad Child Adolesc Psychiatry* 2004; **43**: 232–240.
71. Bush G, Valera E, Seidman L. Functional neuroimaging of attention-deficit/hyperactivity disorder: A review and suggested future directions, *Biol Psychiatry* 2005; **57**: 1273–1284.

72. Bush G, Luu P, Posner M. Cognitive and emotional influences in anterior cingulate cortex, *Trends Cogn Sci* 2000; **4**: 215–222.

73. Bush G, Vogt B, Holmes J, Dale A, Greve D, Jenike M. Dorsal anterior cingulate cortex: A role in reward-based decision making, *Proc Natl Acad Sci USA* 2002; **99**: 523–528.

74. Nigg J. *What Causes ADHD?* New York, NY: Guilford Press, 2006.

75. Mick E, Biederman J, Prince J, Fischer M, Faraone S. Impact of low birth weight on attention-deficit hyperactivity disorder, *J Dev Behav Pediatr* 2002; **23**: 16–22.

76. Mick E, Biederman J, Faraone S, Sayer J, Kleinman S. Case-control study of attention-deficit hyperactivity disorder and maternal smoking, alcohol use, and drug use during pregnancy, *J Am Acad Child Adolesc Psychiatry* 2002; **41**: 378–385.

77. Kreppner J, O'Connor T, Rutter M. Can inattention/overactivity be an institutional deprivation syndrome? *J Abnorm Child Psychol* 2001; **29**: 513–528.

78. Nigg J. Is ADHD a disinhibitory disorder? *Psychol Bull* 2001; **127**: 571–598.

79. Sprich S, Biederman J, Crawford M, Mundy E, Faraone S. Adoptive and biological families of children and adolescents with ADHD, *J Am Acad Child and Adolesc Psychiatry* 2000; **39**: 1432–1437.

80. Faraone S, Doyle A. The nature and heritability of attention-deficit/hyperactivity disorder, *Child Adolesc Psychiatric Clin N Am* 2001; **10**: 299–316.

81. Spencer TJ, Biederman J, Mick E. Attention-deficit/hyperactivity disorder: Diagnosis, lifespan, comorbidities, and neurobiology, *Ambulatory Pediatrics* 2007; **7**: 73.

82. Faraone S, Perlis R, Doyle A. Molecular genetics of attention-deficit/hyperactivity disorder, *Biol Psychiatry* 2005; **57**: 1313–1323.

83. Brookes K, Xu X, Chen W, *et al.* The analysis of 51 genes in DSM-IV combined type attention deficit hyperactivity disorder: Association signals in DRD4, DAT1 and 16 other genes, *Mol Psychiatry* 2006; **11**: 934–953.

84. Sheehan K, Lowe N, Kirley A, *et al.* Tryptophan hydroxylase 2 (TPH2) gene variants associated with ADHD, *Mol Psychiatry* 2005; **10**: 944–949.

85. Walitza S, Renner TJ, Dempfle A, *et al.* Transmission disequilibrium of polymorphic variants in the tryptophan hydroxylase-2 gene in attention-deficit/hyperactivity disorder, *Mol Psychiatry* 2005; **10**: 1126–1132.

86. Abikoff H, Hechtman L, Klein R, *et al.* Social functioning in children with ADHD treated with long-term methyphenidate and multimodal psychosocial treatment, *J Am Acad Child Adolesc Psychiatry* 2004; **43**: 820–829.

87. Abikoff H, Hechtman L, Klein R, Weiss G, Fleiss K. Symptomatic improvement in children with ADHD treated with long-term methylphenidate and multimodal psychosocial treatment, *J Am Acad Child Adolesc Psychiatry* 2004; **43**: 802–811.

88. Hechtman L, Abikoff H, Klein R, *et al.* Children with ADHD treated with long-term methylphenidate and multimodal psychosocial treatment: Impact on parental practices, *J Am Acad Child Adolesc Psychiatry* 2004; **43**: 830–838.

89. Hechtman L, Abikoff H, Klein R, Weiss G, Respitz C, Kouri J. Academic achievement and emotional status in children with ADHD treated with long-term methylphenidate and multimodal psychosocial treatment, *J Am Acad Child Adolesc Psychiatry* 2004; **43**: 812–819.
90. Pliszka SB. *AACAP Pocket Cards: Managing Attention Deficit/Hyperactivity Disorder Version 3.0.* Washington, D.C.: American Academy of Child and Adolescent Psychiatry, 2006.
91. Sallee FR, McGough J, Wigal T. Donahue J, Lyne A, Biederman J. Guanfacine extended release in children and adolescents with attention-deficit/hyperactivity disorder: A placebo controlled trial, *J Am Acad Child Adolesc Psychiatry* 2008; **48**(2): 155–165.
92. Weiss B, Laties V. Enhancement of human performance by caffeine and the amphetamines. *Pharmacol Rev* 1962; **14**: 1–36.
93. Greely H, Sahakian B, Harris J, *et al.* Towards responsible use of cognitive-enhancing drugs by the healthy, *Nature* 2008; **456**(7223): 702–705.
94. Rapoport J. Dextroamphetamine. Its cognitive and behavioral effects in normal and hyperactive boys and normal men, *Arch Gen Psychiatry* 1980; **37**: 933–943.
95. Rapoport J, Buchsbaum T, Zahn H, Weingartner C, Ludlow C, Mikkelsen E. Dextroamphetamine: Cognitive and behavioral effects in normal prepubertal boys, *Science* 1978; **199**: 560–563.
96. Joshi SV. Psychostimulants, atomoxetine, and alpha-agonists. In: Steiner H, Ed. *Handbook of Mental Health Interventions in Children and Adolescents.* San Francisco, CA: Jossey-Bass, 2004: pp. 258–287.
97. Kratochvil CJ, Newcorn JH, Arnold LE, *et al.* Atomoxetine alone or combined with fluoxetine for treating ADHD with comorbid depressive or anxiety symptoms, *J Am Acad Child Adolesc Psychiatry* 2005; **44**: 915.
98. Wender EH. Managing stimulant medication for attention-deficit/hyperactivity disorder: An update, *Pediatr Rev* 2002; **23**: 234–236.
99. Greenhill LL, Pliszka SR, Dulcan MK, and the Workgroup on Quality Issues. Practice parameter for the use of stimulant medications in the treatment of children, adolescents and adults, *Supplement to J Am Acad Child Adolesc Psychiatry* 2002; **41**: 26S–49S.
100. Pliszka SR, and the Texas Consensus Conference Panel on Medication Treatment of Childhood Attention-Deficit/Hyperactivity Disorder. The Texas children's medication algorithm project: Report of the Texas consensus conference panel on medication treatment of childhood attention-deficit/hyperactivity disorder. Part I. *J Am Acad Child Adolesc Psychiatry* 2000; 908–919.
101. Pliszka SR, and the Texas Consensus Conference Panel on Medication Treatment of Childhood Attention-Deficit/Hyperactivity Disorder. The Texas children's medication algorithm project: Report of the Texas consensus of conference panel on

medication treatment of childhood attention-deficit/hyperactivity disorder. Part II. *J Am Acad Child Adolesc Psychiatry* 2000; 920–927.

102. Behrman R, Kliegman R, Jenson H. *Nelson Textbook of Pediatrics,* 17th edition. Philadelphia, PA: Saunders, 2004.
103. Rojas NL, Chan E. Old and new controversies in the alternative treatment of attention-deficit hyperactivity disorder, *Ment Retard Dev Disabil Res Rev* 2005; **11**: 116–130.
104. Chan E. The role of complementary and alternative medicine in attention-deficit hyperactivity disorder, *J Dev Behav Peds* 2002; **23**(1): S37–S45.
105. Richardson A. Omega-3 fatty acids in ADHD and related neurodevelopmental disorders, *Int Rev Psychiatry* 2006; **18**: 155–172.
106. Prince J. Pharmacotherapy of attention-deficit hyperactivity disorder in children and adolescents: Update on new stimulant preparations, atomoxetine, and novel treatments, *Child Adolesc Psychiatric Clin N Am* 2006; **15**: 13–50.
107. Wisor JP. Dopaminergic role in stimulant-induced wakefulness, *J Neurosci* 2001; **21**: 1787.
108. Cephalon Inc. Cephalon reports no benefit from Provigil in study of adults with ADHD: Plans for label expansion into other indication on track [press release]. Westchester, PA, 2000.
109. Rugino TA, Copley TC. Effects of modafinil in children with attention-deficit/hyperactivity disorder: An open-label study, *J Am Acad Child Adolesc Psychiatry* 2001; **40**: 230–235.
110. Taylor FB, Russo J. Efficacy of modafinil compared to dextroamphetamine for the treatment of attention-deficit/hyperactivity disorder in adults, *J Child Adolesc Psychopharmacol* 2000; **10**: 311–320.
111. Taylor FB, Russo J. Efficacy of modafinil compared to dextroamphetamine for the treatment of attention-deficit/hyperactivity disorder in adults, *J Child Adolesc Psychopharmacol* 2000; **10**: 311–320.
112. Turner DC, Clark L, Dowson J, Robbins TW, Sahakian BJ. Modafinil improves cognition and response inhibition in adult-attention-deficit/hyperactivity disorder, *Biol Psychiatry* 2004; **55**: 1031–1040.
113. Wigal SB, Biederman J, Swanson JM, Yang R, Greenhill LL. Efficacy and safety of modafinil film-coated tablets in children and adolescents with or without prior stimulant treatment for attention-deficit/hyperactivity disorder: Pooled analysis of 3 randomized, double-blind, placebo-controlled studies, *Primary care companion to the Journal of clinical psychiatry* 2006; **8**: 352.
114. Ratner S, Laor N, Bronstein Y, Weizman A, Toren P. Six-week open-label reboxetine treatment in children and adolescents with attention-deficit/hyperactivity disorder, *J Am Acad Child Adolesc Psychiatry* 2005; **44**: 428.
115. Mozes T, Meiri G, Ben-Amity G, Sabbagh M, Weizman A. Reboxetine as an optional treatment for hyperkinetic conduct disorder: A prospective open-label trial, *J Child Adolesc Psychopharmacol* 2005; **15**: 259.

116. Laws HF, Heil SH, Bickel S, Faries D, Badger G. Subjective responses to LY139603 (tomoxetine) and methylphenidate. In: *41st Annual NCDEU Meeting*. Phoenix, AZ, 2001.
117. Leurs R, Blandina P, Tedford C, Timmerman H. Therapeutic potential of histamine H, receptor agonists and antagonists, *Trends Pharmacol Sci* 1998; **19**: 177–183.
118. Schweitzer JB, Holcomb HH. Drugs under investigation for attention-deficit/hyperactivity disorder, *Current Opinion Investigational Drugs* 2002; **3**: 1207–1211.
119. Wesnes KA, Garratt C, Wickens M, Gudgeon A, Oliver S. Effects of sibutramine alone and with alcohol on cognitive function in healthy volunteers, *Br J Clin Pharmacol* 2000; **49**: 110–117.
120. DeVeaugh-Geiss J, Conners CK, Sarkis EH, *et al.* GW320659 for the treatment of attention-deficit/hyperactivity disorder in children, *J Am Acad Child Adolesc Psychiatry* 2002; **41**: 914.
121. Tedford CE, Pawlowski GP, Khan MA, Phillips JG, Yates SL. Cognition and locomotor activity in the developing rat: Comparisons of histamine H, receptor antagonists and ADHD therapeutics, *Abstract Soc Neurosci* 1996; 22.
122. Akhondzadeh S, Tavakolian R, Davari-Ashtiani R, Arabgol F, Amini H. Selegiline in the treatment of attention deficit hyperactivity disorder in children: A double blind and randomized trial, *Progress Neuro-Psychopharmacol Bio Psychiatry* 2003; **27**: 841.
123. Mohammadi MR, Ghanizadeh A, Alaghband-Rad J, Tehranidoost M, Mesgarpour B, Soori H. Selegiline in comparison with methylphenidate in attention deficit hyperactivity disorder children and adolescents in a double-blind, randomized clinical trial, *J Child Adolesc Psychopharmacol* 2004; **14**: 418.
124. Levin-Epstein M. A new way to deliver psychiatric meds, *Behavioral Healthcare* 2006; **26**: 22.
125. Wilens TE, Spencer TJ. The stimulants revisited, *Child Adolesc Psychiatric Clinics North Am* 2000; **9**: 573 603.
126. Wilens TE, Waxmonsky J, Scott M, *et al.* An open trial of adjunctive donepezil in attention-deficit/hyperactivity disorder, *J Child Adolesc Psychopharmacol* 2005; **15**: 947.
127. Levin ED, Rezvani AH. Development of nicotinic drug therapy for cognitive disorders, *Eur J Pharmacol* 2000; **393**: 141–146.
128. Wilens T, Biederman J, Spencer T, Bostic JQ, Prince J, Monuteaux BA. A pilot controlled clinical trial of ABT-418, a cholinergic agonist, in the treatment of adults with attention-deficit/hyperactivity disorder, *Am J Psychiatry* 1999; **156**: 1931–1937.
129. Wilens TE, Biederman J, Wong J, Spencer TJ, Prince JB. Adjunctive donepezil in attention deficit hyperactivity disorder youth: Case series. *J Child Adolesc Psychopharmacol* 2000; **10**: 217.
130. Rezvani AH. Cognitive effects of nicotine, *Bio Psychiatry* 2001; **49**: 258.
131. Potter AS. Effects of acute nicotine administration on behavioral inhibition in adolescents with attention-deficit/hyperactivity disorder, *Psychopharmacol* 2004; **176**: 183.

132. Mohammadi MR, Kashani L, Akhondzadeh S, Izadian ES, Ohadinia S. Efficacy of theophylline compared to methylphenidate for the treatment of attention-deficit hyperactivity disorder in children and adolescents: A pilot double-blind randomized trial, *J Clin Pharmacy Therapeutics* 2004; **29**: 139.
133. Froelich J, Doepfner M, Lehmkuhl G. Effects of combined cognitive behavioral treatment with parent management training in ADHD, *Behavioral Cognitive Psychotherapy* 2002; **30**(1): 111–115.
134. Wilens T. ADHD treatment with once-daily OROS methylphenidate: Interim 12-month results from a long-term open-label study, *J Am Acad Child Adolesc Psychiatry* 2003; **42**: 424.
135. Safren S. Cognitive-behavioral approaches to ADHD treatment in adulthood, *J Clin Psychiatry* 2006; **67**: 46–50.
136. Elliott G. Treating ADHD: Lessons from the MTA. In: *Psychiatry Grand Rounds.* Stanford, CA, 2007.
137. Lock J. Psychotherapy in children and adolescents: An overview. In: Steiner H, Ed. *Handbook of Mental Health Interventions in Children and Adolescents: An Integrated Developmental Approach.* San Francisco, CA: Jossey-Bass, 2004.
138. Erickson S, Achilles G. Cognitive behavioral therapy with children and adolescents. In: Steiner H, Ed. *Handbook of Mental Health Interventions in Children and Adolescents: An Integrated Developmental Approach.* San Francisco, CA: Jossey-Bass, 2004.
139. Hinshaw S. Attention-deficit/hyperactivity disorder: The search for viable treatments. In: Kendall PC, Ed. *Child and Adolescent Therapy: Cognitive-Behavioral Procedures*, 2nd edition. New York, NY: Guilford Press, 2002: pp. 88–128.
140. Pfiffner L. Psychosocial treatment for children with ADHD. In: *9th Annual Stanford Symposium on Developmental Approaches to Psychopathology.* Palo Alto, CA,: 2006.
141. Pfiffner L, Barkley R, DuPaul G. Treatment of ADHD in school settings. In: Barkley RA, Ed. *Attention-Deficit Hyperactivity Disorder: A Handbook for Diagnosis and Treatment*, 3rd edition. New York, NY: Guilford Press, 2006; 547–589.
142. Frankel F, Myatt R. *Children's Friendship Training.* New York, NY: Routledge, 2003.
143. Cunningham C, Cunningham L, Martorelli V. Effects of primary division, student-mediated conflict resolution programs on playground aggression, *J Child Psychol Psychiatry* 1998; **39**: 653–662.
144. Cunningham C, Cunningham L. Student-mediated conflict resolution programs. In: Barkley RA, Ed. *Attention-Deficit Hyperactivity Disorder: A Handbook for Diagnosis and Treatment*, 3rd edition. New York, NY: Guilford Press, 2006; 590–607.
145. Chronis A, Lahey B, Pelham W, Kipp H, Baumann B, Lee S. Psychopathology and substance abuse in parents of young children with attention deficit/hyperactivity disorder, *J Am Acad Child Adolesc Psychiatry* 2003; **42**: 1425–1432.

146. Forgatch M, Bullock B, Patterson G. From theory to practice: Increasing effective parenting through role-play. In: Steiner H, Ed. *Handbook of Mental Health Interventions in Children and Adolescents: An Integrated Developmental Approach.* San Francisco, CA: Jossey-Bass, 2004; 782–813.
147. Sonuga-Barke E, Daley D, Thompson M, Laver-Bradbury C, Weeks A. Parent-based therapies for preschool attention-deficit/hyperactivity disorder: A randomized controlled trial with a community sample, *J Am Acad Child Adolesc Psychiatry* 2001; **40**: 402–408.
148. Ota K, DuPaul G. Task engagement and mathematics performance in children with attention-deficit hyperactivity, *School Psychology Quarterly* 2002; **17**: 242–257.
149. DuPaul G, Volpe R, Jitendra A, Lutz J, Lorah K, Gruber R. Elementary school students with ADHD: Predictors of academic achievement, *J School Psychol* 2004; **42**: 285–301.
150. Kratochvil C, Turgay A, Weiss M, *et al.* In: *Joint Annual Meeting Scientific Proceedings* 2005: 136.
151. Pliszka SR. Non-stimulant treatment of attention-deficit/hyperactivity disorder, *CNS Spectrums* 2003; **8**: 253–258.
152. Faraone SV, Biederman J, Roe C. Comparative efficacy of Adderall and methylphenidate in attention-deficit/hyperactivity disorder: A meta-analysis, *J Clin Psychopharmacol* 2002; **22**: 468–473.

Chapter 11

Aggression

Niranjan Karnik and Hans Steiner

1. Introduction

Recent history has included events such as those at Virginia Tech University in Blacksburg, which tragically fell victim to a young 23-year-old student who killed himself, and 32 other individuals in a brief but highly lethal murder spree. This shocking act of aggression had roots that likely ran deep into this young man's history. He not only showed functional speech delays as a young child that raised the question of a developmental disorder of communication and language, but then as he entered school in the context of immigration from South Korea, he faced bullying and social isolation by peers. Later as he became older the patterns of social isolation and rejection continued and his anger grew to rage, which became evident in his writing. This rage eventually reached a point where he sought and legally obtained several guns that he then used to commit a calculated act of murder and suicide.

This trajectory shows the developmental nature of aggression and one terrible pathway through which it can unfold if left unchecked by skilled psychiatric intervention. The case also depicts a common reaction to problems, such as are encountered in this case: ignoring the antecedents of maladaptive aggression in the hopes that they will disappear. Cases like this can be found at many points in history and in all cultures. It is the ready access to guns in this country that makes these individuals so lethal.

Another case provides a stark contrast. In March 2007, a news station in Central Florida reported the following headline "Six-year-old's arrest triggers controversy." The accompanying story describes how a kindergarten student was taken to a local jail, charged with one felony and two misdemeanors. This young girl reportedly became "violent, throwing chairs, striking a teacher, and crying and wailing uncontrollably."[1] At some point in the process, school officials believed that they had a potentially dangerous situation on their hands and summoned the police, as per their protocol, to assist and the police charged and then took this young into custody. The story mirrors other stories that occasionally emerge in the news media that depict uncontrollably violent children and their interactions with law enforcement. At the heart of these tragic stories lies our confusion regarding the concept of childhood aggression. In contradistinction to our first case, authorities overreact in ways that are not helpful and even result in escalation of the situation. Is this a moral failing or a disorder? Should this be punished or treated? Do we have a diagnostic label for this? Is it adequate? Many questions arise, and not all of them have good answers, as of this writing.

The study of aggression and antisocial behavior is a field that historically resides in several different literatures which often remain in parochial isolation; criminology, psychology, sociology, jurisprudence and psychiatry all have data regarding these phenomena, but there is a pronounced split in how to best approach this topic. As a result, the field is not unified, and the research is of highly varying quality. The current nosology sometimes incriminates those that are victims of circumstance and at the same time also often fails to identify those youth who are at highest risk of producing harm, and to be persistent in these actions one fact is certain: aggression, disruptive, and antisocial behavior are the most common presenting behavioral complaints to pediatric and child psychiatric clinics.[2–5] Families and caregivers often turn to physicians to help understand why their children engage in aggressive behaviors and what can be done to reduce these behaviors. Developmental psychiatry introduces the perspective that, to a certain extent, aggression is a normal and valid form of behavior that typically has its most prevalent and unbridled expression within a particular developmental window from toddlerhood to school age. Behaviors that fall outside of this window or that exceed predicted norms in frequency or intensity merit closer scrutiny and examination.

Problems with disruptive behavior and aggression are among the most threatening, prevalent, and serious in psychiatry. The reason that our data are of such varying quality is due to the fact that, for complex historical, political, and methodological reasons, the study of disorders of aggression has proceeded in fits and starts. First, the founding fathers of modern psychiatry (such as Freud, Jung, Janet, Charcot, Kraepelin, and Bleuler) had almost no interest in the subject. Their interests lay with disorders of anxiety, mood, and psychosis. Second, declaring aggression to be in the realm of mental disorders has always attracted a great deal of suspicion and political attention. Some have argued that categories like conduct disorder are flawed because they are socially determined.[6] Finally, no other set of problems requires a deep conceptual analysis to prevent the pathologization and medicalization of morals as do problems in which a highly social phenomenon (anger and aggression almost always involves "the other") which serves a supremely adaptive function (such as defense of one's own person and limit setting to personal injury). All these factors historically combined to make our field shy away from the concerted study of aggression and its disorders, especially as the biological underpinnings of aggression are concerned.[7] But it is precisely these new insights of neuroscience and the social sciences that are currently paving the way to a more accurate and useful conceptualization, taxonomy, and treatment. In this chapter, we draw heavily on these new insights to improve the confusing state of disorders of aggression and their treatment. The dialectic between phenomenology and practice, and the insights of several basic sciences may well serve as one model on how to improve the future nomenclatures in psychiatry.

1.1. *Normal developmental patterns of aggression*

In the course of childhood development, aggression is a normal behavioral pattern that emerges in the context of children learning about the social world. It is one strategy for testing the limits of the social and interpersonal context that they inhabit. Aggression in this sense is a strategy like tasting, touching, asking, and playing. We can expect that aggression decreases as the child matures, and as they are able to substitute increasingly more effective and age appropriate strategies to act on their own behalf or in their own defense. Unfortunately, we do not have available to us a complete set of studies with age appropriate instruments and informed by similar constructs. In fact, there is a dichotomy of aggression, which is supported by clinical and preclinical data to be discussed below, which is of considerable interest and import, but has not been studied systematically across the entire age span. The concepts of emotionally "hot" and "cold" aggression arc reflected in hundreds of years in legal thinking, and appears under several different labels in a wide range of nomenclatures trying to subtype aggression.[8] These two subforms of aggression most likely have important implications for diagnosis and treatment.[9,10] The best one can glean from available data and clinical experience, the developmental progressions of these two forms differ in the ways indicated. Hot aggression peaks early on in life, subsides, returns in early adolescence, and then steadily declines as we age. By contrast, cold aggression comes on line as we develop planning and thinking capacities, far beyond the abilities of a preschooler. Again, it peaks in early adolescence, and then subsides steadily over time.[11–13]

For children, aggression emerges at times from senses of frustration or limit testing. Despite its normalcy, it is a behavior that should not be ignored; on the contrary, it requires understanding and attention. Younger children who act aggressively need to learn frustration tolerance, and that there are limits to behaviors. They also need to understand that there are repercussions for behaving in certain ways. Viewed is this light, aggression then becomes a basic tool for the child to understand social rules. While touching and playing are socially acceptable, in excess or at an inappropriate time, they can be seen as inappropriate. Aggression is the inverse force in some ways. It is generally seen as unacceptable, but there are times when it may be appropriate or understandable (Box 1).[14,15]

Box 1. Developmentally normative aggression case examples

Jenny is a three year old who attends a preschool. She has periods of time when she gets frustrated with tasks or activities. She usually simply stops working and then refuses to cooperate with the teacher or other students for 10–15 min. Last week, she grew particularly frustrated with a drawing she was trying to do, and in anger threw her markers at another child in the class who was doing very well at the activity. The teacher after witnessing this, pulled Jenny aside, and told her that throwing markers was not acceptable in the class and placed her in a time out. As part of the time out, she had to tell the teacher how she thought the other child felt when the markers were flying toward her. Jenny became very quite and whispered "scared." The teacher complimented her on her accurate empathy. (hot aggressive act)

Bobby is an eight-year old boy growing up in a in a middle class family with two parents and an older 12-year-old sister. He did not show any major developmental or academic problems. His mother grew mildly concerned about his constant seeking of candies and sugary foods. Bobby had gained some weight and the parents had been directed by their pediatrician to try to modify his diet. His parents forbade him from eating any candy. The child did not like this new rule, but did not risk protest in order not to appear "bad." However, Bobby, while at a shopping center with his mother, was stopped by a security guard after he was observed stealing candies and putting them in his pockets unbeknownst to his mother. This was the first time something like this ever happened with Bobby who was ordinarily an obedient and easy to parent child. The parents had a serious discussion with Bobby about stealing and its implications. They also asked that in the future Bobby should tell them if he disagreed with a rule so that a compromise could be considered. (cold aggressive act).

Studies from the Oregon Social Learning Center (OSLC) based on the work of Gerald Patterson have traced some fascinating features of aggression and it origins within complex familial structures. In the 1970s, Patterson theorized that at the root of learning about the age appropriate expression and use of aggression is a cycle between parent and child. As demands get issued, the child can either obey or not. Typically, the cycle of demand and resistance to authority starts as soon as the child learns that there are certain functions that the parent cannot control. Such behaviors usually emerge around the age of two or three, as the child begins to walk (remove himself or herself) or control other functions (such as bowel or bladder, eating, chewing, *etc.*). Patterson described the key construct as being an interaction of "parent inept discipline" and "child antisocial and coercive behavior." The OSLC researchers theorized that at a certain point in the process of parenting a child, some families took one of two pathways into poor parenting (Fig. 1). One pathway that might be described as the "permissive parent" begins when the child refuses to obey the parent (*i.e.* "please put your toys away — no I am too tired; I do not want, etc."). In the face of this resistance, the parent then desists and allows the child to continue to disobey, or worse, completes the demanded task for the child. The child learns that he or she is more powerful than the parent, and then begins to more routinely disobey and resist parental demands and limit setting. The parents' permissiveness has just reinforced coercive behavior on the part of the child. The net outcome is that the child fails to learn about pleasing others, compromise, and age-appropriate use of aggression and resistance. While this may not immediately lead to dire consequences in the family, problems with fulfilling demands, compromise and rules are sure to impact the child adversely as soon as they step out of the family of origin. This will likely be especially true as they enter school and are asked to conform to a more structured setting with a steady stream of demands that must be met efficiently and swiftly lest the child be left behind in learning and emotional growth. Failure at school and learning then compounds the problems with internalizing the proper adaptive space for and use of aggression.

The second pathway into maladaptive aggression is in many ways diametrically opposed to the permissive parent described above. The cycle begins again with the child refusing to obey the parent's wishes. In this pathway the parent uses their physical force and often even violence against the child to compel him or her to obey their will. The child learns from this that when faced with conflicting demands, aggression is an appropriate and legitimate response, especially when one is in charge and is the stronger partner in the dyad. Through modeling of aggression the parent teaches the child to use force on others especially as they get older and more capable of using this technique, and as a power gradient is present. In the aggressive act, the original demand is usually forgotten or not carried out because the child is hurt, confined, or otherwise removed. The net effect of this cycle is that demands do not get fulfilled,

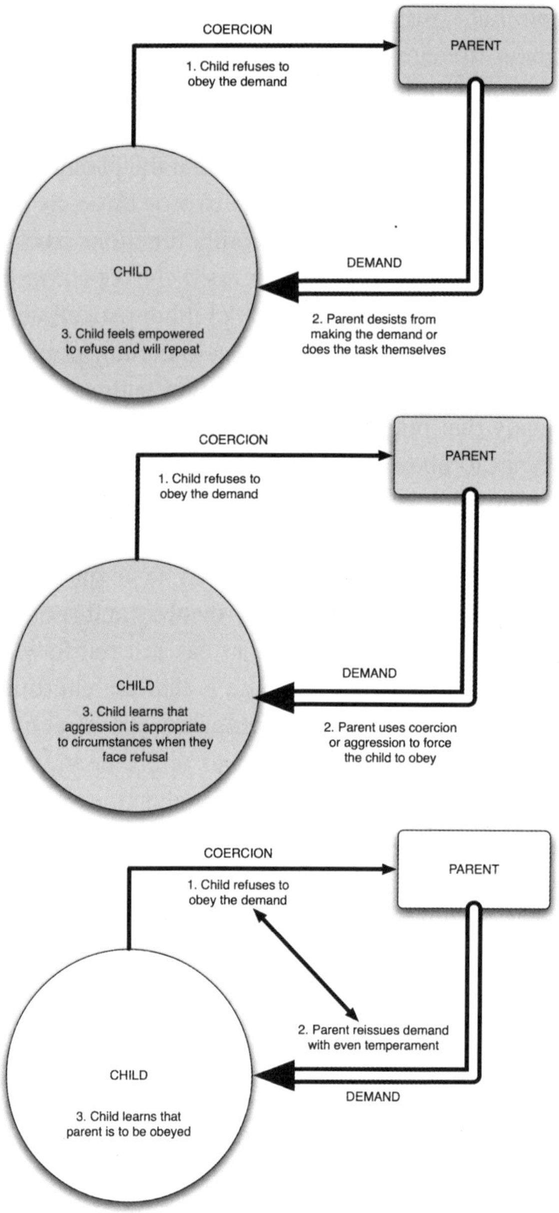

Fig. 1: Schematic of patterns of behaviors and cycles that lead to negative behaviors.

and there is no learning about compromise, negotiation, and proper space for normative aggression.

The most appropriate pathway and preferred technique that we term the "even tempered parent" begins once again with the child refusing to obey the parent's wishes. In this case the parent reissues the request with a firm but even tempered tone, making the request clear and powerful by the sheer force of their insistence, the weight of their presence, and the reliance on the fact that children, in principle, want to please those to whom they are attached and who take care of them properly. The child may still refuse but the parent simply repeats the cycle, and may use behavioral reinforcers that indicate to the child that they cannot leave or move on to something more fun until the child does what he or she needs to. From this, the child will eventually learn that the parent is to be obeyed. If there are extenuating circumstances, they will eventually be voiced, considered, and factored into a negotiated timetable or compromise.

Several studies by members of the OSLC have now confirmed these general structures and that a relationship exists between coercive parenting style, problematic temperament on the part of the child, parental poverty, and substance use disorders in the production of child antisocial behavior.[16] The OSLC has also developed a very effective form of treatment that they term Parent Management Training — Oregon Model (PMTO). They have been able to show demonstrable effects of teaching parents how to move from coercive styles of parenting toward more positive strategies which increase family stability and decrease antisocial and aggressive patterns.[17]

1.2. *Maladaptive aggression*

Connor[13] in a recent monograph on aggression and antisocial behavior argues for a new definition of maladaptive aggression. Based on a synthesis of the current clinical and preclinical research on aggression, he argues that maladaptive aggression has four elements, the presence of any of which should trigger suspicion that a psychopathological substrate might have to be considered. First, maladaptive aggression occurs outside of expectable social context. For example, a child who walks over to another child during a church service and hits him in the face. Such an event emerges without any clear context, and serves no clear function. Church is ordinarily a sedate and calm venue without any context for violence or aggression.

Second, maladaptive aggression occurs independent from expectable antecedent social cues. For example, an adolescent starts verbally fighting with a passenger on the bus who was quietly reading his own newspaper. Here, there is no antecedent trigger. The passenger did not interact with the youth. Such aggression emerges surprisingly and often appears to have little connection to actions on the part of the victim.

According to Connor's schema, the third element to maladaptive aggression is disproportionate in intensity, frequency, duration, or severity. In other words, the aggressor acts in ways which seems to be completely at odds with the trigger or context. For example, a student calls another student by a derogatory name. This second student then viciously attacks the first student, and beats him to the point of being unconscious. In this example, the aggressive sequence starts with some mild verbal aggression by the first student. The second student responds with a certain degree of maladaptive aggression by beating the student so significantly.

The final element of maladaptive aggression is that it does not terminate appropriately, even though the victim signals defeat and apology. In the last example, it is clear that the second boy continues to harm the first despite it being clear that the first student cannot defend himself. Other examples might include a boy who verbally berates a girl who inadvertently stepped in line in front of him and then apologizes and moves behind him in line. He continues to berate her verbally despite her appropriate response, and he seems unable to contain himself or terminate his aggression.

This schema moves our understanding of maladaptive aggression more toward aggression being psychopathological and internally driven. The assumption is that while we need to understand the context of aggression to judge whether it is maladaptive or not, the roots of psychopathological aggression lie predominantly in a more internally and functionally psychological place.

1.3. *Comparative nosology*

August Aichorn as director of the Vienna Boys Reform School first brought the plight of criminality, youth, and aggression to foreground by publishing his book Wayward Youth in the 1930s.[18] His conceptualization emphasized the developmental nature of these processes, and potential for rehabilitation in helping these children regain a role in society. His work was expanded by Fritz Redl, a Viennese analyst who taught at Wayne State University and was extremely effective in designing behavioral interventions that were dynamically informed, but effective translations of aggressive acts into therapeutic communications.[19,20]

There is a significant tension in the current nomenclature emanating from this early period where a split developed between the criminological classification of delinquent acts and the psychiatric conceptualization of the delinquent mind. Criminology has emphasized an approach that classifies the acts of aggression and conduct disorder along a continuum based on the severity of the act and links these to various legal definitions of criminal acts. The person deserving of "criminological treatment" is the one who has been convicted. Treatment is closely linked to punishment and deprivation of rights. The advantage of this system is that it is simple to use because it is based primarily on the act itself, the finding of *mens rea* and of conviction. Culpability and responsibility are assumed to be always relevant, and there is no struggle to investigate the etiological roots, and weigh responsibility against biopsychosocial risk.

Modern psychiatry instead takes the view that aggression and disruptive behaviors are emergent over time; that clusters of maladaptive aggression are syndromal disorders whose roots lie in the developmental experiences and biological predispositions of an individual. When the result of the individual's trajectory is one that proceeds in an antisocial or criminal path, where aggression has ceased to serve its adaptive purpose, the interventions must necessarily be therapeutic and rehabilitative to stem future acts and to break the cycle of aggression and disruptive behavior. Most importantly, the individual's diagnosis no longer depends on the legal outcome of whether or not the person is found culpable. Fulfilling certain predefined criteria can lead to intervention, treatment, and rehabilitation. The limits between personal responsibility and disorder have been moved into the direction of the latter. There is some unease among our criminological and legal colleagues regarding this outcome, but it seems a necessary step, as we argue, due to our developing increasingly deeper understandings of the neuroscience of aggression. Where the future lines will be drawn between responsibility and rehabilitation remains to be seen, and will no doubt be a matter of intense debate.

Historically, the *Diagnostic and Statistical Manual of Mental Disorders* (DSM) developed criteria for the diagnosis of conduct disorder and aggression in the second edition of the DSM-II in 1968.[21] At this point, disruptive behavior disorders compromised three categories: undersocialized aggressive reaction of childhood or adolescent, the runaway reaction of childhood, and the group delinquent reaction of childhood. This marked a significant change from the prior edition of DSM-I which only had a diagnosis for sociopathic personality. This diagnosis did not extend to children. DSM-III expanded the subtypes and first introduced the term conduct disorder into the official nomenclature building on the subtypes in DSM-II. This edition of the DSM outlined four general variants of disorder: socialized, undersocialized, aggressive, and not aggrcssive.[22]

These early attempts at subtyping form the beginnings of work that is now culminating at this moment through multiple lines of neuroscience and psychological research. The subtypes of aggression seem to have validity and point to varied pathogenetic underpinnings, different neuroscientific bases, and consequent treatments. These issues are discussed in detail later in this chapter.

The 1987 revision which marked a significant change in DSM-III further defined the category of conduct disorder by identifying the most common variants of the previous classification: solitary, aggressive, group type, and undifferentiated.[23] The comparison of these definitions reveals the basic feature of conduct disorder; a pattern of behavior by an individual that violates age appropriate and socially appropriate behavior often characterized by aggression. Current definitions that include aggression are highly varied in terms of their taxonomies and their approach to understanding this phenomenon in children.

Table 1: Current Nosological Categories by System

Diagnostic & Statistical Manual, 4th Edition Text Revision	*International Classification of Diseases,* 10th Edition
Conduct disorder, adolescent-onset	Conduct disorder confined to the family context
Conduct disorder, childhood-onset	Unsocialized conduct disorder
Oppositional defiant disorder	Socialized conduct disorder
Disruptive behavior disorder, not otherwise specified	Oppositional defiant disorder
	Other conduct disorders
	Conduct disorder, unspecified

In contrast to the DSM approach which emphasizes multiple comorbid diagnoses, the *International Classification of Disease*, 10th edition (*ICD-10*)[24] takes a principal diagnosis approach and then places other diagnoses as secondary (Table 1). Such an approach has the advantage of helping to focus treatment on what clinicians see as the major symptoms that need to be addressed. With aggression, which can be highly multifactorial and also a symptom of many psychiatric illnesses, it is important to thoroughly exclude other possible causative factors through a detailed history and exam before establishing a primary diagnosis in the disruptive behavior disorders or conduct disorder clusters.

In many respects, the ICD-10 system is a more cogent system that better acknowledges both normative patterns of aggression as well as overlays well with the emerging neuroscience of aggression. The ICD-10 is also more sensitive to the effect of context on the emergence of maladaptive aggression. While the DSM-IV acknowledges many of these issues in the descriptions of the disorders, the diagnostic categories themselves are limited in their utility when trying to ascertain etiology and plan for treatment. Part of the failure of these systems of classification is that they do not sufficiently incorporate the criteria for maladaptiveness described above or the neuroscience of aggression described below. This puts them dangerously close to medicalizing moral standards or can lead to the pathologization of normal behaviors. Nevertheless, both systems are much better than legal categories of delinquency and criminality which put courts in the position of deciding which youth get treatment and what the outlines of this treatment entails.

2. Epidemiology

As noted earlier, disruptive behavior disorders are a normative process in childhood. The National Institute of Child Health and Human Development (NICHD) Early Child Care Research Network[11] found that physical aggression which started relatively high at age two gradually went down over the course of early development kindergarten and then grades 1 to 3 in elementary school.

This early time period appears to be developmentally sensitive. The NICHD Early Child Care Network in a recent work found that although parenting was by far the strongest predictor of childhood behavior, early child-care experiences could have a stressful effect on children and that this stress often results in elevated levels of aggression at later ages.[25] These findings illustrate the largely normative epidemiological patterns of childhood aggression and disruptive behaviors. The one limitation of these studies is that they focused on physical aggression when there are many other subtypes of aggression that are developmentally evident and often normal.

Disruptive behaviors are the most common referring complaint for pediatric psychiatric consultation and often accounts for between 25 and 90% of requests in some clinics. This stands in contrast to the general population prevalence of disruptive patterns which varies between 1.5 and 20%, again depending on definitions and methods of data collection.[13] Notably, these behaviors, at least in their overt form, are highly skewed toward males with male-to-female ratios ranging between 3:1 and 5:1.[26] Recent research is beginning to uncover a different pattern for girls, and it is becoming evident that social aggression and more covert forms of aggressive behavior may be present for females.[27,28] It is quite likely that our studies of aggression in children may underreport these types of aggression relative to the more traditional forms of physical aggression and disruptive behaviors seen in boys.

A subset of these children go on to develop maladaptive patterns of disruptive behaviors which merit clinical attention. Current estimates show that in a general population sample, using DSM-IV criteria, roughly 1.8% of children meet criteria for oppositional defiant disorder (ODD) while 3.2% will meet ICD-10 standards for ODD.[29] Psychiatric epidemiologists have noted that the ICD-10 definition more effectively captures children who are having clinically significant behavioral issues. Conduct disorder (CD) appears to also be present in about 2% of children at any given time but age of these is markedly older than those with ODD.[29] Using the ICD standard, we can see that a cohort of children may progress from ODD to CD. Strict DSM-IV criteria do not capture this transition well. The finding of 2% seems to be a relatively stable number with a study from the British National Child Mental Health Study finding CD at a rate of 2.1% in boys and 0.8% in girls.[30]

3. Diagnosis

For this section and the following clinical ones, please refer to two recent AACAP practice parameters, on ODD;[5] and CD.[31]

3.1. *Clinical history*

The cornerstone to any assessment of children for aggression is a detailed clinical history. Such history should focus on the presenting issue, and then seek to gain a developmental perspective of how this symptom has emerged over the youth's development. It is important to ask about factors that exacerbate aggression and those that may ameliorate it. Attention should be paid to all the major domains of child psychiatric evaluation including screening for pervasive developmental disorders, mood and anxiety disorders, sleep problems, neurological symptoms (especially seizure events), educational history, and potential trauma and abuse.

Such history needs to be done in a working relationship with the youth and his or her family. Often it can be difficult to establish a working relationship with the youth as the initial contact can be adversarial. Thus, efforts must be made to establish rapport with the youth. As this process is taking place, consideration needs to be given to the context of the aggression. For example, a boy who lives in the midst of significant community of gang violence and is often targeted when he walks down the street could be understood to be living in a different context of violence when he repeatedly gets into fights with members of other gangs in the neighborhood. In contrast we might see the context of violence differently around a young girl who is engaged in significant social and physical violence along with her friends against a new girl in the high school.

In evaluating aggression in children and adolescents, clinicians should make certain to obtain collateral information from parents, teachers, and/or primary care providers. Such information is useful because children with disruptive behaviors will sometimes avoid full disclosure of symptoms and history. In obtaining a history, collateral informants can also provide essential history about early childhood development and temperament.

A final component to the initial history is a detailed evaluation of alcohol and drug abuse patterns. Honest appraisal of this is sometimes impossible depending on the youth, but the clinician may need to order routine drugs screens to evaluate current patterns and also help reinforce sobriety for clinical work. The knowledge of which substances are being used can help to steer diagnosis and subtyping of aggression. Reactive, affective, defensive, or impulsive (RADI) aggression tends to favor alcohol and cannabis abuse, while proactive, instrumental, or planned (PIP) aggression often combines with the use of all classes of drugs including cocaine, heroin, and other highly potent substances.

3.2. *Clinical exam*

The clinical exam should focus on the present state of the child, and getting a clear picture of how present state emotions may relate to broad trait emotions.[32] This distinction helps to separate those emotions that vary rapidly moment-to-moment and are affected by environmental stimuli (state) from emotions that form a more generalized underlying phenomenon over which experience occurs for larger segments of time (trait). These emotions appear to be substantially different for children with aggressive patterns. In addition, any clinician evaluating children with histories of aggression should attempt to ascertain whether the child may be having thoughts of self-harm or harm toward others that in extreme forms may advance to suicidality or homicidality. Assessment of these indices may, if found to be present, require emergent hospitalization to protect the minor or others from harm and to initiate treatment.

3.3. *Laboratory and imaging studies*

Currently, there is no laboratory or imaging study that can accurately identify or diagnosis disruptive behaviors. Certain laboratory tests may be in order as part of a broader psychiatric work-up and evaluation. Some providers routinely screen blood chemistries, complete blood counts, thyroid, and heavy metals. These studies may also be done by primary medical providers as part of routine pediatric care. Urine toxicology can be very helpful in ascertaining if a youth is abusing substances that may have a relationship to aggression.

Imaging studies need not be routinely ordered, and functional studies only have a role in academic research at the present time. Their predictive value is limited and requires highly specialized neuroradiologists for interpretation. Should the child have other neurological evidence of lesion or seizure activity then imaging may be merited to rule out a primary neurological disorder. Referral to a neurologist would be prudent at this stage for a more extensive work-up for mass lesions, cerebral palsy, epilepsy, or vasculitis.

3.4. *Family history*

Family history is an essential component of any evaluation for aggression. Family history of aggression may raise the possibility of a biological trait or highlight maladaptive intrafamilial relationships that are leading to aggression. Additionally, family substance abuse and dependence histories can be useful in ascertaining familial risk of substance use disorders, and also point toward the availability of certain classes of substances in the youth's household and neighborhood. As part of a complete family history, it can be useful to take a parenting history and try to get some idea of the techniques that were used to discipline, educate, and raise the child.

3.5. *Psychometric tests*

Numerous psychometric instruments have been developed to assess aggression and its component psychological properties.[5,8] Commonly used systems like the Achenbach System of Empirically Based Assessment (CBCL and YSR) and the Behavior Assessment System for Children, Version 2 (BASC-2) both have aggression subscales which can be used to identify children and adolescent who may be having difficulties with aggression. Use of these can compliment a sound history and clinical exam. As part of this evaluation, we advocate that a lifetime history of aggression be used. The Brown-Goodwin Lifetime History of Aggression is particularly suited to this type of evaluation and can help understand the longer context of aggressive and violent behaviors.[33] Following this history, more recent acts can be considered and classified. Symptoms can then be tallied and measured using broader gauged psychometrics which can assess psychiatric morbidity across the spectrum of experience. Finally, testing with regard to personality styles and adaptation can be assessed as these will help the provider to understand the underlying basis upon which the aggressive behaviors may be presenting and also highlight important treatment strategies.

3.6. *Formulation*

Our approach to the treatment of aggressive youth requires an accurate formulation. This step involves the synthesis of clinical history, exam data, and any relevant studies to try to understand what the principal diagnosis is and what the target symptoms are. An accurate formulation will take a biopsychosocial perspective and combine this with a developmental view of the youth. This then leads to the selection of intervention strategies that are appropriate in the clinical situation. Collaboration with other providers may be necessary and should be initiated at an early stage to maximize cooperation and to avoid duplication of services.

When addressing aggression, there are several key decision points to be made in developing a rational formulation. First, a decision needs to be made as to whether aggression is maladaptive or not. In other words, we need to consider whether the aggressive acts make sense given the developmental context that the youth is growing up in. Does the aggression exceed normal patterns? Is it isolated to particular contexts where the child feels threatened (abuse or domestic violence) or is threatened (war, conflict)? Is the aggression limited to specific triggers or people, or does it pervade the child and family's life on a daily or highly regular basis?

Consideration then needs to be given to whether other diagnoses may be triggering the aggression. Could the child's symptoms be better explained by bipolar disorder or does the child have features suggestive of autism, and might these diagnostic clusters better explain the origins of the youth's aggression? Other major diagnoses need to be considered before proceeding down the formulation algorithm. In the case of autism, for example, it may be the child's inability to communicate their needs well that may produce aggressive patterns.

Next, consider the subtype of aggression that characterizes the behavior. Is the aggression "cold" in nature and have characteristics of proactive, instrumental, or planned (PIP) violence? This subtype would lack empathy or remorse for the act. Conversely, does the aggression show a reactive nature that is "hot" and have characteristics of defensive, impulsive, or affective symptoms? The reason for such subtyping is that these different forms of aggression might respond differentially to treatment.

By accurately subtyping the aggression, consideration can then be given to the causal loops that underlie the disruptive patterns. If the child shows excess activation that is then leading to reactivity and impulsive acts, then we can use agents like atypical antipsychotics, mood stabilizers or beta-blockers to address this underlying physiology. If the youth shows an inability to self-regulate then consideration could be given to agents that focus on GABA or dopamine, like divalproex, psychostimulants, or atomoxetine. Addressing "cold" or PIP aggression would take a different path and we detail these strategies more in the next section.

3.7. *Differential diagnosis and comorbidities*

The goal of differential diagnosis is to find a principal diagnosis that can be treated with highly specific interventions which then resolves problems associated with the diagnosis. Special care must be taken as one approaches disruptive disorder, as aggression is so commonly found in a whole range of disorders[34] which may require radically different treatments.

In contrast, the DSM comorbidity model allows for the coexistence of multiple disorders. Reporting within the DSM model will automatically lead to high levels of comorbidity. While this may be helpful in some ways, when designing treatments for youth we should attempt to assign primacy as best as we can. This is all the more important as we are beginning to have increasingly specific treatments that target some but not all forms of psychopathology. The treatment of primary disorders will sometimes lead to resolution of comorbidities. The resolution of attention problems with the treatment of bipolar disorder and the reduction of aggression with stimulant treatment in ADHD are prime examples of the value of this process. Still, it is possible that certain disorders persist even after our most concerted attempt at clarification of primary disorder and despite our best attempts at intervention. It is in these scenarios that we should reserve the term comorbidity.

Attention deficit hyperactivity disorder

The most common of disorders with disruptive patterns is ADHD (see Chap 10 of this volume). The central characteristic of this disorder is sustained disruption of attention regulation that is not a component of CD or ODD. This characteristic helps to distinguish ADHD from CD or ODD. In terms of establishing a differential and primary diagnosis, if attentional symptoms predominate then ADHD should be suspected. Aggressive symptoms that remain despite improvement and treatment of ADHD may then raise the possibility of comorbidity. Addressing comorbidity in these scenarios requires more than simply utilizing medications. Clinicians should seek to optimize medications that may have been initiated for ADHD but then engage families in other treatments such as Parent Management Training (PMT) as described and developed by the OSLC (see section earlier in this chapter).

Mood and anxiety disorders

Mood and anxiety disorders in children and adolescents can often present with disruptive patterns.[5,9] The central symptom of these disorders is dysregulation of affect, mood, and excess anxiety. As a rule, exclusive CD and ODD are not anxious or depressed, although if their problems persist then these comorbid disorders can develop.[10–12] If anything, ODD and CD may have as their predominant affect acute anger and chronic irritability. While irritability may be a component of other childhood mood and anxiety disorders, ODD and CD will have these symptoms in a non-phasic pattern that often characterizes mood and anxiety symptoms.

When looking at comorbidities, several studies have documented that mood and anxiety disorder are also present in significant numbers among young offenders.[13–15] A good history and timeline will help the clinician identify whether the mood and anxiety symptom predate or antedate the disruptive behaviors. Incarceration in juvenile hall can easily lead to both mood and anxiety symptoms especially given how difficult and taxing the experience can be for a juvenile who has never encountered such settings.

Social phobia and separation anxiety present special cases that can lead to aggressive patterns in children. Consideration should be given to the timeline and sequence of presentation to tease apart whether these disorders could potentially be primary disorders or whether they are truly comorbid with the disruptive behavior.

Post-traumatic stress disorder

As a subset of anxiety disorders, PTSD deserves special attention given the degree to which this condition can cause disruptive behaviors or be comorbid with them. Our studies have also show that high rates of PTSD exist among incarcerated youth[16,17] and these may be particularly morbid with dissociative symptoms present in many children.[18,19] The trauma spectrum disorders are increasingly found to respond to specialized interventions,[20–22] and can occur long after disruptive behavior disorders have their onset.

Substance use disorders

Likewise, it is easy to understand how substance use disorders coincide with disruptive disorders. Given the high degree of comorbidity between these groups of disorders[23,24] it is important to distinguish the leading edge. If the substance use significantly predates the onset of aggressive symptoms, then it is likely that substance treatment should be the primary focus and the aggression should be monitored to see if it improves as the substance use diminishes. Another aspect to monitor is whether the individual is committing acts while using substances. Conversely, the disruptive patterns may have led the child or adolescent into social situations where exposure to substances is common. In such situations, the degree to which the disruptive or CD patterns drive substance use may be important to ascertain. Finally, routine testing for drugs should be considered since history alone may not be sufficient.

Psychosis, mental retardation and pervasive developmental disorders

Among psychiatric comorbidities, a final set of concerns may arise about psychosis, mental retardation, and pervasive developmental disorders. For psychosis, the degree of overlap outside of substance-induced psychosis with disruptive behaviors may be small given the rates of primary psychotic disorders in the general population. Distinguishing this from primary disruptive patterns is best done on the degree to which the core symptom of primary psychosis is being out of touch with reality. Certainly aggression and disruptive patterns can emerge in such contexts but the initial goal should be treatment of the psychosis and then observation of whether their aggressive symptoms improve. For mental retardation and pervasive developmental disorders, the core symptoms revolve around impaired language skills, lack of connection to social situations and ignorance of social conventions. Such features are not part of the primary disruptive pattern and are relatively easy to distinguish.

Medical and neurological conditions

Consideration should also be given to potential medical sources of these behaviors. Prospective data from population-based studies have shown that any chronic pediatric illness is more likely to result in externalizing behaviors and potential disruptive patterns.[25–27]

CNS injury and neurological disorders are especially common and can originate from a variety of diseases. Lead poisoning, or other heavy metals, can result in neurological problems that then display with behavioral dysregulation. In addition, malnutrition and disorders of metabolism can also in rare instances produce effects on the body that result in disruptive patterns. Finally, chronic and neurological illnesses of various types can make children feel poorly and produce outward symptoms of disruptive behaviors that are driven by their internal sensation of illness. Children often lack a framework to understand the somatic processes in their bodies and may instead present with behavioral manifestations. Lewis and her colleagues have, over the past 20 years, documented an amazing degree of comorbidity between violence, aggression, and neuropsychiatric injury. She has found that a large proportion of severely aggressive offenders have traumatic brain injuries, severe mental retardation, and epilepsy. In aggregate, these central nervous system (CNS) insults may have roots in the significant degree of childhood violence and abuse that many extreme offenders have been subject to at developmentally critical periods.[28–31]

Impulse control disorders

In addition to these disorders, there are a set of impulse control disorders in the DSM-IV which span a wide gambit of problems likely with different etiologies. These include intermittent explosive disorder (IED), pathological gambling, kleptomania, trichotillomania, and pyromania. We find the grouping of these disorders to be somewhat problematic. They lack a cohesive etiology that binds them, and their grouping lacks any internal unity.

Gambling and pyromania hold a special interest for our taxonomy of aggression and disruptive behaviors because they have both been linked to antisocial patterns and because each disorder could at times be a subset of conduct disorder as currently defined. The literature on gambling especially with regard to children and adolescents is rather small. This is likely a reflection of the fact that pathological gambling more significantly affects adults and late adolescence while its roots may lie in childhood.[32,33] The few epidemiologic studies on this topic have found that among students in grades between 7 and 13 in Canada, 6% had gambling problems within the past year and another 7.5% were at-risk for gambling.[60]

Unsurprisingly, male gender, substance abuse, maladaptive peers, family history of gambling, and other impulsive behavior all are known risk factors for adolescent gambling.[61]

Firesetting or pyromania likewise has a small literature for children and adolescents. Here, the connections to future antisocial patterns have been more clearly raised[34–37] although the etiological pathways are poorly defined. Recent studies have found that firesetting youth have more stress at home, often have single-parent families, present with higher levels of depression, report more aggressive thoughts, and display more delinquent behaviors than their peers.[66] Other studies have likewise found increased antisocial patterns, elevated levels of suicidality, significant drug use, and perceived failure at school as distinguishing firesetters from nonfiresetters.[67] Clearly, a developmental perspective is needed to understand the relationship between pyromania and antisocial or aggressive acts, and in order to contextualize these patterns to usefully understand their relationship to the child's or adolescent's life.

It is not clear at this juncture if these syndromes are separate disorders or whether they are better kept nosologically under the rubrics of disruptive behavior disorders. Aggressive acts in the child and adolescent age range are usually highly diverse, and often include the acts discussed in these diagnostic labels. One of the points the literature on juvenile delinquency has repeatedly made is that a great deal of delinquency (and by extension disruptive behavior disorders) are "nonspecialized" and opportunistic in nature. This means that prematurely lumping them into discrete disorders may not serve us well. There are also few special interventions other than those directed at disruptive behavior disorders to treat these behaviors. Aligning them with hotly and coldly aggressive patterns holds more promise for a more productive research agenda and future development of specific interventions.

Personality disorders

While we are hesitant to lay diagnoses of personality disorders on youth under the age of 18, we do recognize that the roots of personality disorders do likely reach into childhood. It therefore seems prudent from a research perspective to look at personality characteristics as they unfold over time while still holding the admonishment in the DSM-IV against diagnosing personality disorders at an early age. Eppright and colleagues in a sample of 100 youth found that 87% of those detained met criteria for conduct disorder and that among those 86% met criteria for antisocial personality disorder.[68] Our group has recently examined this question in a sample of 790 incarcerated youth and likewise found wide evidence of personality disorders among this population. We also find that those with antisocial, borderline, or narcissistic personality disorders have significantly more anger and irritability, distress and aggressive and delinquent behavior, as well as significantly less restraint than their counterparts not meeting criteria for these diagnoses.[38,39] This is an expanding area of research and we believe that we will continue to learn more about the development of personality as we move forward with these types of studies. Whether or not the 18-year cutoff criterion will stand the test of time is not known.

4. Pathogenesis

Aggression originates from a complex series of interactions and systems that have neurobiological, psychological, and social underpinnings. It is important to remember that all of these systems are dynamic throughout life, and that especially in childhood these systems develop significantly and in continuous interaction with one another. The etiology of maladaptive aggression and disruptive disorders are complex interactions of social and biological forces,[71] combining in a dynamic relationship to produce a clinical outcome.

4.1. *Psychobiological subtypes of aggression*

Evidence from the neurobiology and psychology of aggression increasingly demonstrates that there are two major phenotypes of aggressive behavior. One phenotype has been termed Planned, Instrumental, or Proactive (PIP), and the second is known as Reactive, Affective, Defensive or Impulsive (RADI). These two forms correspond to known differences in the psychobiology of aggression and each most likely responds to very different interventions. PIP is often termed "cold" aggression and corresponds to what most investigators see as an early form of psychopathic aggression. It is remorseless, calculated, and lacking in a moral decision-making structure. Currently, there is a high likelihood that PIP aggression does not exist along a single neuronal architecture, and instead emerges through multiple pathways at multiple sociopsychobiological levels.

Conversely, RADI or "hot" aggression is an emotionally charged form that often is poorly thought out and highly reactive to situational stimuli; this form of aggression is known to have links to serotonin, dopamine, norepinephrine, and GABA systems and to be rooted in neuronal architecture of the limbic system (an activation locus) and the prefrontal cortex (a controlling and shaping locus). RADI aggression is by far the more common form of aggression, and is seen in multiple contexts. Children with RADI aggression often commit acts of unplanned and poorly considered aggression, and will often show remorse for their acts afterwards. They are the children who are likely to easily get into fights when they perceive an immediate insult or threat to themselves.

As much as the situation permits, attempts to differentiate these forms of aggression should be undertaken, as this will guide treatment strategies and outcome expectations. It is highly likely that each of these forms of aggression will have different interventions to target the specific nature of the aggression, and given the emerging differentiation of pathways leading to each form of aggression we would expect that different interventions would be necessary.

4.2. *Neurobiological*

There is a substantial literature amassing on the effects of neurobiological factors on the risk of developing aggression and disruptive behaviors. Studies of conduct-disordered youth have implicated several neurotransmitters including serotonin,[40,41] noradrenaline, and dopamine.[74] It is therefore not surprising that there have also been implications concerning several genetic types linked to these neurochemical systems including the monoamine oxidase A (MAO-A)[75] and serotonin transporter genes (5-HTT) through different pathways. Interestingly, Caspi and colleagues have shown that depression tied to early life stress can be a moderated by polymorphisms at the 5-HTT site.[76] More recent studies have shown similar effects on the development of depression in children who have histories of maltreatment.[77] This has led to the intriguing hypothesis and working model that gene–environment interactions are mutually effect generating and potentially have significant impacts on psychiatric illness.[78]

The neurobiological studies in aggregate support the distinction of PIP and RADI aggression with different pathways being implicated in these two forms of aggression. For RADI it appears that the basic threat circuits often have overactivation of the amygdala, hypothalamus, and periaqueductal gray which link to the medial and orbital frontal cortex regions. In contrast, PIP aggression seems to be linked to cortical circuits tied to more goal-directed behavior and may have a component of underarousal which drives this system.[7,42]

Further understandings of the ways through which children come to act in antisocial and disruptive ways are sure to emerge in coming years from the fields of neuroscience and social cognitive science. For example, research by Bill Greenough's group at Illinois has shown the plasticity of neuronal pathways, and has begun to show the powerful effects that result from social and environmental stimuli.[80]

4.3. *Psychological and educational*

A host of psychological correlates exist for the development of aggression and disruptive behaviors including childhood temperament, learning disabilities, neuropsychological lateralization and localization, and particular personality traits.

Breslau and colleagues have recently found an association between intelligence and being able to have resiliency in the face of traumatic events. She found that children at age six who had intelligence quotients greater than 115 were much less likely to be exposed to either assaultive or non-assaultive violence. These youth also had a decreased risk for the development of PTSD.[81] These findings are especially relevant when we consider the high rates of PTSD and dissociative symptoms in this population.[19,43]

Learning disabilities have been well documented in the delinquent population,[83] most of whom also fulfill criteria for one of the externalizing disruptive behavior disorders. A national survey of juvenile corrections systems has suggested that as many as 38% of the juveniles incarcerated had a specific learning disability.[84] This is compared to estimates that within the non-incarcerated population, the rate of specific learning disabilities is somewhere between 5 and 10%.[85] A portion of the literature examines the link between learning disabilities and psychiatric disorders. Sundheim and Voeller reported that children with language disorders are four times more likely to have externalizing disorders than children without language disorders. It is estimated that between 15 and 20% of children and adolescents with learning disabilities will also have ADHD.[86]

It is increasingly recognized that there is a link between externalizing disorders and learning disabilities, particularly deficits in verbal abilities. Studies have suggested that among children or adolescents diagnosed as having CD, or young adults diagnosed as having personality disorder, approximately one-third have an undiagnosed or poorly treated learning disability.[87] In a study by Baker and Cantwell involving 600 children with language disabilities, 50% received a DSM diagnosis, including: conduct disorder, ADHD, oppositional defiant disorder, affective disorder, or adjustment disorder.[88]

Brier concluded that there is likely a multifactorial explanation; that LD is a risk factor for delinquent behavior, but that other factors come into play as well. He stated that individuals with LD are more likely than non-LD individuals to display several of the language, social perception, and social relationship difficulties that have been found to contribute to the development of antisocial behavior. Important factors contributing include early conduct problems, ADHD, low IQ, parent criminality, alcoholism, parental deficiency, and a lack of motivation to achieve.[89]

In studies by our group, we find that the subtypes of aggression seem to correspond to known psychological adaptive styles.[90] It appears that PIP aggression is characterized by a low degree of self-control and low levels of activation at times. PIP youth seem to show a pattern of habitual underarousal, low self-regulation, and an inability to process emotions well,[44,45] having unusual reactions to emotion expressed through facial characteristics.

In contrast, RADI aggression shows low self-control and high activation or distress. We have also found that adolescents with the RADI type of aggression often have high levels of anxiety and mood symptoms.[82] Youth with RADI aggressive patterns in our studies seem to have difficulty disaggregating the emotional experiences of sadness, anger, and fear especially when faced with stressful experiences.[32] This conflation of emotions seems to be dependent on prior trauma and that some trauma experiences, especially in their severity and number, are more potent than others.

4.4. *Social and environmental*

Three major domains of social experience have been found to impact the development of conduct disorder and antisociality in youth–family, peer, and the neighborhood. Parental criminal behavior is a strong predictor for the development of conduct issues in children. This effect likely has some biological component in that children are likely to share the same stress and anxiety associated genetic polymorphisms MAO-A and 5-HTT with their parents. Nevertheless, the major impact of familial effects likely comes from compromised parenting. There is strong evidence that lack of parenting including absences, poor supervision, and ineffective parenting all lead to increased aggression, impulsivity, and other conduct-related behaviors. Parent–child relations are not the only familial influences that impact children. Divorce, separation, and conflictual relationships are predictive but seem to not have as much impact as parenting style and temperament. Familial effects seem to recede in importance as children pass through puberty.[5]

Peer influences also act to affect the etiology of childhood aggression and disruptive patterns. These influences appear to act late and may be among thc more highly gendered of the effects.[27] Nevertheless, for some youth aggression becomes a way of life through affiliation with gangs and other antisocial groups. Such affiliations often substitute for the protective role that family should play and that for a variety of reasons has not been able to function.

The social context of aggression is undoubtedly important. Socioeconomic status and poverty have both been shown to interact with parenting capabilities and risk factors for the development of childhood aggression. We have been far slower to appreciate the effect of ethnic health disparities as a macrostructural force on the development of childhood psychopathology. Health care disparities for underserved and minority populations are a well-established finding in medical practice and outcomes. The 2003 Institute of Medicine (IOM) report on health disparities noted that there are documented differences in care for cardiovascular illness, cancer, cerebrovascular disease, and mental illness.[93] Despite these general findings, little is understood about the specific causes of disparities or their effects. Documenting the ways that disparities impact the lives of individuals and their communities is one component of the agenda for health disparities research.

In addition to the IOM report, the 2001 supplement to the Surgeon General's report on mental health concluded that despite relatively equal prevalence of psychiatric illness between ethnic groups, minorities continue to experience poorer quality of care and restrictions on access to care. It also found that minority groups are disproportionately represented in vulnerable groups like the homeless and incarcerated, and that these factors contribute to decreased access and care.[94]

Prevalence studies of incarcerated youth have generally found that these youth are at higher risk for psychiatric illness than the general population.[13,46–48] Studies from our group when examining the mental health needs of juveniles in the California Youth Authority in 2001 found continued high rates of psychiatric morbidity even at nine months postincarceration. This has led to concerns being raised about the quality and availability of psychiatric care for children in juvenile justice settings.[98]

Over 90% of the youth met criteria for conduct disorder and 85% met criteria for a substance use disorder. As Table 1 shows, large numbers of these youth have a diagnosable psychiatric disorder and there is a significant amount of comorbidity with most juveniles having three or more diagnoses based on DSM-IV criteria. In addition, over 40% of girls and 20% of boys met criteria for a personality disorder when excluding antisocial personality disorder.[49,50] Other research from our group has found that youth in the juvenile justice system have high rates of PTSD which are often accompanied by dissociative symptoms.[19,43]

The degree to which the results of the study showed strong gender effects was surprising. Most studies of incarcerated or delinquent youth focus on males, and hence little data has been amassed to indicate the degree of morbidity among girls. The CYA study was one of the first major opportunities to report on girls, and the findings found increased rates of psychiatric diagnoses as well as increased morbidity. Girls had double the rates of the anxiety disorder and nearly three times the rates of boy's depressive disorders.

Abram and colleagues found that incarcerated Caucasian youth had higher rates of substance and psychiatric disorders than African-Americans[95] but given the absolute numbers of minority children in prisons, the numbers of ethnic youth may be greater. Data collected on a population of incarcerated youths in the California Youth Authority indicate that wards tend to underutilize mental health services.[98] This is consistent with the general finding of lower lifetime utilization of mental health services among detained youth versus youth receiving community mental health services.[100]

Despite the generally lower levels of self-reported psychopathology,[101] minority youth are more likely to be seen as having aggressive and violent risks and are more likely to face involuntary commitment.[102] Research on general populations of children and adolescents finds that ethnic minorities seek psychiatric services less frequently than their Caucasian counterparts.[103] There is also evidence that suggests that African-American males are treated less frequently for psychiatric disorders.[51,52] African-American children are more likely than equivalently impaired Caucasian peers to enter the juvenile justice system rather than the mental health system.[105] In addition, African-American youth are less likely to receive prescription drugs than Caucasian youth.[106] Specifically, there is a wide racial disparity with psychotropic drug prescriptions. African-American children are 2.5 times less likely to receive methylphenidate than Caucasian children.[107]

Despite these findings, observers often perceive ethnic minorities as possessing more psychopathology than Caucasians. Externalizing behavior is generally thought to be more common in African-American children than Caucasian children.[108] Research has shown that Mexican American boys are more frequently perceived to be "aggressive" and "acting out" than Caucasian boys, while the latter group is frequently described as "neurotic."[109] Studies on attention-deficit and hyperactivity disorder indicate that African-American boys are rated higher on inattention, hyperactivity-impulsivity symptoms, factors reflecting externalizing behavior, and an antisocial factor (including items related to lying, stealing, and destructiveness) than their Caucasian counterparts.[53,54] Such factors can contribute to the development of aggression due to social and environmental forces *via* distorted perceptions and differential expectations.

4.5. *Developmental course*

As noted earlier, aggression is a normative process in early childhood.[55,56] Developmentally, most children have a peek of aggressive behavior around ages 2–3 which corresponds with a period of socialization where children are trying to learn normative patterns of behavior. As children progress through toddlerhood, aggression should gradually deescalate and begin to resolve.

Tremblay and colleagues have described the pathways for maladaptive aggressive children in several of the longest longitudinal studies available.[57–59] They find three major groups of aggressive children out of community samples. The majority of children (over 80%) do not exhibit excessive aggression. Roughly 6% exhibit reactive aggression (or what we term RADI) while about 3.5% present with non-reactive (PIP) aggression, and the final 10% show a combined form with elements of both. They found that the non-reactive pathway is characterized by children with low physiological arousal and a withdrawn temperament.

The parents of these children tend to use reward seeking and modeling, and the resulting children's behavioral patterns tend to emphasize physical aggression. The reactive pathway in contrast has children who tend to be less tentative, more emotionally reactive, active and withdrawn. The parents of these children tend to be aversive and lacking intimacy. The children's behavioral pattern tends to show anxiety and physical aggression.

For a small subset of children, aggression becomes maladaptive and often takes on the characteristics of ODD. Children in this subset will through toddlerhood and young childhood begin to show patterns of vindictive and oppositional behavior. These children will resist authority and show a lack of respect for usual social rules that goes far beyond normal limit testing.

Unchecked, these patterns of behavior can advance to conduct disorder as children enter adolescence and latency. At this point, peer influences enter significantly into the dynamics of these aggressive patterns. It is at this point that the two forms of aggression begin to more clearly differentiate. The current taxonomy in the DSM and the ICD does not capture this bifurcation. This has lead a group of expert researchers, clinicians, and educators (Stanford-Howard Workgroup on Juvenile Impulsivity and Aggression) to propose a new taxonomic spectrum, which is discussed in detail elsewhere[8] and depicted below in Fig. 2. Each one of these spectra shows a continuum from adaptive to maladaptive aggression, culminating in syndromal disorders. In this schema, CD and ODD are separate forerunners of adult psychopathology within each spectrum. Adult forms of hot and cold aggression receive new labels, differentiated by more acute (intermittent explosive disorder; psychopathy) or chronic, lower grade presentations personality disorders. This schema would require a redefinition of labels currently employed in the DSM, or a new definition if not included in the current version.

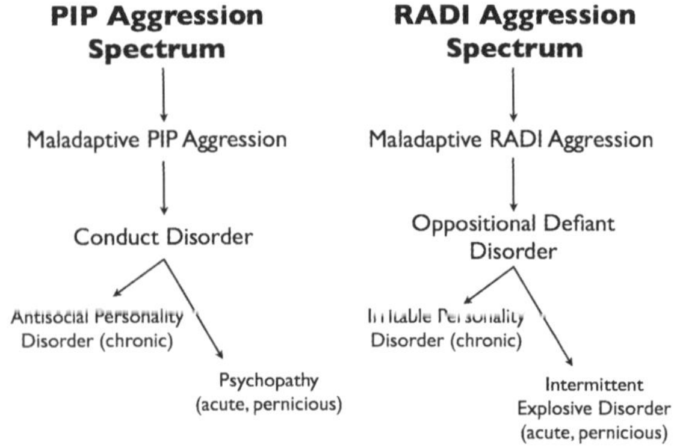

Fig. 2: AACAP/Stanford/Howard Workgroup on Juvenile Impulsivity and Aggression Proposed Taxonomy of Disruptive Behaviors.

The group felt though that such an effort would be worthwhile and lead to taxa that have more immediate implications for research and clinical practice than the existing ones.

RADI or "hot" aggressive children will have periods of reactive aggression to perceived threats from the environment. These children will often have difficulty regulating their emotions and may exhibit significant anxiety as well as elevated states of arousal. Untreated, this form of aggression may advance to a pattern of intermittent explosive disorder in adulthood (Fig. 2).

More problematic in adolescence is the emergence of PIP or "cold" aggression. This form of aggression is characterized as remorseless and calculated in nature. Such children are often seen as "budding" psychopaths whose cruelty toward animals or minor criminal transgressions escalate to violence toward other people. These children are rare but they are nonetheless volatile and have the potential to exact significant social costs by hurting other children and adults, or by committing significant acts of violence. PIP-aggressive youth often have lengthy criminal histories, are difficult to engage in therapeutic interventions, and will likely require long-term structured environments to have any degree of rehabilitative potential.

5. Relevance for Primary Care

Primary care providers will often be the presenting site for problems with aggression in children and adolescents. Pediatricians, general practitioners, family medicine, and other primary care providers will often be the individuals to whom families will arrive seeking advice and treatment. Primary care providers will benefit from the broad understanding of aggression outlined in this chapter. They should always initially assess the youth and families for safety. In the event that there is acute danger or threat from aggression that puts the youth or others at risk then these youth should be immediately referred to a higher level of care with a capability of maintaining security. Screening for the presence of guns and weapons is an important aspect of the primary care evaluation. Assuming that the child or adolescent is safe to remain in the outpatient setting, the primary care provider can certainly give general advice about behavioral strategies for addressing aggression. Should these interventions prove ineffective or insufficient or if the severity of the aggression is complex or significant enough, then the primary care provider should seek consultation and make referrals to mental health professionals who have experience and qualifications to work with children and adolescents. Psychiatric and/or psychological referrals can be an excellent starting point as aggression is a common presenting problem in mental health settings.

6. Interventions and Outcomes[a,b]

When examining interventions for aggression, it is not sufficient to take them all in aggregate and simply say that this or that intervention or program is the way to treat these youth. As with most complex psychiatric illnesses, multimodal approaches are likely to yield the best outcomes.[61,62] It is important to note that the best interventions are multimodal and should intervene at multiple levels simultaneously. Broadly defined, the interventions literature is very large and heterogeneous. That being said, many of the interventions are creative and deserving of attention.

6.1. *Prevention*

Prevention as a strategy requires that providers have knowledge of major clinical issues and public health concerns. Our group actively participates in educational and outreach activities to bring a greater understanding of aggression to families, schools, primary care providers, and mental health professionals. We try explaining, in audience appropriate ways, how these groups might conceptualize and engage with violence prevention in their own communities as well as methods for addressing aggression. We also try to encourage all of these constituents to consider how our emerging understanding of aggression can help change their practices.

The evidence base for such initiatives is limited but some reports are prescient. In this regard, Runyan and colleagues describe one such intervention program created as part of the US National Training Initiation in Injury and Violence Prevention called PREVENT (Preventing Violence Through Education, Networking and Technical Assistance).[116] While the focus of the training is quite broad, the advantage that it offers is a systemized way for educating professionals about the empiric approaches to violence and provides a framework for understanding the nature of violence within a social-ecological model. Such education is a necessary part of creating systems of care and for prevention of the development of environments from which young offenders are likely to emerge.

Among the various levels of intervention for young offenders, primary prevention has had the least number of studies largely due to the need for long follow-up intervals and large sample sizes. The AACAP/Stanford/Howard Workgroup on Juvenile Impulsivity and Aggression identified five programs that

---

[a,b] Portions of this section on treatment and interventions were published previously as 60. Karnik NS, Steiner H. Evidence for interventions for young offenders, *Child Adolesc Mental Health.* 2007. These sections are reproduced here with permission.

have empirically validated outcomes data.[9] The notable findings for these interventions are that they all had some degree of decreased arrest, delinquency, and aggression in multiyear follow-up, one as far out as 27 years from the intervention. Only one study of the five found no difference from controls at 10-year follow-up. All of these interventions targeted very young children, most under age 4, and only the Chicago Child–Parent Center for under age 9.[63–65] All of these programs utilized a combination of family and education services and supports as well as parent skills training on a daily or weekly basis. In many respects, we could class the majority of these interventions under the rubric of family interventions since that is the unit of intervention, and the focus is on high-risk children.

6.2. *Social and community*

Interventions at the community and social level have shown some degree of success and are among the most novel and creative areas for further research. This area which we have termed "sociotherapy" marks a major focus on the social and contextual environment around young offenders.[61,66]

Callaghan and colleagues used qualitative research methods to track the mental health interventions of two Young Offender Teams (YOTs) in the United Kingdom.[121] The teams were constituted of representatives of the various agencies involved in addressing young offenders including police, educational, psychological, medical, and judicial branches of the government. By combining these separate institutions into one team, the participants generally found that they were able to overcome their disciplinary view of the child and instead focus on the best intervention strategies available using the resources of their various agencies more effectively. Such approaches are increasingly necessary in addressing the needs of young offenders especially in systems with large multifaceted bureaucracies which can at times work against one another instead of focusing on the needs of the child.

Yet another important avenue for further research and interventions lies in gang prevention programs. Programs like the Gang Violence Prevention Project in Chicago utilize a combination of community mobilization and outreach to youth to help prevent the aggregation of maladaptive and antisocial patterns.[122] Such interventions are time consuming and often require large-scale programs to support them. Nevertheless, the advantage of these programs is that they make use of multiple stakeholders as done with the YOTs in the United Kingdom.

6.3. *Family*

In our clinic, we favor parent management training (PMT) for the treatment of aggression and most especially to help them understand how to address ODD.[67,68]

This approach emphasizes educational techniques to help parents understand their child's aggression and uses behavioral modification strategies to reduce the child's aggression. In essence, this is a means for introducing evidence-based parenting strategies to families that may have maladaptive patterns.

A significant number of studies have targeted the family as the unit of intervention. Among the most established methods for family intervention is termed Multisystemic Treatment (MST). This form of treatment utilizes a high-intensity case management approach with specially trained therapists following small numbers of families and having a high degree of availability. Therapists work toward empowering the family and drawing in collateral support from other family members, friends, and community members over several months. Borduin and colleagues have conducted a series of studies on this method in the treatment of young offenders.[69–71] In their long-term follow-up study of 176 youths who were on average over 10 years out from the intervention they found substantially lower rates of recidivism, arrests, and days of confinement. Despite these generally positive results, Littell and colleagues, who conducted a detailed metaanalysis, were unable to establish conclusively that MST was advantageous to standard treatment.[128]

Another intervention at the family level is Multidimensional Treatment Foster Care (MTFC) which uses an intensive model of foster care to in one sense reparent and resocialize young offenders. The program relies on having foster parents who follow a highly structured approach to monitoring and rewarding behaviors from the young offender. The children and their families participate in individual and family therapy during the program, and also have intensive case management. Foster parents receive additional support through group meetings and program support.[72–76] Such approaches are especially useful when the custodial parents of the child are especially impaired, and perhaps poor candidates for MST or PMT. The availability of these major modalities for treatment at the family level constitutes good empirically based arms of intervention at this level.

6.4. *Individual*

Among all the therapies we have outlined and levels of care we have identified, the research on individual modalities remains the weakest and least clearly explicated. We believe that this is the result of the fact that young offenders are embedded in powerful social and family networks, and that these forces are ecologically salient and prevent any single individual-level intervention from yielding a robust result. Nevertheless, in our experience, individual therapy combined judiciously with the use of medications when indicated for comorbid psychiatric conditions can lead to reducing triggers in the environment for young offenders.[43,62,77]

The aggregate data on juvenile aggression and conduct disorder indicates that there are two major pathways to delinquency, both of which appear to be differentiated at the neural level.[7] Our current focus seems to implicate the amygdala, orbitofrontal cortex, and frontal cortex regions as exhibiting changes that correspond to maladaptive aggression. Such changes are the first steps in understanding the neurobiology of aggression, and as our tools improve we are likely to gain more specificity in targeting regions. It should be emphasized that our understanding of this biology does not yet indicate a causal source or etiology. It is likely that some individuals have a genetic risk, but as with most psychiatric disorders, this risk only becomes expressed in relation to certain environmental stimuli and stressors. In the case of young offenders, it is important to be mindful of the high rates of trauma exposure at very young ages that have the potential to affect neuronal development. It is also unclear whether these changes are reversible over time with targeted treatments and interventions.

Our approach to these youths is defined by the predominance of symptoms in one or the other aggressive pathway.[78,79] We believe that RADI youth often benefit from psychopharmacological and psychotherapeutic strategies that reduce their impulsivity, anxiety, and reactivity.[137] We know that these children often have high levels of PTSD.[17,18,43] and we theorize that this combined with mood and anxiety symptoms place these children in a high state of activation which potentially leads them to be overly responsive to their environment and aggressively reactive to perceived threats.[138] Preliminary studies from our group show that some youth with PTSD and conduct disorder may respond to divalproex sodium to help reduce their symptoms.[48]

With PIP youth, our approach emphasizes the development of moral reasoning and emotional skills development. These are the youth who likely need long-term and concerted systems of care to prevent them from becoming the most problematic and recalcitrant adult offenders. Some of these children will benefit more substantively from highly structured environments and possible residential care which utilizes the therapeutic perspectives we have outlined. Structured environments can create circumstances where these youth can be positively encouraged to develop a better reasoning system but also enables providers to address with consequences instances of proactive aggression when they arise.

From a psychotherapeutic perspective it is still unclear which therapeutic modalities are likely to be beneficial to young offenders in either pathway, especially when the subtyping of aggression is taken into account. The interventions literature shows some benefit from anger management programs.[77,80,81]

6.5. *Psychopharmacology*

The psychopharmacology of aggression is a complex field but one which can yield substantial benefits for children and adolescents. As described earlier, one of the key steps in evaluating a child for treatment is to determine the subtype of aggression that is taking place (PIP versus RADI). Along with this is a determination of whether the aggression is acute or chronic. In the context of acute aggression, consideration may need to be given as to whether hospitalization is needed to secure the child from harming himself or herself, and harming others. In the acute context, medications can be used to reduce aggression. Common medication formulas used with the inpatient setting might include haloperidol, ativan, and benedryl in combination given intramuscularly or intravascularly to speed delivery and effect. There are now intramuscular preparations of olanzapine and ziprasidone which can also be used to address immediate and threatening aggression or violence. These products should be used only in settings where, if needed, continuous medical monitoring such as electrocardiographic, respiratory, and blood pressure can be done. While generally considered safe, the rapid delivery of these medications at high doses to address violent or aggressive behaviors can lead to complications such as acute dystonia, neuroleptic malignant syndrome, or QTc prolongation which may need medical support to monitor and address.

In the outpatient sphere, acute aggression may take the form of a child who has been acting out more substantially for the past several days due to a limited social stressor. In these situations, behavioral and social interventions would likely take precedence over pharmacologic ones, but in the event that the clinician feels it is necessary to use an agent to break the immediate cycle of aggression either atypical antipsychotics or benzodiazepines, used judiciously, might be considered.

A more typical pathway has parents or caretakers reporting chronic aggressive behavior. In these instances understanding the roots of this aggression becomes more central. If the aggression is taking place in the context of another diagnosis then treating this diagnosis becomes the first-line treatment for the aggression. For example, in the case of a young child who has depression, they may present with significant oppositionality, sleep disturbance, and aggression. This child, who used to be very cooperative and kind, now appears mean spirited and targets his siblings with significant aggression when things do not go his way. He also acts out against his parents at times. The approach to this child should be to address the depression that may involve pharmacological strategies. An antidepressant like fluoxetine that successfully addresses the underlying depression should also bring resolution to the aggressive symptoms.

One of the subfields that has produced a great deal of research on aggression and comorbid conditions is in treating youth with mental retardation (MR).[141]

Atypical antipsychotics like risperidone and olanzapine have been shown to be effective in treating disruptive youth who have MR with moderate to good response rates and effect sizes.[82–86] Similarly, both methylphenidate and sodium valproate have been shown to be effect in treating children with comorbid MR and disruptive behavior disorders.[87,88]

Some medications have already shown benefits as demonstrated in the response of children to treatment with divalproex sodium for aggression using the modified overt aggression scale as the measure. Overall aggression decreased significantly ($p < 0.05$), as well as verbal aggression ($p < 0.01$), irritability ($p < 0.01$), and assualtiveness against others ($p < 0.01$). Such studies show to key points. First, they point to the responsiveness and utility of using pharmacological agents as one element of an integrated treatment plan to stabilize behavior and allow new modes of behavioral and social intervention to take hold for the family and child. Second, these pharmacological studies may give us a hint of the neurobiological systems that can become imbalanced by understanding the receptor activities of the various compounds that are effective in reducing aggression and violent behavior. There are now wide arrays of compounds and agents that can be used to treat aggression, and guidelines have been published to assist clinicians in making prudent choices.

Among the most comprehensive reviews available is the Treatment Recommendations for the Use of Antipsychotics for Aggressive Youth (TRAAY).[89,90] TRAAY provides 14 recommendations on how to treat acute and chronic aggression, and gives an algorithm on how the clinician can make choices when using these medications. The recommendations advise clinicians to conduct a thorough diagnostic evaluation and begin psychosocial, education, and/or crisis interventions as the first step. They then urge clinicians to use appropriate pharmacological interventions for primary disorders that may be causing the aggression before moving to antipsychotics for the aggression. When starting antipsychotics, TRAAY advises clinicians to start with low doses and increase doses slowly. While ensuring an adequate trial clinicians need to monitor for side effects, and try to avoid using multiple medications. Should one medication fail, they urge clinicians to taper it and then start another while continuing to monitor the aggression and continue the non-pharmacological strategies.

Pharmacologically, we believe that RADI youth have the potential to benefit from medications when they are used as part of an integrated treatment strategy that includes individual and family therapy. We have extensively reviewed this topic and will not enumerate all the specific agents here.[137] Two classes of medication do deserve mention here because of their recent and emerging data. Our research indicates that anticonvulsants[91–94] and atypical antipsychotics[89,90,95] appear to show early efficacy and potential for helping RADI youth to gain better control of their behaviors. Consensus guidelines exist for the use of these agents in the treatment of aggression and conduct disorder.[89,96,97]

Since a review by our group of medication interventions for young offenders was published,[137] two new studies have emerged which deserve brief mention in order to update the current research base on the use of medications. Several studies examine the role of medications in the treatment of aggression as a comorbid factor to illnesses, such as bipolar affective disorder or mental retardation. Very few studies have examined aggression in the context of primary conduct disorder. Findling and colleagues have continued to research the uses of atypical antipsychotics for the treatment of aggression in children. In their most recent set of studies, they find that quetiapine is well tolerated and efficacious at moderate doses for children.[98,99]

As an example of pharmacotherapy in this population, the response of incarcerated juveniles, subtyped by PIP or RADI, was examined after treatment with low-or high-dose divalproex sodium.[94,100] PIP aggression failed to respond to either condition while RADI aggression had almost no response or a potentially negative response in terms of worsening self-restraint in the low-dose condition but at therapeutic doses these same youth had marked reduction in activation and increases in self-restraint.

7. Practice

Our clinic is a typical tertiary care clinic which receives new referrals as well as referrals for consultation from with our system and community. A special feature of our clinic is the close cooperation we have with community agencies, such as high-risk alternative schools, county juvenile justice settings, state juvenile justice detention, and screening facilities, and government task forces that are charged with improving the care services for youth. We are also active in providing forensic consultation in selected cases and regularly receive youth for evaluation from family court.

We evaluate and treat patients across the entire life span, although most of our patients are in the adolescent or young adult range. There is a preponderance of males (65%) but we have a substantial number of females. Individuals usually receive a carefully assembled package of psychometric tests, a clinical interview, and collateral contacts with family, schools, and forensic entities. Typical evaluations take between 1 and 4 diagnostic and testing sessions, and findings are presented to the patient and family in a separate session. Forensic authorities and schools are included as appropriate. Follow-up is usually coordinated with semistructured and structured settings and primary care physicians. The following cases may give a typical flavor of our practices.

Johnny is a 13-year-old boy who was observed by his grandmother sexually fondling his younger sister. Following this event and in the course of a child protective services investigation, he was hospitalized due to his report that he was hearing command auditory hallucinations telling him to hurt himself and others. After his hospitalization, he was transferred to a local children's shelter with diagnoses of psychosis disorder, not otherwise specified and impulsive disorder, not otherwise specified. At this point, the supervising social worker in consultation with the grandmother determined that Johnny should be removed from the house and placed in a group home due to concerns about the safety of the other children in the household, and grandmother's inability to continue to care for Johnny with a pattern of escalating behavior including fire starting, anger, fighting, and both verbally and physically threatening behavior prior to the event with his sister.

One day after being transferred to the group home, Johnny reported to the staff that he was angry, frustrated, and having thoughts of harming himself and others. He proceeded to scratch his arm and wrist, and endorsed suicidal thoughts. He was readmitted to the hospital. During this hospitalization, he was started on escitalopram for depression, dysphoric mood, and intermittent suicidal ideation.

This young man presents with a constellation of behaviors consistent with a diagnosis of disruptive behavior disorder, not otherwise specified, and comorbid major depression. He has symptoms of reactive aggression, difficulty controlling his temper, fire starting, difficulty with authority, and sexual aggressiveness. He does not appear to have a primary psychosis or schizophrenia.

Johnny has several positive characteristics and traits. He cares deeply for his siblings and most especially his younger brother. He was noted by his grandmother and social worker to have a generous spirit. During our examination we found him to be friendly and open, and he continues to have an ability to form relationships with people around him. When in emotional control, he shows good humor and spirit.

His symptoms appear to have started after his removal into foster care with subsequent placement with grandmother and he appears to have weathered this transition more poorly than his siblings. He perceives the situation as one in which his older brother already had a solid relationship with their grandmother. Johnny feels that there was a degree of favoritism present in the household, although this appears more likely to be the result of degrees of comfort that his older brother had with their grandmother. The other four siblings were forced to adjust not only to the loss of the removal from their parent's lives but also to a new setting. Since this shift, Johnny has had significant disputes with his grandmother and appears to have been unable to bring his behavior under control.

When questioned about past sexual or physical trauma, Johnny refused to answer questions. Collateral information gathered from his grandmother and court documents indicates that there is a high potential that Johnny was abused at an early point in his life; likely when he was living with his biological mother. The root of his behavior toward his sister likely resides, in part, with his diagnosis of disruptive behavior disorder but may also have more complex connections to a past history of sexual and/or physical abuse that Johnny likely experienced.

Johnny's testing showed high degrees of distress and low restraint, He displayed greater than average acting out, passive aggression, withdrawal, dissociation, omnipotence, sublimation, denial, and suppression. Our studies also showed that he had a very high level of anger and frustration, as well as guilt over what he has done and the situation that he now finds himself in. These characteristics are consistent with a reactive aggressive pattern. Also, troubling was his high degree of depression with elevated levels of suicidal ideation.

Due to the need for individual and community safety, adolescents with these symptoms require a high level of care. It would benefit Johnny to continue in individual psychotherapy, with a target of helping him to understand the ways that his behaviors manifest and trying to give him methods for coping with his anger and frustration. We have found that cognitive behavioral therapeutic techniques work well for children like Johnny.

Pharmacologically, escitalopram was a good choice due to its antidepressant qualities and potential to address the underlying depression that may have been driving the disruptive patterns. Given that the aggressive behaviors continued despite some resolution of the depressive symptoms, consideration could next be given to adding an agent specifically for aggression. We advised a trial of divalproex to address the reactive aggression that he displayed, and should he show good stability on this mood stabilizer, then the escitalopram could be discontinued.

We advised that Johnny should be continued in a residential treatment program due to his suicidal ideation and risk for harm to himself or others. We also thought it is prudent to expand contact with his father. Johnny and his grandmother both noted that Johnny has always relied on his father, and should he be able to demonstrate that he is a positive influence then Johnny might benefit therapeutically. We also advised that it would be prudent to involve the father in some type of family therapy at a later point. Should the father be unavailable, then he may benefit from contact with a child advocate with whom he could form a long-term relationship.

It seemed clear to us that Johnny's situation worsened with contact with his mother. It appears that both prior to his removal to foster care and following, each contact with his mother lead to subsequent disruption and strife in the household. Johnny's grandmother noted that his mother often took him on the streets prior to his removal to foster care, and this exposure to drugs and violence likely hurt Johnny and may have led to many of his present behaviors.

Educationally, he has an ability to focus on tasks when in emotional control. Due to the number of schools Johnny has attended, it was difficult to get an accurate impression of the degree to which his psychiatric issues may be impacting his educational performance. While at the residential treatment center, assuming pursued a dedicated educational plan. We found no evidence of learning or physical disability. Due to his prolonged period of depression, Johnny met the criteria for educational disability, and obtained special education services which helped to support his overall rehabilitation and treatment.

Through a combination of social service interventions, pharmacology, individual therapy, and family therapy, Johnny was able to come to terms with his past trauma including the sexual abuse he suffered at the hands of one of his mother's drug dealers. He later went to live with his father and has made good strides in trying to rebuild relationships with his siblings and grandmother, all of whom have been open to his return to the family. His school performance has gradually improved over a 2-year period and he is now performing at grade level after years of being behind. His prognosis for continued stability is quite good.

The following case of a 14-year-old girl, Jane, may serve as a good example from our female population. Her mother, who worked as a nurse, referred Jane for care. The girl had been in several fights at school (all without weapons) that had led to the threat of expulsion from her middle school. The family had recently moved to the San Francisco Bay Area because of the father's job as a manager at a large retailer. This was the seventh move for the family since Jane was born. Jane has five younger siblings who have all done well in school. There was a family history of depression in both parents and unspecified anxiety disorder without treatment in one of the younger brothers.

The girl arrived with the following array of diagnoses; conduct disorder, bipolar disorder, ADHD, learning disability (reading subtype), separation anxiety disorder, social phobia, and rule out substance abuse. She was treated with methylphenidate, quetiapine, risperidone, lithium, gabapentin, escitalopram, and alprazolam; all at suboptimal doses and without much compliance due to the dosing requirements.

There was little question that her aggression was quite maladaptive. Her outbursts were almost always following provocation of one sort or another, and usually involved bullying with sexual references by boys around her. She was an attractive mid-pubescent girl who denied any sexual activity, contact, or desire largely due to her family being of strict Catholic origin.

In analyzing her patterns of aggression, it became rapidly clear that they were almost always at school and involved other boys and sometimes girls. The triggers were invariably after some derogatory comment regarding Jane's moral character.

She would respond with a wrestling attack that was usually weakly resisted by the victims and seemed to be openly enjoyed by many. The patient herself was not aware of the sexual undertones of the provoked assaults. All of her previous evaluations had never explored the character of the aggression. The girl had been examined cursorily and medications were prescribed rapidly. When the mother reported a lack of efficacy, more medications were added or others introduced.

In a careful developmental timeline, it is clear that this was a temperamentally difficult child from a very early age with significant separation problems in kindergarten. As these problems subsided, her mood worsened and she entered a precocious puberty. She never fulfilled criteria for depression or bipolar disorder and best as could be ascertained, her problems were driven by being the object of bullying and provocation.

We simplified her medication regimen to divalproex and escitalopram, and then optimized the dose. The main intervention was with the family and the schools to find a way to stop the provocations. The school proved to be less than effective or helpful, and the family chose to move Jane to a smaller private school campus which met her educational needs better.

Six years later, the patient is off all medications. She wants to remain so because she aspires to a career in law enforcement. She has graduated from college and is enrolled in a police academy for training. She is particularly interested in providing services to young women from diverse and challenging backgrounds so that they can become effective at handling themselves. She has also achieved the rank of black belt in karate.

Our patients are usually quite challenging and require a carefully assembled team to fulfill all their needs. Overall, more than half of our patients recover and go on to lead healthy and productive lives. Many of them need the support and help offered in semistructured and structured settings to get them started, but the mainstay of their longer-term treatments are individual and family sessions along with judicious and targeted psychopharmacology.

8. The Next Five Years

Aggression and disruptive behavior research has come a significant distance in part due to recent advances in the neurosciences more generally. It is clear that the RADI aggression is rooted in dysregulation of the threat detection systems of the brain and at times its overresponsiveness. The neuroscience of PIP is beginning to be understood in adults but it is much less well defined in children. In children, there are likely competing neuropsychological circuits that are developmentally emergent during childhood, including empathy and response reversal, that play a key role in the development of control mechanisms that reduce aggression.

In order to understand the nature of PIP and RADI in children, there is a great need for taxanomic and epidemiologic work using these new labels. To some extent all the prior studies available are now obsolete because they fail to distinguish these two essential subgroups under the broad labels of ODD, CD, and aggression. These prior studies give us the broad contours of how aggression emerges, but only by subtyping can we see the degree to which different pathways underpin these final pathways and then develop treatment strategies that are appropriate to each type. The assumption would be that the "hot" RADI aggression responds to medication, while "cold" PIP aggression requires more structured approaches. We need to be careful in making these jumps because in the ADHD literature we know that both overt and covert aggression respond to some extent to medication.[160]

We also know that present studies of aggression likely overestimate the treatment effects size of medications due to the settings in which the studies are conducted. In our recent study of the effects of divalproex sodium in a community sample as compared to our prior work among incarcerated youth, we find a much lower response rate to medications.[161] We theorize that this is the case because most children in outpatient studies lack the significant structured treatments that are inherent within incarcerative and inpatient settings. Such studies present the challenging notion that we may be underestimating the effects of the various sociotherapies.[162]

Sociotherapies are not universally efficacious and must be structured with care to what is currently known about the structure of programs. Lipsey, in a 1992 metaanalysis of interventions for delinquency, found that community-based interventions tied to schools and other community elements worked better than other levels of interventions. He also found behaviorally focused and highly structured approaches generally did better than traditional case management and counseling.[163] Such findings suggest that inpatient settings, while providing a high degree of structure, may not provide the lasting benefits that community-based interventions can provide. In our future research protocols, we must begin to better measure the sociotherapeutic effects especially in the context of medication and other biological interventions lest we ascribe too much effect to medications.

After we rework our understandings of the effects of subtypes of aggression, and begin to better account for the effect of sociotherapies, then we need to reexamine our approach to diagnosis and treatment pathways. In this regard, it is especially important for us to collaborate with our colleagues in forensics to update the knowledge base for interventions, rehabilitation, and jurisprudence. These revised models will place new questions forward about the degree to which children can exercise free will and the extent to which they can be responsible for their own actions. Such questions have already emerged and had some effect on changing the ways that we consider aggression ad violence committed by youth. The neurobiological understanding of the adolescent mind helped to influence the US Supreme Court to bar the death penalty for those under the age of 18 in *Roper v. Simmons.*[164]

Finally, we are faced with a growing problem of disparate care faced by millions of youth. Increasingly those who have resources can access care and those who do not find their choices limited. This had held to a broad realization that disparities are a large and growing concern across multiple fields of medicine and health care.[93] Among these areas, mental health care disparities are particularly striking,[94] especially when trying to understand the pathways related to juvenile aggression. In this realm, the implications for youth are significant. Those youth who present with disruptive patterns at an early age who then get early access to care are likely to have continued follow-up with the medical and mental health care systems, which can support families and their children to move toward more positive outcomes. This is especially true when we incorporate the developmental understandings of aggression outlined in this chapter.

Conversely, when individuals who exhibit these same behaviors at an early age do not have access to care, we can expect that their problems will worsen. Aggression on the part of the child is likely to escalate, and with it family stress will also increase. As we have outlined these cycles of worsening behavior and increase family stress, unchecked, will feed one another. Without outside support, many of these children and families will likely encounter the police or justice system as the children begin to exhibit aggressive and disruptive patterns across multiple contexts of school and community, but by then the momentum generated over years of maladaptive behaviors become more entrenched and difficult to undo. When seen in this light, addressing health care disparities and access to care becomes a key component to addressing aggression, disruptive, and antisocial behaviors.

References

1. Six-year-old's arrest triggers controversy. 2007; Local television news website. Available at: http://www.baynews9.com/content/36/2007/3/30/235384.html. Accessed on April 4, 2007.
2. Briggs-Gowan MJ, Horwitz SM, Schwab-Stone ME, Leventhal JM, Leaf PJ. Mental health in pediatric settings: Distribution of disorders and factors related to service use, *J Am Acad Child Adolesc Psychiatry* 2000; **39**(7): 841–849.
3. Dulcan MK, Costello EJ, Costello AJ, Edelbrock C, Brent D, Janiszewski S. The pediatrician as gatekeeper to mental health care for children: Do parents' concerns open the gate? *J Am Acad Child Adolesc Psychiatry* 1990; **29**(3): 453–458.

4. Horwitz SM, Leaf PJ, Leventhal JM. Identification of psychosocial problems in pediatric primary care: Do family attitudes make a difference? *Arch Pediatr Adolesc Med* 1998; **152**(4): 367–371.
5. Steiner H, Remsing L. Practice parameter for the assessment and treatment of children and adolescents with oppositional defiant disorder, *J Am Acad Child Adolesc Psychiatry* 2007; **46**(1): 126–141.
6. Huffine CW. Conduct disorder should be eliminated from the diagnostic and statistical manual of mental disorders, *Adolescent Psychiatry* 2002; **26**: 215.
7. Blair RJ, Karnik NS, Coccaro EF, Steiner H. Taxonomy and neurobiology of aggression. In: Ash P, Benedek E, Scott C, Eds. *Principles and Practices of Child and Adolescent Forensic Mental Health*. Washington, DC: American Psychiatric Publishing, Inc., 2009.
8. Connor DF. *Aggression and Antisocial Behavior in Children and Adolescents: Research and Treatment*. New York: Guilford Press, 2002.
9. Hughes CW, Emslie GJ, Crismon ML, *et al.* Texas children's medication algorithm project: Update from Texas consensus conference panel on medication treatment of childhood major depressive disorder, *J Am Acad Child Adolesc Psychiatry* 2007; **46**(6): 667–686.
10. Pardini DA, Loeber R. Interpersonal and affective features of psychopathy in children and adolescents: Advancing a developmental perspective introduction to special section, *J Clin Child Adolesc Psychol* 2007; **36**(3): 269–275.
11. McBurnett K, Raine A, Stouthamer-Loeber M, *et al.* Mood and hormone responses to psychological challenge in adolescent males with conduct problems, *Biol Psychiatry* 2005; **57**(10): 1109–1116.
12. Beyers JM, Loeber R. Untangling developmental relations between depressed mood and delinquency in male adolescents, *J Abnorm Child Psychol* 2003; **31**(3): 247–266.
13. Teplin LA, Abram KM, McClelland GM, Dulcan MK, Mericle AA. Psychiatric disorders in youth in juvenile detention, *Arch Gen Psychiatry* 2002; **59**(12): 1133–1143.
14. Vermeiren R, De Clippele A, Deboutte D. A descriptive survey of Flemish delinquent adolescents, *J Adolesc* 2000; **23**(3): 277–285.
15. Wasserman GA, McReynolds LS, Fisher P, Lucas C. Psychiatric disorders in incarcerated youths, *J Am Acad Child Adolesc Psychiatry* 2003; **42**(9): 1011.
16. Koopman C, Carrion V, Butler LD, Sudhakar S, Palmer L, Steiner H. Relationships of dissociation and childhood abuse and neglect with heart rate in delinquent adolescents, *J Traumatic Stress* 2004; **17**(1): 47–54.
17. Carrion VG, Steiner H. Trauma and dissociation in delinquent adolescents, *J Am Acad Child Adolesc Psychiatry* 2000; **39**(3): 353–359.
18. Plattner B, Silvermann MA, Redlich AD, *et al.* Pathways to dissociation: Intrafamilial versus extrafamilial trauma in juvenile delinquents, *J Nerv Ment Dis* 2003; **191**(12): 781–788.

19. Steiner H, Carrion V, Plattner B, Koopman C. Dissociative symptoms in post-traumatic stress disorder: Diagnosis and treatment, *Child Adolesc Psychiatr Clin N Am* 2003; **12**(2): 231–249, viii.
20. Cohen JA. Treating traumatized children: Current status and future directions, *J Trauma Dissociation* 2005; **6**(2): 109–121.
21. Cohen JA, Mannarino AP, Zhitova AC, Capone ME. Treating child abuse-related post-traumatic stress and comorbid substance abuse in adolescents. *Child Abuse & Neglect* 2003; **27**(12): 1345–1365.
22. Steiner H, Saxena KS, Carrion V, Khanzode LA, Silverman M, Chang K. Divalproex sodium for the treatment of PTSD and conduct disordered youth: A pilot randomized controlled clinical trial, *Child Psychiatry Hum Dev* 2007; **38**(3): 183–193.
23. Wilson JJ, Karnik NS, Haapanen R, Redlich AD, Plattner B, Steiner H. Substance dependence and psychopathology among incarcerated adolescents. Forthcoming.
24. Wilson JJ, Rojas N, Haapanen R, Duxbury E, Steiner H. Substance abuse and criminal recidivism: A prospective study of adolescents, *Child Psychiatry Hum Dev* 2001; **31**(4): 297–312.
25. McDougall J, King G, de Wit DJ, *et al.* Chronic physical health conditions and disability among Canadian school-aged children: A national profile, *Disabil Rehabil* 2004; **26**(1): 35–45.
26. Cadman D, Boyle M, Offord DR. The Ontario Child Health Study: Social adjustment and mental health of siblings of children with chronic health problems, *J Dev Behav Pediatr* 1988; **9**(3): 117–121.
27. Cadman D, Boyle M, Szatmari P, Offord DR. Chronic illness, disability, and mental and social well-being: Findings of the Ontario Child Health Study, *Pediatrics* 1987; **79**(5): 805–813.
28. Lewis DO, Pincus JH. Epilepsy and violence: Evidence for a neuropsychotic-aggressive syndrome, *J Neuropsychiatry Clin Neurosci* Fall 1989; **1**(4): 413–418.
29. Lewis DO, Pincus JH, Bard B, *et al.* Neuropsychiatric, psychoeducational, and family characteristics of 14 juveniles condemned to death in the United States, *Am J Psychiatry* 1988; **145**(5): 584–589.
30. Lewis DO. Neuropsychiatric vulnerabilities and violent juvenile delinquency, *Psychiatr Clin North Am* 1983; **6**(4): 707–714.
31. Yeager CA, Lewis DO. Mental illness, neuropsychologic deficits, child abuse, and violence, *Child Adolesc Psychiatr Clin N Am* 2000; **9**(4): 793–813.
32. Messerlian C, Derevensky J, Gupta R. Youth gambling problems: A public health perspective, *Health Promot Int* 2005; **20**(1): 69–79.
33. Turchi RM, Derevensky JL. Youth gambling: Not a safe bet, *Curr Opin Pediatr* 2006; **18**(4): 454–458.

34. MacKay S, Henderson J, Del Bove G, Marton P, Warling D, Root C. Fire interest and antisociality as risk factors in the severity and persistence of juvenile firesetting, *J Am Acad Child Adolesc Psychiatry* 2006; **45**(9): 1077–1084.
35. Dadds MR, Fraser JA. Fire interest, fire setting and psychopathology in Australian children: A normative study, *Aust N Z J Psychiatry* 2006; **40**(6–7): 581–586.
36. Chen YH, Arria AM, Anthony JC. Firesetting in adolescence and being aggressive, shy, and rejected by peers: New epidemiologic evidence from a national sample survey, *J Am Acad Psychiatry Law* 2003; **31**(1): 44–52.
37. Kolko DJ, Day BT, Bridge JA, Kazdin AE. Two-year prediction of children's firesetting in clinically referred and nonreferred samples, *J Child Psychol Psychiatry* 2001; **42**(3): 371–380.
38. Tracy DL, Karnik NS, Soller MV, Haapanen R, Blair RJ, Steiner H. Impact of personality disorders on psychopathological variables in incarcerated delinquents. Paper presented at the Annual Meeting of the American Academy of Child & Adolescent Psychiatry 2006; San Diego, California.
39. Tracy DL, Karnik NS, Soller MV, Haapanen R, Steiner H. Personality disorders in incarcerated delinquents: Results of a structured interview study (SID-P). Paper presented at the American Psychiatric Association Annual Meeting 2006; Toronto, Canada.
40. Lee R, Coccaro E. The neuropsychopharmacology of criminality and aggression, *Can J Psychiatry* 2001; **46**(1): 35–44.
41. Swann AC. Neuroreceptor mechanisms of aggression and its treatment, *J Clin Psychiatry* 2003; **64**(Suppl. 4): 26–35.
42. Blair RJ. The roles of orbital frontal cortex in the modulation of antisocial behavior, *Brain Cogn* 2004; **55**(1): 198–208.
43. Steiner H, Garcia IG, Matthews Z. Post-traumatic stress disorder in incarcerated juvenile delinquents, *J Am Acad Child Adolesc Psychiatry* 1997; **36**(3): 357–365.
44. Blair RJ. Applying a cognitive neuroscience perspective to the disorder of psychopathy, *Dev Psychopathol* Summer 2005; **17**(3): 865–891.
45. Blair RJ. Responding to the emotions of others: Dissociating forms of empathy through the study of typical and psychiatric populations, *Consciousness Cognition* 2005; **14**(4): 698–718.
46. Abram KM, Teplin LA, McClelland GM, Dulcan MK. Comorbid psychiatric disorders in youth in juvenile detention, *Arch Gen Psychiatry* 2003; **60**(11): 1097–1108.
47. Domalanta DD, Risser WL, Roberts RE, Risser JM. Prevalence of depression and other psychiatric disorders among incarcerated youths, *J Am Acad Child Adolesc Psychiatry* 2003; **42**(4): 477–484.
48. Wasserman GA, McReynolds LS, Lucas CP, Fisher P, Santos L. The voice DISC-IV with incarcerated male youths: Prevalence of disorder, *J Am Acad Child Adolesc Psychiatry* 2002; **41**(3): 314–321.

49. Steiner H, Humphreys K, Redlich A, Silverman M, Campanaro A. *The Assessment of the Mental Health System of the California Youth Authority: Report to Governor Gray Davis.* Palo Alto: Stanford University School of Medicine, December 31, 2001.
50. Steiner H, Redlich A. Child psychiatry and juvenile justice. In: Lewis M, Ed. *Child Psychiatry.* New York: Williams & Wilkins, 2002, pp. 1417–1425.
51. Cuffe SP, Waller JL, Cuccaro ML, Pumariega AJ, Garrison CZ. Race and gender differences in the treatment of psychiatric disorders in young adolescents, *J Am Acad Child Adolesc Psychiatry* 1995; **34**(11): 1536–1543.
52. Lewis DO, Balla DA, Shanok SS. Some evidence of race bias in the diagnosis and treatment of the juvenile offender, *Am J Orthopsychiatry* 1979; **49**(1): 53–61.
53. Epstein JN, March JS, Conners CK, Jackson DL. Racial differences on the Conners Teacher Rating Scale, *J Abnorm Child Psychol* 1998; **26**(2): 109–118.
54. Reid R, DuPaul GJ, Power TJ, *et al.* Assessing culturally different students for attention deficit hyperactivity disorder using behavior rating scales, *J Abnorm Child Psychol* 1998; **26**(3): 187–198.
55. Arsenio WF. *Trajectories of Physical Aggression from Toddlerhood to Middle Childhood: Predictors, Correlates, and Outcomes.* Boston, Massacuesetts; Oxford: Blackwell Publications, 2004.
56. Campbell SB, Spieker S, Burchinal M, Poe MD. Trajectories of aggression from toddlerhood to age 9 predict academic and social functioning through age 12, *J Child Psychol Psychiatry* 2006; **47**(8): 791–800.
57. Dodge KA, Lochman JE, Harnish JD, Bates JE, Pettit GS. Reactive and proactive aggression in school children and psychiatrically impaired chronically assaultive youth, *J Abnorm Psychol* 1997; **106**(1): 37–51.
58. Dodge KA, Pettit GS, Bates JE. Socialization mediators of the relation between socioeconomic status and child conduct problems, *Child Dev* 1994; **65**(2 Spec No.): 649–665.
59. Vitaro F, Brendgen M, Tremblay RE. Reactively and proactively aggressive children: Antecedent and subsequent characteristics, *J Child Psychol Psychiatry* 2002; **43**(4): 495–505.
60. Karnik NS, Steiner H. Evidence for interventions for young offenders, *Child Adolesc Mental Health* 2007.
61. Steiner H. *Handbook of Mental Health Interventions in Children and Adolescents: An Integrated Developmental Approach.* 1st edition San Francisco, CA: Jossey-Bass Publishers, 2004.
62. Steiner H, Karnik NS. New approaches to juvenile delinquency: Psychopathology, development, and neuroscience, *Psychiatric Times* 2006: 15–17.
63. Reynolds AJ, Chang H, Temple JA. Early childhood intervention and juvenile delinquency. An exploratory analysis of the Chicago Child-Parent Centers, *Eval Rev* 1998; **22**(3): 341–372.

64. Reynolds AJ, Ou SR, Topitzes JW. Paths of effects of early childhood intervention on educational attainment and delinquency: A confirmatory analysis of the Chicago Child-Parent Centers, *Child Dev* 2004; **75**(5): 1299–1328.
65. Reynolds AJ, Temple JA, Ou SR. School-based early intervention and child well-being in the Chicago Longitudinal Study, *Child Welfare* 2003; **82**(5): 633–656.
66. Karnik NS. The social environment. In: Steiner H, Ed. *Handbook of Mental Health Interventions in Children and Adolescents: An Integrated Developmental Perspective*. San Francisco: Jossey-Bass, 2004.
67. Barkley RA, Edwards G, Laneri M, Fletcher K, Metevia L. The efficacy of problem-solving communication training alone, behavior management training alone, and their combination for parent-adolescent conflict in teenagers with ADHD and ODD, *J Consult Clin Psychol* 2001; **69**(6): 926–941.
68. Webster-Stratton C, Reid MJ, Hammond M. Treating children with early-onset conduct problems: Intervention outcomes for parent, child, and teacher training, *J Clin Child Adolesc Psychol* 2004; **33**(1): 105–124.
69. Borduin CM. Multisystemic treatment of criminality and violence in adolescents, *J Am Acad Child Adolesc Psychiatry* 1999; **38**(3): 242–249.
70. Curtis NM, Ronan KR, Borduin CM. Multisystemic treatment: A meta-analysis of outcome studies, *J Fam Psychol* 2004; **18**(3): 411–419.
71. Schaeffer CM, Borduin CM. Long-term follow-up to a randomized clinical trial of multisystemic therapy with serious and violent juvenile offenders, *J Consult Clin Psychol* 2005; **73**(3): 445–453.
72. Chamberlain P, Reid JB. Comparison of two community alternatives to incarceration for chronic juvenile offenders, *J Consult Clin Psychol* 1998; **66**(4): 624–633.
73. Chamberlain P, Weinrott M. Specialized foster care: Treating seriously emotionally disturbed children, *Child Today* 1990; **19**(1): 24–27.
74. Eddy JM, Chamberlain P. Family management and deviant peer association as mediators of the impact of treatment condition on youth antisocial behavior, *J Consult Clin Psychol* 2000; **68**(5): 857–863.
75. Leve LD, Chamberlain P, Reid JB. Intervention outcomes for girls referred from juvenile justice: Effects on delinquency, *J Consult Clin Psychol* 2005; **73**(6): 1181–1185.
76. Liddle HA, Dakof GA, Parker K, Diamond GS, Barrett K, Tejeda M. Multidimensional family therapy for adolescent drug abuse: Results of a randomized clinical trial, *Am J Drug Alcohol Abuse* 2001; **27**(4): 651–688.
77. Trupin EW, Stewart DG, Beach B, Boesky L. Effectiveness of a dialectical behaviour therapy program for incarcerated female juvenile offenders, *Child Adolesc Ment Health* 2002; **7**(3): 121–127.
78. Karnik NS, McMullin MA, Steiner H. Disruptive behaviors: Conduct and oppositional disorders in adolescents, *Adolesc Med Clin* 2006; **17**(1): 97–114.

79. Karnik NS, Steiner H. Disruptive behaviour disorders. In: Klykylo WM, Kay JL, Eds. *Clinical Child Psychiatry*, 2nd Edition. West Sussex: John Wiley & Sons Ltd., 2005.
80. Lochman JE. Cognitive-behavioral intervention with aggressive boys: Three-year follow-up and preventive effects, *J Consult Clin Psychol* 1992; **60**(3): 426–432.
81. Zun LS, Downey L, Rosen J. The effectiveness of an ED-based violence prevention program, *Am J Emerg Med* 2006; **24**(1): 8–13.
82. Janowsky DS, Barnhill LJ, Davis JM. Olanzapine for self-injurious, aggressive, and disruptive behaviors in intellectually disabled adults: A retrospective, open-label, naturalistic trial, *J Clin Psychiatry* 2003; **64**(10): 1258–1265.
83. Snyder R, Turgay A, Aman M, Binder C, Fisman S, Carroll A. Effects of risperidone on conduct and disruptive behavior disorders in children with subaverage IQs, *J Am Acad Child Adolesc Psychiatry* 2002; **41**(9): 1026–1036.
84. Turgay A, Binder C, Snyder R, Fisman S. Long-term safety and efficacy of risperidone for the treatment of disruptive behavior disorders in children with subaverage IQs, *Pediatrics* 2002; **110**(3): e34.
85. Aman MG, De Smedt G, Derivan A, Lyons B, Findling RL. Double-blind, placebo-controlled study of risperidone for the treatment of disruptive behaviors in children with subaverage intelligence, *Am J Psychiatry* 2002; **159**(8): 1337–1346.
86. Buitelaar JK, van der Gaag RJ, Cohen-Kettenis P, Melman CT. A randomized controlled trial of risperidone in the treatment of aggression in hospitalized adolescents with subaverage cognitive abilities, *J Clin Psychiatry* 2001; **62**(4): 239–248.
87. Pearson DA, Santos CW, Roache JD, *et al.* Treatment effects of methylphenidate on behavioral adjustment in children with mental retardation and ADHD, *J Am Acad Child Adolesc Psychiatry* 2003; **42**(2): 209–216.
88. Lindenmayer JP, Kotsaftis A. Use of sodium valproate in violent and aggressive behaviors: A critical review, *J Clin Psychiatry* 2000; **61**(2): 123–128.
89. Pappadopulos E, Macintyre Ii JC, Crismon ML, *et al.* Treatment recommendations for the use of antipsychotics for aggressive youth (TRAAY). Part II, *J Am Acad Child Adolesc Psychiatry* 2003; **42**(2): 145–161.
90. Schur SB, Sikich L, Findling RL, *et al.* Treatment recommendations for the use of antipsychotics for aggressive youth (TRAAY). Part I: A review, *J Am Acad Child Adolesc Psychiatry* 2003; **42**(2): 132–144.
91. Khanzode LA, Saxena K, Kraemer H, Chang K, Steiner H. Efficacy profiles of psychopharmacology: Divalproex sodium in conduct disorder, *Child Psychiatry Hum Dev* Fall 2006; **37**(1): 55–64.
92. Rana M, Khanzode L, Karnik N, Saxena K, Chang K, Steiner H. Divalproex sodium in the treatment of pediatric psychiatric disorders, *Expert Rev Neurother* 2005; **5**(2): 165–176.
93. Saxena K, Silverman MA, Chang K, Khanzode L, Steiner H. Baseline predictors of response to divalproex in conduct disorder, *J Clin Psychiatry* 2005; **66**(12): 1541–1548.

94. Steiner H, Petersen ML, Saxena K, Ford S, Matthews Z. Divalproex sodium for the treatment of conduct disorder: A randomized controlled clinical trial, *J Clin Psychiatry* 2003; **64**(10): 1183–1191.
95. Findling RL, Steiner H, Weller EB. Use of antipsychotics in children and adolescents, *J Clin Psychiatry* 2005; **66**(Suppl. 7): 29–40.
96. Steiner H, Dunne JE. Summary of the practice parameters for the assessment and treatment of children and adolescents with conduct disorder, *J Am Acad Child Adolesc Psychiatry* 1997; **36**(10): 1482–1485.
97. Steiner H. Practice parameters for the assessment and treatment of children and adolescents with conduct disorder. American Academy of Child and Adolescent Psychiatry, *J Am Acad Child Adolesc Psychiatry* 1997; **36**(10 Suppl.): 122S–139S.
98. Findling RL, Reed MD, O'Riordan MA, Demeter CA, Stansbrey RJ, McNamara NK. A 26-week open-label study of quetiapine in children with conduct disorder, *J Child Adolesc Psychopharmacol* 2007; **17**(1):1–9.
99. Findling RL, Reed MD, O'Riordan MA, Demeter CA, Stansbrey RJ, McNamara NK. Effectiveness, safety, and pharmacokinetics of quetiapine in aggressive children with conduct disorder, *J Am Acad Child Adolesc Psychiatry* 2006; **45**(7): 792–800.
100. Padhy R, Saxena K, Remsing L, Khanzode L, Steiner H. Divalproex sodium treatment in high and low activation conduct disorders, *J Clin Psychiatry*, Under review.

Chapter 12

Diagnosis, Development, and Treatment of Substance Use Disorders among Adolescents and Young Adults

Anna Lembke, Keith Humphreys, and Rudolf Moos

1. Introduction

Understanding substance use disorders requires a broader understanding of adolescence. The majority of adults with substance use disorders began using substances as teenagers and young adults. Many developmental and contextual factors contribute to the progression from substance use to substance abuse and dependence. After an overview of evolutionary conservation, epidemiology, and diagnostic considerations, we review selected theoretical perspectives of development: the epigenetic model, the social development model, social control theory, social learning theory, behavioral economics, and stress and coping theories. We then discuss treatment interventions, and present a clinical case to illustrate the Stanford approach to adolescents and young adults with substance use disorders. Finally, we explore how public policy could improve upon treatment options in the future.

2. Evolutionary Conservation

One characteristic of complex organisms, including humans, is the ability to rapidly learn which behavioral responses enhance the likelihood of survival. From infancy onwards, humans can distinguish which behaviors please caregivers, lead to relief from hunger and pain, *etc*. Many learned associations become emotionally valenced. For example, a blanket and a cup of hot cocoa at grandma's house on a wintry day not only meets a physical need, but may also generate subjective feelings of well-being and fond memories of prior similar experiences. Activation of various neuroreceptors in the brain is essential to the formation of these emotionally valenced learned associations of behaviors to consequences that promote or threaten survival. Because this neurobehavioral system helps humans learn and repeat behaviors that lead to food, sex, warmth, and positive social interactions, it conveys a significant survival advantage and has therefore been evolutionarily conserved.

Unfortunately, throughout human evolution, a number of plants (*e.g.* tobacco, cocoa) have contained chemicals that convey no survival advantage but nonetheless stimulate the same brain receptors, emotional reactions, and neural pathways. In recent centuries, modern chemistry has created many more such substances, either by refining plant products (*e.g.* heroin from the poppy plant) or by generating them *de novo* (*e.g.* methamphetamine). At the risk of anthropomorphizing, these substances have significant power to "trick" the human brain. Because the same opiate receptors are triggered by an orgasm as by a shot of morphine, the brain may mistake a morphine shot as a behavior that is essential to survival. After the injection, the individual may feel the happiness, joy, and relief of doing something essential to survival, which is not in fact grounded in reality. Through repeated use of morphine, the individual's brain and psyche may have as strong a desire for morphine as they previously had for sex. The process by which an evolutionary function is commandeered in such a fashion is known as exaptation.[1] Understanding this process illuminates why addicted individuals might neglect eating and sleeping for their substance, and why they have such intense motivational and emotional forces fixated on substances that objectively have no survival benefit.

3. Epidemiology

Youth substance use is a major public health problem in the United States. According to the 2004 National Survey on Drug Use and Health (NSDUH), 22,506,000 (9.4%) people in the United States are addicted to illicit drugs or alcohol, and 9,068,000 of those individuals are between the ages of 12 and 25. Although the majority of youths who experiment with substances do not go on to develop a substance use disorder, the majority of people who develop a substance use disorder began using substances in adolescents or young adulthood. The average age of first use among the current 2.2 million marijuana users was 18 years, with 63.8% under 18. Almost all (86.9%) alcohol users were under 21 when they first drank. About two-thirds (67.8%) of cigarette smokers were under 18 when they initiated smoking.[2]

The contribution of environment and social development to adolescent substance use problems is reflected in the epidemiology of substance use. Among people aged 12 to 17, rates of current illicit drug use varied according to racial and ethnic groups. American Indian and Alaska Native youths (26.0%) had the highest rate of illicit drug use, followed by mixed race youths (12.2%), white youths (11.1%), Hispanic youths (10.2%), black youths (9.3%), and Asian youths (6.0%). Young adults aged 18–22 enrolled in full-time college were more likely than their peers (*i.e.* persons not enrolled in college and those in part-time college) to drink alcohol, binge drink, and drink heavily.[2] The most disturbing trend in the last half-decade has been the escalation in non-medical use of psychotherapeutic drugs. Between 2003 and 2004 those aged from 18 to 25 showed a significant increase in the use of pain relievers, such as hydrocodone (vicodin) (from 15 to 16.5%), oxycodone-acetaminophen (percocet) (from 7.8 to 8.7%), and oxycodone (oxycontin) (from 3.6 to 4.3%). In 2004, the non-medical use of pain relievers was the category of substance use which showed the largest number of new users.[2]

According to the 2004 NSDUH, the past year prevalence of major depressive episode was highest among those aged 18 to 25 (10.1%), and those with a major depressive episode were more likely to suffer from substance dependence or abuse. In 2004, 22.5% of youths aged 12–17 began receiving treatment or counseling for emotional or behavioral problems, which is more than in 2002 (19.3%) or 2003 (20.6%).[2]

The net effect of these trends is that mental health care providers will see and treat increasing numbers of young people who have serious substance use problems; and many of these youths will be abusing prescription medications. The research suggests that adolescents who abuse prescription drugs, most often obtain these drugs without consent from adult prescriptions, rather than having been directly prescribed the substances. These new dynamics mandate involvement of family members in the treatment of adolescent substance use. Providers need to be aware that this new generation of substance users is abusing prescription medications than any generation preceding it.

4. Diagnosis

4.1. *Diagnostic criteria*

The Diagnostic and Statistical Manual of Mental Disorders, fourth edition, defines "substance" as "a drug of abuse, a medication, or a toxin."[3] We are speaking here primarily of drugs of abuse, including medications which are used as drugs of abuse, but not toxins. We focus on substance use disorders (substance dependence and substance abuse), although substance-induced disorders (psychosis, depression, etc) are also addressed.

The DSM-IV denotes specific substances or categories of substances as "drugs of abuse": alcohol, amphetamines and other sympathomimetics, cannabis, cocaine, hallucinogens, inhalants, nicotine, opioids, phencyclidine, and other arylcyclohexlamines, and sedative/hypnotic/anxiolytics. For substances not included in this list, *e.g.* ecstasy, the code for "other substances" is used.[3]

The DSM-IV coding system adheres closely to the International Statistical Classification of Diseases and Related Health Problems, Tenth Revision (ICD-10), as developed by the World Health Organization. The codes and terms of DSM-IV and ICD-10 are fully compatible, with virtually no gaps in translation, thanks to the close cooperation of the American Psychiatric Association and the World Health Organization.

"Substance dependence" can be applied to all classes of substances specifically mentioned above. "Substance abuse" applies to all classes of substances except nicotine. The cardinal features of substance dependence are tolerance, withdrawal, and/or compulsive use in any 12-month period (Table 1). Although tolerance and withdrawal are common features of dependence, these physiologic symptoms are not required to meet criteria for dependence, a common misperception. The cognitive and behavioral symptoms alone can qualify an individual for this diagnosis. Once the lifetime criteria for dependence have been met for any given substance, this diagnosis always takes precedence over a substance abuse diagnosis.[3]

Substance abuse is characterized by repeated use with negative social consequences in any 12-month period. What differentiates substance abuse from dependence is the absence of tolerance and withdrawal, and much less time spent seeking and using in a compulsive manner. However, the differences between these two diagnostic categories are not empirically validated, and do not represent progression of disease from one diagnostic category to another.[4]

4.2. *Applicability to adolescents*

The criteria for substance use disorders are based on clinical and research experience with adults. When the same diagnostic criteria are applied to young people, they appear to be at least minimally valid in that adolescents with substance dependence, substance abuse, and no alcohol problems, differ on external measures of involvement with alcohol.[5,6] However, developmental differences between adults and children may diminish the sensitivity and specificity of the diagnostic benchmarks in youths.

Table 1:

Criteria for Substance Abuse and Dependence

Substance abuse
A maladaptive pattern of substance use leading to clinically significant impairment or distress, as manifested by one (or more) or the following, occurring within a 12-month period:

1. recurrent substance use resulting in failure to fulfill major role obligations at work, school, or home
2. recurrent substance use in situations in which it is physically hazardous
3. recurrent substance-related legal problems
4. continued substance use despite having persistent or recurrent social or interpersonal problems caused or exacerbated by the effects of substance

The symptoms have never met criteria for substance dependence for this class of substance.

Substance dependence
A maladaptive pattern of substance use, leading to clinically significant impairment or distress, as manifested by three (or more) of the following, occurring at any time in the same 12-month period:

1. tolerance, as defined by either of the following:
   (a) need for markedly increased amounts of the substance to achieve intoxication or desired effect
   (b) markedly diminished effect with continued use of the same amount of the substance
2. withdrawal, as manifested by either of the following:
   (a) the characteristic withdrawal syndrome for the substance
   (b) the same (or closely related) substance is taken to relieve or avoid withdrawal symptoms
3. the substance is often taken in larger amounts, or over a longer period of time than was intended
4. there is a persistent desire or unsuccessful efforts to cut down or control substance use
5. a great deal of time is spent in activities necessary to obtain the substance, use the substance, or recover from its effects
6. important social, occupational, or recreational activities are given up or reduced because of substance use
7. the substance use is continued despite knowledge of having a persistent or recurrent physical or psychological problem that is likely to have been caused or exacerbated by the substance

For example, adolescents tend to drink less frequently than adults, but consume alcohol in larger amounts when they do drink[7]; a fact which could potentially impact the assessment of "time spent in activities" related to use. Withdrawal, another important criterion of substance dependence, does not tend to occur until after years of heavy use, so may have limited utility among younger individuals with substance use disorders.[8] Tolerance is also a problematic criterion in young people. Some adolescents who endorse "markedly increased amounts of the substance to achieve intoxication or desired effect," are in fact light drinkers, increasing from one to three drinks'; whereas other adolescents begin by drinking a larger amount of alcohol, six drinks, due to the social situation, and so in a sense bypass the tolerance phase altogether.[8]

Alcohol is illegal in the under-21 population. For an adolescent to obtain alcohol therefore usually involves a layer of complexity and time that is not present in the adult group. Since accessibility and legality impact adolescent drinking, certain diagnostic criteria, such as "alcohol related legal problems," potentially take on a different meaning in young people. Simply consuming alcohol is by definition a "legal problem" in this age group.

Contextual considerations are particularly important with younger people. Adolescents are keenly sensitive to social pressures, and substance use at this vulnerable age may be a response to environmental pressures combined with a lack of internal and external resources to resist these pressures, rather than an indicator of compulsive use.[8] In fact, when contextual factors are taken into account in assessments of tolerance and time spent using alcohol, the prevalence of alcohol use disorders is markedly altered in adolescent community samples.[9]

Developmental differences between adults and children, and the importance of social context in adolescents, complicate the diagnostic validity of substance use disorders in young people. Markers of compulsivity, and legality, just to name a few, need to be carefully considered when assessing adolescents and young adults for addictive disorders.

5. Differential Diagnosis and Comorbidities

5.1. *Primary versus substance-induced mental disorders*

Distinguishing primary mental disorders from those that are substance-induced is one of the biggest diagnostic challenges in treating patients with substance use disorders. Substance intoxication, withdrawal, and abstinence syndromes, can all mimic primary mental disorders. For example, amphetamine intoxication can look exactly like paranoid psychosis, alcohol intoxication can mimic bipolar mania, and withdrawal from all substances of abuse generates dysphoria, which if prolonged can resemble major depression.

DSM-IV made a major advance over its predecessor by carefully considering substance-induced mental disorders. In the earlier DSM-III, substance-induced mental disorders were lumped together with mental disorders due to a general medical condition. Both these categories were considered "organic" brain problems. Organic problems were thought to be rooted in biological processes, and were differentiated from other forms of mental illness, which were called "nonorganic" or "functional." The DSM-IV eliminated the terms "organic" and "functional," and established separate categories for substance-induced mental disorders, mental disorders due to a general medical condition, and other "primary" mental disorders.[3]

The DSM-IV also makes some effort to guide the clinician in distinguishing substance-induced mental disorders and primary mental disorders. "In evaluating whether the symptoms of a mental disorder are the direct physiological effect of substance use, it is important to note the temporal relationship between the onset and offset of substance use and the onset and offset of the symptoms or the full syndrome." (p. 210).[3] The DSM-IV text gives four weeks of abstinence as a general time frame in which substance-induced psychiatric symptoms should resolve. Although research on this subject is limited, Brown and Schuckit studied adult patients who met criteria for alcohol dependence and/or major depression, and showed that at least four weeks of abstinence were required before substance-induced versus primary depression could be differentiated.[10]

Periods of extended sobriety under 24-h careful monitoring are a luxury most clinicians do not have in daily practice. In fact, the four-week time frame may be too long or too short for a given individual addicted to a given substance. Given sparse empirical data and limited clinical resources, we clinicians are usually forced to try to tease apart substance-induced and primary mental disorders on the basis of incomplete information. We are often left to make treatment plans without being sure if the psychiatric symptoms are primary or secondary.

Riggs and Davies have recommended the use of a lifetime timeline to help with diagnostic formulations in adolescents.[11] The lifetime timeline should include major life events throughout the development of the individual, such as childhood abuse, school performance, major family disruptions, *e.g.* divorce, *etc.*; as well as the onset of substance use and psychiatric symptoms, and the relationship, if any, between the two. The timeline is a means by which the clinician can begin to integrate the psychosocial and biological phenomena that may be driving the substance use, and vice versa.

The art of distinguishing primary from substance-induced mental disorders is further complicated by the pervasive cultural norm of invoking the self-medication hypothesis. Many patients and providers have come to embrace the paradigm of "self-medication," which loosely defined puts forth that the primary reason for substance use is to alleviate psychiatric symptoms. Yet, substantial evidence contradicts this idea: *e.g.* a large, prospective study of adolescents found that substance use and sex among boys and girls ($N = 13{,}491$, grades 7 to 11) predicted an increased likelihood of depression, and not the other way around.[12] The self-medication hypothesis furthermore fails to account for all the other factors that may be contributing toward substance use,[13] not the least of which are the inherent effects of the substance themselves. Some patients have come to justify substance use for themselves as a necessary evil in the absence of effective treatment for mental illness. If physicians do not remain skeptical in the face of the self-medication hypothesis, they are at risk to overdiagnose primary mental disorders, undertreat addictive disorders, and contribute to the patient's bulwark of denial.

In our practice, we tend to discourage the self-medication ethos. We try to avoid the "self-medication" language with patients, and to emphasize that independent of causal factors, aggressive treatment of a substance use disorder will support rather than detract from successful treatment of a psychiatric illness. The latter assertion is well supported by the literature, which clearly establishes that dual diagnosis patients, *i.e.* those with comorbid substance use and primary mental disorders, experience a worsening of their psychiatric symptoms in the face of ongoing substance use.[13] A substance use disorder should be treated whether or not it is "due to" another cooccurring disorder.

5.2. *Remuneration and diagnosis*

Despite the fact that substance use disorders are perhaps the leading public health problem facing the United States, many insurance companies do not adequately compensate providers or hospitals for treating substance-related problems, except for specific "carve-outs," which cover very limited protocols, such as acute detoxification. In the adult population, only eight psychiatric diagnoses are reimbursed on par with other major medical illnesses. Substance use disorders are not among them. Strikingly, in children (up to age 17), primary substance use is one of only two psychiatric illnesses which is not reimbursed on par with medical illnesses. (The other is pervasive developmental disorders.)

Some insurance companies or state- and government-sponsored insurance systems only cover substance use treatment if the patient is also found to have a primary mental illness. As discussed above, differentiating primary from secondary mental disorders in substance using patients is challenging. When faced with the added factor of knowing that treatment for substance use disorders will not be administered due to lack of coverage, or if administered, not compensated after the fact, providers may feel pressured into listing a primary mental disorder, even if the evidence does not support it. Thus, the physician is potentially ethically compromised in order to care for his/her patients. In addition, the ensuing medical record is inaccurate, and perpetuates falsehoods, which are neither good for patients nor for our broader understanding of these disorders. Aligning treatment and financial incentives will be central to providing better care in the future.[14]

6. Developmental Pathways and Pathogenetic Models

Several theories have been formulated to try to understand the progression toward substance use and misuse among youth. Theories range in focus from the macrocosm of social systems, to the microcosm of family interactions: *e.g.* the social development model emphasizes social bonding and social norms, whereas the epigenetic model cites temperament and self-control factors as primary. More specific theories that have highlighted the role of social context factors in the development of substance use and misuse include social control, social learning, behavioral economics, or behavioral choice, and stress and coping theories.[15,16]

6.1. *Epigenetic model*

The epigenetic model posits that specific underlying components of temperament, such as high activity level, impulsivity and novelty seeking, and negative emotionality, raise the risk of substance use and misuse. Because these aspects of temperament result in greater demands for self-regulation and make it harder to acquire self-control skills, they tend to interfere with the development of supportive relationships with parents and teachers. Moreover, highly active youngsters who lack persistence and problem-solving skills are prone to helplessness and anger and to seek novel or sensation-arousing experiences. Low self-control is also associated with other proximal risk factors, such as life stressors and affiliation with social networks of non-normative peers, which predispose youngsters to substance use and misuse. In contrast, some aspects of temperament, such as positive emotionality and the ability to focus attention on a task, underlie the development of good self-control and, in turn, proximal factors that protect against substance use, such as a higher level of cognitive and social development, academic competence, and expectations about harmful effects of substances.[17]

6.2. *Social development model*

The social development model asserts that temperament and other personal characteristics affect problem behavior and substance misuse because they alter the socialization process. This model posits that social bonding in primary socialization settings, such as the family, peer groups, and school, typically results in youngsters learning conventional norms and engaging in acceptable behavior. It assumes that secondary sources of socialization, such as religious organizations, neighborhood, and community, also tend to have positive influences on youngsters, and that they exert their effects primarily through their impact on the family, peer groups, and school. However, active socialization processes, such as observation and modeling of others using substances, can promote deviant norms and behavior. Moreover, personal factors, such as impulsivity, novelty seeking, and externalizing disorders, are associated with less bonding with family and school and more bonding with deviant peers, which lead to the development of antisocial attitudes, conduct disorders, and substance misuse.[18]

6.3. *Social control theory*

According to social control theory, strong bonds with family, school, religion, and other aspects of traditional society motivate youngsters to engage in responsible behavior, refrain from substance misuse, and reduce their susceptibility to influences from deviant peers. When such bonds are weak or absent, youngsters are less likely to adhere to conventional standards of behavior and tend to associate with antisocial, substance using peers and to engage in problem behavior, such as misuse of alcohol and drugs. The main cause of weak social bonds and rebellion against existing social standards is social disorganization and inadequate monitoring of behavior, including families that lack cohesion and structure, low levels of support and supervision in school and social settings, and disorganized neighborhoods with rampant poverty and crime.[19]

6.4. *Social learning theory*

According to social learning theory, modeling and observational learning shape expectations and behavior. Substance use is a function of adult and peer modeling of the use of substances, positive norms about use, and the easy availability of alcohol and drugs. Learning begins with observing and imitating role models' substance-specific behaviors, continues with social reinforcement and expectations of positive consequences from substance use, and culminates in substance use and misuse. Watching parents and peers use alcohol and drugs can instill positive expectancies for the effects of these substances and provide models that show how to obtain and use them.[20]

6.5. *Behavioral economics or behavioral choice theory*

This theory posits that the key elements of the social context are the alternative rewards provided by activities other than substance use. These rewards protect individuals from exposure to substances and opportunities to use them, as well as from escalating and maintaining substance use. Lack of effective access to rewards from educational pursuits, religious involvement, and participation in conventional activities promotes the choice of other reinforcing behaviors, such as substance use. For example, physical activity and substance use both elevate mood and decrease anxiety, which may make them functionally similar and substitutable. Involvement in physical activities also encompasses social affiliation with individuals who do not use alcohol or drugs and reinforces a youngster's decision to refrain from using these substances.[21]

6.6. *Stress and coping theory*

According to this theory, the stressors that stem from social disorganization, especially in family, peer, school, and neighborhood settings, lead to alienation and distress. Family stressors, such as physical and sexual abuse, continual conflict, and lack of cohesion and structure, create alienation and distress. Life stressors may also generate anxiety by challenging a youngster's desired self-image, such as when a failure at school arouses doubts about self-competence. The theory assumes that stressors are most likely to impel substance use among impulsive youngsters with poor coping skills who try to avoid facing problems and experiencing negative affect. For these youngsters, substance use is a form of avoidance coping to reduce alienation and dysphoria which, if successful, reinforces substance use.[22]

6.7. *Parental bonding and monitoring*

Consistent with social control theory, disruptions in parenting lead to a lack of nurturance and control that impair the bonding process and increase the likelihood of youngsters' alienation and distress. Disturbances of family management processes, such as ongoing parent–child conflict and lack of support, erratic and inconsistent discipline, and inadequate parental monitoring, raise the likelihood of youngsters' substance use, are associated with earlier initiation of use, and predict accelerated growth in use. For example, lack of parental monitoring predicts the onset of regular weekly alcohol consumption and progression to heavy episodic (five or more drinks on one occasion) drinking, as well as the onset of illicit drug use. Youngsters who are poorly supervised and have many drug-using peers are an exceptionally high-risk group.[23,24] When a youngster engages in substance use or misuse, mutual influence processes occur. As parents try to manage a child's substance use, they may become less supportive and institute strict rules and discipline, thereby alienating the child and stimulating rebellious behavior. In a maladaptive spiral, parents sometimes strengthen family control and restrict independence in a vain attempt to keep the youngster's behavior within acceptable limits. In a continuation of this downward spiral, escalating substance use may lead to a decline in parental support and monitoring. Thus, in part, parent–youth conflict is a response to parents' attempts to influence and control the youngster's initial problem behavior.

6.8. *Parental and sibling norms and modeling*

Through a process of social learning and the development of expectancies, parents' and other family members' influence the likelihood of youngsters' substance use and misuse. Parents' positive attitudes about youngsters' alcohol and drug use, and parental modeling of alcohol and drug use, predict adolescents' positive expectancies about substances and initiation and growth of substance use. Parental norms that fail to discourage underage drinking lead to more positive cognitions about alcohol that foreshadow the initiation and growth of alcohol use.[25,26]

Siblings may also play an important role in the initiation and growth of a youngster's substance use. Adolescents with older siblings who use substances are much more likely to use substances themselves. Exposure to sibling substance use contributes to earlier affiliations with substance-using peers and provides easier access to alcohol and drugs. Sibling substance use also increases the likelihood of youngsters' drinking to cope with the tension and alienation associated with stressful life events. In fact, a strong bond between antisocial siblings may contribute to the development of a shared deviant social network and amplify the risk of substance misuse and other problem behavior.[27,28]

6.9. *Family-based stressors*

Youngsters who experience a high level of negative life events are more likely to engage in substance use and show a sharper rise in use. Many of these negative events are associated with parent–child conflict, physical and sexual abuse, and parental separation and divorce, and are part of the syndrome of growing up in a high-risk family. Life stressors may shake youngsters' beliefs in the predictability of events and the relevance of conventional norms and lead to alienation and distress, loosening of family bonds, more interaction with peers who use drugs, and coping with negative affect through substance use. In addition to the direct role of affect regulation or tension reduction in the development of adolescent substance use, affective factors may raise the likelihood that youngsters will develop coping motives that predispose them to engage in substance misuse.

These risk factors have been integrated into a three-stage model that combines aspects of social learning and stress and coping theories: (1) Parental modeling of substance use, low levels of parental support and supervision, and lack of commitment to conventional goals lead to youngsters' initial experimentation with substances. (2) Resulting association with deviant, substance-using peers promotes an escalation of substance use. (3) Parental and peer substance use, emotional distress, and deficits in coping skills foreshadow use of substances to cope with stressors and transition into problem use.[29]

6.10. *Friends' norms and modeling*

Through their relationships with peers, youngsters are exposed to three forms of social influence that may increase their substance use: explicit offers of substances, social modeling, and perceptions of friends' and other youngsters' substance use. In general, explicit offers to try substances, social modeling driven by friends' actual substance use, and perceptions of friends' positive attitudes and substance use are predictably related to increases in youngsters' substance use and misuse. In addition, when more students in a school use alcohol and drugs, youngsters perceive that these substances are more acceptable and available and are more likely to use them. Peer influences seem to be especially strong among youngsters who are heavy substance users and when they occur in a social context in which alcohol and/or drug use are highly prevalent.[30,31]

Since mutual choice is involved in friendship formation, the association between a youngster's substance use and his or her friends' substance use depends on selecting and maintaining like-minded friendships (social selection), as well as on the influence of existing friends (social causation). Social selection contributes to peer group similarity in substance use; once formed, friendships tend to reinforce common behaviors and may operate as a stabilizing influence on substance use. In this regard, there is a positive, bidirectional association between adolescents' and peers' substance use. Adolescents who report more peer substance use subsequently engage in more use themselves (social causation); adolescents who engage in more substance use subsequently tend to report more peer substance use.[32,33]

6.11. *Life stressors*

Youngsters who experience uncontrollable life change events often have a sense of helplessness and lack of self-efficacy, which spawns feelings of alienation and anomie. Uncontrollable life events experienced in adolescence are directly related to subsequent substance use; such life events are also indirectly related to substance use because they produce depression and lack of control, which increase the likelihood that youngsters will use substances to try to raise their mood. Youngsters who rely more on passive or indirect coping strategies, such as anger and helplessness, are more likely to associate with peers who use substances and to increase their own substance use. These effects of coping tend to be stronger when youngsters experience more life stressors, which are related to higher initial levels of substance use and to greater increases in use. Moreover, the use of alcohol and drugs to alleviate distress foreshadows heavy substance use and abuse.[34,35]

6.12. *Bonding and monitoring as protective factors*

Adolescents who have stronger bonds to family, school, and community are less susceptible to negative influences from friends, less likely to associate with peers who use substances, and less likely to use substances themselves. Effective parenting is especially important in moderating peers' potential negative influences. For example, among adolescents whose parents are relatively low on authoritative parenting, friends' drug use tends to lead to higher levels of own drug use. In contrast, for adolescents whose parents are high on authoritative parenting, friends' drug use may be less influential. Effective parenting may enhance adolescents' internalization of parental norms and make them less susceptible to deviant peer norms and behaviors.[36]

In addition to parents, disapproval of substance use by other important reference groups, such as best friends, other students at school, and other adults in the community, can counteract the influence of substance-using peers. Even when best friends approve of drinking, disapproval from other reference groups is associated with a lower likelihood of drinking. Moreover, schools can serve a key social monitoring or social control function. Students in an involving and structured school milieu with well-articulated rules are less likely to begin to use substances or to transition into heavy substance use. Friends' drug use is likely to have less influence in school and other social contexts in which most peers are not using substances.[37,38]

Religious involvement also involves protective processes, including a network of social support based on shared values, a sense of meaning and purpose, negative beliefs and expectations about substances, and a tendency to rely more on approach than avoidance coping. Religious beliefs are associated with stable sources of socialization, such as parents and friends who tend not to use alcohol or drugs, attendance at a school with structured substance-free social activities, and participation in rewarding communal activities that limit opportunities for substance use. Religious involvement can help youngsters cope with life stressors, shield them from the opportunity to try drugs, and strengthen resistance once the opportunity to try drugs has occurred.[39,40]

6.13. *Personal factors*

The most salient personal risk factors involved in the development of substance use and misuse are youngsters' risk taking and impulsivity, emotional distress, novelty seeking, susceptibility to social influence, and positive expectations of substance use. With respect to temperament, *e.g.* parent–child conflict appears to have an especially strong influence on increasing substance use among more active and impulsive youngsters characterized by negative emotionality (*i.e.* those who are at higher temperamental risk). Parent–child conflict seems to have less influence on substance use among youngsters at less temperamental risk; *i.e.* those who are more task oriented and characterized by positive emotionality.[41]

6.14. *Risk-taking and impulsivity*

Youngsters with high levels of emotional distress are more likely to drink heavily and to escalate into other substance misuse, which is consistent with the idea that youngsters use substances to cope with distress. Increases in risk taking also heighten the odds of heavy drinking, which supports the idea that lack of inhibition (impulsivity, seeking novelty) is associated with adolescent alcohol misuse. More broadly, the cooccurrence of personal and environmental risk factors tends to increase the likelihood of sustained rises in problematic substance use. The influence of friends who use substances tends to be more robust when an adolescent is more inclined toward risk taking and less inclined to perceive substance use as potentially harmful. The positive association of impulsivity and lack of inhibition with substance use, is even stronger when combined with low parental control, more interaction with deviant peers, and more life stressors.[34,42]

As described earlier, epigenetic models posit that some temperament characteristics, such as high activity levels and emotional distress, inhibit the development of self-control skills, because they decrease attention to relevant environmental cues and lead to less effective parenting practices. For example, a child's high activity level may create more demands on parents, who in turn have less ability to provide support. Accordingly, young adolescents with a highly active temperament are more likely to seek novel stimulation, to have less self-control and less parental support, and to experience more life stressors and employ less adaptive modes of coping, which are associated with a higher likelihood of substance misuse. In contrast, young adolescents who have a temperament characterized by positive mood tend to have more self-control and support, which are associated with less novelty seeking, more adaptive coping, fewer associations with substance-using friends and, ultimately, less substance use.[43]

6.15. *Susceptibility to social influence*

Personal characteristics associated with high susceptibility to social influence include extroversion, low self-esteem, and a lack of personal convictions, placing credence on other people's values and behavior, looking to others for guidance, interpersonal vulnerability and being easily upset by criticism, and preference for a follower rather than a leader role. Youngsters who are more attuned to social rewards tend to be more exposed to peer substance use and are more likely to overindulge in alcohol and drug use. Susceptibility to peer influence is a powerful risk factor for substance misuse and contributes to subsequent exposure to peers' alcohol use.[44]

Youngsters who are not members of a close-knit peer group may be more susceptible to peer influence and more likely to become substance users than are youngsters who are group or clique members. Relative social isolation may be associated with more substance use because it produces boredom and alienation and because isolates are not constrained by conventional social processes.[45]

6.16. *Cumulative risk and resistance models*

Risk factor models typically encompass a broad array of personal and social influences that, consistent with the theories reviewed earlier, tend to be associated with a heightened likelihood of the development of substance misuse. Some of these models also consider resistance or protective influences that help to explain why some youngsters who are exposed to many risk factors thrive nonetheless. According to problem behavior theory, *e.g.* both personality and social context factors are predictably associated with alcohol and drug problems. It is the combination of more risk and fewer protective factors that tend to accelerate the likelihood of becoming a heavy drinker and of developing other problem behaviors.[46]

7. Treatment Interventions

7.1. *Prevention*

Billions of dollars have been expended on drug use prevention programs, and at least tens of millions of dollars have been expended to evaluate them. In the main, the results have been less than overwhelming. A major review by the National Research Council[47] found that the mostly widely-employed programs such as Drug Abuse Resistance Education (DARE), life skills training, and other educationally oriented programs, have a collective average effect size of 0.03, which although statistically significant is disappointingly close to zero. This finding is not particularly surprising when one realizes that typical prevention programs last less than 12 h, whereas the typical teenager watches thousands of hours of television (including countless ads for beer, wine, and pills).

The contextual-developmental understanding of substance use we offer in this chapter would lead one to predict that prevention programs will be most effective if they (1) attempt to change young people's enduring life contexts, and (2) conceptualize drug abuse as a problem embedded in a broad negative developmental pathway. This developmental pathway broadly speaking includes lack of early family cohesion and monitoring, social bonding with deviant peers, and poor emotional regulation, frequent dysphoria, with a tendency toward impulsivity and/or aggressiveness.

Trying to prevent substance use by teaching a young person drug refusal skills, *etc*., makes the assumption that 10 or 20 h of individual instruction can overcome thousands of hours of parent and/or peer modeling; television, movies, and videogames that promote use; as well as a broad cultural climate that conveys in countless ways the value of immediate gratification.[48] An ecological framework acknowledges that each individual's knowledge and skills influence response to the environment, but changing the environment leads to more lasting behavior change in more people.

A significant change in the school environment will affect children each day for many days. (Going to school may be the only activity children engage in as much as they do consuming electronic media.) Key examples of programs that have been effective in reducing substance use are programs that improve teacher's ability to manage their classrooms, to discipline effectively, and to increase student cooperation and reduce social rejection. Schoolwide efforts that establish a climate of predictability and mutual helping may also create an environment that reduces substance use problems. The NRC report showed that the average effect size for such environmentally focused programs is more than four times that of individually focused programs, making one wonder why the former of such programs continue to command the lion's share of school resources.

An ecological framework also leads us to see heavy drug use not as a distinct disorder, but as part of a cluster of behaviors that constitute a negative developmental trajectory. This developmental trajectory has some shared genetic and social influences.[49] Programs that promote emotion self-regulation, behavioral management, and positive social interaction could reduce drug use more than programs that exhort students not to use drugs.

A potent example supporting both of the above two observations is the "good behavior game" of Kellam and colleagues.[50] This intervention reorders the classroom environment substantially by having teachers form teams of students who receive rewards for engaging in good behavior. As the rewards are team based, peer pressure tends to work to reduce problem behavior rather than intermittently reinforce it as often happens in standard classrooms. A randomized study showed that even years after the students had left those classrooms, they had lower rates of teacher-rated aggression and cigarette smoking compared to children assigned to standard classrooms, even though the game explicitly conveyed nothing about smoking.

7.2. *Psychosocial treatment*

We focus here on psychosocial and behavioral interventions for substance use disorders in young people, rather than pharmacotherapy, primarily because there is a paucity of pharmacotherapy research for substance use disorders in youth. Furthermore, youths with cooccurring substance use and mental illness are typically excluded from pharmacotherapy trials for mental illness. One exceptions is a placebo-controlled trial using pemoline for attention-deficit/hyperactivity disorder (ADHD) in non-abstinent adolescents, which showed improvement of the ADHD, with no change in the substance use.[51]

Several controlled trials have looked specifically at different types of psychosocial and behavioral interventions in young people with substance use problems, most of which were adapted from adult treatment models. Numerous prevention programs have been geared toward youths, but to date very few developmentally tailored programs have been created and empirically validated. The treatment interventions for adolescents which have so far proven to be most effective, are those which transform the social context, in particular the family and school environments. Unfortunately, these programs are also the most complex, with multiple components and providers; and therefore not favored by the current health care financing system. In response to economic pressures, researchers are also exploring simpler, more cost-effective regimens for adolescent substance use disorders, such as motivational interviewing.

Stanton did a metaanalysis to review all the drug abuse outcome studies that included a couples/family therapy treatment condition, including programs with young patients.[52] They reviewed 1501 cases involving approximately 3500 patients and family members, and found that family therapy was superior to couples or individual therapy, peer counseling, or family psychoeducation. For adolescents, family therapy was even more effective than a multilevel intervention that included court-ordered school monitoring, curfews, and meetings with probation officers.[53] This metaanalysis underscores the importance of changing the interpersonal dynamics and structure of the family environment, an ecologically informed approach, which trumps skills training, education, and punitive measures. Furthermore a "non-blaming" stance toward families is more effective than confrontation, and also keeps patients and families from abandoning treatment.

Interventions which have proven effective in young people with alcohol use disorders also include family therapies with both family and community components.

Some preliminary evidence also shows that pharmacologic treatment of cooccurring psychiatric disorders in adolescents with alcohol use disorders enhances alcohol use outcomes.[54]

Motivational interviewing is potentially a more cost-effective approach to the problem of youth substance use, and can be administered across different health care settings, including primary care and psychiatric office settings.[55] It adopts a non-authoritarian approach which encourages people to take responsibility for their choices current and future, as well as provides advice about the direction to change and ways to achieve it. Motivational interviewing has preliminary evidence of reducing alcohol related problems in adolescents.[56]

In 1997, the NIAAA formally initiated a program of research to promote the creation of effective developmentally tailored treatments for adolescents with alcohol use disorders. As many as 20 studies are currently underway, including family-therapy, cognitive behavioral therapy, brief motivational therapy, and guided self-change therapy. Results will be available over the next several years.

8. Our Clinical Experience — Practice-Based Evidence

Here at Stanford University Hospital and Clinics, we do not have a formal substance use disorder program, despite the fact that we are a major medical center. The reasons for this glaring absence are complex and beyond the scope of this chapter, but have been alluded to in previous sections, *e.g.* see "Remuneration and Diagnosis." Hence, our practice relies heavily on external referral services, from residential treatment programs to 12-step mutual help groups; and our patient population consists largely of individuals seeking treatment for psychiatric and/or medical problems other than substance use. The plight we find ourselves in, *i.e.* not having a dedicated substance use program, is one that we share with many other medical centers and clinics across the country, and so we hope our methods of practice are applicable to other practitioners in the field.

One of the biggest clinical challenges we face is convincing our addicted patients that they do indeed have a substance use problem. The adolescents and college-age youths in our practice are mostly undergraduate college students at Stanford or other colleges and universities in and around the Bay Area. They typically present to our clinic from the inpatient service or are brought in by parents. We collaborate closely with student mental health service providers, who send students our way when they suspect a cooccurring mental illness in addition to an addictive disorder, or when the overall clinical picture is very severe and hospitalization may be required. The most common chief complaint of the youth we see is not substance use, but rather a psychiatric symptom, most commonly depression and/or anxiety. Seldom do our adolescent patients come seeking help for substance use *per se*, and they are often resistant to the idea that their substance use is problematic. Therefore, the first interview is crucial. We must open a discussion of the substance use problems, while maintaining an adequate therapeutic alliance.

We explore a clinical case in depth to illustrate our treatment approach. The patient will herein be referred to as "MS." Identifying details of this patient's person and history have been changed without substantively changing the case, in order to protect her privacy.

MS was a 19 year old, Caucasian, female, Stanford University student referred to our outpatient treatment clinic from the campus health center for assessment and treatment of "mood swings" and "insomnia" for at least the past two months. She had been feeling "very sad," particularly in the last three weeks, with bouts of crying, difficulty completing her schoolwork, and thoughts of suicide, but no specific plan to take her life. She also reported excessive sleep, often not getting out of bed until midday, and episodes of overwhelming anxiety, during which she would begin to hyperventilate and "feel overwhelmed." In addition to symptoms of depression and anxiety, MS described a pattern of mood fluctuation, in which for up to three days at a time she could feel happy, even euphoric, with high energy, increased talkativeness, decreased sleep, and decreased need for sleep; i.e. not feeling tired even if she had only slept three hours the night before. MS also described some high-risk behaviors at these times: excessive spending and unprotected sex with multiple partners. Her last episode of elevated mood was over three weeks ago.

The history that the patient initially presented was highly suggestive of a mood disorder, possibly bipolar affective disorder. She endorsed current depression, and described that three weeks prior she had been having brief episodes of hypomania/mania. Certainly, the high risk sexual behaviors immediately alert the clinician to offer a test for HIV and other sexually transmitted diseases; to get a pregnancy test as part of the initial treatment plan; and to encourage protected rather than unprotected sexual contact.

In order to differentiate a substance-induced mood disorder from a major depressive or bipolar affective disorder, we employ several techniques during the history taking that we have found useful. We take a complete substance use history early in the interview, separate from the psychiatric history, focusing on age of onset and patterns of relapse and remission, as well as any sustained periods of sobriety and past treatment interventions. Only after these separate lines of questioning are complete do we explore the possible relationship between symptoms and substance use. This method allows us to have a more objective view of the relationship between substance use and psychiatric symptoms, than if the patient were simply asked "Do you get depressed first, and then start drinking, or do you start drinking, and then get depressed?" In our experience, a question asked in that way will more likely than not get a response that attributes substance use to the psychiatric illness. This is not because patients are intentionally duplicitous, but rather because the human brain is seeking to order the world, and to ascribe a rational cause to an irrational behavior. Further, because substance use is stigmatized, framing use as a side effect of illness may alleviate shame in the patient's mind. If separate lines of questioning are pursued, and the patient is able to give enough detail in their history, the clinician may be able to deduce a pattern that may provide a more valid reflection of reality.

MS first began using substances at age 15, when she started smoking marijuana two to three times per month. At age 17 she began to drink alcohol heavily, and at age 18 began snorting cocaine. For the past four to five months, she reported drinking much more than usual for her, drinking at least four times a week, typically consuming between five and seven drinks in a single sitting, and habitually drinking to the point of blacking out. She reported drinking even more if there were parties in the dormitories. She had tried to cut back on her own in the last couple of months, but had been unable to do so. She also reported that once she began drinking, even if she only intended to have one or two, she found she was not able to stop drinking. She admitted she planned her entire day, and even her week, around going out and drinking, and that it was the only thing she looked forward to all day long. She stated that she lived in a sorority, and that her entire social life revolved around going out and "partying" with her friends. When asked about other drugs currently, she admitted to rare marijuana use, about one to two times a month, and habitual cocaine use up until three weeks ago, when she "stopped cold turkey." Prior to three weeks ago, she had been snorting one to two lines during the week, and up to four or five lines per night on the weekends. She also smoked approximately five cigarettes a day, but could smoke up to a pack in a single sitting if she had been drinking heavily. "Then I smoke until my throat hurts."

The patient's substance use over the 12 months prior to her intake appointment, meets criteria for alcohol dependence, nicotine dependence, and possibly cocaine dependence as well. Further information would be needed to clarify the nature of her cocaine use. As pertains to her chief complaint, "mood swings" and "insomnia," the history reveals that all of her symptoms of depression and hypomania could be substance induced. The hypomanic symptoms may well have been due to intoxication with cocaine and/or alcohol, and the depressive symptoms to withdrawal from both substances. It is clinically significant that she stopped cocaine three weeks ago, around the same time that her mood became consistently more depressed. Withdrawal from cocaine in the three weeks, as well as the absence of the intense euphorogenic effects of cocaine intoxication, may well have contributed to the more intense depression that prompted her to seek treatment. Next, we try to get more details about the age of onset and patterns of relapse and remission of her "mood swings."

MS stated that her mood swings started in high school, fluctuating wildly up and down, but that she never sought or received professional treatment for this problem, and that it never impaired her function. She was not sure whether her mood swings were tied in any way to her menstrual cycle. She then volunteered, without our asking, that her mood problems pre-dated her substance use problems, because she was not drinking in high school. She also stated that she believed she began drinking to "self-medicate" her depression. This information was at odds with the substance use history she had given earlier, in which she stated that alcohol and marijuana use began at age 15, around the time she would have matriculated into high school. When asked about this discrepancy, she demurred by saying that in fact she would go for several months at a time without drinking or using marijuana in high school, and still had mood problems.

It is unclear whether her periods of sobriety in high school were really long enough to rule out substance-induced phenomena. Furthermore, high school itself is a time fraught with mood instability for many teenagers. Mood fluctuations during this time without any signs of role impairment, potentially represent normal adolescence, particularly if accompanied by an unstable home environment and intermittent substance use. However, we must take seriously the possibility that she indeed has a primary mood disorder. We do that by leaving open the possibility of this diagnosis, but remaining skeptical in the face of the discrepant evidence she presents. We feel that the weight of the retrospective evidence must be very good to favor a primary mental disorder diagnosis in the absence of sustained sobriety, because retrospective evidence in and of itself is potentially biased. Drinking in response to sadness tends to elicit more sympathy than becoming sad after drinking, and patients may present the former narrative to avoid disapproval.

As in the case of many patients, we will not be able to differentiate substance-induced mood disorder from primary mood disorder at the first interview. More definitive information will have to come from prospective monitoring during a period of sustained sobriety (per DSM-IV "rule of thumb" >4 weeks.) The diagnoses we would list after this initial encounter would include the following: (1) Mood disorder, not otherwise specified, (with a differential diagnosis which would include but is not limited to substance-induced mood disorder, major depressive disorder, bipolar affective disorder, premenstrual dysphoric disorder, dysthymia, etc); (2) Alcohol dependence; (3) Nicotine dependence; (4) Cocaine abuse versus dependence; and (5) Rule out marijuana use disorder.

The first diagnosis, mood disorder NOS, encompasses her current chief complaint, and indeed her reason for seeking treatment, and leaves open the possibility that she has a primary mental disorder in addition to substance use disorders. It also has the practical advantage of being reimbursable by the insurance company, while not ethically compromising the provider. The diagnosis of alcohol dependence comes next, as this appears to be her substance of choice, and the one with the longest period of addiction.

Third is nicotine dependence, a diagnosis that is too often left off by mental health care providers.[57] We feel strongly that nicotine dependence should be included, when applicable, for a number of different reasons. Nicotine addiction is the highest contributor toward morbidity and mortality in this country, taking up to 350,000 lives every year. There is evidence to suggest that quitting smoking at the same time as quitting drinking leads to better abstinence outcomes for both disorders. It is important for mental health care provider to identify nicotine dependence as a health care issue and to discuss treatment options, lest they covertly communicate that smoking is not a problem. The last diagnosis, cocaine abuse versus dependence, is suggested by the limited history obtained, but more history would be necessary to definitely make the diagnosis. We include it so as not to forget that her substance use escalated to include another illicit substance.

As we begin to clarify diagnoses and work toward an early treatment intervention, we ask about social context, as environmental factors are crucial toward understanding why adolescents use substances, and how we can help them break the cycle of addiction.

MS and her younger brother were raised by her parents in a fairly affluent middle class community. She stated there was not any overt sexual or physical abuse as a child, but her early home life had always been troubled and chaotic. Her father was an "alcoholic" and her mother "a bulimic who binges and purges every night." Her parents' relationship was overtly tumultuous, and they had initiated divorce proceedings in the year prior to MS seeking treatment. MS had always excelled in school, despite the limited support at home. In fact, school was her refuge from an unhappy home life. Her primary social support, from her early teens on, consisted of deviant peers. Since starting at Stanford University, she was actively involved in a sorority, and her primary extracurricular activity was her social life: "partying with my friends." She reported having a boyfriend, who also drank and used drugs, as well as several other casual sex partners. She had very limited contact with her parents or brother, and avoided returning home as much as possible, spending school vacations in the dorms or with friends. She presented as a very attractive, healthy, well-groomed teenager, whose physical appearance and general presentation gave no hint of the problems she was experiencing, or of the pattern of substance use she described.

MS's developmental trajectory is characteristic of the childhoods commonly described by adolescents who become involved in early problematic substance use. Although the information we have on her development is incomplete, it is enough to begin to understand what environmental factors led to her current clinical presentation. Her early life narrative is consistent with social developmental theories, including social control, social learning, behavioral choice, and stress and coping. As described by social control theory, *MS*'s substance use problems developed out of an absence of family bonding and cohesion, limited monitoring at home, and an early reliance on deviant peers for support. As per social learning theory, her parents modeled addictive behavior patterns in the home first, her father to alcohol, and her mother to food; and she subsequently affiliated with peers who normalized habitual substance use. Behavioral choice theory suggests that success in school may have served as a protective factor for MS, providing her with an alternative reward to getting high. The stress and coping theory implies that MS's early alienation and stress at home left her without the basic skills for affect regulation, such that the only coping skill she ever mastered was substance use.

In addition to understanding MS's life narrative, and the forces that contributed to her substance use disorder, it is essential to have a good grasp of the current social and contextual factors that may be perpetuating her substance use. Social selection and social causation theories have demonstrated that adolescents who use substances tend to socialize with other youths who use substances. At the time of her clinical presentation, MS was living in a sorority where using substances was the normative common culture, and she had a boyfriend who also habitually used substances. She continued to have minimal or no contact with her parents and brother, and avoided going home on vacations. After years of strife, her parents were officially going through a divorce.

Now that we have a working diagnosis, and some sense of MS's developmental trajectory and current social context, we discuss some early treatment intervention techniques that we have found useful. Our intervention is focused on establishing a therapeutic alliance, openly discussing factors that might be contributing toward substance use, and introducing the notions of abstinence and "cutting back" on substance use. Although we evolved these techniques through trial and error in our own practice, the approach resembles that of motivational interviewing in its emphasis on listening and collaboration, rather than a didactic, paternal stance.

In our attempts to establish a therapeutic alliance with our adolescent patients, we try very hard not to replicate the nagging insistence of exhausted, worried, and overwhelmed parents/teachers/friends who repeatedly tell them to stop using substances. Instead, in addition to gathering a careful history, we ask patients to think aloud about the impact their substance use has had on their lives, the upsides and the downsides. We listen intently to what patients perceive as good about using substances, in order to open the door to a freer discussion of what is bad about it. We then read aloud the diagnostic criteria from the DSM, and let the patient know that these are some of the problematic behaviors that are associated with an addictive pattern of substance use. We ask patients if they believe the criteria apply, and also let them know which criterion we think aptly describe them and why.

As we move toward suggesting a trial of abstinence or decreased substance use, we first embark on a detailed discussion of the environmental factors which contribute toward the patient's substance use. With adolescent patients in particular, we often hear the phrase: "I use because all my friends do." In the case of MS, she lived in a sorority with a reputation for partying, and had a circle of friends, including a boyfriend, with whom she habitually drank to get drunk. In other words, the network of people at the center of her life used substances. It is essential to explore with SUD patients how the relationships in their lives would be affected if they stopped using substances. Not uncommonly, removing the major shared activity, *i.e.* substance use, can threaten the foundation of the relationship. We try to acknowledge that stopping substance use may have a destabilizing effect on the patient's social milieu. Likewise, we ask patients to identify who in their lives might help them stop using substances, and encourage them to seek out settings in which substances are not used, which may range from religious communities to athletic teams to study groups.

Patients tend to normalize substance use by arguing that everyone around them is doing the same thing. It is helpful to introduce the idea that their perception may not be reality, by explaining that they have self-selected a group of high users, when in fact most kids of their age are not using substances with the same frequency and amount. We impart this perspective with the help of a self-administered computer survey, which is available to anyone on the Internet, takes no more than five minutes to complete, and is free of charge (http://www.CheckYourDrinking.net). This survey tells patients how their substance use compares to the national average. Patients are genuinely surprised to learn that, *e.g.* the average 19 year old consumes a mere fraction of the amount of alcohol they are consuming.

Once we have "wondered aloud" with patients about their substance use, explored the social context of their substance use, and attempted to challenge their denial around "normal substance use"; we make our first suggestions for change. For outpatients with the strongest denial and the least readiness for change, we agree to temporarily withhold definitive judgment about the presence of a substance use disorder, and suggest an agreed upon period of abstinence, as a kind of test of the patient's control over substances. With this approach we learn from the results together, and avoid patients lying to us, as well as appearing to say "I told you so." If patients experience significant withdrawal as they try to abstain from or reduce substance use, we prescribe medication to ease the withdrawal and thereby maximize chances of their ongoing commitment to the goal, and/or recommend hospitalization for the acute withdrawal phase.

For those who are not successful in their trial of abstinence the first time around, but are making the effort to stop or reduce substances, we continue to encourage them and work with them, even as we gently introduce the idea of visiting a 12-step group like Alcoholics Anonymous (AA). Some patients immediately resist AA by declaring that it is "too religious" for them. We have found several strategies useful in such situations. One is to clarify that AA is a spiritual program with no set religious beliefs, and as a result includes many atheists and agnostics as well as Muslims, Christians, and Jews. A second useful strategy is to inform the patient that there are multiple self-help groups available that include no spiritual component, for example SMART recovery. If the patient is horrified, this usually means that the objection to "religion" is more accurately described as an objection to taking steps to reduce substance use, and should be explored as such in session. On the other hand, if the patient shows genuine interest, we are not rigid in insisting on AA as the only way, as long as the patient regularly attends SMART recovery (or Secular Organization for Sobriety) and works actively to change substance use behavior.

We continue to follow and monitor our patients closely as they begin 12-step meetings. We use the language of AA and other 12-step groups, and ask patients at every appointment how meetings are going, which step they are working on, and how the relationship with their sponsor is working out. For a detailed description of AA and other self-help groups, please see Ref. 58. We believe that by being knowledgeable about the 12 steps and inquiring about patients' progress in the language of 12 steps, we reinforce their participation in and enthusiasm for this type of intervention. AA and other 12-step groups also encourage participants to develop relationships with same-age peers who are not using substances.

We also continually explore and monitor psychiatric symptoms. Whether dysphoria, insomnia, anxiety, or psychosis; it is sometimes enough to educate patients about substance-induced psychiatric problems, and reassure them that with sustained abstinence or significant substance reduction, many or all symptoms will resolve. We have seen this to be the case over and over again in clinical practice, and the empirical literature certainly supports this idea. If the patient comes to us already on a reasonable psychotropic regimen for a mental disorder but complaining of psychiatric symptoms, we will typically not change this regimen until the patient has achieved a period of sobriety or reduction, (2–4 weeks), and we have more clarity about the source of the disturbing symptoms. If sustained sobriety is achieved, we are able to reevaluate the patients' diagnosis prospectively. Sometimes this results in getting the patient off of psychotropics altogether, whereas at other times we need to initiate psychotropic medications.

MS readily agreed to a trial of abstinence, in the hope that her insomnia and mood swings would improve, and because she acknowledged that her substance use was out of control. We gave her a limited prescription of desyrel, a non-addictive sleep aid, to help with early withdrawal and promote abstinence, and to respond to her initial chief complaint of "insomnia." We also warned her about more serious withdrawal symptoms, such as delirium tremens and seizure, although we did not feel she was at risk for these. We often refer to the Clinical Institute Withdrawal Assessment of Alcohol Scale, Revised (CIWAR), used to screen medical and surgical patients for the risk of developing alcohol withdrawal syndrome. It can be found on the web at http://medapps.stanford.edu/detox/

She missed her next follow-up appointment scheduled for a week later, stating that she had forgotten it, but said she was doing better, had drastically reduced her alcohol consumption, and was not using any other substances except for occasional nicotine. We emphasized how important it was for her to come in and see us, and indeed the next week she did make her appointment. Her mood seemed upbeat, and she reported that she was sleeping better than she had in years, and her mood was much steadier. She had decided to tell everyone in her sorority, and her boyfriend, that she had to stop drinking and using drugs; and to her great surprise, they were very supportive. Her boyfriend apparently commented that he liked her "better off drugs," because she was not "so loopy." Life was looking up, and we continued the same treatment plan encouraging her try to further reduce her alcohol consumption down to nothing, and to even try and abstain from cigarettes, which she was smoking at the rate of 3 or 4 per week.

Several weeks later MS called before her appointment, stating that her sleep had gotten worse again, although still not as bad as before she initially presented, and her mood was low. She had not been using substances, but found herself getting progressively more depressed. Since it was almost four weeks from her initial appointment and she reported reduction/abstinence from substances, we started her on a trial of antidepressant therapy. She responded well, with improvements in sleep, mood, and anxiety. She remained largely abstinent from substances, and when she did use, used only alcohol and/or nicotine in moderation. She continued to struggle with affect regulation and self-esteem, and for these issues we referred her to psychotherapy and a skills training group, which emphasized distress tolerance and mindfulness meditation. At the time of this writing, she was 8 months into treatment and still doing well. We continue to see her on a monthly basis.

9. Conclusion and a Look into the Future

With this chapter we have tried to present some of the most important themes of adolescent and young adult substance use disorders, while emphasizing an ecological framework for understanding this devastating problem. We have touched upon recent epidemiologic trends, the most disturbing of which is the increased use among adolescents of prescription medications for non-medicinal purposes. We have discussed diagnostic challenges: the difficulty of using diagnostic categories which are based on adult patterns of substance use, and may have limited applicability to adolescents; the perennial problem of distinguishing primary from substance-induced mental disorders, particularly in a culture steeped in notions of self-medication; and the negative impact that financial constraints can have on accurate diagnosis. We have reviewed numerous developmental pathways, many of which point to family and peer interactions as central to maladaptive patterns of development; hence our belief that context is central both to the development of psychopathology, and to healing. Our review of treatment considerations consists primarily of behavioral treatments. Our clinical case presentation reflects the college-age patient population that we see, and illustrates the unique challenges of treating individuals who present for treatment, but do not self-identify as having a substance use disorder, in a treatment setting without a designated substance use disorder treatment program.

In terms of what the future holds, and how public policy may change current practice, the 2010 Affordable Care Act mandates that health insurance exchanges must cover mental health and substance abuse treatment at the same level as other types of health care. This policy change will help youths by providing more financial coverage for substance-related problems. It may also induce more people to open treatment programs for adolescents.

Acknowledgment

Preparation of this chapter was supported in part by the Department of Veterans Affairs Health Services Research and Development Service and NIAAA grant AA15685. The views expressed here are the authors' and do not necessarily reflect the views of the Department of Veterans Affairs.

References

1. Gould SJ. Exaptation: A crucial tool for evolutionary psychology, *J Social Issues* 1991; **47**: 43–65.
2. Office of Applied Studies. Overview of findings from the 2004 national survey on drug use and health. In: *Administration*. S.A.A.M.H.S, Ed. Rockville, MD: Office of Applied Studies, 2005.

3. American Psychiatric Association. *Diagnostic and Statistical Manual of Mental Disorders*. Washington, DC: American Psychiatric Association, 2000.
4. Lemke S, Schutte KK, Brennan PL, Moos RH. Sequencing the lifetime onset of alcohol-related symptoms in older adults: Is there evidence of disease progression? *J Stud Alcohol* 2005; **66**: 756–765.
5. Lewinsohn PM, Rohde P, Seeley JR. Alcohol consumption in high school adolescents: Frequency of use and dimensional structure of associated problems, *Addiction* 1996; **91**: 375–390.
6. Winters KC. Treating adolescents with substance use disorders: An overview of practice issues and treatment outcome, *Subst Abus* 1999; **20**: 203–225.
7. Deas D, Riggs PD, Langenbucher J. Adolescents are not adults: Developmental considerations in alcohol users, *Alcoholism: Clin Exp Res* 2000; **24**: 232–237.
8. Chung T, Martin CS, Winters KC. Diagnosis, course, and assessment of alcohol abuse and dependence in adolescents. In: Galanter M. Ed. *Recent Developments in Alcoholism, Vol. 17: Alcohol Problems in Adolescents and Young Adults: Epidemiology, Neurobiology, Prevention, Treatment.* New York, NY: Springer, 2005.
9. Chung T, Martin CS, Armstrong TD, Labouvie EW. Prevalence of DSM-IV alcohol diagnoses and symptoms in adolescent community and clinical samples, *J Am Acad Child Adolesc Psychiatry* 2002; **41**: 546–554.
10. Brown SA, Inaba RK, Gillin JC, Schuckit MA, Stewart MA, Irwin MR. Alcoholism and affective disorder: Clinical course of depressive symptoms, *Am J Psychiatry* 1995; **152**: 45–52.
11. Riggs PD, Davies RD. A clinical approach to integrating treatment for adolescent depression and substance abuse, *J Am Acad Child Adolesc Psychiatry* 2002; **41**: 1253.
12. Hallfors DD, Waller MW, Bauer D, Ford CA, Halpern CT. Which comes first in adolescence — sex and drugs or depression? *Am J Prev Med* 2005; **29**: 163–170.
13. Mueser KT, Drake RE, Wallach MA. Dual diagnosis: A review of etiological theories, *Addict Behav* 1998; **23**: 717–734.
14. Libby AM, Riggs PD. Integrated substance use and mental health treatment for adolescents: Aligning organizational and financial incentives, *J Child Adolesc Psychopharmacol* 2005; **15**: 826–834.
15. Kandel D, Ed. *Stages and Pathways of Drug Involvement: Examining the Gateway Hypothesis.* Cambridge, UK: Cambridge University Press, 2002.
16. Petraitis J, Flay BR, Miller T. Reviewing theories of adolescent substance use: Organizing pieces in the puzzle, *Psychol Bull* 1995; **117**: 67–86.
17. Wills TA, Sandy J, Yaeger A. Temperament and adolescent substance use: An epigenetic approach to risk and protection, *J Personality* 2000; **68**: 1127–1151.
18. Oetting E, Donnermeyer J. Primary socialization theory: The etiology of drug use and deviance, *Substance Use & Misuse* 1998; **33**: 995–1026.

19. Foshee V, Bauman K. Parental and peer characteristics as modifiers of the bond-behavior relationship: An elaboration of control theory, *J Health Social Behav* 1992; **33**: 66–76.
20. Maisto S, Carey K, Bradizza C. Social learning theory. In: Leonard K, & Blane, H, Eds. *Psychological Theories of Drinking and Alcoholism.* New York, NY: Guilford Press, 1999.
21. Audrain-Mcgovern J, Rodriguez D, Tercyak K, Epstein L, Goldman P, Wileyto E. Applying a behavioral economic framework to understanding adolescent smoking, *Psychol Addict Behav* 2004; **18**: 64–73.
22. Cooper ML, Russell M, Skinner JB, Frone MR, Mudar P. Stress and alcohol use: Moderating effects of gender, coping and alcohol expectancies, *J Abnormal Psychol* 1992; **101**: 139–152.
23. Chilcoat HD, Anthony JC. Impact of parent monitoring on initiation of drug use through late childhood, *J Am Acad Child Adolesc Psychiatry* 1996; **35**: 91–100.
24. Reifman A, Barnes G, Dintcheff B, Farrell M, Uhteg L. Parental and peer influences on the onset of heavier drinking among adolescents, *J Stud Alc* 1998; **59**: 311–317.
25. Colder C, Chassin L. The psychosocial characteristics of alcohol users versus problem users: Data from a study of adolescents at risk, *Dev Psychopathol* 1999; **11**: 321–348.
26. Getz J, Bray J. Predicting heavy alcohol use among adolescents, *Am J Orthopsych* 2005; **75**: 102–116.
27. Bullock B, Dishion T. Sibling collusion and problem behavior in early adolescence: Toward a process model for family mutuality, *J Abnormal Child Psychol* 2002; **30**: 143–153.
28. Windle M. Parental, sibling, and peer influences on adolescent substance use and alcohol problems, *Appl Dev Sci* 2000; **4**: 98–110.
29. Power T, Stewart C, Hughes S, Arbona C. Predicting patterns of adolescent alcohol use: A longitudinal study, *J Stud Alcohol* 2005; **66**(1): 74–81.
30. Barnes G, Welte J, Hoffman J, Dintcheff B. Shared predictors of youthful gambling, substance use, and delinquency, *Psychol Addict Behav* 2005; **19**: 165–174.
31. Li F, Barrera M, Hops H, Fisher K. The longitudinal influence of peers on the development of alcohol use in late adolescence: A growth mixture analysis, *J Behav Med* 2002; **25**: 203–315.
32. Krohn M, Lizotte A, Thornberry T, Smith C, Mcdowall D. Reciprocal causal relationships among drug use, peers, and beliefs: A five-wave panel model, *J Drug Issues* 1996; **26**: 405–428.
33. Sieving R, Perry C, Williams CL. Do friendships change behaviors, or do behaviors change friendships? Examining paths of influence in young adolescents' alcohol use, *J Adolesc Health* 2000; **26**: 27–35.

34. Colder C, Campell RT, Ruel E, Richardson J, Flay BR. A finite mixture model of growth trajectories of adolescent alcohol use: Predictors and consequences, *J Consult Clin Psychol* 2002; **70**: 976–985.
35. Wills TA, Sandy J, Yaeger A, Cleary S, Shinar O. Coping dimensions, life-stress, and adolescent substance use: A latent growth analysis, *J Abnormal Psychol* 2001; **110**: 309–323.
36. Mounts N, Steinberg L. An ecological analysis of peer influence on adolescent grade point average and drug use, *Dev Psychol* 1995; **31**: 915–922.
37. Erickson K, Crosnoe R, Dornbusch SM. A social process model of adolescent deviance: Combining social control and differential association perspectives, *J Youth Adolesc* 2000; **29**: 395–425.
38. Fitzgerald J, Arndt S. Reference group influence on adolescent alcohol use, *J Alc Drug Educ* 2002; **47**: 42–56.
39. Chen DY, Dormitzer C, Bejarano J, Anthony JC. Religiosity and the earliest stages of adolescent drug involvement in seven countries of Latin America, *Am J Epidemiol* 2004; **159**: 1180–1188.
40. Miller L, Davies M, Greenwald S. Religiosity and substance use and abuse among adolescents in the national comorbidity survey, *J Am Acad Child Adolesc Psychiatry* 2000; **39**: 1190–1197.
41. Wills TA, Sandy J, Yaeger A, Shinar O. Family risk factors and adolescent substance use: Moderation effects for temperament dimensions, *Dev Psychol* 2001; **37**: 283–297.
42. Windle M, Wiesner M. Trajectories of marijuana use from adolescence to young adulthood: Predictors and outcomes, *Dev Psychopathol* 2004; **16**: 1007–1027.
43. Wills TA, Duhamel K, Vaccaro D. Activity and mood temperament as predictors of adolescent substance use: Test of a self-regulation mediational model, *J Personality Social Psychol* 1995; **68**: 901–916.
44. Schulenberg J, Maggs J, Dielman T, Leech S, Kloska D, Shope J. On peer influences to get drunk: A panel study of young adolescents, *Merrill-Palmer Quarterly* 1999; **45**: 108–142.
45. Dishion T, Capaldi D, Spracklen K, Li F. Ecology of male adolescent drug use, *Dev Psychopathol* 1995; **7**: 803–824.
46. Jessor R, Donovan J, Costa F. *Beyond Adolescence: Problem Behavior and Young Adult Development.* Cambridge, UK: Cambridge University Press, 1991.
47. National Research Council. *Informing America's Policy on Illegal Drugs: What We Don't Know Keeps Hurting Us.* Washington, D.C.: National Academy Press, 2001.
48. Bickel WK, Johnson MW. Junk time: Pathological behaviour as the interaction of evolutionary and cultural forces. In: Vuchinich RE. Heather N, Eds. *Choice, Behavioural Economics and Addiction.* Oxford, UK: Elsevier, 2003.

49. Hesselbrock VM, Hesselbrock MN. Developmental perspectives on the risk for developing subtance abuse problems. In: Miller WR, Carroll HM, Eds. *Rethinking Substance Abuse: What the Science Shows and What We Should Do About It.* New York, NY: Guilford, 2006.
50. Furr-Holden CDM, Ialongo NS, Anthony JC, Petras H, Kellam SG. Developmentally inspired drug prevention: Middle school outcomes in a school-based randomized prevention trial, *Drug Alcohol Depend* 2004; **73**: 149–158.
51. Riggs PD, Mikulich SK, Hall SM. Effects of pemoline on ADHD, antisocial behaviors, and substance use in adolescents with conduct disorder and substance use disorder. *Proceedings of the College on Problems of Drug Dependence, Sixty-Third Annual Scientific Meeting.* Scottsdale, AZ, 2001.
52. Stanton MD. Getting reluctant substance abusers to engage in treatment/self-help: A review of outcomes and clinical options, *J Marital Fam Ther* 2004; **30**: 165–182.
53. Henggeler SW, Pickrel SG, Brondino MJ. Multisystemic treatment of substance-abusing and dependent delinquents: Outcomes, treatment fidelity, and transportability, *Ment Health Serv Res* 1999; **1**: 171–184.
54. Cornelius JR, Clark DB, Bukstein OG, Kelly TM, Solloum IM, Wood DS. Fluoxetine in adolescents with comorbid major depression and an alcohol use disorder: A 3-year follow-up study, *Addict Behav* 2005; **30**: 807–814.
55. Miller WR, Toscova RT, Miller JH, Sanchez V. A theory-based motivational approach for reducing alcohol/drug problems in college, *Health Educ Behav* 2000; **27**(6): 744–759.
56. Tevyaw TO, Monti PM. Motivational enhancement and other brief interventions for adolescent substance abuse: Foundations, applications and evaluations, *Addiction* 2004; **99**(Suppl. 2): 63–75.
57. Himelhoch S, Daumit G. To whom do psychiatrists offer smoking-cessation counseling? *Am J Psychiatry* 2003; **160**: 2228–2230.
58. Humphreys K. *Circles of Recovery: Self-Help Organizations for Addictions.* Cambridge, UK: Cambridge University Press, 2004.

Chapter 13

Somatoform Disorders

Richard J. Shaw, Rebecca S. Bernard, and David R. DeMaso

1. Introduction[a]

It is relatively common for children and adolescents to experience physical symptoms that cannot be readily explained and thus fall in the realm of the diagnosis of a somatoform disorder. Epidemiologic catchment area studies suggest that up to 12% of the general population may be affected.[1] The central feature of somatoform disorders is the presence of physical symptoms that are not fully explained by a general medical condition, often referred to as "somatization."[2] Unexplained somatic symptoms may be classified into categories that include musculoskeletal complaints, sensory motor deficits, visceral sensations, visceral pain, and chronic fatigue.[3] Common somatic complaints in children and adolescents include headaches, recurrent abdominal pain, limb pain, fatigue, dizziness, and chest pain.

1.1. *Definition*

A number of different models have been used to conceptualize the process of somatization. Some researchers have defined somatization as a pattern of seeking medical help for physical symptoms which the individual perceives as being attributed to a physical disease but which cannot be fully explained by

[a]This chapter has been adapted from previously published chapters on Pediatric Pain and Somatoform Disorders, published in: Shaw RJ, DeMaso DR (2006), *Clinical Manual of Pediatric Psychosomatic Medicine: Mental Health Consultation with Physically Ill Children and Adolescents* and Somatoform Disorders, published in Shaw RJ, DeMaso DR, Eds. *Textbook of Pediatric Psychosomatic Medicine*, Washington DC: American Psychiatric Publishing, Inc., 2010 Used with permission.

pathophysiologic mechanisms.[4] Others focus on the individual's ability or, more appropriately, inability to tolerate and express psychological distress. This distress tends to be conveyed through somatic complaints.[5] Researchers purport that somatization is a universal phenomenon in young children because they do not have the cognitive or linguistic abilities to understand and express how they are feeling.[6] The assumption in most cases is that there may be a physical basis for the child's symptoms, but that the intensity of the symptoms has become exaggerated.[2] Somatization is more prevalent in cultures that are accommodating of disabilities due to physical illness but not accepting of disability due to psychological symptoms.

Somatic symptoms are often seen as a form of psychological defense against intrapsychic distress, referred to as "primary gain." Primary gain is an unconscious process that serves to restore psychological equilibrium, but in the process distorts reality and can lead to physical disability. Once present, symptoms may be consciously used to achieve potential interpersonal benefits, a process referred to as "secondary gain." Because diagnoses of somatoform disorders are made on the basis of the exclusion of physical health conditions, they tend to promote an "either/or" approach which carries the risk of overlooking potentially treatable general medical conditions that may coexist with psychological distress.[7]

1.2. *Epidemiology*

Studies of primary care pediatric populations report relatively low rates of patients who meet full criteria for a somatoform disorder, but large numbers of patients with clinically significant somatic symptoms.[7] For children and adolescents, community surveys have identified four major symptom clusters of recurrent somatic complaints: cardiovascular, gastrointestinal, pain/weakness, and pseudoneurological.[8] Young children often report recurrent headaches and abdominal pain as well as feeling fatigued and experiencing gastrointestinal symptoms.[9] Recurrent abdominal pain accounts for 5% of pediatric office visits and headaches have been reported in 20–55% of all children. During adolescence, 10% of the population report frequent headache, chest pain, nausea, and fatigue.[10] In early childhood, there is no significant difference in prevalence rates between males and females. By adolescence, the prevalence of somatic complaints is five times greater in females than in males.

1.3. *Health care utilization*

Patients with somatoform disorders are a source of significant health care costs, and may undergo unnecessary and potentially harmful medical interventions.[11]

Studies have shown that somatization significantly increases utilization of both outpatient and inpatient medical care, and that annual medical care costs may be double those of non-somatizing patients.[12] Adults with somatoform symptoms tend to have higher levels of role impairment, more missed days of work, and higher rates of unemployment. In children and adolescents with a history of somatization, there is a greater likelihood of school absences, poor academic performance, and frequent emotional and behavioral difficulties, including a link with symptoms of depression and anxiety.[13] Barsky *et al.*[12] have estimated that the total incremental cost of somatization in the United States is approximately $256 billion per year.

2. Developmental Factors

Young children in general have greater difficulties with the verbal expression of emotional distress and it is considered developmentally appropriate for such distress to be expressed through physical symptoms.[2] Thus, a certain degree of somatization can be considered normal.[14] In fact, the *Diagnostic and Statistical Manual for Primary Care (DSM-PC)* includes a category of symptoms known as "Somatic Complaints Variation," which is described as the universal experience of discomfort and complaints that does not interfere with everyday functioning, including recurrent abdominal pain, headaches, and "growing pains."[15] For example, young children who are anxious about attending preschool may express their anxiety through headaches, stomachaches, or other physical symptoms. It is only as they get older that children develop a greater awareness of their emotions and increased ability to express their emotions through words and behavior. By contrast, younger children are more likely to make use of immature defenses, including somatization.[16,17] This developmental step generally results in the reduction of the child's need to use somatic symptoms as a way to express emotions.[2] Children who are overwhelmed by their physical symptoms and who have little training in the recognition and expression of their emotions may persist with their tendency to use somatic complaints as a way to express their feelings. Additionally, children who have been severely abused are more likely to use physical symptoms to express emotional trauma.

From a developmental perspective, pediatric somatoform symptoms are often expressed differently at different ages. For example, young children experience affective distress in the form of somatic sensations which initially tend to be monosymptomatic, with recurrent abdominal pain and headaches predominating in early childhood. However, symptoms of limb pain, fatigue, and neurological symptoms emerge with increasing age.[10]

Developmental theories can shed some light on the appearance of unexplained somatic symptoms. By age 6 or 7, children have become more aware of their feelings of anxiety. For children who develop in an environment that permits verbalization of emotions, the expression of anxiety should develop relatively normally. However, children whose families discourage verbalization of feelings or who have experienced high levels of trauma, are more likely to somatize in response to intense anxiety.[18]

3. Risk Factors for Pediatric Somatization

There are multiple factors that place children and adolescents at risk for developing somatic symptoms or disorders. Specifically, genetic and familial factors, demographic and sociocultural factors, childhood physical illness, stressful life events, personality traits and coping styles, learned complaints, and psychiatric comorbidity have all been associated with pediatric somatization.

3.1. *Genetic and familial factors*

3.1.1. *Genetic*

Rates of somatization are higher among families than in the general population. Monozygotic twin studies have found a concordance rate of 29% for somatization disorders.[19] Similarly, 10–20% of first-degree relatives of patients with somatization disorder meet criteria for this disorder. Further support of a genetic etiology is evidenced by the familial link between somatization disorders and other psychiatric disorders. Family members of youngsters with somatization disorders have higher rates of anxiety and depressive disorders.[14] One hypothesis is that genetic factors may lead to personality traits that predispose certain individuals to somatize, particularly when combined with environmental risk factors.[4] More recently, researchers have proposed that serotonergic amino acids, specifically decreased plasma concentrations of tryptophan, a precursor of serotonin, or perhaps elevated plasma levels of bradykinin, may be implicated in somatization.[20,21]

3.1.2. *Familial*

Parental modeling and the familial culture regarding the expression of emotion may play roles in pediatric somatization. Studies have noted a potential link between parental medical symptoms and the expression of somatic symptoms during childhood.[19] Children who observe their parents utilizing somatic symptoms to express emotional distress appear to use these same strategies, especially those families that discourage the emotional expression of distress.[22]

Yet another role that families may play in the development and maintenance of somatic symptoms stems from family systems theory. Somatic symptoms may draw attention away from a significant parent–child conflict.[2] Symptoms may even provide a way for a parent to meet their own unresolved needs for attention by their interactions with pediatric care providers or through sympathy and attention from friends and family members. The concept of "enmeshment" refers to the blurring of intergenerational boundaries with overinvolved and hyperresponsive family interactions. Minuchin *et al.*[23] postulated that family enmeshment, overprotectiveness, rigidity, and lack of conflict resolution predisposed family members to the development of somatization. It has been suggested that children in such families with significant degrees of conflict may develop somatic complaints as a mechanism to avoid any emotional expression that may exacerbate familial stress.

There also has been interest in the concept of attachment, specifically insecure patterns of attachment, and its relationship with somatization. Adults who endorsed insecure attachment styles have been found to be more likely to present with medically unexplained physical symptoms.[24] Additionally, adolescents with a tendency toward somatization tend to report lower perceptions of parental affection.[25] Waldinger *et al.*[24] suggests that individuals with somatization may minimize the expression of negative affect and instead focus on physical symptoms, and care seeking for unexplained medical complaints.

3.2. *Demographic and sociocultural factors*

3.2.1. *Demographic*

Somatic symptoms have been related to age, birth order, gender, and ethnic background. There is a high frequency of somatic complaints in younger children, according to most studies.[2] Young children are more likely to experience distress during pain episodes or painful procedures partly due to their less mature coping skills.[26] Studies have indicated that first-born children seem to have lower pain thresholds which may in part be due to greater reinforcement of pain complaints that may occur with first time parents. Adolescent girls generally report lower pain tolerance, more pain complaints, and increased general somatic symptoms compared to boys.[25] Studies on the use of defense mechanisms also have shown that females tend to have higher rates of somatization.[16] Differing general role expectations between boys and girls stemming from cultural and societal expectations have been hypothesized to lie behind this difference.[27]

3.2.2. *Sociocultural*

Culture and ethnicity play important roles in determining how much expression of pain is acceptable, the level of pain to which an individual should respond, and strategies used to provide soothing and comfort as well as ways in which individuals demonstrate their response to pain.[26] Individuals of lower socioeconomic status and/or who live in rural areas demonstrate higher rates of somatoform disorders.[28] Local cultural ideas about acceptable and credible ways to express distress may play a role. For example, falling down with loss or alteration in consciousness, or fainting, has historically been a culturally sanctioned manner to express distress and is a feature in a variety of culture-specific syndromes.

3.4. *Childhood physical illness*

Although the data is mixed and retrospective, there does appear to be a connection between childhood physical illness and the latter development of somatization. Hypochondriacal adults have reported being sick more often as children as well as missing school more often for health reasons.[29] Persistent childhood abdominal pain has been associated with multiple somatic complaints in adulthood.[30] Approximately, 66% of men and 75% of women who reported frequent somatic symptoms as adults reported frequent somatic symptoms during high school.[31] Children who tend to somatize appear to have a greater susceptibility to physical diseases and increased sensitivity to their internal states.[2] For example, children with irritable bowel syndrome have heightened sensitivity in their gastrointestinal tract. Patients with recurrent abdominal pain that does not have a definitive medical diagnosis similarly may have identifiable alterations in gastric motility and sensitivity, including increased transit times or exaggerated utility responses to multiple stimuli, including stress and food.[32]

3.5. *Stressful life events*

Early adverse life experiences may contribute to the development of adult somatization. In particular, individuals with histories of childhood trauma (including sexual, physical, and emotional abuse) appear to be at increased risk.[24] Severe forms of child sexual abuse have been associated with higher rates of somatization.[4] Between 33 and 55% of adult patients with non-epileptic events have reported a history of childhood sexual abuse.[33]

Stress is thought to exacerbate physical symptoms in children with and without somatization.[2] School-related stressors, family stressors, and stressors related to the illness may play important roles in the development and/or exacerbation of somatic symptoms. In fact, the following factors were significantly correlated with somatic symptoms in Finnish high school students: illness or physical injury within the family, family conflict, breakup with a boyfriend/girlfriend, and parental absence.[34] Adult patients with hypochondriasis retrospectively have recalled higher level of conflict between parents, increased traumatic sexual experiences in childhood, and increased victimization by violence when compared to a group that does not have somatic complaints.[29]

3.6. *Personality traits and coping styles*

3.6.1. *Personality traits*

Somatoform symptoms have been found to be more common in children who are conscientious, sensitive, insecure, anxious, and in those who strive for high school achievement.[2] The tendency to withdraw from others in response to pain, the capacity to cope independently, and the ability to seek social support underlies how children and adolescents cope when they are in pain. Increased pain behavior has been noted in patients with difficult temperaments (*e.g.* increased reactivity, decreased adaptability, low sensory threshold, negative mood, and greater intensity of reactions).[26]

Somatic complaints in adults have been linked to what has been termed "somatosensory amplification" or the tendency to experience normal somatic sensations as "intense, noxious and disturbing."[35] These patients tend to be hypervigilant to their own bodily sensations, to overreact to these sensations, and to interpret them as indicating physical illness.[35] EEG examinations of evoked potentials suggest that somatizing patients are not able to discriminate between relevant and irrelevant physical stimuli and have an inability to habituate to repetitive stimuli.[36]

3.6.2. *Coping style*

There are a variety of conceptualizations of children's coping styles. Patients may be classified based on their habitual tendency to approach or avoid new situations.[37] Similarly, individuals may manifest coping styles that are either problem focused (directly trying to alter a stressor or external circumstance) or emotion focused (trying to regulate their emotional response to a stressor). Neither one of these coping styles is necessarily associated with better adaptation, but the critical dimension appears to be whether or not the child has the freedom to use the specific approach that is most comfortable and successful in stressful situations. It can be helpful for the patient in some circumstances to confront stressful medical information by seeking out information, while in other situations the ability to use distraction is adaptive (*e.g.* during a painful procedure). A patient's coping style can be maladaptive. For instance in conversion disorder, individuals generally have difficulties dealing with confrontation and interpersonal conflict, and tend to use avoidance, denial, and repression as coping strategies.[38]

3.7. *Learned complaints*

Many cases of somatization have an antecedent true underlying general medical condition that may then be reinforced by parental and/or peer attention. Reinforcement for physical symptoms may come in multiple ways (*i.e.* the prescription of medications, missing school, and attention from family members). In assuming a sick role, children may elicit concern and attention from parents and/or be excused from school and extracurricular activities, which may in turn reinforce their somatic complaints and make them reluctant to give up these symptoms. Continued increased parental attention and/or avoidance of unpleasant school pressures may only further reinforce the symptom. There may be reinforcement related to removal from a stressful home environment. Physicians may unwittingly reinforce physical symptoms by their focus on diagnostic procedures and treatment.

3.8. *Psychiatric comorbidity*

There is an association between somatization and a number of psychiatric disorders including depression and anxiety. Major depression has been identified in 30–60% of patients with chronic pain and in 48–90% of patients with somatization.[39] Depression also has been found in 54–88% of patients presenting with conversion symptoms.[39] Thus, depression appears to be a powerful contributing factor to the development and maintenance of somatic symptoms.[25] Children, particularly girls, with somatization symptoms have higher rates of depression and anxiety.[13]

Although depression may be secondary to the physical illness or its treatment, the presence of a depressive disorder increases the risk of developing chronic pain conditions. There are studies that have shown that as many as 60% of patients with depression report pain symptoms.[40] Additionally, there is a strong relationship between pain and anxiety. Pain often results in symptoms of anxiety, while anxiety may decrease the pain threshold and increase the sensation of pain.[41] Recurrent abdominal pain in children and adolescents is thought to have a strong association with symptoms of anxiety, and to a lesser extent depression.[42] It is not certain whether there is a causal relationship between recurrent abdominal pain and anxiety, or whether there is a shared common risk factor or pathophysiology.[43]

4. Model of Pediatric Somatization

Figure 1 outlines a model of pediatric somatization that details the pathways associated with the development of somatic symptoms and the risk factors described above. Physical symptoms may be generated by authentic physical illness and/or as an indirect result of psychological distress. Although the tendency to experience emotional distress in the form of physical symptoms is a universal characteristic in younger children, it may persist beyond what is considered developmentally appropriate as a result of genetic, temperamental, or environmental factors. This tendency in older children, adolescents, and adults is called "alexithymia."[6] It is defined as a difficulty in verbally expressing psychological distress and is associated with the expression of anxiety and distress through complaints of physical symptoms.

Physical symptoms may be promoted and given more attention by the individual through the process of somatosensory amplification described and defined earlier as the tendency to amplify the experience of normal somatic sensations and

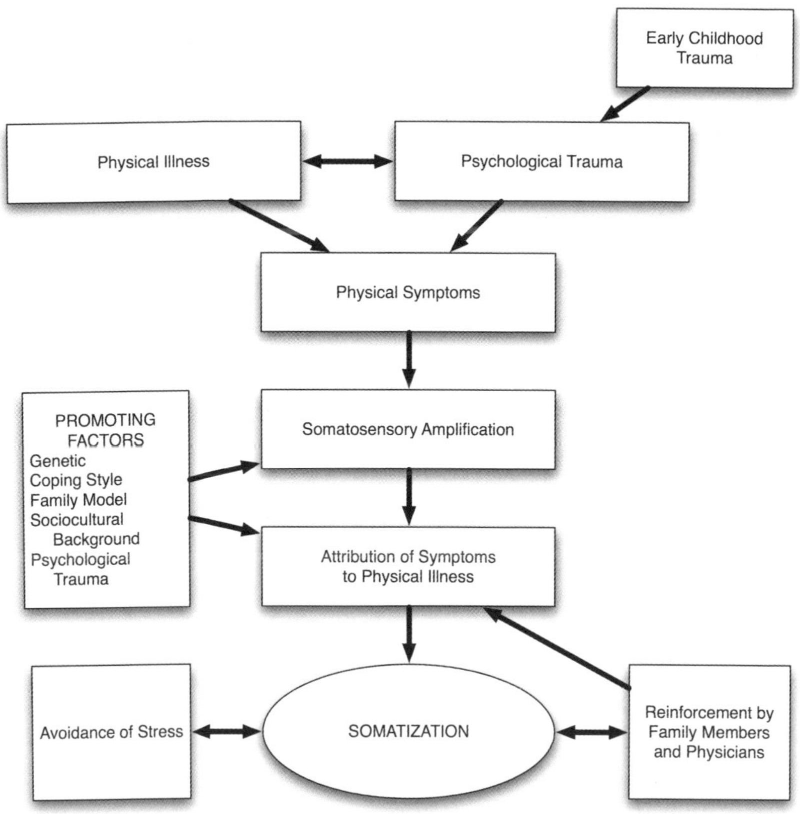

Fig. 1: Developmental model of pediatric somatization.

to interpret these sensations as having a potential pathological basis.[35] In somatoform disorders, these physical symptoms are frequently reinterpreted and attributed to medical illness. Patients who have had a prior traumatic physical illness (*e.g.* cancer) may be particularly prone to scan their bodies for physical symptoms and interpret these symptoms, often incorrectly, as heralding illness recurrence. This pathway continues toward clinically significant somatization and the diagnosis of a somatoform disorder.

The process of somatization may be reinforced by attention from caregivers and physicians and/or avoidance of stressful situations (*e.g.* attending school or competitive athletics) as a consequence of their illness behavior. These feedback loops may help establish a pattern of the illness behavior that persists beyond the original reason for the symptom, whether it was physiological or psychological in nature. Psychological trauma may play an important role in amplifying symptoms and fostering somatoform symptoms. Treatment interventions are targeted at each step or pathway in this model (Fig. 2).

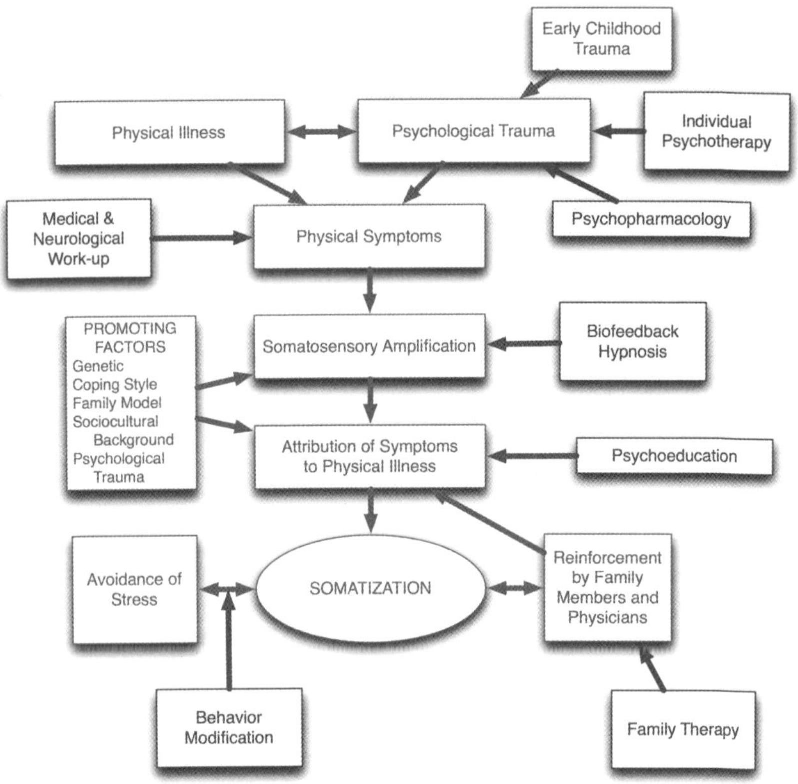

Fig. 2: Treatment approaches to pediatric somatization.

Recent imaging studies have the potential to help explain some of the neural mechanisms involved in somatization. Further, MRI studies of patients with conversion disorder have shown decreased or absent activation in the contralateral sensorimotor cortex during sensory or motor tasks.[44,45] Lower rates of cerebral glucose metabolism have also been demonstrated in patients with somatization disorder.[46] There is debate as to whether these neuroimaging studies suggest an exclusion of sensorimotor representations from awareness through attentional processes, or whether the findings might better be explained by the modulation of such representations by primary affective or stress-related factors.[45]

5. The Somatoform Disorders

In the *Diagnostic and Statistical Manual of Mental Disorders* 4th Edition, Text Revision (DSM-IV-TR), somatoform disorders are characterized by the presence of one of more physical complaints for which an adequate medical explanation cannot be found.[28] The symptoms are severe enough to cause significant distress or impairment in functioning and result in the family seeking medical help (Table 1).

The International Statistical Classification of Disease and Related Health Problems, 10th Revision (ICD-10)[47] similarly defines the main features of somatoform disorders as "the repeated presentation of physical symptoms together with persistent requests for medical investigations, in spite of repeated negative findings and reassurances by doctors that the symptoms have no physical basis. If any physical disorders are present, they do not explain the nature and extent of the symptoms or the distress and preoccupation of the patient." The ICD-10 lists somatization disorder, undifferentiated somatoform disorder, hypochondriacal disorder, persistent somatoform pain disorder, and other somatoform pain disorder, all of which match with their DSM-IV-TR counterparts. The ICD-10 differs from the DSM-IV-TR by its inclusion of the diagnosis, somatoform autonomic dysfunction, and by its exclusion of body dysmorphic disorder which has been hypothesized to have features more in common with obsessive-compulsive disorder.

5.1. *Somatization disorder*

5.1.1. *Definition*

Somatization disorder is a chronic debilitating illness characterized by the presence of multiple somatic complaints that cannot be adequately explained on the basis of physical or laboratory investigations. The combination and number of

Table 1: Selected Medical Differential Diagnosis for Somatoform Disorders

Acquired immune deficiency syndrome
Acquired myopathies
Acute intermittent porphyria
Angina
Basal ganglia disease
Brain tumors
Cardiac arrhythmias
Chronic systemic infections
Creutzfeldt-Jakob disease
Guillan-Barre syndrome
Hyperparathyroidism
Hyperthyroidism
Lyme disease
Migraine headaches
Multiple sclerosis
Myasthenia gravis
Narcolepsy
Optic neuritis
Periodic paralysis
Polymyositis
Seizure disorders
Superior mesenteric artery syndrome
Systemic lupus erythematosis

pain, gastrointestinal, sexual/reproductive, and pseudoneurological symptoms required over a several year time period and the inclusion of criteria, which are appropriate only for postpubertal and/or sexually active patients, mitigate against the diagnosis of the somatization disorder in childhood and adolescence.[9] As a result, it is likely that this disorder has been underdiagnosed in children who are more likely to meet DSM-IV-TR criteria for an undifferentiated somatoform disorder.

5.1.2. *Epidemiology*

The lifetime prevalence of DSM IV TR somatization disorder in adults is estimated to be between 0.2 and 2% for women, and less than 0.2% in men.[28] Epidemiologic catchment area studies show a 10:1 female-to-male ratio in the lifetime prevalence.[48] Women with somatization disorder outnumber men by 5–20 times. Somatization disorder is more commonly observed in families where there is a relative with the same disorder and in children who have been exposed to sexual abuse. Adults often date the onset of their symptoms to adolescence. While no data exists regarding the prevalence of somatization disorder in childhood, surveys examining pediatric somatic complaints have identified polysymptomatic "somatizers."[4] Although the criteria used to define those with frequent unexplained somatic complaints vary, prevalence rates of 4.5–10% in boys and 10.7–15% in girls have been reported.[4]

5.1.3. *Clinical features*

The full DSM-IV-TR somatization disorder criteria are rarely reported in childhood. There is commonly a history of evolving recurrent unexplained physical complaints. Headaches, fatigue, muscle aches, abdominal distress, back pain, and blurred vision are commonly reported.[8] Prepubertal children are more likely to report headache and abdominal pain, while limb pain, fatigue, and muscle aches appear to increase with age. Specific symptom constellations may result in the diagnosis of syndromes such as irritable bowel syndrome, chronic fatigue, or fibromyalgia. Somatic symptoms are strongly associated with psychological distress, as well as comorbid mood and anxiety disorders.[7] These patients tend to be high utilizers of pediatric services. Comorbid anxiety and depressive symptoms are common as well as conduct or substance-related disorders.

5.2. *Conversion disorder*

5.2.1. *Definition*

Conversion disorder is defined by the presence of one or more neurological symptoms that cannot bc medically explained after thorough investigation. Thc hallmark of conversion is that the disruption in neurological function does not follow known neurologic anatomic pathways. The DSM-IV-TR specifies that symptoms must be associated with psychological factors that include conflicts or other stressors that precede the development or worsening of the conversion symptom. The symptom must not be consciously feigned, and must produce clinically significant distress or impairment in functioning. The symptoms must be viewed as abnormal within the individual's own culture. Although the DSM-IV-R classified conversion disorder as a somatoform disorder, it is important to note that the International Statistical Classification of Diseases and Related Health Problems, 10th revision (ICD-10)[47] locates conversion disorder as one of the dissociative disorders, with a presumed different etiological mechanism. Some authors have noted that dissociative symptoms are much more frequent in conversion disorder, in contrast to the other somatoform disorders.[49]

The term "conversion" derives from the psychoanalytic concept that the somatic symptom is the result of an unconscious resolution of a psychological conflict—commonly a sexual or aggressive impulse—in which the mind "converts" psychological distress into a physical symptom. The resulting reduction in anxiety may explain in part the phenomenon of "*la belle indifférence*," or the apparent lack of concern sometimes observed in patients with conversion disorder. Primary gain is obtained by keeping the conflict out of consciousness and minimizing anxiety. The symptom allows the partial expression of the forbidden wish, but in a disguised form, so that the patient does not need to consciously confront the unacceptable impulse. Secondary gain in the form of increased attention from caregivers or being excused from various pressures or responsibilities may also contribute to the development or continuation of conversion symptoms.

5.2.2. *Epidemiology*

Conversion disorder is the most common type of somatoform disorder in childhood. The incidence varies between 0.5–10% in pediatric patients.[9] Conversion disorder is three times more common in adolescents than preadolescents, and rarely occurs in children younger than five years. Females tend to outnumber males in adolescence, while the ratio is more equal in younger children. Conversion disorder is more common in rural populations, among those from lower socioeconomic status, and in adolescents who are under pressure to perform in academic or athletic settings. The incidence of conversion disorder is increased following physical or sexual abuse.

5.2.3. *Clinical features*

Patients with conversion disorders may present with motor and/or sensory symptoms as well as loss of consciousness. "Motor symptoms" include abnormal movements, disturbances in gait, weakness, paralysis, and tremors. "Sensory symptoms" include anesthesia and paresthesia, commonly in one of the extremities, as well as deafness, blindness, and tunnel vision. Patients may present with symptoms of "*seizures*," referred to as conversion "seizures," pseudoseizures, non-electrical seizures, or non-epileptic events. Functional neuroimaging studies suggest that conscious active inhibition in selected areas of the brain may be responsible for the neurologic symptoms.[39]

Symptom onset is generally acute. Individual conversion symptoms are generally short lived, remitting within two weeks in most hospitalized patients.[28] Good prognostic factors include sudden onset, an easily identifiable stressor, good premorbid adjustment, and absence of comorbid physical or psychiatric illnesses. Patients with conversion seizures have a poorer prognosis than those with paralysis or blindness. The recurrence of symptoms is not uncommon, occurring in 20–25% of cases within one year.[28] Comorbid mood and anxiety disorders, including separation anxiety disorder, are common. Stressful family events (*e.g.* recent divorce, current marital conflict, or death of a close family member) are common.[50] Estimates of the presence of concomitant epilepsy in patients with conversion seizures vary widely, although recent data suggests that 10% of patients may have both diagnoses. Other important physiologic disorders include daydreaming, inattention, movement disorders, and parasomnias.[51] Some studies have suggested that up to 30% of patients diagnosed with conversion symptoms were subsequently discovered to have had a misdiagnosed general medical condition.[39]

5.3. *Pain disorder*

5.3.1. *Definition*

In the DSM-IV-TR psychological factors can play an important role in the onset, severity, exacerbation, or maintenance of pain as well as causing significant distress or functional impairment.[28] Pain disorders are divided into: (1) disorders associated with psychological factors, in which emotional factors alone are judged to play a major role; (2) disorders associated with psychological factors and a general medical condition, in which both together are deemed to have important roles; and (3) disorders entirely related to a general medical condition. The first two are coded as mental disorders on axis I and the latter are coded on axis III.

5.3.2. *Epidemiology*

Between 25 and 44% of children and adolescents report somatic pain complaints which are generally transient in nature. Headaches and limb pains are more frequently seen in the 11–13 year age group whereas older adolescents are most likely to report headaches, chest pain, and abdominal pain. Approximately 10–20% of children younger than 10 years report recurrent headaches, and the frequency of migraine headache increases significantly after puberty, particularly in adolescent girls.[52] Community based studies suggest that 75% of adolescents experience abdominal pain, and that 13–15% experience pain on a weekly basis.[53] Most of these patients do not have underlying disease but require an evaluation and treatment to provide reassurance. Complaints of recurrent abdominal pain complaints have been reported in 10–25% of school-age children and adolescents, and account for 2–4% of pediatric office visits.[54] The gender ratio is equal in early childhood, but girls are more symptomatic in later childhood and adolescence.[55] Symptoms of pain increase significantly in patients with underlying physical conditions. Approximately 25% of pediatric cancer patients report daily pain episodes, while pain is a common symptom in 60% of children with HIV.[56]

5.3.3. *Clinical features*

Recurrent abdominal pain is common with a variety of presentations. These disorders have been classified by the Committee on Childhood Functional Gastrointestinal Disorders, Multinational Working Teams to Develop Criteria for Functional Disorders (Rome II) into five subgroups: functional dyspepsia, irritable bowel syndrome, functional abdominal pain, abdominal migraine, and aerophagia.[57] Symptoms may fit into a well-defined clinical entity or present as a more poorly defined clinical syndrome.[32] It is believed that pediatric recurrent abdominal pain may progress into adult gastrointestinal disorders (*e.g.* irritable bowel syndrome).[54] Recurrent abdominal pain is significantly associated with psychopathology including anxiety and depression.[42]

5.4. *Hypochondriasis*

5.4.1. *Definition*

Hypochondriasis is a preoccupation with the idea that one has or may have a serious disease despite medical reassurance. This preoccupation is based on the misinterpretation of physical symptoms or signs, and is severe enough to cause clinically significant distress or functional impairment, but is not of delusional intensity.[28] The disorder must last at least six months to meet DSM-IV-TR criteria. In contrast to other forms of somatization, it is the significance attached to various symptoms, rather than the physical symptoms themselves, which produces distress.

5.4.2. *Epidemiology*

Although it is believed that hypochondriasis may have its onset during adolescence, the onset of symptoms is much more common in early to middle adulthood with men and women equally affected. The full syndrome of hypochondriasis is fairly rare with a prevalence of approximately 0.2–0.8% in adult populations, although some studies suggest rates of 3–9% in primary care or medical settings.[7]

In adults, prevalence rates of 4–6% have been reported in a general clinic population.[19] Many patients in primary care present with acute symptoms of hypochondriasis that resolve spontaneously with reassurance from their physician. By contrast, very little data is available regarding the incidence or prevalence of hypochondriasis in children and adolescents.

5.4.3. *Clinical features*

Patients with hypochondriasis present with a set of core symptoms that include a fear of disease, the conviction of having a disease, and bodily preoccupation or absorption associated with multiple somatic complaints.[58] Patients often complain of poor relationship with their physicians, feelings of frustration and anger, and are prone to "doctor shopping." Patients with hypochondriasis are particularly prone to "somatosensory amplification" and may experience significant secondary gain as a result of their ability to adopt the sick role. Complications may arise as the result of exposure to unnecessary treatments and procedures. Adolescents may manifest subclinical forms of the disorder, *e.g.* an unrealistic concern that one has AIDS or cancer.[14] Hypochondriasis is commonly associated with both mood and anxiety disorders and has features in common with OCD.

5.5. *Body dysmorphic disorder*

5.5.1. *Definition*

Body Dysmorphic Disorder (BDD) is characterized by an excessive preoccupation with a defect in appearance. This defect is either imagined or is too minor to warrant the degree of concern and distress felt by the individual. Symptoms cannot be better accounted for by another psychiatric illness.

5.5.2. *Epidemiology*

Although there are no pediatric epidemiological data, estimates of the adult prevalence ranges from 1.9% in a non-clinical sample to 12% in psychiatric outpatients.[59] Disease onset is believed to most often occur during adolescence or early adulthood, although childhood cases have been reported. Patients may wait a mean of six years before seeking treatment.[60] Unlike many other somatoform disorders, the ratio of men to women is nearly equal. Many people with the disorder do not seek psychiatric help, but rather seek treatment from dermatologists and plastic surgeons, which may influence efforts to study the psychological aspects of this disorder.

5.5.3. *Clinical features*

While any body part or aspect of physical appearance may be a source of concern and several body parts may be involved simultaneously, concerns generally focus on the patient's face or head (*e.g.* size or shape of the nose, eyes, lips, teeth, or other facial features, thinning hair or excessive facial hair, acne, wrinkles, or scars). Patients may spend hours per day checking the defect, or engage in excessive grooming or exercising to minimize or erase the defect, or even become housebound. This disorder shares much in common with OCD. Both disorders are characterized by the presence of intrusive thoughts and repetitive behaviors, as well as the need to seek reassurance. Those individuals with BDD who are successful in obtaining surgery may continue to be concerned about the perceived defect, or may shift the focus of attention to other aspects of their appearance.[60] Substantial comorbidity exists between BDD and depression, OCD, social phobia, delusional disorder, anorexia nervosa, gender identity disorder, and narcissistic personality disorder. Up to 20% of affected patients have histories of attempted suicide.[19]

6. Assessment

The biological, psychiatric, and social dimensions need to be evaluated both separately and in relation to each other in all somatoform disorders. Patients should have a complete and comprehensive medical workup to rule out serious medical illness combined with an effort to avoid unnecessary and potentially harmful tests and procedures. Ideally, if somatization is suspected, psychiatric consultation should be included early in this workup process. Campo and Fritz[61] noted that when somatization was presumed, the likelihood of subsequently discovering a previously undiagnosed physical disease is less than 10%. Nevertheless, certain physical illnesses are commonly overlooked and should be carefully considered as part of the diagnostic work up (Table 1). It is important to note that the presence of physical illness does not definitively exclude the possibility of pediatric somatization. Methods such as video-EEG monitoring, which has been increasingly used to investigate seizure disorders, may also help with the differential diagnosis. The lack of EEG changes during seizure-like behavior makes conversion disorder a likely diagnosis.[52]

The following factors should be considered in a comprehensive assessment: inconsistent findings in the medical evaluation, the presence of psychosocial stressors, the presence of comorbid depressive or anxiety disorders, a past history of somatization in the child and/or family, a symptom model of illness behavior in the family, and the presence of secondary gain or reinforcement. The presence of any one risk factor does not conclusively prove the presence of a somatization disorder; however, psychiatric and social risk factors can increase the diagnostic likelihood.[55]

6.1. *Differential diagnosis*

The primary differential diagnosis is that between somatoform disorder and a general medical condition. Assessment should always start with and include a thorough and complete medical evaluation. However, it is also important to consider differential diagnosis with respect to a number of possible psychiatric diagnoses. Mood and anxiety disorders, for example, frequently include the presence of physical symptoms which tend to remit with treatment of the primary mood or anxiety symptoms and which appear distinct from physical complaints seen in pain or somatization disorders. Similarly, concerns about physical appearance that suggest body dysmorphic disorder may be present in individuals with obsessive compulsive-disorder or the somatic subtype of delusional disorder. Additional diagnoses to consider include both malingering as well as factitious disorder, such as Munchausen syndrome or factitious disorder by proxy. Malingering can be distinguished from somatoform disorders by looking at the motivation for the symptoms. Individuals who are malingering will intentionally produce or exaggerate physical symptoms in order to receive some external reward. Individuals with factitious disorder on the other hand are not motivated by external rewards but instead have an intrapsychic need to remain in the sick role. In factitious disorder by proxy, it is necessary to identify the falsification of physical symptoms or induction of illness in a child by the caregiver.

6.2. *Standardized assessment instruments*

Psychometric instruments offer another way to assess somatic symptoms.[5] The Minnesota Multiphasic Personality Inventory[62] has been used to detect malingering and characterological problems in adult patients.[5] The Children's Somatization Inventory (CSI),[63] a 35-item self-report scale, has child and parent versions and provides information about somatic symptoms occurring in a child over the two weeks prior to assessment.[61] It may be used in children as young as seven years of age. Factor analysis performed on the CSI yields four factors: pseudoneurological symptoms, cardiovascular symptoms, gastrointestinal symptoms, and pain/weakness, resembling the diagnostic categories for somatization disorder. This instrument can be complemented with the Functional Disability Inventory,[64] a 15-item scale also with parent and child versions, which assesses the functional disability over the past two weeks caused by a child's physical health problems. This scale correlates with both school absences and reports of somatic symptoms.[61]

7. General Approaches to the Treatment of Somatoform Disorders

Treatment outcome studies on pediatric somatoform disorders are quite limited in number, partially due to the difficulties in the recruitment of subjects. There is little data from evidence-based treatment studies, in particular randomized controlled studies, and much of the existing data supporting treatment efficacy is based on small case series or case reports. However, it is generally believed that the effective treatment of pediatric somatoform disorders needs to incorporate a number of different treatment modalities that target the factors that are believed to be associated with the development of somatization. These interventions and their place within the developmental model of pediatric somatization are outlined in Fig. 2. Interventions may, for example, include education about the mechanisms of somatization, behavioral interventions to change patterns of reinforcement, psychotherapy to address familial or intrapsychic conflicts, and techniques such as hypnosis or biofeedback to help with the development of alternative coping skills.

7.1. *Education of the family/psychoeducation*

Education of the patient and the family about the diagnosis of a somatoform disorder begins with an "informing conference" between the primary care (or treating) physician and family.[9] It is important in this meeting that the treating physician present the medical and psychosocial findings to the patient and the family in a supportive and nonjudgmental manner as well as acknowledge the child's suffering and the parents' difficulties in dealing with their disabled child. In the treatment of somatoform disorders, it is helpful to establish realistic goals that emphasize improvements in functioning, rather than the illusion that the symptoms can be completely removed. By contrast, it may be necessary to emphasize that treatment does not lead to an immediate interruption in the physical symptoms, and that initially the family may need to learn to live with the child's somatic symptoms. However, it should be explained that medically unexplained symptoms are common and real with available effective treatment options.

7.2. *Role of the primary care physician*

Care of the patient with a somatoform disorder should be centralized to one primary care physician. Reassurance that a serious or life threatening illness is not present is necessary but generally insufficient to alleviate the anxiety of the patient.[61] To help allay this anxiety, primary care physicians can schedule frequent, brief, and ongoing medical visits in anticipation of health concerns.[65] Efforts should be made to avoid unnecessary tests or investigations which have to potential to reinforce somatic symptoms. This practice has been shown to reduce overall health care utilization and to improve patient satisfaction. It may also be helpful to educate the primary care physician. For example, there have been a number of randomized studies in adult patients showing the benefits of sending a written consultation letter to educate the referring physician about somatoform disorders and their recommended management.[7]

7.3. *The rehabilitation model*

A rehabilitation model approach provides a useful framework for the treatment of patients with somatoform disorders.[66] This perspective shifts the focus away from finding a cure for symptoms, and instead emphasizes a return to normal functioning.[61] The patient becomes an active participant in his/her recovery which means that the sick role must be relinquished. Parents must be encouraged to view their child as capable, strong, and competent rather than passive, helpless, and fragile. Success is measured by the ability to return to school, and the resumption of normal social and recreational activities. Treatment involves setting up a regular, predictable schedule with discouragement of daytime rest or avoidance of school. Parents need education and support to persist with what the children may perceive as unfair or unsupportive treatment by their parents until they are able to see the long-term benefits of the treatment. It is frequently important to involve school personnel as part of the wider treatment program. Patients with chronic and entrenched symptoms may require an inpatient rehabilitation treatment approach. It is not uncommon for some patients to have increased frequency of psychiatric symptoms as their somatic symptoms resolve.

Treatment approaches include the use of intensive physical and occupational therapy that emphasizes the recovery of function which also offer face saving remedies for the patient. Physical therapy may be particularly helpful in restoring function in cases of conversion disorder.[5] This approach can be combined with a behavioral modification program, with incentives for improvements in functioning, while removing secondary gain for illness behavior. In severely disabled patients, it may be preferable to recommend admission to an inpatient treatment program that specializes in the treatment of somatoform disorders. Another useful option to consider is that of partial hospitalization. These approaches have the benefit of temporarily removing the child from the home environment where the family may be playing an unwitting role in reinforcing the child's symptoms.

8. Cognitive Behavioral Therapy

Cognitive behavioral therapy (CBT) approaches have been shown to be particularly effective in the management of somatoform disorders. In CBT, attention is drawn to the factors that increase worries about health, including excessive focus on physical symptoms or the misinterpretation of these symptoms. This may include cognitive restructuring, which involves teaching techniques to help modify automatic thoughts and distortions of perceived physical symptoms as indicating medical illness. Cognitive strategies may also help address learned behavioral responses to stress, or the tendency to model behavior on family models of illness. A variety of self-management strategies have also been employed in treatment of somatoform disorders in children and adolescents including relaxation training, self-hypnosis, and biofeedback.[61]

8.1. *Hypnosis*

Hypnosis, which may be used as a diagnostic technique in conversion disorder, may also be used as a treatment technique by providing the patient with a face-saving method of obtaining control over their symptoms.[67] Hypnosis may be useful in reducing symptoms of physiological and emotional arousal, and may be used to help distract the individual and divert attention away from physical symptoms. Guided imagery and hypnosis are commonly used as part of a pain management intervention.[68]

8.2. *Biofeedback*

Biofeedback refers to the procedure in which physical parameters such as muscle tension or temperature are continuously monitored and fed back to the patient, who then attempts to alter the parameter. Biofeedback may have a very useful role in helping reduce physiological and emotional arousal. Although the measurement and control of physiologic responses are usually not thought to be under voluntary control, biofeedback is based on the principle that it is possible to amplify and transform the response in such a way that it can be monitored and understood by the patient. Muscle tension and finger temperature are the most common physical functions measured in the treatment of pain. Biofeedback uses electrical equipment that allows the use of auditory and visual feedback from a physiological function (*e.g.* muscle contraction or relaxation). The patient's increased ability to monitor and control the muscle tension is then applied in controlling or altering the physiological process thought to cause the pain sensations.[69] Biofeedback results in an increased sense of mastery and control for patients who are generally enthusiastic and receptive to this intervention.

8.3. *Behavior modification*

Behavior modification programs may also play a key role as part of the treatment program. Operant conditioning is used to increase the reinforcement the child receives for healthy behavior and to reduce reinforcement received for somatization.[4] There should be reinforcement of healthy behavior, but also for reduced complaints about symptoms, such as participation in pleasant activities when the child is symptom free. Behavior modification programs with incentives for greater functioning and decreased attention to illness behavior and symptoms may play an important role in helping break cycles of secondary gain and reinforcement.

8.4. *Evidence supporting the efficacy of cognitive behavioral therapy*

8.4.1. *Hypochondriasis*

Brief individual cognitive behavioral therapy has been found to be an effective treatment for adult patients with hypochondriasis in a number of randomized controlled trials. Techniques have included efforts to assess patient illness beliefs, explain the role of selective perception in the development of illness fears, and modify misinterpretations of bodily sensations.[7] Techniques have also incorporated stress management and relaxation and attention exercises to change patterns of somatosensory amplification. There appear to be greater benefits from symptom-focused strategies as opposed to general stress management.

8.4.2. *Body dysmorphic disorder*

There is evidence from randomized controlled studies that CBT in either individual or group formats may be useful in the treatment of body dysmorphic disorder in adult patients. For example, CBT has been used successfully in the treatment of both BDD and recurrent abdominal pain.[59,70] Treatment studies have incorporated psychoeducation, progressive muscle relaxation, systematic desensitization, and cognitive strategies to correct automatic thoughts.[7] Treatment has been associated with improvements in measures of self-esteem and psychological functioning in some studies, and effects were maintained several months after completion of treatment.

8.4.3. *Conversion disorder*

There is a notable absence of randomized controlled studies for the treatment of conversion disorder in both adult and pediatric patients. Techniques that have been reported include behavioral approaches with incentives for increased functioning. The successful use of hypnosis as a treatment modality has been described in many uncontrolled case studies that include pediatric patients.[7,71,72] Although there are no rigorous controlled studies to support the use of hypnosis in pediatric patients, one study of adult outpatients with conversion disorder diagnoses randomly assigned to hypnosis or a waiting list found significantly greater clinical improvement at three months with hypnosis.[73] However, a second study involving a comprehensive treatment approach with or without hypnosis showed no added benefits with hypnosis.[72] Case reports and small case series also support the use of biofeedback, amobarbital interviewing, behavioral reinforcement, and family therapy treatments that combine physical therapy and stress management appear to have greater benefits. However, it may be difficult to interpret some of these data given the high rate of spontaneous remission of symptoms in conversion disorder.[7]

8.4.4. *Somatization disorder*

There is very little data on the use of CBT in the treatment of either adult or pediatric patients with somatization disorder. There have been a few randomized controlled studies showing the benefits of group CBT, with a focus on psychoeducation, relaxation, and stress management, in samples of adult patients, but no studies of individual therapy.[74]

9. Psychotherapy

Both individual and family therapies have been found useful in the treatment of patients with somatization disorder and have resulted in reduced health care expenditures.[19] The primary goals of treatment are identifying potential psychosocial stressors, developing insight into the potential impact of these stressors, and establishing ways to cope with stress.

9.1. *Individual psychotherapy*

Insight-oriented psychotherapy may have a role in the treatment of children with conversion disorder. The concept of psychotherapy may be introduced by informing patients that the goal of treatment initially is to help the child adjust to the stress of their illness and to learn new coping strategies. In individual psychotherapy, patients are encouraged to express their underlying emotions, and to develop alternative ways with which to express their feelings of distress. Individual psychotherapy can play an important role in helping change a child's erroneous cognitions about their ability to resume functioning. It is helpful to explore potential sources of stress and gain understanding into the emotional factors that may perpetuate pain behaviors. Common developmental issues (*e.g.* separation anxiety) often require further analysis and treatment.

9.2. *Family therapy*

Family therapy can be helpful in changing family members' views of the patient's physical impairment and helplessness. As they cease to see the somatizing patient as permanently or severely ill, parents and siblings may stop reinforcing illness behavior. Also, important family stressors or dysfunctional family dynamics that are relevant in terms of the etiology of the child's symptoms may be revealed. Family therapy is designed to help the family support healthy, functional behaviors and reduce support for pain behaviors, but also to address family conflicts that may be causing stress for the child or interfering with efforts to cope with pain.

10. Psychopharmacology

There is little literature pertaining to pharmacological treatment of somatoform disorders in the pediatric population. Clinical experience suggests that mood and anxiety disorders will respond to medications even when somatization complicates the picture.[14] Although data are not available for pediatric patients, some adult studies suggest that antidepressants may be helpful with certain somatic symptoms, such as functional gastrointestinal disorders.[61] Benzodiazepines may ameliorate distress and anxiety in anxious somatizing patients.[61] There has been one open label study of general somatoform disorders including adult patients with somatization disorder, hypochondriasis, and conversion disorder that suggested an almost two-thirds response to a 2-week trial of treatment with fluvoxamine.[75] SSRIs have also been found to be helpful in the treatment of irritable bowel syndrome.[32]

10.1. *Hypochondriasis*

Hypochondriasis is a frequent presenting symptom of other primary psychiatric disorders such as panic disorder or depression and in these cases is referred to as secondary hypochondriasis. Treatment of the underlying disorder frequently leads to resolution of the hypochondriacal symptoms. More recently, data have suggested that primary hypochondriasis may also be responsive to pharmacologic interventions. There have been a number of case reports demonstrating the efficacy of clomipramine and the SSRIs for adult patients with hypochondriasis.[76] There are also a number of uncontrolled open-label studies showing benefits with both SSRIs and tricyclic antidepressants. These studies have shown efficacy in patients both with and without diagnosed psychiatric comorbidity such as depression. There is one published report of a placebo-controlled trial of SSRIs for adult patients with hypochondriasis that suggests potential benefits.[77] Data from these studies should be interpreted with the caution that somatization symptoms frequently fluctuate in severity independently of treatment.

10.2. *Pain disorder*

Tricyclic antidepressants, such as amitryptyline and nortriptyline, and serotonin norepinephrine reuptake inhibitors, such as venlafaxine and duloxetine, have been used as adjuncts in the pharmacological treatment of pain.[78] In patients with pain disorders who clearly have comorbid diagnoses of depression, it is reasonable to choose either venlafaxine or duloxetine as primary antidepressant agents. Although there has been interest in the use of the selective serotonin reuptake inhibitors, they have generally not been found to be as effective in pain treatment with the exception of one recent trial of citalopram to treat recurrent abdominal pain.[43] Several of the anticonvulsant agents, including neurontin, carbamazepine, clonazepam, and phenytoin have been widely used in the treatment of migraine and neuropathic pain and divalproex sodium has been used for migraine prophylaxis. Other agents used as adjunctive medications in the treatment of pain syndromes include membrane stabilizing agents, psychostimulants, antipsychotics, and clonidine.

10.3. *Body dysmorphic disorder*

There are several case reports and small open clinical trials regarding the treatment of body dysmorphic disorder in childhood.[79,80] Selective serotonin reuptake inhibitors were found to be effective in reducing preoccupation with appearance and improving functioning. There have also been at least two published, controlled pharmacological studies on body dysmorphic disorder in adult patients, using clomipramine, desipramine, and SSRIs.[76]

11. Prognosis

Although few prospective studies exist addressing this issue, some data suggest that certain types of somatization may persist from childhood into adulthood. For example, 25–50% of adults who had recurrent abdominal pain as children continue to suffer from similar symptoms in adulthood.[61] Body dysmorphic disorder and hypochondriasis are felt to be chronic, unremitting illnesses. By contrast, most conversion disorders are thought to resolve within a few months of diagnosis, although symptoms may recur. Shorter duration of illness is generally associated with better outcomes. Many patients will undergo spontaneous remission of their symptoms although treatment is thought to hasten recovery and is necessary for patients with chronic or more entrenched symptoms. Patients particularly resistant to treatment may have had more active reinforcement of the symptoms by family members, or have experienced benefits in the form of secondary gain.

12. Future Directions

Interest in the systematic study of pediatric somatoform disorders has grown in recent years, but is still in its infancy. There is still a significant lack of knowledge related to even simple data on the incidence and prevalence of these conditions. Efforts are being made to address some of these deficits including the recent initiative to develop a multisite randomized prospective clinical trial of pediatric non-epileptic seizures.[81] Developments in neuroimaging technology hold out the promise of increased understanding of the mechanisms and pathophysiology of clinical phenomena such as conversion symptoms.[44] It is likely that future systems of diagnostic classification may undergo several refinements as our knowledge of these disorders increases.[82] Insights from such studies may also help to reduce the tendency to dichotomize patients into either medical or psychiatric categories.

Treatment of pediatric somatoform disorders is clearly another area where further work is needed. Future work will require multisite investigations using manualized treatment interventions that must be applicable to and replicable by clinicians who encounter these patients. Yet another issue that will require attention is that of advocacy for this patient population. Treatment for children or adolescents with somatoform disorders is often complex and the ability to access appropriate treatment is often limited by the lack of clinicians who have the expertise or motivation to treat this very challenging group of patients. Existing inpatient psychiatric treatment facilities are often not appropriate venues for the somatoform patient, yet medical insurance companies are generally unwilling to fund treatment within a medical facility. This is true even given the few studies that have demonstrated the enormous financial costs of this patient population.[12] Academic medical centers will need to continue efforts to define, describe, and develop effective evidence-based treatments that can then be exported to the community.

References

1. Escobar JI, Rubio-Stipec M, Canino G, Karno M. Somatic Symptom Index (SSI): A new and abridged somatization construct. Prevalence and epidemiological correlates in two large community samples, *J Nerv Ment Dis* 1989; **177**: 140–146.
2. Haugaard JJ. Recognizing and treating uncommon behavioral and emotional disorders in children and adolescents who have been severely maltreated: Somatization and other somatoform disorders, *Child Maltreat* 2004; **9**: 169–176.
3. Ballas C, Staab JP. Medically unexplained physical symptoms: Toward an alternative paradigm for diagnosis and treatment, *CNS Spectrums* 2003; **2**: 20–26.
4. Campo J, Fritsch S. Somatization in children and adolescents, *J Am Acad Child Adolesc Psychiatry* 1994; **33**: 1223–1235.
5. Abbey SE. Somatization and somatoform disorders. In: Levenson JL, Ed. *The American Psychiatric Publishing Textbook of Psychosomatic Medicine,* Washington DC: American Psychiatric Publishing Inc, 2005: pp. 271–296.
6. Stoudemire A. Somatothymia. *Psychosomatics* 1991; **32**: 365–381.
7. Loopier KJ, Kirmayer LJ. Behavioral medicine approaches to somatoform disorders, *J Consult Clin Psychol* 2002; **70**: 810–827.
8. Garber J, Walker LS, Zeman J. Somatization symptoms in a community sample of children and adolescents: Further validation of the children's somatization inventory, *Psychol Assess* 1991; **3**: 588–595.
9. DeMaso DR, Beasley PJ. The somatoform disorders. In: Klykylo WM, Kay JL, Ruber DM, Eds. *Clinical Child Psychiatry,* Indianapolis: Wiley; 2005, pp. 429–444.
10. Silber TJ, Pao M. Somatization disorders in children and adolescents, *Pediatr Rev* 2003; **24**: 255–264.
11. Servan-Schreiber D, Kolb R, Tabas G. The somatizing patient, *Prim Care* 1999; **26**: 225–242.
12. Barsky AJ, Orav J, Bates DW. Somatization increases medical utilization and costs independent of psychiatric and medical comorbidity, *Arch Gen Psychiatry* 2005; **62**: 903–910.
13. Campo JV, Jansen-McWilliams L, Comer DM, Kelleher JJ. Somatization in pediatric primary care: Association with psychopathology, functional impairment, and use of services, *J Am Acad Child Adolesc Psychiatry* 1999; **38**: 1093–1101.
14. Fritz GK, Fritsch S, Hagino O. Somatoform disorders in children and adolescents: A review of the past ten years, *J Am Acad Child Adolesc Psychiatry* 1997; **36**: 1329–1338.
15. American Academy of Pediatrics. *Diagnostic and Statistical Manual for Primary Care (DSM-PC) Child and Adolescent Version.* Elk Grove Village, IL: American Academy of Pediatrics, 1996.

16. Steiner H, Araujo KB, Koopman C. The response evaluation measure (REM-71): A new instrument for the measurement of defenses in adults and adolescents, *Am J Psychiatry* 2001; **158**: 467–473.
17. Araujo KB, Medic S, Yasnovsky J, Steiner H. Assessing defense structure in school-age children using the response evaluation measure-71-youth version (REM-Y-71), *Child Psychiatry Hum Dev* 2006; **36**: 427–436.
18. Gemelli R. *Normal Child and Adolescent Development.* Washington DC: American Psychiatric Publishing, Inc, 1996.
19. Kaplan HI, Sadock BJ, Grebb JA. Somatoform disorders. In: *Kaplan and Sadock's Synopsis of Psychiatry: Behavioral Sciences/Clinical Psychiatry,* 7th edition. Baltimore: Williams and Wilkins, 1994: pp. 617–631.
20. Fukuda K. Somatization disorder and bradykinin, *Psychiatry Clin Neurosci* 2003; **57**: 609.
21. Rief W, Pilger F, Ihle D, Verkerk R, Scharpe S, Maes M. Psychobiological aspects of somatoform disorders: Contributions of monaminergic transmitter systems, *Neuropsychobiology* 2004; **49**: 24–29.
22. Stuart S, Noyes R. Attachment and interpersonal communication in somatization, *Psychosomatics* 1999; **40**: 3–43.
23. Minuchin S, Rosman BL, Baker L. *Psychosomatic Families: Anorexia Nervosa in Context.* Cambridge, MA: Harvard University Press, 1978.
24. Waldinger RJ, Schulz MS, Barsky AJ, Ahern DK. Mapping the road from childhood trauma to adult somatization: The role of attachment, *Psychosom Med* 2006; **68**: 129–135.
25. Rhee H, Holditch-Davis D, Miles MS. Patterns of physical symptoms and relationships with psychosocial factors in adolescents, *Psychosom Med* 2005; **67**: 1006–1012.
26. Schechter NL. The development of pain perception and principles of pain control. In: Lewis M, Ed. *Child and Adolescent Psychiatry: A Comprehensive Textbook, 3rd Ed.,* Philadelphia: Lippincott, Williams and Wilkins; 2002, pp. 404–413.
27. Dahlquist LM, Switkin MC. Chronic and recurrent pain. In: Roberts MC, Ed. *Handbook of Pediatric Psychology,* 3rd edition, New York: The Guilford Press; 2003, pp. 198–215.
28. American Psychiatric Association. *Diagnostic and Statistical Manual of Mental Disorders,* 4th edition, Text Revision. Washington DC: American Psychiatric Association, 2000.
29. Barsky AJ, Wool C, Barnett MC, Clearly PD. Histories of childhood trauma in adult hypochondriacal patients, *Am J Psychiatry* 1994; **151**: 397–401.
30. Hotopf M, Mayou R, Wadsworth M, Wessely S. Childhood risk factors for adults with medically unexplained symptoms: Results from a national birth cohort study, *Am J Psychiatry* 1999; **156**: 1796–1800.

31. Poikolainen K, Aalto-Setala T, Martunnen M, Tuulio-Henriksson A, Lonnqvist J. Predictors of somatic symptoms: A five year follow up of adolescents, *Arch Dis Child* 2000; **83**: 388–392.
32. Zeiter DK, Hyams JS. Recurrent abdominal pain in children, *Pediatr Gastroenterol Nutr* 2002; **49**: 53–71.
33. Salmon P, Al-Marzooqi SM, Baker G, Reilly J. Childhood family dysfunction and associated abuse in patients with nonepileptic seizures: Towards a causal model, *Psychosom Med* 2003; **65**: 695–700.
34. Poikolainen K, Kanerva R, Loonqvist J. Life events and other risk factors for somatic symptoms in adolescence, *Pediatrics* 1995; **96**: 59–63.
35. Barsky AJ, Goodson JD, Lane RS, Cleary PD. The amplification of somatic symptoms, *Psychosom Med* 1988; **50**: 510–519.
36. James L, Gordon E, Kraiuhin C, Meares R. Selective attention and auditory event-related potentials in somatization disorder, *Compr Psychiatry* 1989; **30**: 84–89.
37. Byrne D. The repression-sensitization scale: Rationale, reliability, and validity, *J Pers* 1961; **29**: 334–349.
38. Risch MD, Morris GL, Allen L, Lathrop L. Psychological treatment of nonepileptic events, *Epilepsy Behav* 2001; **2**: 277–283.
39. Hurwitz TA. Somatization and conversion disorder, *Can J Psychiatry* 2004; **49**: 172–178.
40. Koenig TW, Clark MR. Advances in comprehensive pain management, *Psychiatr Clin North Am* 1996; **19**: 589–611.
41. Green WH, Kowalik SC. Psychopharmacologic treatment of pain and anxiety in the pediatric patient, *Child Adolesc Psychiatr Clin North Am* 1994; **3**: 465–483.
42. Dorn LD, Campo JC, Thato S, Dahl RE, Lewin D, Chandra R, Di Lorenzo C. Psychological comorbidity and stress reactivity in children and adolescents with recurrent abdominal pain and anxiety disorders, *J Am Acad Child Adoles Psychiatry* 2003; **42**: 66–75.
43. Campo JV, Perel J, Lucas A *et al.* Citalopram treatment of pediatric recurrent abdominal pain and comorbid internalizing disorders: An exploratory study, *J Am Acad Child Adolesc Psychiatry* 2004; **43**: 1234–1242.
44. Ghaffar O, Staines WR, Feinstein A. Unexplained neurologic symptoms: An fMRI study of sensory conversion disorder, *Neurology* 2006; **267**: 2036–2038.
45. Vuilleumier P. Hysterical conversion and brain function, *Prog Brain Res* 2005; **150**: 309–329.
46. Hakala M, Vahlberg T, Niemi PM, Karlsson H. Brain glucose metabolism and temperament in relation to severe somatization, *Psychiatry Clin Neurosci* 2006; **60**: 669–675.
47. WHO. *International Statistical Classification of Diseases and Related Health Problems, Version 10.* Geneva: World Health Organization, 2007.
48. Schwartz M, Landerman R, Geprge LK, Blazer DG, Escobar JI. Somatization disorder. In: Robins LN, Regier DA, Eds. *Psychiatric Disorders in America,* New York: The Free Press, 1991, pp. 220–257.

49. Guz H, Doganay Z, Ozkan A *et al.* Conversion and somatization disorders: Dissociative symptoms and other characteristics, *J Psychosom Res* 2004; **56**: 287–291.
50. Wyllie E, Glazer JP, Benbadis S, Kotagal P, Wolgamuth B. Psychiatric features of children and adolescents with pseudoseizures, *Arch Pediatr Adolesc Med* 1999; **153**: 244–248.
51. Kotagal P, Costa M, Wyllie E, Wolgamuth B. Paroxysmal nonepileptic events in children and adolescents, *Pediatrics* 2002; **110**: e46.
52. Hämäläinen M, Masek BJ. Diagnosis, classification, and medical management of headache in children and adolescents. In: Schechter NL, Berde CB, Yaster M, Eds. *Pain in Infants, Children and Adolescents,* 2nd edition, Philadelphia: Lippincott Williams and Wilkins, 2003, pp. 707–718.
53. Hyams JS, Burke G, Davis PM, Rezepski B, Andrulonis PA. Abdominal pain and irritable bowel syndrome in adolescents: A community-based study, *J Pediatrics* 1996; **29**: 220–226.
54. Robins PM, Glutting JJ, Shaffer S, Proujansky R, Mehta D. Are there psychosocial differences in diagnostic subgroups of children with recurrent abdominal pain? *J Pediatr Gastrenterol Nutr* 2005; **41**: 216–220.
55. Fritz GK, Campo JV. Somatoform Disorders. In: Lewis M, Ed. *Child and Adolescent Psychiatry: A Comprehensive Textbook,* 3rd edition, Philadelphia: Lippincott Williams and Wilkins, 2002, pp. 847–857.
56. Galloway KS, Yaster M. Pain and symptom control in terminally ill children, *Pediatr Clin North Am* 2000; **47**: 711–746.
57. Rasquin-Weber A, Hyman PE, Cucchiara S *et al.* Childhood functional gastrointestinal disorders, *Gut* 1999; **45**: S2:60–68.
58. Folks DG, Feldman MD, Ford CV. Somatoform disorders, factitious disorders, and malingering. In: Stoudemire A, Fogel BS, Greenberg DB, Eds. *Psychiatric Care of the Medical Patient,* 2nd edition, Oxford: Oxford University Press, 2000, pp. 459–476.
59. Allen A, Hollander E. Body dysmorphic disorder, *Psychiatr Clin North Am* 2000; **23**: 617–628.
60. Phillips KA. Body dysmorphic disorder: The distress of imagined ugliness, *Am J Psychiatry* 1991; **148**: 1138–1149.
61. Campo JV, Fritz G. A management model for pediatric somatization, *Psychosomatics* 2001; **42**: 467–476.
62. Butcher JN, Dahlstrom WG, Graham JR, Tellegen A, Kaemmer B. *Minnesota Multiphasic Personality Inventory-2: Manual for administration and scoring.* Minneapolis: University of Minnesota Press, 1989.
63. Walker LS, Garber J, Greene JW. Psychosocial correlates of recurrent childhood pain: A comparison of pediatric patients with recurrent abdominal pain, organic illness, and psychiatric disorders, *J Abnorm Psychol* 1993; **102**: 248–258.

64. Walker LS, Greene JW. The functional disability inventory: Measuring a neglected dimension of child health status, *J Pediatr Psychol* 1991; **16**: 39–58.
65. Kroenke K, Rosmalen JGM. Symptoms, syndromes, and the value of psychiatric diagnostics in patients who have functional somatic disorders, *Med Clin N Am* 2006; **90**: 603–626.
66. Lock J, Giammona A. Severe somatoform disorder in adolescence: A case series using a rehabilitation model for intervention, *Clin Child Psychol Psychiatry* 1999; **4**: 1359–1045.
67. Maldonado JR, Spiegel D. Medical hypnosis. In: Stoudemire A, Fogel BS, Greenberg DB, Eds. *Psychiatric Care of the Medical Patient,* 2nd edition, Oxford: Oxford University Press, 2000, pp. 73–90.
68. Kuttner L, Solomon R. Hypnotherapy and imagery for managing children's pain. In: Schechter NL, Berde CB, Yaster M, Eds. *Pain in Infants, Children and Adolescents,* 2nd edition, Philadelphia: Lippincott Williams and Wilkins, 2003, pp. 317–328.
69. McGrath PJ, Dick B, Unruh AM. Psychologic and behavioral treatment of pain in children and adolescents. In: Schechter NL, Berde CB, Yaster M, Eds. *Pain in Infants, Children and Adolescents,* 2nd edition. Philadelphia: Lippincott Williams and Wilkins, 2003, pp. 303–316.
70. Sanders MR, Shepherd RW, Cleghorn G, Woolford H. The treatment of recurrent abdominal pain in children: A controlled comparison of cognitive-behavioral family intervention and standard pediatric care, *J Consult Clin Psychol* 1994; **62**: 306–314.
71. Bloom PB. Treating adolescent conversion disorders: Are hypnotic techniques reusable? *Int J Clin Hyp* 2001; **49**: 243–256.
72. Moene FC, Spinhoven P, Hoogduin KA, van Dyck R. A randomized controlled clinical trial of a hypnosis-based treatment for patients with conversion disorder, motor type, *Int J Clin Exp Hypn* 2003; **51**: 29–50.
73. LaFrance WC Jr, Devinsky O. The treatment of nonepileptic seizures: Historical perspectives and future directions, *Epilepsia* 2004; **2**: S45:15–21.
74. Kroenke K, Swindle R. Cognitive-behavioral therapy for somatization and symptom syndromes: A critical review of controlled clinical trials, *Psychother Psychosom* 2000; **69**: 205–215.
75. Noyes R, Happel R, Muller B *et al.* Fluvoxamine for somatoform disorders: An open trial, *Gen Hosp Psychiatry* 1998; **20**: 339–344.
76. Fallon BA. Pharmacotherapy of somatoform disorders, *J Psychosom Res* 2004; **56**: 455–460.
77. Fallon BA, Schneier FR, Marshall R *et al.* The pharmacotherapy of hypochondriasis, *Psychopharm Bull* 1996; **32**: 607–611.
78. Carter GT, Sullivan MD. Antidepressants in pain management, *Curr Opin Investig Drugs* 2002; **3**: 454–458.
79. El-khatib ME, Dickey TO. Sertraline for body dysmorphic disorder, *J Am Acad Child Adolesc Psychiatry* 1995; **34**: 1404–1405.

80. Hollander E, Cohen LJ, Simeon D. Fluvoxamine treatment of body dysmorphic disorder, *J Clin Psychopharmacol* 1994; **14**: 75–77.
81. LaFrance WC Jr, Alper K, Babcock D *et al.* Nonepileptic seizures treatment workshop summary, *Epilepsy Behav* 2006; **8**: 451–461.
82. Mayou R, Kirmayer LJ, Simon G, Kroenke K, Sharpe M. Somatoform disorders: Time for a new approach in DSM-V, *Am J Psychiatry* 2005; **162**: 847–855.

Chapter 14

Eating Disorders in Children and Adolescents

James Lock and Kathleen Kara Fitzpatrick

1. Introduction

Eating disorders are one of the most common psychiatric problems in children and adolescents.[1] They can also be among the most serious because of the interplay between the psychological and medical aspects of serious malnutrition, binge eating, overweight, and purging.[2] Unfortunately, our scientific understanding of the cause, risk factors, and treatments of these disorders lags behind that of other mental disorders.

2. Epidemiology

The DSM-IV describes three diagnosable eating disorders, which include anorexia nervosa (AN), bulimia nervosa (BN), and eating disorder not otherwise specified (EDNOS).[3] Of these three, AN exhibits the most serious symptoms, greatest relapse rate, and highest mortality rates, which in the opinion of most clinicians renders it the most serious of the three. Bulimia nervosa, however, is more prevalent, as it affects between 1 and 3% of the population and exhibits the highest incidence of any eating disorder among the affected male population.[1] The third diagnosis, EDNOS, is the least precise of the diagnostic categories and serves as the category for eating problems that are not AN or BN. It is at the same time the most heterogeneous and most common. Many studies suggest that those with EDNOS are more similar to those with AN and BN than different and that EDNOS should not be considered a subthreshold type disorder because evidence suggest that these patients are just as ill as those who are diagnosed with AN or BN.[4,5]

The prevalence and incidence of AN are difficult to estimate because both are highly contingent on the nature of the studied population.[1,6] The prevalence of sub-threshold AN (patients meeting all but one criteria for AN, according to the DSM-IV) is higher than that of diagnosable AN, for which estimates of point prevalence fall within 0.1 to 0.9% of the population. Estimates tend toward the higher end of this range if the studied population resides in an industrialized Westernized country; however, there is evidence of increased incidence of eating problems in Asia.[7] This, however, does not mean that AN is "culture-bound," as studies have shown that although AN remains more common in higher SES groups it is found among almost all socioeconomic statuses and demographics.[8] In females, the onset of AN can be as young as seven with most cases occurring during adolescent years, with peaks at 14 and 18 years of age, which are traditionally the ages at which adolescents enter high school and college, respectively.[9] Affected males constitute approximately 5 to 10% of the AN patient population and generally experience the onset of AN somewhat later than women. The true percentage of AN patients who are male, however, is likely to be higher, as males with diagnosable eating disorders are less likely to seek professional help.[10]

The incidence of AN seems to have been increasing over the past 50 years, however, the following factors might be a product of an increasing AN: (1) population of young women, (2) number of AN patients that seek clinical attention, (3) awareness of the disease, and (4) ability to detect and understand symptoms.[11] According to a study reported by Lucas *et al.* the incidence of AN for women 15 through 24 years old shifted quite dramatically from 7/100,000 in 1935–1939 to 26.3 in 1980–1984, but remained constant for women over 24-years old.[12,13] A similarity between AN and BN is that each claims around nine female victims for every one male victim; however, several differences exist when the epidemiology of each is examined. The prevalence of BN is much higher, ranging from 1 to 3%, and usually onsets in middle adolescence or late adulthood, somewhat later than the onset of AN.[14] BN also appears to be more "culture bound," as it is prevalent only among populations that are live by or are exposed to Western ideals about body weight and shape. The availability of food is also a requirement to the onset of BN. It has been suggested by Keel and Klump that in BN, Westernization and poor body image are highly associated with one another.[15] The fact that AN is equally prevalent in non-Western and Western societies, if and only if the AN criterion requiring poor body image for a diagnosis is disregarded, also appears to support this postulate.

The prevalence and incidence of EDNOS is much harder to estimate than either BN or AN because of (1) the highly individual quality of each case, (2) difficulty in detecting certain symptoms of EDNOS, (3) the larger number of men that fall into this category combined with the misconception that men are more "immune" to eating disorders, and (4) the difficulty of assigning such a diagnosis with vague requirements.[16] In many cases, doctors give the EDNOS diagnosis to children whose disordered eating patterns have been detected early and might meet all but one requirement for the diagnosis of AN or BN. A subset of EDNOS is non-purging bulmia or binge eating disorder (BED).

Binge eating disorder (BED) (non-purging bulimia) has recently been proposed as being a separate diagnostic entity. This is because there is a growing consensus that the features, treatment, and prognosis of BED differ substantially from that of BN.[17] BED responds to a wider range of treatments and has an overall better prognosis than does BN. About 40–50% of diagnoses of EDNOS with a BED subcategory are male and the overall prevalence of BED in random samples is 0.7 to 4%. This range of percentages, however, escalates from 15 to 50% if the sample populations are drawn from participants in weight loss programs. BED is similar to BN in that late adolescence and early adulthood are the characteristic ages of onset of this seemingly chronic disease. More recently, some researchers have suggested that there is likely a diagnostic entity of "purging only" disorder, wherein the patient does not binge eat and does not have AN.[18]

3. Diagnosis

For a diagnosis of anorexia nervosa (AN), the DSM-IV requires that the following four major components all be evident characteristics of a patient: (1) body weight of less than 85% of that expected, for the patient's height and gender, due to weight loss, and strong refusal to maintain body weight at or above his/her expected weight; (2) even though unhealthily underweight, the patient harbors a marked fear of becoming fat or gaining weight; (3) the patient experiences body image disturbance, the degree to which one is underweight is not perceived as a serious health problem, and an unreasonably large emphasis on weight and/or shape as criteria for self-evaluation; (4) and amenorrhea in post-menarchal females.[3] The DSM-IV also lists two subtypes of AN, one of which is called the "binge-eating/purging type" and is characterized by recurrent episodes of binge eating and purging (whether self-induced vomiting or other compensatory behaviors) while fulfilling the requirements for anorexia outside of these episodes. The second category, known as the "restricting type," does not require binge eating or purging. ICD-10 criteria for AN are generally similar to those provided by the DSM-IV-TR, although the ICD-10 provides greater behavioral specifications and laboratory findings for differential diagnosis. For example, the ICD-10 criteria provide behavioral examples of weight-loss strategies. Further, the ICD-10 provides a framework for the role of low weight in endocrine disturbance and the importance of assessing HPA dysfunction, which often manifest as changes in menstrual functioning among females and decreased sexual interest and potency in males. The ICD-10 also suggests evaluation of growth hormone, cortisol and thyroid levels in support of diagnoses.

Of the three diagnosable eating disorders, AN was the first to be recognized as a serious medical condition and is, with little dispute, the most serious of the three.[19] Severe cases of AN may lead to death usually due to cardiac arrest or irreversible medical complications (*e.g.* osteoporosis). Both of these outcomes are generally results of prolonged physiological malnutrition, which triggers organ systems to reduce their activity to solely the most essential functions, and can also lead to heart and organ muscle mass reduction.[2] Preserved for as long as possible are brain and heart function, but with the progression of AN, low blood pressure and low heart rate ensue as cardiac muscle weakens, which might be irreversible and lead to death. Shrinkage in brain tissue has been proven to occur during an episode of AN, with incomplete although substantial reversal with renourishment.[20] The other major cause of death is suicide, which accounts for about half of the deaths associated with AN. The overall increased mortality rate is about 1% per year of illness, culminating in mortality rates of between 10 and 15% in most studies.[21] Less severe physiological factors include reduction of peripheral blood flow, leading to intolerance to low temperatures, dry skin, hair loss, and growth of lanugo (fine hair that conserves warmth) on various parts of the body. In post-pubertal women, menstrual cycles become irregular or completely cease, and infertility occurs. Of all these physical pathologies, the most permanent is calcium loss from the bones, which is inclined to persist after weight recovery, depending on age of onset, the severity of weight loss, and the duration of low weight. This can potentially lead to osteopenia or in worse cases, osteoporosis, which is an especially worrisome problem in children whose bone growth can decelerate and/or cease and in young adolescent females who deposit most mineral in their bone between the ages of 12 and 20 years.

A diagnosis of BN, according to the DSM-IV (APA, 1994), requires the patient meet the following criteria: (1) binge eating during a discrete period of time, during which a subjective sense of lack of control over eating prevails, and after which inappropriate compensatory behaviors for weight control are employed, (2) and that these episodes of binge eating and purging occur at least twice a week for a minimum of three months.[3] The DSM-IV specifies two subtypes of BN, which serve to define the nature of the compensatory behavior in which a BN patient engages after an episodic binge. The "purging type" mainly utilizes vomiting, laxatives, and diuretics, whereas the "non-purging type" lists severe dieting or fasting, vigorous exercise, and abuse of diet pills as possibilities. Either of these forms of BN may occur during an episode of AN, yet, the diagnosis will still be AN. As with AN, ICD-10 criteria are consistent with the

DSM-IV-TR, although they provide greater illumination of the types of compensatory behaviors, including specific mention of issues such as insulin manipulation among diabetic patients. Interestingly, the ICD-10 also includes obsessive preoccupation and "irresistable craving" for food, while the DSM-IV-TR focuses largely on behavioral characteristics of binge eating episodes.

Many characteristics that are not listed in the DSM-IV, and hence not required for diagnosis, are also associated with BN. These characteristics are arguably just as important because of how helpful they are in detecting patients and in determining the prognosis, medical treatment, psychotherapy, and the medical urgency of the disorder. Common symptoms that physically affect the patient are hypokalemia, hypochloremia, hyponatremia, metabolic alkalosis, tooth decay, esophageal erosion, and fatigue. Bulimic patients can be extremely difficult to detect because, unlike AN, they often exhibit a weight that fluctuates within a normal range and few of the aforementioned physical manifestations are identifiable without a medical examination.[2] A few key psychological symptoms of BN include placing an abnormally large emphasis on weight and/or shape in determining self-evaluation, impulsivity, personality deficits, interpersonal problems, and irritability. Other common psychiatric comorbidities include major depression, substance abuse, and dependence and personality disorders.

As noted, Eating Disorder Not Otherwise Specified (EDNOS) is the most frequently given diagnosis. It generally is a "catch all" category to include disordered eating that does not fulfill the requirements for either AN or BN.[3] The DSM-IV lists examples that can be applied to many broader cases, *e.g.* a female who exhibits all qualities of AN but menstruates regularly or only meets one to three of the four requirements for AN. Another example is an AN patient who has lost a significant amount of weight but is currently overweight or in a normal weight range. A diagnosis of EDNOS can also be valid if the patient engages in bingeing and purging less frequently than twice a week, purging occurs after meals that would be considered neither a subjective nor objective binge-quantity of food, or if the patient regularly chews and spits large quantities of food without swallowing.

A subset of EDNOS is BED, currently listed in the appendix of DSM IV as a research diagnosis.[3] The simplest way of describing BED is to understand the symptoms of BN and eliminate the inappropriate compensatory behaviors that normally occur immediately following the episode of binge eating. Researchers and clinicians are still debating the key criteria for BED. Most people with serious binge eating problems have frequent episodes of eating what others would consider an abnormally large amount of food and frequent feelings of being unable to control what or how much is being eaten. Other characteristic behaviors of a patient has BED include eating much more rapidly than usual, eating until uncomfortably full, eating large amounts of food, even when not physically hungry, eating alone out of embarrassment at the quantity of food being eaten, and feelings of disgust, depression, or guilt after overeating. Major complications of BED include diseases that accompany obesity. These include diabetes, high blood pressure, high cholesterol levels, gallbladder disease, heart disease, and certain types of cancer. People with BED are typically distressed by their binge eating, and most try to control it on their own, but success is generally ephemeral. Some binge eaters miss work, school, or social activities to binge eat. Obese people with binge eating disorder often feel badly about themselves, are preoccupied with their appearance, and may avoid social gatherings. Binge eaters are often successful at hiding these issues, usually to the extent that close family members and friends are oblivious to the truth. Debate about whether BED deserves its own categorical diagnosis in the DSM is ongoing but it appears likely that future iterations of the DSM will include BED as a separate eating disorder diagnosis. Of particular importance in future DSM iterations for BED is the clarification of the frequency and intensity criteria required for diagnosis.

For children and adolescents, there are considerable problems with the utilization of the current diagnostic systems. Neither DSM nor ICD make sufficient concessions to the developmental realities of symptom presentation in young persons.[22] Data suggest that eating disorders, like most other medical and psychiatric disorders, differ somewhat early in development in younger persons. Significant problems arise in trying to apply DSM criteria to children and young adolescents. The suggested weight criteria of a BMI of 17.5 is reasonable enough for documenting low weight in an adult, but for children, this can be a normal BMI; instead, age-adjusted BMI must be used. The requirement of three missed menstruations is problematic for girls who have just begun to menstruate because of common unpredictability of the periodicity of cycles in this age group.[23] Many children and many adolescents do not have the capacity for taking the perspective on their behaviors and thoughts (abstract thinking) required to formulate their behaviors and thoughts such as "wishing to be thin" or "over exercise" or experiencing their body image as distortion. In addition, many who begin to binge eat or purge may begin the behaviors at a relatively low frequency, but just as *in situ* cancer cells require intervention, so do these conditions. Changes reflecting these developmental modifications are expected to be included in future iterations of the DSM-V.

3.1. *Differential diagnosis*

Despite the difficulties of diagnosing children and adolescents using current diagnostic systems, there are important medical and psychiatric conditions that should not be confused with eating disorders. It is important not to confuse malnutrition secondary to severe neglect with AN. Also, weight loss in the context of depression, swallowing phobia, psychotic disorder (paranoid ideation about food poisoning usually), or obsessions and behaviors about germs and food in the context of OCD need to be carefully distinguished from classic eating disorders. Rumination and chronic vomiting secondary to stomach pain or psychosomatic pain is not best considered a classic eating disorder. A host of medical problems can cause eating disorder like symptoms. Thyroid disease, cancers, and malabsorbtion disorders need to be ruled out in all cases of anorexia.[24] Brain tumors, liver, and adrenal diseases can cause symptoms similar to AN and BN as well and should be screened using routine laboratories such as CBC and liver function tests.[25] MRI of the head is sometimes indicated if pseudotumor cerebri is on the differential for a person with purging behavior. As can be appreciated, because of the complexity of both the evaluation and differential diagnoses of eating disorders, it is common for clinicians who have a large practice of patients with eating disorders to work in a team that includes a pediatrician or internist with experience and knowledge of such patients and with differential diagnostic procedures.

3.2. *Comorbidity*

Another complicating factor with diagnosing eating disorders is the reality that many people with eating disorders also have other psychiatric problems. For example, in AN, many have anxiety disorders (about 40–60%) including OCD.[26,27] It is sometimes difficult to ascertain in these situations if the obsessions and compulsions about eating and weight are due to a specific elaboration of OCD or are truly AN. A careful history in cases where OCD is a true comorbidity, usually reveals other areas where there is definite obsessive and compulsive thoughts and behaviors besides weight and eating but that is similar in intensity and irrationality. In the case of BN, depressive disorders are common cooccurring psychiatric problems. Luckily, both CBT and antidepressants can be useful for symptoms of both diagnoses, although doses of antidepressant are higher in BN than major depression. Clinicians who treat eating disorders, even those in young children and adolescents, should expect to also treat these comorbid conditions. In many instances, these comorbid conditions persist even after recovery from the eating disorder.

4. Pathogenesis

The pathogeneses of AN, BN, and EDNOS are challenging to study, as unlike many purely biological afflictions, there are usually several factors that contribute to the development of an eating disorder. To add to its complexity, many of these factors are intangible and a linear approach to understanding these diseases usually constitutes only part of the answer. Many psychosocial factors are known to contribute to the onset, perpetuation, and exacerbation of AN.[28] As a result, the development of AN rarely occurs overnight. The most common pathway that an individual experiences in developing AN starts with a diet, in which the intentions were solely, for instance, to get into better shape or feel healthier. The reason this course might lead to AN is that this dieting, in a specifically susceptible population, becomes an obsession, and the patient discards his/her original healthy goal for the destructive characteristics of AN. Eventually, the incessant weight loss escapes any control that the patient had. As some AN patients attempt to emerge from this destructive weight loss spiral, they realize that they have lost control and their ingrained drive to continue dieting actually controls them. The AN patient may develop a fixation on the size of a specific body part, on a certain calorie quota, or the exact number that appears on the scale. This mentality, which is characteristic of a vast number of afflicted patients, drives the development, maintenance, and/or progression of AN.

Significant psychological stressors are a major source triggering the onset of many psychiatric disorders like AN and BN. A trigger can exist in the form of a life transitional period, such as going to college, parental divorce/separation, the death of a loved one, or even the dissolution of a friendship or intimate relationship. History of sexual and/or physical abuse are also known risk factors for AN and BN. Triggers that seem trivial may also occur, such as being harassed or called "fat" by a peer, sibling, and sometimes parent. For BN, low self-esteem, sensitivity to peer rejection, perfectionism, interpersonal deficits, and impulsivity are all factors that might lead to its development and prolongation.

Patients who develop characteristics of the restricting type of AN usually are somehow able to eat in secret and/or deceive their relatives and friends that, indeed, they are engaging in healthy eating. Excuses such as illness, pickiness, food allergies, ideals (*e.g.* vegetarianism), and a claim of previous food consumption are common when AN patients are confronted with their unhealthy eating habits. If an AN patient is successful, he/she will gradually decrease daily portions in efforts to further reduce weight. Understandably, this manner of behaving would galvanize the patient to plummet increasingly further into the disease and increased risk of medical consequences.

Development of the binge purge type of AN and BN are slightly different from the restricting type of AN. In this case, patients may use laxatives, diuretics, enemas, excessive exercise, and vomiting to control their weight. A lifestyle that includes unavoidable meals, social outings, and mandatory events in which eating is an expectation is likely to lead to the development of this subtype of AN. It is interesting to note that males afflicted with AN are more likely to develop behaviors that align with this subtype of AN. The reason for this may be that it is much less acceptable, in many cultures, for men to restrict their eating patterns than for women. For those with BN, restricted eating and dieting behaviors serve as similar triggers for episodes of uncontrolled eating and subsequent compensatory behaviors to relieve discomfort or anxiety regarding weight gain.

4.1. *Biological origins of eating disorders*

Family aggregation studies have found evidence that AN is familial and that genetics might be credible for more than 50% of the heritable risk for becoming afflicted with AN.[29,30] An exact mechanism for the genetic basis of AN is unclear, but this elevated heritability risk is probably linked to inherited vulnerabilities for temperament and anxiety.[31] Heredity estimates are similar for BN and unknown in EDNOS.[32] Although the study of the neurobiology of eating disorders remains somewhat unexplored, a few ways in which this area has been examined are detection for presence of certain regulatory peptides of appetite, testing for activity of neurotransmitters, and use of neuroimaging to determine how brain structure and function correlate with AN.

The dysregulation of serotonin (5-hydroxytryptamine or 5-HT) pathways seems to contribute an important role in the pathogenesis of eating disorders.[33] Disturbances to functional serotonin pathways are heavily associated with many behavioral characteristics that are known to correlate with AN. For example, dysfunctional serotonin pathways can lead to impulsivity, obsessive-compulsivity, anxiety, depression, fear, rumination, and disturbed appetite regulation. In patients afflicted with AN, BN, and those who are recovering from either, the activity of 5-HT has been found to be hindered.[34] Additionally, for patients currently afflicted, low concentrations of 5-HT metabolites in the cerebrospinal fluid seem to be characteristic of this population.[35] As of yet, no specific conclusions about the link between abnormalities in the serotoninergic neurotransmitter system have been formulated, but interest in the dopaminergic system has more recently increased.[36] The fact that AN patients tend to overreact when presented with novel stimuli (*e.g.* sucrose) has led to theory that AN patients exhibit hypersensitive dopaminergic systems, which dictates obsessive-compulsive thinking, enjoyment, and the reward system. Patients with BN show abnormalities in the orbital-frontal serotonergic circuits, which are known to contribute to behavioral dyscontrol.

Other recent studies offer indirect evidence for the presence of a neural basis of eating disorder pathogenesis. fMRI investigations of AN patients have shown differences in their activation responses to stimuli, such as food.[37] Also, studies that included PET and SPECT scans demonstrated that AN patients show neurotransmitter and more commonly, neurotransmitter receptor, abnormalities. Neuroimaging studies have disclosed the presence of enlarged sulci and decreased brain mass in AN patients that have reached the acute malnourished phase. Malnutrition and elevated cortisol are currently blamed for these phenomena and studies show that recovered patients may never fully regain their grey matter mass completely after recovery. Other neurobiological aspects that propel the development and maintenance of both AN and BN, in this case, are neurocognitive abnormalities, such as problems with attention, working memory, mental inflexibility, response inhibition, divided attention, and executive functioning.[38] Many of these symptoms prolong recovery by making an AN patient resistant to treatment and unable to follow longer or insight oriented treatment sessions.[39]

4.2. *Social factors*

One's surroundings have proven to play an extremely important role in triggering the onset of AN, BN, and other disordered eating patterns, especially in the extremely susceptible adolescent population. Pressures to be thin and in shape, especially for females and gay males, are ubiquitous. Examples of ways in which these pressures manifest themselves are media presentations that portray unreasonable ideals of beauty, peer, and sometimes parental pressure.[40] Non-western countries exhibit increased rates of AN and BN when first exposed to Western media, as demonstrated in a study in which the observed incidence of AN among a population of ethnic Fijian adolescent girls increased with the introduction of the television, which broadcasted Western channels, in the mid-1990s.[41]

Destructive weight loss will occur as a result of media infiltration when the ideals portrayed are overvalued. Within those who engage in this weight loss, there are only a few who experience weight loss comparable to that of AN. This provides evidence for the duality of AN, as a patient must not only be exposed to media with unrealistic ideals of beauty but also must exhibit the personality traits, such as perfectionism, obsessive-compulsivity, and the tendency to suppress emotions. BN develops along similar paths, with overvaluation of shape and weight concerns, coupled with personality traits but with greater emotional lability and impulsivity rather than the emotional suppression triggering restrictive eating and binge/purge cycles. Low self-esteem also plays an important role in the development of AN, as the negative energy from self-loathing can sometimes be directed to weight and appearance and lead to an obsession with becoming perfect. Also, before the onset of AN, it is typical for parents of patients to describe their children's lives as having few problems and full of high achievement, but many triggers can alter the direction that a patient originally channeled his or her obsessive energy.

4.3. *Psychological concerns*

Males tend to have the same presentation as females during the course of AN, but some suggest they have better prognosis than females.[42] Males with AN are also usually more concerned with attaining a low body fat percentage rather than a low weight, like females, which is likely driven by the increasingly leaner and muscular male ideal that has been portrayed since the 1980s.[43–45] Furthermore, males who identify as bisexual or homosexual appear in some studies to be more likely to exhibit disordered eating patterns characteristic of AN or BN, and likewise more likely to be diagnosed with either disorder.[46]

Another possible developmental pathology of AN and BN occurs during the transition to puberty.[47] Puberty accompanies physical, especially endocrinological, social, and cognitive changes that can sometimes result in anxiety, depression, and hence the onset of an eating disorder. The journey to adolescence represents an immense amount of change, such as separation from patents, assuming new roles according to gender, acquiring autonomy, all of which can be frightening and lead to the onset of AN and BN. The behaviors of both serve to stifle physical changes that occur as a result of puberty in order to revert to a preadolescent state and avoid this transition.

Family environment has been suggested as adding to the risk for developing an eating disorder. Few systematic data are available to support that there are specific family interaction styles or characteristics that are specific risks for eating disorders. Limited data on the level of criticism in a family suggest that higher levels of criticism (expressed emotion), may make using some form of therapy more difficult and increase dropout from treatment.[48,49]

5. Relevance for Primary Care

Primary care physicians are typically the first health care workers to engage with suspected cases of eating disorders. Parents or patients themselves may present with eating concerns, or health practitioners may become concerned when they see changes in weight or see concerning data on laboratory findings. Pediatricians and family health practitioners may be best placed to identify eating disordered behavior, as they may see patients more frequently and have an understanding of the patient's weight and height changes and typical development. In addition, child and family practitioners can also be responsive to family questions about eating, health, shape, weight, and development. As such, these practitioners are in a position of great importance for the early identification of disordered eating behaviors. Primary care physicians involved in the care of children and adolescents should pay particular attention to weight loss, as well as failure to make expected weight and height gains. In addition to weight, inquiring about eating habits, changes in appetite and amounts being eaten should be part of standard assessment procedures and, where possible, asked of both parents and youths. Finally, particularly in youth who are sensitive to issues of weight, primary care physicians should be mindful of advising their patients around diet and nutrition, with an emphasis on well-rounded, healthy eating, rather than specific dietary rules. Similar issues arise in adulthood, although with these patients there may be a greater emphasis on-going management of medical sequela.

6. Interventions

There are many types of treatments used to address eating disorders in children and adolescents as well as a range of treatment intervention settings. Family therapy, individual therapy, group therapy, and medications are used both separately and in combination with one another. Treatment settings include traditional outpatient settings as well as more restrictive setting to control eating-related behaviors such as hospital, day hospital, and residential treatments. In addition, treatment often includes other professionals working in a collaborative team, consisting of a psychotherapist, child psychiatrist, and a dietician and a pediatrician.

The current evidential base for interventions for eating disorder is small but growing.[50] For BN in adults, considerable evidence is available to support specific treatments; in contrast, for AN in adults there is little evidence that anything is helpful.[51,52] Studies of adults with AN are fraught with severe attrition problems leaving the data from most studies uninterpretable.[53] In children and adolescents, few studies have been conducted.[50] For AN, family treatment of various types appear to be useful, although large randomized studies that compare treatments are not yet available. For adolescent BN, there are two studies suggesting that adolescents respond to specific treatments (CBT and family therapy), but these studies are small and need replication.[54,55] Overall, the quality of the evidence in studies for AN is poor according to a recent systematic review.[50] For BN, the quality of the evidence in adult treatment studies using CBT is good.

6.1. *Treatments for adolescents with anorexia nervosa*

6.1.1. *Family approaches*

Although there is a dearth of published clinical trials on treatments for AN, family therapy has been the subject of most of the published studies thus far.[50] Family therapy as an approach for AN was first suggested in the work of Minuchin *et al.* who described family treatment in the context of psychosomatic family process.[56]

Minuchin characterized psychosomatic family process as being inflexible, enmeshed, conflict avoidant, and overprotective and resulted in a milieu wherein psychosomatic illnesses such as AN would develop. Psychosomatic family process lead to the suppression of individual identity and negative emotions, as well as generated alliances between family members that undermined parental authority. Family therapy based on this formulation endeavored to directly challenge these family processes through structural and behavioral interventions. He reported that 86% of the adolescent subjects he treated in a case series of 53 mostly adolescent subjects were recovered at follow-up.[56,57] These results inspired others in the field to explore family therapy using a variety of models as a treatment for adolescent AN. Minuchin's work inspired clinical researchers at the Maudsley Hospital in London to embark on family therapy as a treatment for adolescent AN.[58] These clinical researchers made significant modifications to the approach and discarded the notion of psychosomatic family process as the target of the intervention. Instead, family therapy based on what is sometimes called the Maudsley approach is initially principally focused on behavioral change around eating in order to promote weight gain.[58,59] There is no focus on the theoretical causes of the AN. In contrast to seeing family processes as being at the heart of the problem, therapists instead advise parents that their support and commitment are of critical importance, and that they can and must take up the task of refeeding their child including prevention of severe dieting, purging, over exercise, and other related problems of AN. Initial sessions focus exclusively on facilitating strategies for parents to challenge and disrupt these behaviors. The therapist does not instruct parents, but consults with them, thereby encouraging empowerment and an increased sense of self-efficacy. In this way, the treatment depends on the leverage that parents have with their children to effect behavior change. Further, by not blaming the parents or seeing them as the cause of the AN, guilt, which often encumbers families taking necessary steps to change behaviors, is diminished. Effort is made to "externalize" the illness of AN by separating the child from the distorting preoccupations and behaviors of the disorder in order to allow parents to see their efforts as being directed at an illness as opposed to their child's will as well as to convey to the adolescent that she or he is also not being blamed for the problems that AN is causing for the family.

There are six published RCTs of outpatient family therapy specific for adolescent AN.[60] Five of these trials test a similar model of family therapy that evolved at the Maudsley Hospital in the 1980s. In addition, there are two long-term follow-up studies documenting the maintenance of improvements over time. Thus, there is limited but consistent empirical evidence that Maudsley-type family therapy is efficacious.[61] Outcomes were intermediate to good (47–95%) using this approach. Two studies suggest that if parents are highly critical of their child, the

Maudsley approach is most effective when provided to parents and the affected offspring separately.[48,62,63] Further, two studies suggest that a brief six month 10-session version of the Maudsley family therapy is as effective[62,64] as longer-term therapy. These findings support the notion that when families are effectively empowered early in treatment, they can be highly efficient. At the same time, studies suggest that families where there is a single parent, divorce or separation, longer treatment is more effective.

While these results are encouraging, there remains significant reasons to be cautious about the data in support of family therapy. For example, only a total of 204 adolescent subjects have been enrolled in the five published randomized clinical trials. Effectively this means that the average cell size of comparison treatments is only about 20 per group, too small for most analyses. Further, three of these five trials were conducted at the same site (Maudsley Hospital)[48,62,65] while only two used manual versions of family treatment needed to confidently replicate treatment.[64,66] In addition, other than weight, outcomes used to assess treatment response vary among the studies making comparisons challenging. Finally, only three studies have published outcome data beyond the end of treatment leaving the long-term benefits of the approach uncertain.[66,67] Nonetheless, taken together the empirical base supporting family therapy of the Maudsley type has been considered sufficient for recognition of this modality as a first line of treatment for children and adolescents with AN (*e.g.* National Institute for Excellence, 2004).

6.1.2. *Individual psychological therapies*

Various forms of individual therapy are used in the treatment of anorexia nervosa including cognitive behavioural therapy, psychodynamic therapy, and supportive therapies. For adolescents with AN in particular, the emphasis of such treatments is usually on autonomy, self-assertion, and assistance with overcoming other developmental challenges associated with adolescence.[68] For adolescents, though many therapists who work primarily with adults may not always agree, parents will generally however be involved in some respect with even treatments that are primarily individually focused.[69] The principal rationale that underlies most individual approaches is that adolescents who develop AN do so to try to control and avoid other pertinent issues of adolescence such as peer relationships, separation from parents, and developing more intimate romantic relationships. The intense focus on weight and shape serves as a way to avoid these challenges.[47] In contrast, cognitive-behavioural therapy (CBT), aims at changing eating disorder specific maintaining factors rather than on developmental or psychodynamic concerns.[70]

Although individual therapy is the probably the most common approach used for AN, there are surprisingly few systematic examinations of it effectiveness. The two studies that have employed individual treatment for adolescents with AN have not found robust support of this form of treatment. In one study, family therapy was compared to supportive individual therapy. This study found that although there were significant improvements in both treatment types, family therapy outperformed individual therapy both at the end of treatment and at 5-year follow-up by a significant margin.[65,67] Robin *et al.*[66] compared family therapy to a highly specific focused individual therapy called Ego-Oriented Individual Therapy (EOIT), a form of therapy aimed at supporting individual psychological development.[66] These authors found that at the end of treatment, family therapy was superior in terms of weight restoration and menstrual return, but at one year follow-up there was no difference between the two treatments, with both having about an 80% success rate. Unfortunately, this was a small study and caution is necessary when considering generalizing the findings.

Unfortunately, even though there have been more studies of individual therapy approaches in adults with AN, including CBT, IPT, nutritional counseling, and other forms of psychodynamic therapies, none of these approaches appear to be particularly effective and no data to support their applicability to younger adolescent patients is available.[60] Further, efforts to evaluate treatment types are limited by the availability of manualized protocols developed specifically for children and adolescents.

6.1.3. *In-patient, day program care, and residential care for adolescent AN*

Although many, if not most adolescents with AN can be successfully treated as outpatients, there may be good reasons for utilizing a more intensive treatment setting in somc cases. These settings sometimes provide more consistent medical monitoring when a person is particularly physically ill. Although there is considerable variation in inpatient treatment programs for eating disorders, most contain nutritional rehabilitation, medical intervention, psychoeducation, psychotherapeutic treatment, psychosocial rehabilitation, and family therapies. At the same time, these benefits accrue potential costs as well. They also infringe on the personal liberties of both the patient and the family. Studies conducted to date, although flawed in some respects have not demonstrated systematic benefit over outpatient alternatives.[71–73]

In addition to hospital, intensive day programs for eating disorders have been developed.[74–77] Usually, day programs run from four to seven days per week and consist of supervised meals, a variety of therapeutic groups, and sometimes concurrent individual therapy.[78] Family therapy and medical and pharmacological management are often included. There are also a growing number of residential care programs that typical provide 24 h care for medically stabilized patients.[79] Often patients in these centers have not responded to outpatient treatments or there are no local experts available to provide specialized outpatient care. Stays in such programs often last several weeks to months and the benefits of these relatively high cost treatment programs remain uncertain.

6.1.4. *Psychopharmacologic interventions*

Although commonly prescribed, there is no evidence available that supports the use of any psychopharmacologic agent for the specific problems of AN.[80] Many agents have been preliminarily examined, but because pilot results were discouraging, further study has not been forthcoming. A recent large multisite clinical study of 90 adults with AN found no benefit of adding fluoxetine to CBT for relapse.[81] At this time, despite the common practice of prescribing SSRIs for adolescent eating disorders, there is little evidence to support the practice of using any medication for AN and particularly for adolescents with AN, a population that has yet to be examined with SSRIs. The use of atypical antipsychotics has also been suggested to be useful in adults with AN, but systematic studies of adolescents are pending.

6.2. *Treatments for adolescent bulimia nervosa*

6.2.1. *Cognitive behavioral therapy*

The greatest evidential support is for CBT. The cognitive-behavioral model of BN assumes that the main factors involved in the maintenance of BN are dysfunctional attitudes toward body shape and weight.[82] Such attitudes lead to an overvaluation of thinness and body dissatisfaction. This leads to a range of behavioral attempts to control shape and weight by excessive dieting, exercise, and purging. However, these behaviors result in both psychological and physiological deprivation and this in turn may lower mood. Ultimately, these behaviors lead to increased hunger and to binge eating. Because of fears that weight and shape will be negatively effected by binge eating, purging behaviors are undertaken to compensate for overeating. This is followed by short-term relief, but as the restrictive eating begins anew, a cycle of binge eating and purging is initiated.

CBT for adults with BN has been found more effective than other conditions, including no therapy, non-directive therapy, pill placebo, manualized psychodynamic therapy (supportive-expressive), stress management, and antidepressant treatment.[83] For those completing CBT between 30 and 40% of patients with BN are abstinent, while another 20% are much improved.

However, there have been only two published case series of adolescent subjects with BN treated with CBT designed for adolescent use (CBT-A), both at Stanford.[54,55] These modifications included: (1) increased contact between the therapist and the adolescent in early treatment to promote therapeutic alliance; (2) involvement of parents in supporting treatment; (3) use of concrete examples to illustrate points; and, (4) exploration of adolescent developmental issues (*e.g.* autonomy concerns) in the context of BN. These studies provide preliminary evidence that CBT-A is acceptable and feasible as a treatment for adolescents with bulimia. There is one RCT comparing cognitive-behavioral guided self-care (CBT-GSC) to family therapy.[84] Results suggest that CBT-GSC was both an acceptable and feasible treatment for adolescents with a treatment drop out rate of 29% and an abstinence rate (from both binge eating and purging) at the end of 12 months treatment of 36%, both similar to rates found in more recent adults studies of CBT. However, it is noteworthy that CBT-A used in the Stanford studies includes direct parental involvement and is therefore a different model from the therapist led guided self-care model that was studied by the London group and more similar to typical CBT used in treatment studies of adults with BN.

6.2.2. *Family treatment*

The family-based treatment model for adolescent BN (FBT-BN) is derived from the approach found to be effective for adolescents with AN originally developed at the Maudsley Hospital and subsequently manualized and examined in treatment studies in the United States.[85,86] Although modified from that employed with adolescent AN, the treatment approach shares many characteristics with the original Maudsley family treatment model. For example, FBT-BN assumes that the secrecy, shame, and dysfunctional eating patterns associated with bulimia have negatively affected adolescent development in the bulimic patient and have confused and disempowered parents and other family members. In addition, parental guilt about having possibly caused the illness and anxiety about how best to proceed have further disabled them. FBT-BN is agnostic as to the cause of BN but assumes that the usual progress through adolescence is negatively affected by the disorder. To target these problems, FBT-BN employs a three-stage treatment. In the first stage, treatment aims at empowering parents to disrupt binge eating, purging, restrictive dieting, and any other pathologic weight control behaviors. It also aims to externalize and separate the disordered behaviors from the affected adolescent to promote parental action and decrease adolescent resistance to their assistance. Once abstinence from disordered eating and related behaviors has been achieved, the second stage of treatment begins wherein parents transition control over eating- and weight-related issues back to the adolescent under their supervision. The third stage is focused on the ways the family can help to address the effects of bulimia on adolescent developmental processes both on the adolescent and the family as a whole.

An RCT for adolescents with BN (BN and partial BN) was recently completed at the University of Chicago wherein 80 adolescents aged 12–19 years (M = 16.1, SD = 1.6) were allocated to either manualized FBT-BN or manualized Supportive Individual Psychotherapy (SPT).[86] In sum, categorical outcomes at posttreatment demonstrated significantly more patients in FBT-BN were binge/purge abstinent compared to SPT, suggesting that FBT-BN is superior to SPT. Rates of abstinence were about 30% for the FBT-BN group. Results from another RCT for adolescent BN and partial BN comparing family therapy to CBT-GSC, has been recently completed. No statistical differences on abstinence rates were found between FBT and the comparison treatment (individual CBT GSC) in that study, but Schmidt and colleagues found that abstinence rates comparable to those achieved by family therapy in the Chicago study.[84] One of the main differences between these two studies was the average age of participants. In the University of Chicago study, the mean age of participants was about 16 years, where it was almost 18 years in the study by Schmidt *et al.* This point in emphasized further by the take up rates for the UK study, wherein 25% of eligible participants refused the study because they did not want their families involved in treatment. In contrast, for the younger adolescents studied at the University of Chicago, where only 11% dropped out of treatment and none of these reported involving the family as the reason for discontinuing treatment. These limited data suggest that there may well be an important age effect on treatment choice suggesting that for younger adolescents with BN, family treatment is a reasonable option, but this may be less the case as adolescents reach young adulthood.

6.2.3. *Dialectical behavior therapy and other group therapies*

There is little evidence about group therapy for eating disorders, especially in youth. Some studies have suggested that group DBT might be useful in BN, but data in support of the approach remains preliminary.[87] In general, support groups are often included as part of a treatment program. Some evidence suggests they may be useful for parents who are struggling with isolation and confusion about how to proceed with seeking help for their children with eating disorders. Inpatient support groups are a varied affair. Sometimes they are helpful in supporting change, but they can also be an opportunity for competing for weight loss, sharing techniques for weight loss, and strategies to avoid detection by physicians.

6.2.4. *Antidepressant medications*

Antidepressant medications in the treatment of adults with BN have received intense research attention in adults.[17] A series of double-blind, placebo-controlled trials of antidepressants among adults with BN have been conducted. In almost all the controlled trials, most types of antidepressants have proven superior to placebo in reducing binge frequency. Generally, mood disturbance and preoccupation with shape and weight also show greater improvement with medication than with placebo. However, only one small case series (10 subjects) found that fluoxetine was well tolerated in adolescents in the context of psychotherapy; however, its effectiveness is unknown in this age group.[88]

7. Outcomes

Outcomes for adolescents with eating disorders appear to be generally favorable for the majority of patients. There is no agreed upon definition for recovery for AN.[89,90] On a practical level, a return to normal weight and waning of severe weight loss strategies and psychological preoccupations about weight and shape are considered reasonable benchmarks. Using these diagnosis-specific criteria, for AN patients, the period of recovery appears to be within the first five years after onset. Unfortunately, after that recovery rates are quite low. There are only three long-term studies of treated adolescents with AN. In those studies, it appears that about two-third are recovered from AN. At the same time, although, about one-third of patients continued to suffer from other psychiatric disorders requiring treatment, most commonly anxiety disorders and depressive disorders. Outcomes for BN in adolescents are unknown. The abstinence rates (for binge eating and purging) in adult studies suggest that between 30 and 40% is a reasonable expected recovery rate in treated subjects. Relapse and a chronic waxing and waning course is therefore common. Similar to AN, many BN subjects whose recovery continue to experience other mental health problems including depression, substance abuse, and personality disorders. Many of these problems may well be associated with chronic BN and some argue that earlier effective intervention with adolescents with BN might prevent these poorer outcomes.

8. Our Practice

We endeavor to practice an evidence-based approach to eating disorders in our clinic. The service includes a medical component which provides a "safety net" for our mostly outpatient practice. This component consists of an adolescent medicine physician expert in the assessing and managing the medical complications of eating disorders and may also include a nutritional consult to assist in determining BMI and likely initial caloric requirements for weight gain. For AN, we employ two main approaches: FBT and a modified version of EOIT used in Robin's study, which we have entitled Adolescent Focused Therapy (AFT). For most patients we begin with FBT, although there are a percentage where there are clearly few parental resources or a decided preference for AFT and in those cases we begin with AFT. For BN, we usually use CBT as modified by our clinic for use with adolescents. However, we also use FBT-BN and IPT. We discuss each of these treatments in more detail below in order to illustrate our specific approaches to adolescent patients with eating disorders.

8.1. *Anorexia nervosa*

Our main practice is to use either of the two approaches for which there is currently the best evidence. Thus, for most patients we use FBT, although a significant minority receive AFT. We have reviewed the evidence of any main principles about these approaches above and a published manual is available for FBT and for AN. Therefore, we provide here only a brief overview of these two approaches.

8.1.1. *Family-based treatment*

This treatment sees the adolescent as incapacitated mostly in terms of his/her eating disorder, or inability to maintain an optimal weight for age and height. The principles of FBT are the same across the age range of patients and are therefore applied consistently. The treatment is otherwise respectful of the particular developmental stage of the patient and the appropriate tasks involved with this stage. Therefore, the way in which the treatment strategies around refeeding are explained to the adolescent and his/her family will be adjusted in accordance with the developmental stage of the patient. Whereas a 12 year old may find it less objectionable to have his/her parents take control of his/her eating than an 18 year old, both patients and their parents are reassured that this is a temporary intervention. As soon as weight is restored, control over eating will be returned to the adolescent, and once weight has been restored, the therapist will address the age appropriate adolescent issue(s) outside the terrain of refeeding. A manual describing this treatment is available.[59] Sessions in FBT last 1 h and begin with weekly sessions, which move to every other week in phase 2 and monthly in phase 3 across the six months to one year of treatment.

8.1.2. *Adolescent focused therapy (AFT)*

Adolescent Focused Therapy (AFT) for adolescents with AN is rooted in self-psychology and similar to Ego-Oriented Individual Therapy as described by Robin and colleagues.[66] Self-psychology, as it pertains to this patient group, posits that individuals with AN manifests ego deficits and confuse control with biological needs. AN represents a disruption in normal ego development. In order to recover, patients must develop sufficient ego strength and function to successfully separate and individuate from the family of origin. According to this therapeutic orientation, AN is a maladaptive coping strategy (a psychological defense) against psychic pain. To develop better ego strength, patients must first learn to identify and define their emotions, and later, to tolerate negative (and even positive) affective states rather than numbing themselves with starvation. AFT for AN posits that the illness is both caused by and serves to maintain a disconnection between chronological age, cognitive/intellectual development, and emotional development. Specifically, adolescents with AN are immature in their ability to process a full range of affective states, particularly negative affect. One of the goals of treatment is to bridge the discrepancies between these different aspects of development. In addition, a primary goal of AFT is to foster the patient's separation and individuation from the family of origin. Collateral sessions with parents are used in this treatment, but their use depends on the adolescent's maturity. In AFT, therapists expect that the types of therapeutic tasks and degree of insight that can be accomplished in treatment will vary by age. Sessions in AFT are 45 min in duration. There are usually a number of collateral sessions, where the parents are seen without the patient, the therapist assesses parental functioning, advocates for the patient's needs, and updates the parents on the patient's progress. Parents are specifically told to refrain from managing eating and weight issues but encouraged to support aspects of appropriate adolescent development and individual strengths in the patient. A manual is available describing this treatment.[91]

8.2. *Bulimia nervosa*

8.2.1. *Cognitive-behavior therapy-adjusted for adolescents*

CBT-A was designed specifically for adolescent patients with BN. It is a modified version of the method originally developed by Fairburn, and has been implemented and modified in a number of pilot projects at our center.[54,92] CBT-A follows three stages over six months. Underlining the flexibility of treatment, moving from one phase to another, or introducing procedures from a later phase, are allowed. Major modifications in application of the model for adolescents are: (1) increased contact of therapist with adolescent in early treatment to promote therapeutic alliance; (2) collateral sessions with parents to elicit their support of treatment; (3) use of concrete examples to illustrate points; and (4) exploration of adolescent developmental issues (*e.g.* autonomy concerns) in the context of BN. Although the use of formal cognitive restructuring techniques is permitted, the expectation is that most adolescents will use problem-solving strategies. A manual is available that describes this treatment in detail.[54]

8.2.2. *Family-based treatment for adolescent bulimia nervosa*

FBT for BN was developed as an adaptation from FBT for AN, for the use in an RCT at Chicago.[59] This manual was first piloted with a small number of cases before adjusted for implementation in the RCT. Upon completion of the study, this manual was further refined for publication as a clinician's manual.[93] FBT for BN, as outlined in this manual, proceeds through three phases with 20 sessions over a period of six months. Phase I lasts between two and three months, with sessions typically scheduled at weekly intervals. Toward phase II, sessions are scheduled every second to third week, while monthly sessions are advisable toward the conclusion of treatment (phase III).

8.3. *Other clinical issues*

Although we use manualized treatments for all our subjects, these approaches are not intended to be "lock step" and the manuals are not so rigid as to disallow individualized modification. For instance, it is not uncommon for our clinicians to spend more time with the individual adolescent in FBT as treatment moves beyond the parentally directed weight restoration phase. Similarly, there are times when using AFT, that convening the entire family or the parents and the child is indeed helpful. When these kinds of modifications are made, though, the overall tenets of the approach are maintained so that the overall intent and specificity of the treatment are not compromised.

It is also noteworthy that there are cases, particularly in adolescent BN, where we have done a kind of "pretreatment" using interpersonal psychotherapy approaches to help motivate and prepare the adolescent to invest in the more specific and personally demanding therapy of CBT. The cases where we use IPT like this are those where the adolescent has many other significant problems in his/her life that are relationally based such as family conflict, peer difficulties, and complex and competing psychiatric issues such as depression, substance use and abuse, or cutting behavior. By using IPT to engage the patient on these other issues, it is sometimes possible to clear the way to the specific issues of binge eating, purging, and eating disorder related behaviors.

8.4. *Inpatient treatment*

Because our center receives many tertiary referrals, many adolescents are medically compromised when they first arrive. As noted above, there are existing standards for medical instability in adolescents with eating disorders published by both the Society of Adolescence and the Academy of Pediatrics. Our center uses these guidelines to determine the medical safety of patients in our care of outpatients. When patients are medically unstable, they are hospitalized on an inpatient pediatric medical unit that has a specialized team of nurses, adolescent medicine specialists, child psychiatrists and psychologists, nutritionists, and social worker to treat these medically compromised young patients.

Over the past several years in response to a general change in philosophy based on our increased appreciation of the capacity for parents to help their children with eating disorders after discharge, we have been moving from an adolescent-focused individual model of treatment to a family model of treatment. This shift is driven in part by the increasing scientific evidence supporting the usefulness of families in helping their children with eating disorders that we discussed above. It is also driven in part by the necessity of shorter hospital stays necessitating that parents take up the nursing staff's role of helping adolescents eat enough to gain weight that used to be a part of a longer hospital stay. This shift has necessitated a range of changes in our treatment program, including parent support and psychoeducational meetings, increased assistance and teaching of parents about meals and nutrition, and decreasing our emphasis on promoting adolescents own management of their meals.

There are a variety of changes inherent in making these changes. It is often difficult to empower parents to help their children when all of the medical decisions are of necessity out of their hands due to the critical nature of their child's current physical state. However, a part of this challenge is to clinicians ourselves to take the chance that parents really CAN help their children and we may need to defer our own authority and opinion to make room for them. On a practical level, one of the most challenging problems is involving parents in the program at meal time, in groups, and in other inpatient decision making processes. This has required reorganizing the timing of some groups, changed the focus of many activities away from individual activities and toward family-based ones. At the same time we are doing all this, though, we do not want to lose sight of the needs of the adolescent for support. Hence, there are continued programs and activities focused on them and with their peers in the hospital. The main focus of the hospital program is to prepare the adolescents to move to outpatient treatment. They are expected upon discharge to participate in both medical follow-up with our team and one of the specific therapies described above.

8.5. *Outcome in our clinic*

Our practice is integrated into a research and outcome structure. Hence, we have important information about how our patients do over time. In a group of 86 subjects with AN treated with FBT using BMI as a measure of treatment progress, we found progress from a 84% IBW to 96% IBW on average. These data demonstrate that the manualized treatment works for typical adolescents with AN that present to our treatment center. Similarly, there are significant declines in all subscales on the EDE.[64] One thing of interest is the fact that the restraint subscale, which is a measure of dieting focus and behavior declines the most and the most rapidly. As parents disrupt their child's self-starvation, and behaviors related to it are the initial focus of FBT, it is not surprising to see the rapid decline on this subscale using this treatment approach. However, it is an evidence of the pattern of improvement of adolescent treated in our clinic with AN using FBT.

Because there is a high likelihood that subjects with eating disorders, particularly those with AN may become medically compromised, a safety net for medical safety is a key part of our practice. Our inpatient program is designed primarily to prepare the patient and family for outpatient treatment and to make sure they are medially safe for this. We illustrated the impact of hospitalization rates over time from a group of adolescents with AN who were treated with family therapy at our center. There was a 35% drop in the rate of hospitalization over time. Given the high cost of hospitalization as well as the negative impact it has on adolescent autonomy and family life, this reduction is an important outcome.

Patients with BN also appear to do well who receive CBT adjusted for adolescents and focused on BN. Overall, our abstinence rates in a case series of 40 subjects are similar to those that would be expected in an adult sample. The abstinence rate is over 50% and the binge purge reduction rate is 78%. These data support the use of the manualized version of CBT we employ for adolescent BN, but further systematic study of this approach is critical in order to know if it is the best approach. Unlike AN, we have not had an opportunity as yet to systematically study CBT for BN in adolescents. As noted, no US study to examine this approach has been published even though it appears to be an excellent candidate for such studies because of the efficacy in adults and the preliminary studies from our group.

It would be useful to know how patients who did well in treatment (or did not) fared over time, but such data are not available. Further, patients who dropped out of treatment in our clinic (as is the case in most centers) are not followed up. It is unclear if these adolescents develop chronic BN, or if some spontaneously recover, or respond to another treatment altogether. For those patients who wish to try a different treatment, IPT is offered, but beyond that we refer these adolescents and their families to local providers who offer an eclectic mix on non-specific treatments.

Treatment for eating disorders in the last quarter century has taken its lead from approaches generally initially tailored for adults. In this sense, it is similar to other disorders where psychological and medication treatments were usually first used with adults, whether it be CBT for depression or lithium for bipolar disorder. Unlike these disorders however, the majority of eating disorders onset during late childhood or adolescents. The more chronic and intractable forms of eating disorders are found in adult populations as a result. As with many medical and psychiatric problems, a prolonged course generally leads to a poorer prognosis. Much of the disappointment in eating disorder treatment research, particularly with AN, is in part attributable to treating the disorder so late in its course where interventions of any type are less likely to be effective. In addition, the approaches that are possible and acceptable with adults with eating disorders are not necessarily those that would be most useful for younger patients. Family treatment, appears both developmentally appropriate and effective for adolescents with AN and BN, but may be less so for even younger adults. In contrast, individually oriented CBT may be more suited to adults with AN because it requires judgment, perspective taking, and assessment of options that come with a fully adult brain. It has been said by some that treating eating disorders among younger patients is "easy," and while this is certainly not true, it is true that many more are likely to respond to effective treatment competently delivered earlier in the course of the disorder just as early stage cancer treatment is more likely to lead to a cure than cancers of more advanced stages. The good news is that early intervention is probably the best way to prevent the development of more chronic and intractable eating disorders. The bad news is that we need to find more effective ways to identify these cases earlier and to develop a broader range of treatments to address them.

9. The Next Five Years

The next five years will likely be an exciting time in our clinic and for research into treatment for eating disorders in adolescents. We are involved in two large-scale studies funded by the NIH on psychotherapy treatment for adolescent AN. The first study will have 120 subjects and compares FBT to AFT. We hope to learn if one treatment is truly superior to the other for most patients, but also for whom which each treatment might work best. Another study we are involved in is a six-site study including sites comparing FBT to systemic family therapy. As such, it is a comparison of a behaviorally focused family therapy to a process oriented family therapy.

For BN, we are conducting a study comparing CBT-A to FBT that includes adolescents at Stanford University and the University of Chicago. In addition to these kinds of treatment research efforts, we are examining neurocognitve processes including neuropsychological findings and associated brain processes in adolescents with AN and BN through fMRI and other imaging technology. By understanding more specifically how they operate in children and adolescents with eating disorders, it may be possible to develop and refine treatments.

References

1. Hoek H, Hoeken D. Review of prevalence and incidence of eating disorders, *Int J Eat Disord* 2003; **34**: 383–396.
2. Golden N, Katzman D, Kreipe R, *et al.* Eating disorders in adolescents: Position paper of the society for adolescent medicine: Medical indications for hospitalization in an adolescent with an eating disorder, *J Adolesc Health* 2003; **33**: 496–503.
3. American Psychiatric Association. *Diagnostic and Statistical Manual of Mental Disorders*. 4th edition. Washington, D.C.: American Psychiatric Association, 1994.
4. Crow S, Agras WS, Halmi K, Mitchell JE, Kraemer H. Full syndromal versus subthreshold anorexia nervosa, bulimia nervosa, and binge eating disorder: A multicenter study, *Int J Eat Disord* 2002; **32**: 309–318.
5. Le Grange D, Binford R, Peterson C, *et al.* DSM-IV Threshold versus subthreshold bulimia nervosa, *Int J Eat Disord* (in press).
6. Hoek H, van Harten PN, Hermans KM, Katzman MA, Matroos GE, Susser ES. The incidence of anorexia nervosa on Curacao, *Am Psychiatry* 2005; **162**: 748–752.
7. Lee S. Self-starvation in context: Towards a culturally sensitive understanding of anorexia nervosa, *Soc Sci Med* 1995; **41**: 25–36.
8. McClelland L, Crisp AH. Anorexia nervosa and social class, *Int J Eat Disord* 2001; **29**: 150–156.
9. Halmi K, Brodland G, Loney J. Progress in anorexia nervosa, *Ann Int Med* 1973; **78**: 907–909.
10. Lock J. Fitting square pegs into round holes: Males with eating disorders, *J Adolesc Health* 2008; **44**: 99–100.
11. van Son G, van Hoeken D, Aad I, Bartelds A, van Furth E, Hoek H. Time trends in the incidence of eating disorders: A primary care study in the Netherlands, *Int J Eat Disord* 2006; **39**: 565–569.
12. Lucas AR, Beard CM, O'Fallon WM. 50-year trends in the incidence of anorexia nervosa in Rochester, Minn: A population-based study, *Am J Psychiatry* 1991; **148**: 917–929.
13. Lucas AR, Crowson C, O'Fallon WM, Melton L. The ups and downs of anorexia nervosa, *Int J Eat Disord* 1999; **26**: 397–405.

14. Flament M, Ledoux S, Jeammet P, Choquet M, Simon Y. A population study of bulimia nervosa and subclinical eating disorders in adolescence. In: Steinhausen H, Ed. *Eating Disorders in Adolescence: Anorexia and Bulimia Nervosa*. New York: Brunner/Mazel, 1995; pp. 21–36.
15. Keel PK, Mitchell JE, Miller KB, Davis TL, Crow SJ. Predictive validity of bulimia nervosa as a diagnostic category, *Am J Psychiatry* 2000; **157**(1): 136–138.
16. Fairburn C, Bohn K. Eating disorder NOS (EDNOS): An example of the troublesome eating disorder not otherwise specified (NOS) category in DSM-IV, *Behav Res Ther* 2005; **43**: 691–701.
17. Mitchell J, Agras WS, Wonderlich S. Treatment of bulimia nervosa: Where are we and where are we going? *Int J Eat Disord* 2007; **40**: 95–101.
18. Bulik CM, Hebebrand J, Keski-Rahkonen A, *et al.* Genetic epidemiology, endophenotypes, and eating disorder classification, *Int J Eat Disord* 2007; **40**: S52–S60.
19. Gull W. Anorexia nervosa (apepsia hysterica, anorexia hysterica), *Trans Clin Soc London* 1874; **7**: 222–228.
20. Katzman D, Christensen G, Young A, Zipursky R. Structural abnormalities and cognitive impairment in adolescents with anorexia nervosa, *Seminars Clin Neuropsychiatry* 2001; **6**: 146–152.
21. Sullivan PF. Mortality in anorexia nervosa, *Am J Psychiatry* 1995; **152**: 1073–1074.
22. Workgroup for the Classification of Child and Adolescents Eating Disorders. Classification of child and adolescent eating disturbances, *Int J Eat Disord* 2007; **40**: S117–S122.
23. Cachelin FM, Striegel-Moore RH, Elder KA, Pike KM, Wilfley DE, Fairburn CG. Natural course of a community sample of women with binge eating disorder, *Int J Eat Disord* 1999; **25**(1): 45–54.
24. Rome E, Ammerman S. Medical complications of eating disorders: An update, *J Adol Health* 2003; **33**: 418–426.
25. Rome E, Ammerman S, Rosen D, *et al.* Children and adolescents with eating disorders: The state of the art, *Pediatrics* 2003; **111**: 98–108.
26. Herzog DB, Nussbaum KM, Marmor AK. Comorbidity and outcome in eating disorders, *Psychiatr Clin North Am* 1996; **19**(4): 843–859.
27. Godart N, Flament M, Perdereau F, Jeammet P. Comorbidity between eating disorders and anxiety disorders: A review, *Int J Eat Disord* 2002; **32**.
28. Lock J, Le Grange D. *Help Your Child Beat An Eating Disorder*. New York: Guilford Press, 2005.
29. Bulik CM. Genetic and biological risk factors. In: Thompson J, Ed. *Handbood of Eating Disorders and Obesity*, Hoboken, New Jersey: John Wiley & Sons, 2004; pp. 3–16.
30. Lilenfeld L, WH K, Greeno C, *et al.* A controlled family study of anorexia nervosa and bulimia nervosa: Psychiatric disorders in first-degree relatives and effects of proband comorbidity, *Arch Gen Psychiatry* 1998; **55**: 603–610.

31. Klump K, Bulik CM, Pollice C, *et al.* Temperament and character in women with anorexia nervosa, *J Nerv Ment Dis* 2000; **188**: 559–567.
32. Bulik CM, Sullivan PF, Kendler KS. Heritability of binge eating and broadly defined bulimia nervosa, *Biol Psychiatry* 1998; **44**: 1210–1218.
33. Ferguson C, La Via M, Crossan P, Kaye WH. Are serotonin selective reuptake inhibitors effective in underweight anorexia nervosa, *Int J Eat Disord* 1999; **25**: 11–17.
34. Frank G, Kaye WH, Meltzer CC, *et al.* Reduced 5-HT2A receptor binding after recovery from anorexia nervosa, *Biol Psychiatry* 2002; **52**: 896–906.
35. Kaye WH, Gwirtsman HE, George D, Ebert MH. Altered serotonin activity in anorexia nervosa after long-term weight restoration. Does elevated cerebrospinal fluid 5-hydroxyindoleacetic acid level correlate with rigid and obsessive behaviors? *Arch Gen Psychiatry* 1991; **48**: 556–562.
36. McConaha C, Gaskill J, La Via M, *et al.* An open trial of olanzapine in anorexia nervosa, *J Clin Psychiatry* 2004; **65**: 1480–1482.
37. Frank G, Bailer U, Henry S, Wagner A, WH K. Neuroimaging studies in eating disorders, *CNS Spectrums* 2004; **9**: 539–548.
38. Roberts M, Tchanturia K, Stahl D, Southgate L, Treasure J. A systematic review and meta-analysis of set-shifting ability in eating disorders, *Psychol Med* 2005; **37**: 1075–1084.
39. Tchanturia K, Morris R, Surguladze S, Treasure JL. An examination of perceptual and cognitive set shifting tasks in acute anorexia nervosa and following recovery, *Eat Weight Disord* 2002; **7**: 312–316.
40. Anderson-Fye, Becker AE. Sociocultural aspects of eating disorders. In: Thompson J, Ed. *Handbook of Eating Disorders and Obesity*. Hoboken, New Jersey: John Wiley & Sons, 2004; pp. 565–589.
41. Becker AE, Burnwell RG, SE, Herzog DB, Hamberg P. Eating behaviors and attitudes following prolonged exposure to television among ethnic Fijian adolescent girls, *Br J Psychiatry* 2002; **180**: 509–514.
42. Strober M, Freeman R, Lampert C, Diamond J, Teplinsky C, DeAntonio M. Are there gender differences in core symptoms, temperament, and short-term prospective outcome in anorexia nervosa? *Int J Eat Disord* 2006; **39**: 570–575.
43. Pope HG, Gruber A, Choi P, Olivardia R, Phillips K. Muscle dysphoria: An underrecognized form of body dysmorphic disorder, *Psychosomatics* 1997; **38**: 548–557.
44. Pope HG, Olivardia R, Gruber A, Borowiecki J. Evolving ideals of male body image as seen through action toys, *Int J Eat Disord* 1999; **26**: 65–72.
45. Leit R, Pope HG, Gray J. Cultural expectations of muscularity in men: The evolution of the playgirl centerfolds, *Int J Eat Disord* 2001; **29**: 90–93.
46. Carlat DJ, Camargo CA, Jr., Herzog DB. Eating disorders in males: A report on 135 patients, *Am J Psychiatry* 1997; **154**(8): 1127–1132.

47. Crisp AH. Anorexia nervosa as flight from growth: Assessment and treatment based on the model. In: Garner DM, Garfinkel P, Eds. *Handbook of Treatment for Eating Disorders*. New York: Guilford, 1997, pp. 248–277.
48. Eisler I, Dare C, Hodes M, Russell G, Dodge E, Le Grange D. Family therapy for adolescent anorexia nervosa: The results of a controlled comparison of two family interventions, *J Child Psychol Psychiatry* 2000; **41**(6): 727–736.
49. Szmukler GI, Eisler I, Russell G, Dare C. Anorexia nervosa, parental 'expressed emotion' and dropping out of treatment, *Br J Psychiatry* 1985; **147**: 265–271.
50. Le Grange D, Lock J. The dearth of psychological treatment studies for anorexia nervosa, *Int J Eat Disord* 2005; **37**: 79–81.
51. Agras WS, Walsh BT, Fairburn CG, Wilson GT, Kraemer HC. A multicenter comparison of cognitive-behavioral therapy and interpersonal psychotherapy for bulimia nervosa, *Arch Gen Psychiatry* 2000; **57**: 459–466.
52. Agras WS, Brandt H, Bulik CM, *et al*. Report of the National Institutes of Health workshop on overcoming barriers to treatment research in anorexia nervosa, *Int J Eat Disord* 2004; **35**: 509–521.
53. Halmi CA, Agras WS, Crow SJ, *et al*. Predictors of treatment acceptance and completion in anorexia nervosa: Implications for future study designs, *Arch Gen Psychiatry* 2005; **62**: 776–781.
54. Lock J. Adjusting cognitive behavioral therapy for adolescent bulimia nervosa: Results of a case series, *Am J Psychotherapy* 2005; **59**: 267–281.
55. Schapman A, Lock J. Cognitive-behavioral therapy for adolescent bulimia, *Int J Eat Disord* 2006; **39**: 252–255.
56. Minuchin S, Rosman B, Baker I. *Psychosomatic Families: Anorexia Nervosa in Context*. Cambridge, MA: Harvard University Press, 1978.
57. Rosman B, Minuchin S, Baker L, Liebman R. A family approach to anorexia nervosa: Study, treatment and outcome. In: Vigersky RA, Ed. *Anorexia Nervosa*. New York: Raven Press, 1977, pp. 341–348.
58. Dare C, Eisler I. Family therapy for anorexia nervosa. In: Garner DM, Garfinkel P, Eds. *Handbook of Treatment for Eating Disorders*. New York: Guilford Press, 1997, pp. 307–324.
59. Lock J, Le Grange D, Agras WS, Dare C. *Treatment Manual for Anorexia Nervosa: A Family-Based Approach*. New York: Guilford Publications, Inc., 2001.
60. Bulik CM, Berkman N, Kimberly A, Brownly JS, Lohr K. Anorexia nervosa: A systematic review of randomized clinical trials, *Int J Eat Disord* 2007; **40**: 310–320.
61. Lock J, Le Grange D. Family-based treatment of eating disorders, *Int J Eat Disord* 2005; 38(Supplement): s64–67.
62. Le Grange D, Eisler I, Dare C, Russell G. Evaluation of family treatments in adolescent anorexia nervosa: A pilot study, *Int J Eat Disord* 1992; **12**(4): 347–357.

63. Le Grange D, Eisler I, Dare C, Hodes M. Family criticism and self-starvation: A study of expressed emotion, *J Fam Therapy* 1992; **14**: 177–192.
64. Lock J, Agras WS, Bryson S, Kraemer H. A comparison of short- and long-term family therapy for adolescent anorexia nervosa, *J Am Acad Child Adolesc Psychiatry* 2005; **44**: 632–639.
65. Russell GF, Szmukler GI, Dare C, Eisler I. An evaluation of family therapy in anorexia nervosa and bulimia nervosa, *Arch Gen Psychiatry* 1987; **44**(12): 1047–1056.
66. Robin A, Siegal P, Moye A, Gilroy M, Dennis A, Sikand A. A controlled comparison of family versus individual therapy for adolescents with anorexia nervosa, *J Am Acad Child Adolesc Psychiatry* 1999; **38**(12): 1482–1489.
67. Eisler I, Dare C, Russell GFM, Szmukler GI, Le Grange D, Dodge E. Family and individual therapy in anorexia nervosa: A five-year follow-up, *Arch Gen Psychiatry* 1997; **54**: 1025–1030.
68. Bruch H. *Eating Disorders: Obesity, Anorexia Nervosa, and the Person Within*. New York: Basic Books, 1973.
69. Lock J. Treating adolescents with eating disorders in the family context: Empirical and theoretical considerations, *Child Adolesc Psychiatric Clin North Am* 2002; **11**: 331–342.
70. Pike K, Walsh BT, Vitousek K, Wilson GT, Bauer J. Cognitive-behavioral therapy in the posthospitalization treatment of anorexia nervosa, *Am J Psychiatry* 2004; **160**: 2046–2049.
71. Crisp AH, Norton K, Gowers S, *et al.* A controlled study of the effect of therapies aimed at adolescent and family psychopathology in anorexia nervosa, *Br J Psychiatry* 1991; **159**: 325–333.
72. Gowers S, Weetman J, Shore R, Hussain F, Elvins R. The impact of hospitalisation on the outcome of adolescent anorexia nervosa, *Br J Psychiatry* 2000; **45**: 138–141.
73. Gowers S, Clark A, Roberts C, *et al.* Clinical effectiveness of treatments for anorexia nervosa in adolescents, *Br J Psychiatry* 2007; **191**: 427–435.
74. Gerlinghoff M, Backmund H, Franzen U. Evaluation of a day treatment programme for eating disorders, *European Eat Disord Rev* 1998; **6**: 96–106.
75. Birchell H, Palmer R, Waite J, Gadsby K, Gatward N. Intensive day programme treatment for severe anorexia nervosa — the Leicester experience, *Psych Bull* 2002; **26**: 334–336.
76. Zipfel S, Lowe B, Deter HC, Herzog W. Long-term prognosis in anorexia nervosa: Lessons from a 21-year follow-up study, *Lancet* 2000; **355**: 721–722.
77. Robinson P. Day treatments. In: Treasure JL, Schmidt U, van Furth E, Eds. *Handbook of Eating Disorders*. Hoboken: John Wiley and Sons, 2003.
78. Olmsted M. Day hospital treatment of anorexia nervosa and bulimia nervosa. In: Fairburn CG, Brownell K, Eds. *Eating Disorders and Obesity: A Comprehensive Review*. New York: Guilford Press, 2002, pp. 330–334.

79. Frisch J, Franko D, Herzog DB. Residential treatment for eating disorders, *Int J Eat Disord* 2006; **39**: 434–439.
80. Attia E, Mayer L, Killory E. Medication response in the treatment of patients with anorexia nervosa, *J Psychiatric Practice* 2001; **7**: 157–162.
81. Walsh BT, Kaplan AS, Attia E, *et al.* Fluoxetine after weight restoration in anorexia nervosa: A randomized clinical trial, *JAMA* 2006; **295**: 2605–2612.
82. Fairburn C. A cognitive behavioural approach to the treatment of bulimia, *Psychol Med* 1981; **11**(4): 707–711.
83. Agras WS. Eating disorders. In: Schatzberg AF, Nemeroff CB, Eds. *Textbook of Psychopharmacology.* 3rd edition. Washington, D.C: American Psychiatric Publishing Inc., 2003, pp. 1030–1040.
84. Schmidt U, Lee S, Beecham J, *et al.* A randomized controlled trial of family therapy and cognitive behavior therapy guided self-care for adolescents with bulimia nervosa and related conditions, *Am J Psychiatry* 2007; **164**: 591–598.
85. Dodge E, Hodes M, Eisler I, Dare C. Family therapy for bulimia nervosa in adolescents: An exploratory study, *J Fam Therapy* 1995; **17**: 59–77.
86. Le Grange D, Crosby R, Rathouz P, Leventhal B. A randomized controlled comparison of family-based treatment and supportive psychotherapy for adolescent bulimia nervosa, *Arch Gen Psychiatry* 2007; **64**: 1049–1056.
87. Safer D, Telch CF, Chen E. *Dialectical Behavior Therapy for Binge Eating and Bulimia.* New York: Guilford Press, 2009.
88. Kotler L, Devlin B, Davies M, Walsh BT. An open trial of fluoxetine in adolescents with bulimia nervosa, *J Child Adolesc Psychopharmacology* 2003; **13**: 329–325.
89. Couturier J, Lock J. What constitutes remission in adolecent anorexia nervosa: A review of various conceptualizations and a quantitative analysis, *Int J Eat Disord* 2006; **39**: 175–183.
90. Couturier J, Lock J. What is recovery in adolescent anorexia nervosa? *Int J Eat Disord* 2006; **39**: 550–555.
91. Fitzpatrick K, Moye A, Hostee R, Le Grange D, Lock J. Adolescent focused therapy for adolescent anorexia nervosa, *J Contemp Psychotherapy* 2010; **40**: 31–39.
92. Fairburn CG, Marcus MD, Wilson GT. Cognitive-behavioral therapy for binge eating and bulimia nervosa: A comprehensive treatment manual. In: Fairburn CG, Wilson GT, Eds. *Binge Eating: Nature, Assessment, & Treatment.* New York, NY.: Guildford Press., 1993, pp. 361–404.
93. Le Grange D, Lock J. *Treating Bulimia in Adolescence.* New York: Guilford Press, 2007.

Chapter 15

Autism Spectrum Disorders

Jennifer Phillips, Mendy Minjarez, Emma Mercier, Carl Feinstein, and Antonio Y. Hardan

1. Introduction

The term Autism Spectrum Disorders (ASD) is used synonymously with pervasive developmental disorders (PDD) to refer to autism and the four autistic-like conditions described in the *Diagnostic and Statistical Manual of Mental Disorders*, Fourth Edition, Text Revision (DSM-IV-TR).[1] ASD has moved to the forefront of child psychiatry in recent years, as community awareness has increased and incidence rates continue to grow at an alarming rate. Autism currently ranks as the second most common developmental disability diagnosed in the United States, behind intellectual disability and in front of cerebral palsy, hearing loss, and vision impairment.[2] The need for early diagnosis and intensive behavioral intervention is paramount, but the demand often exceeds the availability of resources. While much remains to be discovered about the etiology of Autism Spectrum Disorders, theories and information not grounded in research are abundant in relation to this disorder, making it difficult for parents to make informed decisions as they seek treatments for their children. The primary aim of this chapter is to provide an update on the current status of research in the neurobiology and genetics of Autism Spectrum Disorders, and discuss current practice parameters for diagnosis and treatment of these conditions.

1.1. *Definition*

Autism Spectrum Disorders are defined by characteristic and pervasive deficits in reciprocal social interactions and communication, as well as the presence of

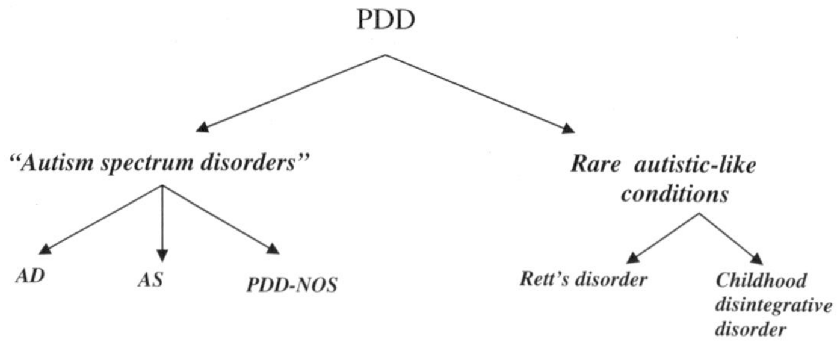

Fig. 1: DSM-IV-TR pervasive developmental disorder.

unusual, restricted, and repetitive behaviors and interests.[1] Social impairments comprise the core deficit in all ASDs. In addition to autism, the DSM-IV-TR lists four other autistic-like conditions that are under the PDD umbrella: Asperger's disorder, Rett's disorder, childhood disintegrative disorder (CDD), and pervasive developmental disorder, not otherwise specified (PDD-NOS). Typically, when clinicians refer to ASD, they are including the three most commonly diagnosed of these conditions: autism, Asperger's disorder, and PDD-NOS (Fig. 1).

1.2. *Historical context*

Autism was first described by Dr. Leo Kanner in 1943, in a paper in which he presented 11 case studies of children that he defined as showing evidence of "extreme autism, obsessiveness, stereotypy and echolalia." In this initial description of autism, Kanner also commented on the families that these children came from, noting the unusually high level of education of both the fathers and mothers and the fact that few parents seemed to be genuinely warm-hearted people. In spite of the possible impact of parental nature, Kanner also specifically noted that the cause of autism was most likely some innate characteristic, rather than a function of the environment. This hypothesis was unfortunately not explored in the years that followed; instead, giving way to years of a focus on the parents, particularly "refrigerator mothers," as the cause of the disorder.

In 1965, Dr. Bernard Rimland established the Autism Society of America, the first advocacy group for parents of children with autism, and began to campaign for a scientific exploration of the disorder and its treatment options. In the late 1980s, the first study of the use of behavioral intervention was published, showing gains in language and social interaction and reduction of repetitive behaviors for children with autism who received intensive behavioral intervention. When this, and other studies that followed, were publicized, they provided hope for many parents, indicating that progress and learning were possible for children who received an autism diagnosis. In 1980, the *Diagnostic and Statistical Manual of Mental Disorders*, Third Edition (DSM-III), classified autism as a developmental disorder, rather than a type of schizophrenia as it had previously been described. The current version of this manual, DSM-IV-TR,[1] classifies autism as a pervasive developmental disorder.

2. Epidemiology

In the past decade, estimates of the prevalence of autism have increased dramatically. The National Institutes of Health (NIH) estimated that autism affected 1 in 500 children in 2000, but increased this estimate to 1 in 250 in 2001. In 2007, the Center for Disease Control (CDC) published its first morbidity and mortality weekly report, based on findings from their Autism and Developmental Disabilities Monitoring Network (ADDM), which reported that during the surveillance years 2000–2002, the prevalence of ASD (including autism, Asperger's, and PDD-NOS) was between 1 in 100 and 1 in 300, with an average prevalence of 1 in 150.[3] In 2009, prevalence results for the surveillance year 2006 were published, noting between 1 in 80 to 1 in 240 children diagnosed with ASD, for an average prevalence of 1 in 110. ASD is more common in boys, with an average prevalence of 1 in 70, while in girls the average prevalence is 1 in 315.[4] Similarly, in 2009 a joint publication from the CDC, the Health Resources and Services Administration (HRSA), and Massachusetts General Hospital reported that an average of 1 in 91 children between the ages of 3 and 17 were diagnosed with an ASD in 2007, as measured by parent telephone survey.[5] Discussions continue about whether this statistical increase is due to an actual increase in the rates of ASD, or whether it reflects issues such as increased awareness and diagnosis, and a broadening definition of ASD or both.[6]

Prevalence of autistic disorder in males versus females is reported at approximately 4.3:1, although this number changes when cognitive abilities are considered, with estimates of 5.5:1 for children without cognitive impairment, and 2:1 when intellectual disability is present.[7,8] Although previous estimates suggested that 70–75% of children with autism also had a diagnosis of intellectual disability, current estimates are lower, with averages of 40–55% reported.[8] Information about prevalence across race is inconsistent, with the most current CDC findings reporting a higher prevalence among non-Hispanic white children than among non-Hispanic black children and Hispanic children.[4]

3. Diagnosis

3.1. *Current diagnostic categories*

Current criteria to diagnose ASDs are drawn from two sources: the *Diagnostic and Statistical Manual of Mental Disorders*, 4th ed., text revision (DSM-IV-TR) and the World Health Organization's International Classification of Diseases (ICD-10). Both classification systems recognize five types of pervasive developmental disorders: autistic disorder, Rett's disorder, childhood disintegrative disorder, Asperger's disorder, and PDD-NOS.

Both the DSM-IV and ICD-10 recognize the complex nature of autistic disorder, requiring symptoms in three areas: (1) social interaction, (2) communication and (3) restricted interests or repetitive behavior, as well as delayed or abnormal development before three years of age. The classification systems are generally in agreement regarding the symptoms of the disorder, with both classifying the onset before the age of three as a necessary condition for diagnosis (Table 1).

Specialists in the ASD field are currently in discussion about a major shift in diagnostic criteria and terminology that will occur with the publication of the DSM-5, currently scheduled for 2013. In February 2010, the DSM-5 neurodevelopmental disorders workgroup submitted the proposed criteria for autism spectrum disorders, although these criteria continue to be discussed and refined.[9] A major proposed shift will be in the use of one diagnosis, "Autism Spectrum Disorder," for all autism spectrum conditions. The proposed diagnostic criteria will no longer separate social and communication deficits, but instead these will be described under the category "social affect." The team also proposed the removal of Rett's disorder, based on the specific etiology of this condition (a known genetic disorder), and the fact that individuals often only have autistic symptoms for a brief time during early childhood. They also proposed removal of the NOS category, while proposing the addition of new categories in areas such as learning disorders and communication disorders to reflect conditions in which children have some social cognitive deficits but do not meet clear criteria for an ASD diagnosis. There will also be a broader description of the developmental spectrum of ASD, including additional information for practitioners about how children present at different stages of development. In addition, severity ratings are being considered. While these suggested changes are still being debated and developed, it is clear that major shifts are occurring in the way that we understand, identify, and diagnose ASD.

Table 1: Diagnostic Criteria for Pervasive Developmental Disorders

Domain	Symptom Criteria	Description
Social interactions	Marked impairment in the use of multiple nonverbal behaviors	• Impairment in social modulation of eye contact • Use of facial expressions to convey emotions may be impaired (*e.g.* blank or limited expressions, not directing expressions to others) • May turn away from others during interactions, not use his/her body to orient to a person during social exchanges • Spontaneous social use of gestures may be limited, such as pointing to express interest
	Failure to develop peer relationships appropriate to developmental level	• Younger children may play alone, have difficulty joining group activities, engage in parallel play when others of their age engage in interactive or make-believe play • Older children may not have an identified friend, choose solitary activities, have difficulty making new friends
	Lack of spontaneous seeking to share enjoyment, interests, or achievements with other people	• Lack of joint attention • Does not show, bring, or point out objects or activities that he/she is interested in, proud of, or engaged in • Difficulty sharing pleasure in accomplishments
	Lack of social reciprocity	• Difficulty maintaining a "back and forth" interaction with another person (turn-taking) • May have difficulty responding to the social overtures of others and do best when interactions are "on his/her terms" • May have difficulty initiating or responding to a social interaction • In older children, may have difficulty understanding empathy and understanding his/her roles in relationships
Communication	Delay in, or total lack of, the development of spoken language	• Any significant early delay in language development (receptive and expressive) • There is no attempt to compensate for the delay with other ways of communicating, like gestures and mime
	Marked impairment in the ability to initiate or sustain a conversation	• This does not apply to children who do not have phrase language • May have one-sided exchanges, talk "at" you rather than with you, have trouble answering open-ended questions

(*Continued*)

Table 1: (*Continued*)

Domain	Symptom Criteria	Description
	Stereotyped and repetitive use of language or idiosyncratic language	• Immediate Echolalia • Use of speech-like jargon • Repeating lines from favorite videos • Scripted or "canned" use of phrases • Pronoun reversal (I/you)
	Lack of varied, spontaneous make-believe play or social imitative play	• Play that is not at a developmentally appropriate age • In young children, lack of interest in social games, such as peek-a-boo • In older children, lack of appropriate pretend play
Restricted/ repetitive behaviors	Encompassing preoccupation with one or more stereotyped and restricted patterns of interest that is abnormal either in intensity or focus	• In younger children, there may be an intense interest in certain videos or toys (*e.g.* trains or cars), in numbers and letters, or in mechanicalobjects such as elevators • In older children, this might include intense interest in certain subjects that he/she knows many facts about, such as marine animals, outer space, *etc.*
	Apparently inflexible adherence to specific, non-functional routines or rituals	• Needing to do things in a particular manner, order, or sequence, and becoming distraught if that order is not followed • Examples: schedule routines, eating routines, placement routines (*e.g.* where furniture is located in the house), dressing routines
	Stereotyped and repetitive motor mannerisms	• Hand flapping • Finger flicking • Spinning • Body posturing (moving the body into unusual and repetitive postures) • Pacing • Running in circles
	Persistent preoccupations with parts of objects	• Interests that seem sensory in nature • Visual examination of parts of toys (*e.g.* the wheels of a car), squinting or peering • Repetitive dropping of objects, or watching objects fall (sand, water, balls, *etc.*) • Lining up or spinning objects

3.2. *Clinical description*

Autistic disorder, Asperger's disorder, and PDD-NOS are the most common of the autism spectrum conditions. Rett's disorder and Childhood disintegrative disorder

(CDD) are much rarer and, although they are classified as pervasive developmental disorders, they differ significantly from the other Autism Spectrum Disorders.

3.2.1. *Autistic disorder*

Autism is characterized by atypical development in three main areas: (1) socialization, (2) communication, and (3) restrictive or repetitive behaviors. Additional associated features are commonly seen in autism, including, but not limited to, sensory issues, sleep and eating disturbances, learning deficits, phobias, temper tantrums, and aggression. Autism must manifest in early childhood (by 36 months of age in DSM-IV-TR), although a final clinical diagnosis may not be made until the preschool or kindergarten years.

Within the diagnosis of autism, there can be vast individual differences in functioning. Children with autism often exhibit uneven cognitive profiles, with deficits in verbal and abstract reasoning skills, and strengths in rote memory and visual-spatial reasoning. They also often have difficulties with adaptive functioning. Some children remain nonverbal, while others develop language abilities but may continue to struggle with social communication skills. Although most children exhibit consistent difficulties from a very young age, patterns of regression have been seen in a subgroup of children diagnosed with autism. This regression typically occurs when the child is between 14 and 24 months of age, and may include a loss of language and/or other acquired skills (*e.g.* play, social interaction) following a period of normal development.[10,11]

Knowing that there is wide variability within this condition, researchers have attempted to differentiate children by their level of cognitive functioning, and from this comes the term "high functioning autism," or HFA.[12] While this is not a separate diagnosis in the DSM-IV-TR, there are distinct differences between children with HFA and children who have autism as well as cognitive deficits. Because children with HFA do not have significant intellectual impairments, their expression of symptoms is often less severe than children with autism who are not high functioning. For example, children with HFA will likely develop better verbal communication skills, but they will still struggle significantly in areas such as vocabulary development and usage, language mechanics, and conversational pragmatics. Children with HFA more closely resemble children with Asperger's disorder in many ways, and as they get older, the distinction becomes even less apparent.

3.2.2. *Asperger's disorder*

In 1944, Asperger described a group of children who exhibited normal intelligence and communication skills, but had deficits in social interaction skills and portrayed a range of stereotyped behaviors.[13] Originally called autistic psychopathy, Asperger's research was not discovered until approximately three decades later, and Asperger's disorder was not introduced into the DSM until the publication of the DSM-IV. Asperger's syndrome is characterized by deficits in social interaction and stereotyped or repetitive behaviors and obsessive interests. Unlike autism, deficits in communication and cognitive capacity are not present, although deficits in adaptive functioning can be seen and occur secondary to social, rather than cognitive impairment. Questions about the distinction between Asperger's disorder and High Functioning Autism (*i.e.* children with autism who do not have a cognitive impairment) exist, although important differences in communication skills have been reported.

3.2.3. *Pervasive developmental disorder, not otherwise specified*

PDD-NOS is a catch-all category which is used in a heterogenous group of children who exhibit symptoms of autism but do not meet full criteria for either Asperger's disorder or autistic disorder.[14] It is more commonly diagnosed than autism. Children with "atypical" autism are also included in this category, and they are defined as such because they may have exhibited a late age of onset, or symptomology that is subthreshold or different from the standard criteria for autism (*e.g.* a child who starts to show symptoms after age three, or who demonstrates social and deficits but no repetitive behaviors or interests). The most common misconception about a diagnosis of PDD-NOS is that it is equivalent to a very mild form of autism. A child can have four or five severe symptoms and meet criteria for PDD-NOS, while another child might meet full criteria for autism with more symptoms that are less severe, and have fewer deficits overall. Treatment options are the same in PDD-NOS as they are in other ASD conditions.

3.2.4. *Rett's disorder*

Identified in 1966 by Andreas Rett, Rett's disorder is associated with normal development for the first 6 to 18 months of life, followed by developmental regression. Although children may demonstrate some autistic-like symptoms, such as loss of social engagement, communication skills, toe walking, and stereotypic hand mannerisms, they also have other traits not associated with autism, such as deceleration of head growth resulting in microcephaly, as well as multiple systemic issues, such as gastrointestinal problems, feeding and swallowing issues, motor problems (including poor coordination and/or trunk movements that may worsen after age 10), and bone density abnormalities. Several comorbid conditions are associated with Rett's disorder, including severe intellectual disability and seizure disorder, which is more common than in autistic disorder. It is also common to see a specific form of stereotypic motor mannerism, comprised on repetitive midline hand movements, such as clapping or wringing of the hands, which affects the purposeful use of the hands. Rett's is more common in females, as male fetuses rarely reach term. Prevalence rates range from 1 in 10,000 to 1 in 20,000 in girls.[15]

Unlike the other pervasive developmental disorders, the cause of Rett's has been identified as a mutation in methyl CpG binding protein 2, or the MECP2 gene in 92% of typical Rett's cases.[15] This gene controls the synthesis of proteins necessary for brain development, methyl cytosine binding protein 2 (MECP2), and the expression of many other genes, leading to more pervasive abnormal gene expression. It appears that the mutation is spontaneous, with less than 1% of cases being inherited, so although prenatal testing is available, having a family history of Rett's disorder does not appear to increase the likelihood of the mutation reoccurring. Additionally, possession of the mutation does not necessarily lead to the development of Rett's disorder, with known occurrences of asymptomatic carriers.

While individuals with Rett's disorder may live into adulthood, there is a higher rate of sudden death than in the general population, reducing their life expectancy.[16] There is no known cure for Rett's disorder. However, as some of the features of this condition include autistic-like symptoms, autism treatment strategies can be employed, including therapies that aim at improving communication, social skills, and behavior. Additionally, management of gastrointestinal and nutritional issues, as well as the use of psychotropic medications to manage mood or behavioral problems, are a common part of the treatment plan.

3.2.5. *Childhood disintegrative disorder*

Also known as Heller's syndrome, CDD, originally referred to as dementia infantilis, is a disorder characterized by apparently normal development during the first two or more years, followed by clear regression in social function, language and behavior, before the age of 10. It was initially described by Heller in 1908, who recorded significant regression in three- and four-year olds subsequent to normal early development.

The symptoms of CDD are similar to those of classic autism, although onset is later, and often more extreme, with regression occurring after significant language and social development has occurred. Regression occurs in at least two of five key areas: (1) language skills (2) social skills and self-care skills, (3) control over bowel and bladder functions, (4) play skills, and (5) motor skills. The cause of this disorder is unknown, and while treatments are similar to those used in autism (*e.g.* behavior therapy), they are less effective, and the prognosis in children with CDD is typically extremely poor. The exact prevalence of the disorder is unknown, although it is estimated at 1.7 per 100,000.[17] This estimate makes CDD at least 60 times less frequent than autism. Like autism, CDD also appears to affect boys more often than girls.

The pathogenesis of CDD is currently unknown, although a number of neurobiological explanations have been proposed but no clear pathophysiological mechanisms have been identified. Small-scale studies have shown abnormal CT scans in about half of the sample, and EEG abnormalities at the same rate as those seen in autism. Further neurobiologic and neuroimaging investigations are needed in order to elucidate the pathophysiology of this disorder.

4. Differential Diagnosis

There are two issues in differential diagnosis with ASD conditions. One is differentiating between the different ASD conditions themselves, and the other is differentiating between other psychiatric and neuropsychiatric conditions. The challenges of accurately differentiating between ASD conditions are part of the reason for the DSM-5 workgroup's proposal to merge these conditions into a single diagnosis of autism spectrum disorder. Part of what complicates differentiation is that we do not have a clear understanding, at this time, of the etiology of the ASDs, apart from Rett's. This will be a key determinant in being able to more accurately clarify whether they represent distinct and different conditions, or whether symptoms should be viewed along a continuum, as is being proposed.

The second issue in differential diagnosis is distinguishing ASD from other psychiatric conditions. Psychiatric comorbidity is common in children with ASD, and there is an increased chance of comorbid conditions as children get older. In some instances, symptoms of other psychiatric conditions are considered to be associated features of the ASD, while in other instances, children meet criteria for a secondary diagnoses. In some cases, other psychiatric disorders share overlapping characteristics with ASD. For example, many children with ASD have executive functioning deficits, such as difficulties with working memory, sustained attention, and adaptability. Similar deficits are also common in children with Attention-Deficit/Hyperactivity Disorder (ADHD). It is also common for children with ASD to demonstrate behavioral challenges, mood dsyregulation, difficulties with sleep and eating patterns, and sensory dysregulation. It is not necessarily the case in these instances that a secondary diagnosis is warranted, as these are considered to be associated features of ASD. However, in some cases, the level of impairment associated with these features is severe enough to warrant a secondary, comorbid diagnosis. A detailed developmental history and a comprehensive mental status examination that includes an assessment of social interactions and reciprocity are essential components to an accurate differential diagnosis of ASD.

Symptoms of depression and anxiety can be common in children with ASD, and in some cases this may be the first way that a child with high-functioning autism or Asperger's may present to a mental health professional. In contrast, some children with ASD may have significant depression or anxiety that presents in a less traditional way, or may be masked due to difficulty effectively communicating emotional states. In both situations, it would require a detailed history to further differentiate these symptoms. Collateral information from parents, caregivers, and school professionals who have the opportunity to observe the child in a wide variety of circumstances may provide the information essential to making the correct diagnosis.

Social phobia is a common differential diagnosis in ASD. Many children with ASD may present with social withdrawal or discomfort that appears to fit the criteria for social phobia. However, while the anxiety they experience in social situations is real, it is driven by their social deficits, and may not dissipate even after attempts to alleviate the anxiety.

Attention-Deficit/Hyperactivity Disorder (ADHD) is another common differential diagnosis for children with ASD. Many of the symptoms of ADHD overlap with ASD, including executive functioning deficits, difficulty with sustained attention and focus, impulsiveness, distractibility, difficulty remaining seated, trouble following simple directions, and high activity level. In most cases, these overlapping symptoms are considered associated features, and a secondary ADHD diagnosis is not warranted. However, in some cases both diagnoses are given in order to target treatments. While the outward behavioral manifestations may be consistent with ADHD, the reason for the behavior may be quite different. For example, a child with ADHD may have difficulty sustaining attention and focus. In ASD, the difficulty may be in what the child focuses on, rather than an inability to focus. Carefully identifying the function or purpose of a behavior is often critical. The function of the behavior may influence both the diagnosis that is rendered and the treatment that is recommended.

Children with ASD often display repetitive behaviors, such as lining up or organizing objects, and can also insist on routines and rituals and become quite upset if those routines are not followed in very particular ways. Based on simple observation, it is often difficult to distinguish these behaviors from those seen in obsessive-compulsive disorder (OCD). However, in OCD there are anxiety-based thoughts that are associated with the compulsive behaviors displayed. In ASD, this is typically not the case. Although the child may insist on these behaviors and show frustration or distress if a behavior is interrupted or a routine is not followed, he/she is typically unable to articulate a reason behind the behavior. In addition, while the child with OCD will often state that they wish they did not engage in the compulsive behavior, the child with ASD often appears to derive pleasure from the activity itself. It may be particularly difficult to make the distinction between OCD and ASD in children who lack strong communication skills. Making the appropriate differential diagnosis may be based on the child's ability to express whether or not intrusive thoughts and fears are present. The appropriateness of specific medical treatments is clearly tied to correct diagnosis.

Another differential diagnosis often considered is psychotic disorder. While some reports described a higher incidence of schizophrenia in individual with autism, no large-scales studies have confirmed these observations. However, several studies have linked several genes to both disorders indicating that autism and schizophrenia probably share some common biologic underpinnings. Clinically, many of the behaviors that children with ASD engage in can appear bizarre and out of touch with reality. For example, some children mumble or talk to themselves. However, rather than responding to voices, they may be engaging in delayed echolalia. Children with ASD are often literal thinkers, and may answer questions about hallucinations and other symptoms of psychosis very concretely, thus appearing to endorse these symptoms when in fact they are not actually present. A careful and thorough mental status exam, along with collateral parent history, is critical to accurately make these distinctions.

Behavioral outbursts and mood dysregulation are extremely common in ASD, and often misunderstood. When extreme behaviors are present, a differential diagnosis of a disruptive behavior disorder, such as oppositional defiant disorder, or even bipolar disorder, may be considered. The true cause of the behavior can be quite different in these different conditions, making accurate differential diagnosis extremely important. In ASD, children often act out behaviorally due to environmental stressors, compounded by their communication and social deficits. Other factors that may impact behavior in ASD include sensory issues, difficulty with transitions, or frustration from not understanding or not being able to express themselves. This is very different from the child with bipolar disorder, whose behavior may be cyclical, or a child with ODD, who does not have any social or communication deficits, but may be reacting to the environment in a negative manner that has been inadvertently learned (Chap. 11). These distinctions may not be readily apparent in children, and will require a careful examination of the nature of the particular behavioral reaction in order to get a better sense of what is driving it, and make an accurate diagnosis.

5. Pathogenesis

Understanding the etiology of Autism Spectrum Disorders is a complex issue, in part due to the complex nature of the spectrum of disorders, and in part due to the delay in exploring biological bases of the disorders while psychodynamic theories of autism prevailed. While Kanner first described autism in 1943, it was not until 1977 that the first systematic study of the prevalence of the disorder in monozygotic and dizygotic twin pairs was published. In this paper, Folstein and Rutter reported a 36% concordance rate for monozygotic twins, and a 0% concordance rate for the dizygotic twin pairs. These results indicated a significant influence of genetics on the development of autism, although their small sample size (only 11 monozygotic and 10 dizygotic twin pairs) and restricted definition of autism suggests that the concordance in both types of twins is higher. More recent studies indicate that the concordance is indeed higher, with concordance between 60 and 90% for monozygotic twins and between 5 and 20% for dizygotic twin pairs.[18]

As research moved away from a neuropsychological theory of autism, a biological basis has been recognized for this disorder in early brain development, with many considering that a complex "three strikes" model will eventually lead us to an explanation of the causes of ASDs. This model posits that a genetic susceptibility is triggered by an environmental event or context at a vulnerable point in development — the cooccurrence of these three strikes leads to a faltering in the development process, and expression of an autism spectrum disorder. In the sections below, we describe the current state of knowledge in relation to the biological and environmental effects that may explain some or all of the causes of Autism Spectrum Disorders.

5.1. *Genetics*

Further exploration into twin concordance for ASD is reported by Roseberg and colleagues (2009) who collected data from 277 twin pairs where at least one had received an ASD diagnosis. For all ASDs, they estimated the concordance for monozygotic twins to be 88%, 86% for male–male twin pairs and 100% for female–female twin pairs. For dizygotic twin pairs, the concordance is estimated to be 30% overall, 40% for male–male, 26% for female–female, and 21% for female–male pairs. When the data is broken down by type of ASD, it is again more complicated, with different diagnoses given to different members of a twin pair (*e.g.* one female monozygotic twin may be diagnosed with autism, while the other is diagnosed with Asperger's), and some twin pairs not receiving any diagnosis (14% of male–male monozygotic twin and 62 to 80% of dizygotic twins have only one twin with an ASD diagnosis) These results indicate some differences in genetic concordance due to sex of the twins, and also influenced by environmental factors. Bohm and Steward[18] argue that attention should be paid to whether the twin pairs shared amniotic sacs and placentas, as this is known to influence concordance of Down's syndrome in twin pairs,[19] pointing to a possible influence of early environment or the expression of genetic mutations.

Family studies also indicate a genetic susceptibility to autism, with prevalence among siblings between 2 and 6%,[20] and reports of siblings of children who receive an ASD diagnosis weakly express aspects of the core features of autism (*e.g.* aloofness, social awkwardness, limited friendships, language difficulties). This expression of the broad autism phenotype also points toward a genetic element in the disorders, and suggest a complex inheritance structure.

While the heritability of autism is acknowledged, the heterogeneity of autism, and associated Autism Spectrum Disorders, as well as the complex inheritance structure, has made indentifying genetic causes a slow process. Progress has been made in the last decade, as more genetic research has advanced, and collaborative resources for the study of autism have increased. Additionally, attempts are being made to identify subtypes of autism, or endophenotypes, based on such characteristics as language ability, gender, or repetitive behaviors, and to identify families with just one affected individual (simplex) and families with two or more first degree relatives with ASD (multiplex) to allow for more focused genetic searches.

Much of the focus of research has been on identifying autism susceptibility candidate genes (ASCG), and identifying and distinguishing between *de novo* (new, noninherited) and heritable copy number variations (CNV) across these ASCGs. As of 2010, at least 15 autistic-susceptible gene loci have received significant consideration,[21] while models have been proposed to account for interaction between ASCGs.[22]

As genes are identified, questions continue to arise, including questions about the large sex differences in ASDs, and how environmental effects influence the development of Autism Spectrum Disorders. The fact that recent large twin studies found concordance rates for monozygotic twins below 100% indicates that while genetics may play a significant role, they are not the only answer to the puzzle of the etiology of autism.[23]

5.2. *Neurobiologic abnormalities*

Multiple approaches, including neuropathologic, neuroimaging, and neuroimmunologic studies, have been used to examine the neurobiologic underpinning of autism. Post-mortem investigations have reported alterations in neuronal organization in the cerebral cortex and subcortical structures. Cerebellar abnormalities have also been reported with loss and atrophy of Purkinje cells.[24] Structural imaging studies have revealed the existence of abnormalities in several brain regions. The most replicated findings include increased total brain volumes that peaks in early childhood[25] volumetric alteration of the amygdala,[26] and reductions of the size of the corpus callosum.[27,28] Diffusion tensor imaging investigations have provided evidence of disruption in several white matter tracts with decreased fractional anisotropy values in the corpus callosum, ventromedial prefrontal cortex, and superior temporal regions.[29] These observations might underlie the aberrant connectivity that has been reported in several fMRI investigations showing an abnormal pattern of activations between different cortical regions during performance of language and memory tasks.[30]

While neuroimaging studies provide insight into gross brain structure and function, investigating molecular systems implicated in brain development and cortical organization are also informative in identifying neuronal pathways with potential role in the pathophysiology of autism. Over the last two decades, a considerable number of studies have been published examining indicating alterations in several molecular systems in autism and a number of examples are discussed here including neurotrophic factors, neurotransmitters, and peptides. Elevations of brain-derived neurotrophic factor, a neurotrophin implicated in cortical plasticity, have been reported in children with Autism Spectrum Disorders when compared to control.[31,32] Immunologic dysfunction have also been found in individuals with autism with studies reporting neuroglial and innate neuroimmune system activation in brain tissue and cerebrospinal fluid of individuals with autism[33] as well as elevated levels of several cytokines.[34]

Abnormalities in serotoninergic, GABAergic, and glutamatergic systems have been reported in autism but consistent findings have not been observed when these peripheral measures of these pathways were examined.[35] Serotonin (5-hydroxytryptamine, 5-HT) which is found in both the gut, where it regulates intestinal movements, and in the central nervous system, where its' numerous functions include regulation of sleep, mood, appetite, learning, and memory, has received significant exploration attention in relation to ASD. The association between elevated levels of serotonin and autism was first described in 1961 in a study that found increased levels of whole blood serotonin in autistic children with autism. These findings have since been replicated in a number of studies, where findings suggest that levels are high for children with autism, and remain high across the age range, while they decrease with age for normal controls. However, studies of urinary excretion, cerebrospinal fluid (CSF), and whole blood tryptophan concentrations have found no difference between autistic and control participants.[36]

Neuropeptides are involved in many aspects of brain function and development, leading to questions about their impact on developmental disorders such as ASD. Research has examined a number of neuropeptides (such as melatonin, secretin and, cortisol), to identify differences in levels in serum, CSF or urine in patients with ASD. While some studies have reported elevated levels of ACTH and low cortisol levels in subjects with autism,[37] others found no differences between the two groups. Studies examining the usefulness of another peptide, secretin, in the treatment of the core features of autism have failed to show any benefits in more than 15 double-blind controlled trials.[38] Finally, oxytocin, a peptide that acts primarily as a neurotransmitter in the brain, has also been implicated in autism with its role in social affiliative behaviors, social recognition, anxiety, and maternal behaviors. Low oxytocin levels and polymoprhisms in its receptors, as well as clinical benefits after oxytocin administration have all been reported in individuals with autism supporting the role that these peptides play in the pathophysiology of autism and open the door to the development of disease-specific treatments.[39]

5.3. *Environmental contributions*

Recently, several environmental factors have been suggested as possibly contributing to the increase in the prevalence of ASD.

Examples of environmental causes are numerous and include infectious etiologies, exposure to toxins such as during vaccination, and excessive ultrasounds during pregnancy. However, to date no scientific data have been published to support any of these hypotheses with emerging evidence supporting the lack of any associations between these factors and autism. For example, no link between immunization and the onset of symptomatology has to date been reported with over 15 studies examining this relationship and none reporting any association.

6. Relevance for Primary Care and Pediatricians

Although many systems might eventually be involved in the treatment of a child with ASD, medical professionals remain at the front line in identifying and referring children with ASD for proper evaluations and follow-up. Training physicians to be aware of early warning signs, the different ways that ASD presents over time, and when to refer for a diagnostic evaluation, is a critical first step in helping children with ASD receive timely and appropriate care.

The first step in identifying autism is systematic developmental surveillance, beginning in early childhood, and usually conducted by the primary care physician. In 2007, the American Association of Pediatrics recommended that all children be screened for autism at their 18-month and 2-year check-ups.[40] These assessments use parent questionnaires and the pediatrician's observations during the appointment, to determine whether the child should be referred for a full diagnostic evaluation by an autism specialist. In 1999, The Academy of Neurology issued practice guidelines for the screening and diagnosis of autism. The practice parameters highlight the importance of routine developmental surveillance, as well as knowledge of the developmental warning signs of autism. Immediate referral to early intervention or the child's local school, as well as to an autism expert for a full diagnostic evaluation should be made if the child fails autism screening, experiences any loss of language or social skills at any time, or fails to meet any of the following behavioral milestones: babbling by 12 months; gesturing (*e.g.* pointing, waving) by 12 months; single spoken words by 16 months; and two-word spontaneous (nonecholalic) phrases by 24 months. Additional early warning signs are listed in Table 2.[41–43]

If a child is referred for a full diagnostic evaluation, the guidelines specify a combination of formal diagnostic procedures by an experienced clinician, as well as a detailed history, neurological evaluation, and formal assessment of the child's developmental profile. Following these guidelines, a full diagnostic evaluation in an autism clinic typically consists of the following: a detailed developmental history, cognitive or developmental assessment, assessment of language and motor functioning, evaluation of adaptive functioning, physical/neurological exam, and a direct play observation of the child. The current standard in autism clinics is direct observation using the autism diagnostic observation schedule.[44] In order to complete a full diagnostic workup, multiple professionals may be involved in the

Table 2: Early Developmental Warning Signs for Medical Practitioners

Age of Child	Warning Signs
0–12 months	• Limited eye contact • Lack of pointing or showing of objects • Failure to look at the face of others • Diminished social responsiveness • Decreased response to the verbalizations of others • Decreased motor or vocal imitation • Problems with arousal • Unusual sensory responses • Failure to assume anticipatory postures • Failure to reach for familiar caregivers • Decreased interest in other children • Lack of interest in simple, social games • Decreased response to name
12–18 months	• Absence of symbolic play • Failure to shift gaze appropriately • Failure to share positive affect • Lack of joint attention • Absence of gestures • Slower rate of verbal communication • Difficulties comprehending language

assessment process. Interdisciplinary team assessments are often comprised of professionals from disciplines such as psychiatry, psychology, developmental pediatrics, neurology, speech-language pathology, and occupational therapy. Following this comprehensive workup, the team is able to not only provide a diagnostic formulation, but also to determine the most appropriate treatments for a given child.

Finally, to help with the screening in primary care settings, a variety of autism screening measures (Table 3) are currently available with young children. In addition, as our understanding of autism in young children continues to advance, new

Table 3: Screening instruments for identifying children at risk of ASD

Test	Target Age Range	Description
Screening Infants and Toddlers		
Checklist for Autism in Toddlers (CHAT; Baron-Cohen, Allen & Gillberg, 1992)	18 months	• 9 item parent report form; 5 item clinician observation • Good specificity but inadequate sensitivity (high number of false negatives) in detecting children diagnosed with autism at 30 months (Baron-Cohen *et al.* 2000) • Available as a free download
Modified Checklist for Autism in Toddlers and Follow-Up Interview (M-CHAT; Robins, Fein & Barton, 1999a and b)	16–30 months	• 23 item parent report form • Additional probes for all items to be used by clinicians when a significant number of ASD indicators are reported • Predictive value consistent with current ASD prevalence rates (Robins, 2008) • Available as a free download in many languages
Quantitative Checklist for Autism in Toddlers (Q-CHAT; Allison *et al.* 2008)	18–24 months	• Revision of the CHAT • 25 item parent report form • Promising preliminary findings
Infant-Toddler Checklist (ITC; Wetherby *et al.* 2002)	9–24 months	• Screen of social communication development • 24 item parent report form • High sensitivity and specificity in detecting toddlers at risk for ASD and other developmental delays (Wetherby *et al.* 2004; Wetherby *et al.* 2008) • Available as a free download

(*Continued*)

Table 3: (*Continued*)

Test	Target Age Range	Description
Early Screening for Autism and Communication Disorders (ESAC; Wetherby *et al.* 2009)	12–36 months	• 47 item parent report form • Promising preliminary findings • In development as a clinical tool
Pervasive Developmental Disorders Screening Test-II, Stage 1 (PDDST-II; Siegal, 2004)	12–48 months	• 23 item parent report form • two additional stages available for use in clinics during diagnostic evaluation
Screening Tool for Autism in Two-Year Olds (STAT; Stone & Ousley, 1997; Stone *et al.* 2004)	25–35 months	• Screening for differentiating autism and other developmental delays once concerns have been identified • Scores based on clinician observations during 12 structured tasks • High degree of sensitivity and specificity
Screening older children		
Social Communication Questionnaire (SCQ; Berument *et al.* 1999; Rutter *et al.* 2003)	four years and older	• Screen of communication and social functioning in children suspected of having an ASD diagnosis • 40 item parent report form • Good sensitivity and specificity in discriminating between ASD and typical development

measures are being created that are more sensitive to early warning signs, and in detecting ASD in younger children.

7. Interventions

7.1. *Overview*

Autism interventions should include a multidisciplinary team of specialists, including educational, medical, behavioral, and allied health professionals (*e.g.* speech and occupational therapists). Current guidelines emphasize that early, intensive intervention is recommended to maximize functioning and enhance prognosis.[45,46] A range of intervention models are currently available, including behavioral, developmental, and combined approaches.[45] These approaches are reviewed in detail in several seminal documents, including *Educating Children with Autism*,[45] *Management of Children with Autism Spectrum Disorders*,[47] and *The National Standards Project*.[48] Parameters for areas to target in intervention and broad intervention considerations, as well as a brief review of intervention models, are outlined below.

7.2. *Areas to target in intervention*

Given that autism is a disorder characterized by deficits in multiple areas, treatment planning involves comprehensive services and supports to address a range of functional domains (Table 4). To adequately address these areas, intervention must by multidisciplinary, intensive, and occur across settings (*e.g.* home, school, community).

Table 4: Intervention targets across domains of functioning

Intervention Target	Description/Examples
Communication skills	Verbal speech output (*i.e.* first words), speech articulation, expanding language beyond requests, conversation skills, augmentative communication (*e.g.* communication devices, picture communication systems)
Engagement and motivation	Willingness to interact, motivation to comply, interest in activities and social interactions, initiating appropriate behaviors, independent engagement in meaningful activities
Attention and imitation	Attending when spoken to, attending to surrounding environment, following verbal instructions, imitating actions, imitating speech
Social skills	Joint attention, eye contact, social conversation, understanding social cues, use of nonverbal social behaviors, perspective taking, empathy
Play/leisure	Turn-taking, sharing, symbolic/make-believe/imaginative play, independent engagement in meaningful leisure activities in home and community settings
Cognitive/academic skills	Basic developmental skills (*e.g.* matching, sorting), academic readiness (*e.g.* numbers, letters, shapes, colors), academic skills appropriate to developmental and grade level, functional academics (*e.g.* time, money, reading signs, *etc.*)
Self-help/life skills (adaptive functioning)	Feeding, toileting, dressing, hygiene (*e.g.* bathing, brushing teeth, caring for hair), household chores (*e.g.* making bed, cleaning up), independent living skills (*e.g.* use of transportation or driving, money management, higher education or job skills, managing housing situation)
Behavioral challenges	Reducing behavior problems (*e.g.* tantrums, aggression), self-injury, self-stimulatory behavior, rigid behavior patterns (*e.g.* insistence on sameness, rituals, routines)
Motor skills	Gross (*e.g.* balance, running, jumping, climbing) and fine (*e.g.* writing, feeding) motor skills

The National Research Council[45] and other more recent practice parameters have proposed a number of important program characteristics for children with autism, including: (1) A focus on early intervention; (2) Intensity of hours (20–45 per week of combined services, 12 months per year); (3) Active family involvement in intervention; (4) Use of highly trained staff; (5) Ongoing assessment using objective assessment measures, resulting in ongoing program modification as needed; (6) Use of a systematic teaching curriculum; (7) A focus on communication and other developmental areas; (8) A systematic emphasis on generalization and maintenance of skills; (9) Individualized programming; (10) Supported and planned transitions; (11) Low student-to-teacher ratio; (12) Opportunities for interaction with typically developing peers when appropriate; and (13) A high degree of structure in programming (*e.g.* predictable routines, visual schedules, clear work space, minimal distractions).

7.3. *Psychotherapeutic approaches*

7.3.1. *Comprehensive early intervention programs*

As children with autism have been diagnosed earlier and earlier, comprehensive intervention programs for very young children have emerged. These programs typically incorporate behavioral, developmental, and/or structured teaching methods (see below), and follow the intervention considerations discussed above. Young children may receive home or center-based services or a combination of these. As they do not yet attend school, the intensity of hours is achieved through a combination of one-to-one or small group autism-specific developmental or behavioral therapy, as well as individual therapies (*e.g.* speech and occupational therapy).

7.3.2. *Educational interventions*

Under the most recent reauthorization of the Individuals with Disabilities Education Act (IDEA),[49] individuals with disabilities are entitled to a free and appropriate education to address not only academic learning, but also skills toward the goal of independent functioning across multiple domains. These may include socialization, adaptive skills, communication, remediation of interfering behaviors, and acquisition of skills that generalize across multiple environments. Given the recommended intensity of interventions for children with autism, many of the necessary services and supports are provided through public school programming for children over the age of three years. Educational interventions often include specific teaching methodology (*e.g.* applied behavior analysis, structured teaching methods, developmentally based methods) embedded in classroom programming to meet the needs of children with autism. In addition to classroom-based programming, speech therapy, occupational therapy, and social skills instruction are often included in educational programs for school age children.

7.3.3. *Autism intervention models*

Applied behavior analysis

Traditionally, ABA-based intervention programs are based on the application of operant procedures during structured one-to-one teaching interactions to target language, social, cognitive, developmental, academic, and play skills using systematic and measurable teaching methodologies. These programs often occur in a discrete trial format with a highly trained behavioral clinician. ABA in its most structured and intensive form is known as discrete trial teaching, which represents one of the earliest and most systematic forms of autism intervention.

Naturalistic behavioral models

Over time, naturalistic behavioral interventions have evolved, whereby operant procedures are functionally embedded within natural contexts to promote learning in the natural environment (*e.g.* pivotal response training; incidental teaching). These modified behavioral programs use the same systematic and measurable ABA-based teaching methodologies; however, the principles are embedded during natural interactions with the child during daily routines and activities. Naturalistic behavioral models are frequently implemented across settings through training of educational specialists, as well as parents.

Structured teaching

Structured teaching, also known, as TEACCH (Teaching and Education of Autistic and Related Communication Handicapped Children),[50] includes a combination of teaching strategies and modifications to the physical environment. These components are incorporated into many educational programs. Structured teaching components include organization of the physical environment, a predictable sequence of activities, and visual supports (*e.g.* visual schedules). TEACCH-based programs focus both on remediating skill deficits to minimize symptoms of autism and necessarily environmental modifications to meet the needs of these students.

Developmentally based programs

Developmental programs (*e.g.* the Denver model; Floortime) target cognitive, communicative, social, and emotional development and are often based on developmental theories, such as Piaget. These interventions take place in developmentally appropriate settings (*e.g.* preschool) through play and relationship-based activities. Advocates of developmental models have argued that traditional behavioral treatment approaches are too circumscribed in their discrete target behavior approach to fundamentally impact symptoms in children with autism.

7.4. *Psychopharmacological interventions*

To date, there are no specific medication treatments that aim at targeting the core features of autism. However, an increasing number of compounds are being identified as potentially helpful in the treatment of this disorder. Most recently, the Food and Drug Administration has approved two atypical antipsychotic agents, risperidone and aripiprazole, in the treatment of irritability and disruptive behaviors associated with autism. The atypical antipsychotic class of medications has been adopted in light of the effectiveness observed with the first-generation antipsychotic agents. While most of the available research supports the efficacy of risperidone and aripiprazole, studies have been published to support the effectivness of other atypical antipsychotic such as olanzapine and quetiapine, although large controlled trials are lacking.

Selective serotonin transporters inhibitors (fluoxetine, sertraline, paroxetine, fluvoxamine, citalopram, and escitalopram) are also widely used in individuals with autism but limited support is currently available to support their usefulness especially in children. Recently, the NIH sponsored a randomized controlled trial with 149 participants with Autism Spectrum Disorders. In this trial, citalopram was compared to placebo for treatment of repetitive behaviors and no difference was found between the two groups. Another study that casts doubt on the effectiveness of SSRIs in patients with autism is the Study of Fluoxetine in Autism (SOFIA), an industry-sponsored trial that evaluated the efficacy and safety of a new low-dose form, melt-in-the-mouth formula of fluoxetine. Although the study showed a decrease in repetitive behaviors with both fluoxetine and placebo, no differences between the two groups were found.

Several other medications have been investigated in autism. Reductions in the rates of hyperactivity have been reported in several trials examining the usefulness of stimulants, such as methylphenidate, in this disorder. Alpha$_2$-adrenergic receptor agonists, such as clonidine and guanfacine, have also been found to be helpful in targeting hyperactivity and impulsivity in children with autism. Naltrexone, an opiate antagonist, was suggested as potentially helpful in targeting the core social and cognitive symptoms, although controlled data are equivocal. Other agents such as anticonvulsants and anxiolytics have been found to be beneficial but randomized controlled trials have yet to be completed. Finally, numerous innovative compounds are promising and include oxcytocin, and glutamatergic modulators. Their usefulness awaits large controlled trials to determine their efficacy and safety in targeting the core features of autism.

Long-term follow-up studies are lacking in the field of autism. No clear guidelines on the use of psychotropic agents have been published to date. Naturalistic longitudinal studies have yet to be completed and treatment studies have examined early interventions for children with autism but they suffer from methodological limitations.

8. Clinical Practice at Stanford University

In the Stanford Autism and Developmental Disabilities Clinic, our team follows current practice parameters for assessment, diagnosis, and treatment of ASD. In 1999, a set of national practice guidelines, created by leading autism specialists across the United States, were published, outlining the manner in which screening and formal diagnostic evaluation of ASD should occur. Diagnostic assessment in our clinic follows these guidelines, which include the following: a thorough review of background information; caregiver history, including developmental, medical, and behavioral history; medical evaluation; direct behavioral observation using standardized diagnostic measures (*i.e.* ADOS); and cognitive and adaptive assessment. Assessments are conducted in a multidisciplinary team, and clinicians work with families to provide direction regarding appropriate treatment approaches. This typically involves feedback on the same day as the assessment, in addition to one or more follow-up appointments to continue to review results of the assessment and recommendations, and to start the family on the process of setting up treatment services.

In addition to providing community referrals when appropriate (*e.g.* educational specialists, social skills groups, support groups, *etc.*), a variety of treatment services are also provided in the clinic setting including individual, parent, and family therapy; training in Pivotal Response Therapy (PRT) in either individual or group format; behavioral consultation with board-certified behavioral analysts; and pharmacotherapy. PRT is an empirically supported treatment model for improving the language, social, and cognitive skills of children with autism. This treatment model relies on scientifically based principles of Applied Behavior Analysis (ABA); however, it expands upon traditional ABA models by embedding treatment strategies in natural and play-based interactions between children and caregivers (*e.g.* parents, teachers, *etc.*).

In 2007, Stanford University developed an autism center (Stanford Autism Center at Packard Hospital) to bring together all the relevant researchers and clinicians working with ASD in the Stanford system. This center funds parent education, translational research, and training for autism specialists. The center hosts an annual symposium geared toward parents, with leading experts in the field invited to present current trends in research and treatments. The center also supports a parent education group which is offered throughout the year (http://childpsychiatry.stanford.edu/ASD.html). This is a low-cost, 10-week series covering important topics for families. For example, classes define and explain different autism treatments, provide information to help navigate the special education system, and teach parents general information about techniques that can be used in the home to address certain behaviors or help advance certain skills.

9. The Next 5 Years

Over the last decade, interest in autism has led to a tremendous increase in our understanding of this disorder. While evidence is mounting to support the heterogeneity of this disorder, the focus has recently shifted to the development of disease-specific treatment. This strategy is promising since it allows the identification of compound that will aim at improving the overall quality of life and functioning level of individuals with autism. Early interventions applying behavioral and developmental strategies are being developed with the goal of targeting core features including social and communication deficits. Elucidating the neurobiology of autism and related disorders will be instrumental in the next decade in yielding insight into the pathophysiology and consequently help in the development of more effective treatment.

References

1. American Psychiatric Association. *Diagnostic and Statistical Manual of Mental Disorders*, 4th edition, Text revision. Washington, DC: American Psychological Association, 2000.
2. Yeargin-Allsopp M, Rice C, Karapurkar T, Doernberg N, Boyle C, Murphy C. Prevalence of autism in a US metropolitan area, *JAMA* 2003; **289**: 49–55.
3. Rice C. Prevalence of autism spectrum disorders — autism and developmental disabilities monitoring network. 14 sites, United States, 2002, *MMWR Morb Mortal Wkly Rep* 2007; **56**: 12–28.

4. Brain-derived neurotrophic factor. Prevalence of autism spectrum disorders — autism and developmental disabilities monitoring network, United States, 2006, *MMWR Morb Mortal Wkly Rep* 2009; **58**.
5. Kogan MD, Blumberg SJ, Schieve LA, *et al.* Prevalence of parent-reported diagnosis of autism spectrum disorder among children in the US, 2007, *Pediatrics* 2009; **124**: 1395–1403.
6. King M, Bearman P. Diagnostic change and the increased prevalence of autism, *Int J Epidemiol* 2009; **38**: 1224–1234.
7. Fombonne E. Epidemiological surveys of autism and other pervasive developmental disorders: An update, *J Autism Dev Disord* 2003; **33**: 365–382.
8. Newschaffer CJ, Croen LA, Daniels J, *et al.* The epidemiology of autism spectrum disorders, *Annu Rev Public Health* 2007; **28**: 235–258.
9. American Psychiatry Association. *DSM-5 Development: 299.0 Autistic Disorder* 2010.
10. Chakrabarti S, Fombonne E. Pervasive developmental disorders in preschool children, *JAMA* 2001; **285**: 3093–3099.
11. Lord C, Shulman C, DiLavore P. Regression and word loss in autistic spectrum disorders, *J Child Psychol Psychiatry* 2004; **45**: 936–955.
12. Ozonoff S, Dawson G, McPartland J. *A Parent's Guide to Asperger's Syndrome and High Functioning Autism*. New York, NY: Guilford Press, 2002.
13. Frith U. Mind blindness and the brain in autism, *Neuron* 2001; **32**: 969–979.
14. Walker DR, Thompson A, Zwaigenbaum L, *et al.* Specifying PDD-NOS, Asperger's syndrome and autism, *J Am Acad Child Adolesc Psychiatry* 2004; **43**: 172–180.
15. Percy AK, Lane JB, Childers J, *et al.* Rett syndrome: North American database, *J Child Neurol* 2007; **22**: 1338–1341.
16. Acampa M, Guideri F. Cardiac disease and rett syndrome, *Arch Dis Child* 2006; **91**: 440–443.
17. Fombonne E. Prevalence of childhood disintegrative disorder, *Autism* 2002; **6**: 149–157.
18. Bohm HV, Stewart MG. Brief report: On the concordance percentages for autistic spectrum disorder of twins, *J Autism Dev Disord* 2009; **39**: 806–808.
19. Matias A, Montenegro N, Blickstein I. Down syndrome screening in multiple pregnancies, *Obstet Gynecol Clin North Am* 2005; **32**: 81–96.
20. Baird G, Simonoff E, Pickles A, *et al.* Prevalence of disorders of the autism spectrum in a population cohort of children in south Thames: The special needs and autism project (SNAP), *Lancet* 2006; **368**: 210–215.
21. Momoi T, Fujita E, Senoo H, Momoi M. Genetic factors and epigenetic factors for autism: Endoplasmic reticulum stress and impaired synaptic function, *Cell Biol Int* 2009; **34**: 13–19.

22. Bill BR, Geschwind DH. Genetic advances in autism: Heterogeneity and convergence on shared pathways, *Curr Opin Genet Dev* 2009; **19**: 271–278.
23. Rosenberg RE, Law JK, Yenokyan G, *et al.* Characteristics and concordance of autism spectrum disorders among 277 twin pairs, *Arch Pediatr Adolesc Med* 2009; **163**: 907–914.
24. Bauman ML, Kemper TL. Neuroanatomic observations of the brain in autism: A review and future directions, *Int J Dev Neurosci* 2005; **23**: 183–187.
25. Redcay E, Courchesne E. When is the brain enlarged in autism? A meta-analysis of all brain size reports, *Biol Psychiatry* 2005; **58**: 1–9.
26. Amaral DG, Bauman MD, Schumann CM. The amygdala and autism: Implications from non-human primate studies, *Genes Brain Behav* 2003; **2**: 295–302.
27. Frazier TW, Hardan AY. A meta-analysis of the corpus callosum in Autism, *Biol Psychiatry* 2009; **66**: 935–941.
28. Hardan AY, Pabalan M, Gupta N, *et al.* Corpus callosum volume in children with autism, *Psychiatry Res* 2009; **174**: 57–61.
29. Barnea-Goraly N, Kwon H, Menon V, Eliez S, Lotspeich L, Reiss AL. White matter structure in autism: Preliminary evidence from diffusion tensor imaging, *Biol Psychiatry* 2004; **55**: 323–326.
30. Minshew NJ, Williams DL. The new neurobiology of autism: Cortex, connectivity, and neuronal organization, *Arch Neurol* 2007; **64**: 945–950.
31. Connolly AM, Chez M, Streif EM, *et al.* Brain-derived neurotrophic fctor and autoantibodies to neural antigens in sera of children with autistic spectrum disorders, Landau-Kleffner syndrome, and epilepsy, *Biol Psychiatry* 2006; **59**: 354–363.
32. Miyazaki K, Narita N, Sakuta R, *et al.* Serum neurotrophin concentrations in autism and mental retardation: A pilot study, *Brain Dev* 2004; **26**: 292–295.
33. Pardo CA, Vargas DL, Zimmerman AW. Immunity, neuroglia and neuroinflammation in autism, *Int Rev Psychiatry* 2005; **17**: 485–495.
34. Molloy CA, Morrow AL, Meinzen-Derr J, *et al.* Elevated cytokine levels in children with autism spectrum disorder, *J Neuroimmunol* 2006; **172**: 198–205.
35. Pardo CA, Eberhart CG. The neurobiology of autism, *Brain Pathol* 2007; **17**: 434–447.
36. McDougle CJ, Erickson CA, Stigler KA, Posey DJ. Neurochemistry in the pathophysiology of autism, *J Clin Psychiatry* 2005; **66**: 9–18.
37. Curin JM, Terzić J, Petković ZB, Zekan L, Terzić IM, Susnjara IM. Lower cortisol and higher ACTH levels in individuals with autism, *J Autism Dev Disord* 2003; **33**: 443–448.
38. Esch BE, Carr JE. Secretin as a treatment for autism: A review of the evidence, *J Autism Dev Disord* 2004; **34**: 543–556.

39. Andari E, Duhamel JR, Zalla T, Herbrecht E, Leboyer M, Sirigu A. Promoting social behavior with oxytocin in high-functioning autism spectrum disorders, *Proc Natl Acad Sci USA* 2010; **107**: 4389–4394.
40. Johnson CP, Myers SM. Identification and evaluation of children with autism spectrum disorders, *Pediatrics* 2007; **120**: 1183–1215.
41. First Signs, Inc. *Concerns About a Child: Red Flags*, 2010.
42. Volkmar F, Chawarska K, Klin A. Autism in infancy and early childhood, *Annu Rev Psychol* 2005; **56**: 315–336.
43. Wetherby A, Woods J, Allen L, Cleary J, Dickinson H, Lord C. Early indicators of autism spectrum disorders in the second year of life, *J Autism Dev Disord* 2004; **34**: 473–493.
44. Lord C, Risi S, Lambrecht L, *et al.* The autism diagnostic observation schedule-generic: A standard measure of social and communication deficits associated with the spectrum of autism, *J Autism Dev Disord* 2000; **30**: 205–223.
45. Lord C, McGee JP. National Research Council, Committee on Educational Interventions for Children with Autism. *Educating Children with Autism.* Washington, DC: National Academy Press, 2001.
46. Myers SM, Johnson CP. Management of children with autism spectrum disorders, *Pediatrics* 2007; **120**: 1162–1182.
47. National Autism Center. 2009 http://specialed.wordpress.com/2009/10/02/national-autism-center-report/
48. US. Congress IDEA 2004 Public Law 108-446 *Individuals with Disabilities ducation Improvement Act of 2004.* Washington, DC: Government Printing Office, 2004.
49. Mesibov GB, Shea V. The TEACCH program in the era of evidence-based practice, *J Autism Dev Disord* 2010; **40**: 570–579.

Chapter 16

Psychiatric Disorders in Individuals with Intellectual Disabilities

Mendy Minjarez, Jennifer M. Phillips, Carl Feinstein, and Antonio Y. Hardan

1. Introduction and Overview

Intellectual disability, or mental retardation, refers to conditions of heterogeneous etiology, arising during the course of development, in which individuals present with significant cognitive impairment coupled with deficits in adaptive functioning. Children and adolescents diagnosed with intellectual disability comprise between one and three percent of the total school-aged population in the United States, and there are about 156 million people worldwide with these conditions, according to the World Health Organization. Intellectual disability is a condition that impacts an individual throughout the lifespan, leading to the need for some degree of support into adulthood in most cases. There is enormous diversity in etiology, phenomenology, and associated medical, psychiatric, and psychosocial features in intellectual disability. In fact, Gillberg referred to intellectual disability as "an administrative cover-all blanket term for a variety of different genetic, social, and specific medical conditions sharing one common feature, that individuals affected test (reliably) below IQ 70."

The associated cognitive, adaptive, and psychosocial deficits that accompany a diagnosis of intellectual disability can be quite limiting. Children and adolescents with mild intellectual disabilities are not categorically different from their cognitively unaffected peers. However, they are at a considerable disadvantage compared to peers in that intellectual abilities affect adaptive functioning, educational achievement, and related activities. Unlike children with mild intellectual disabilities, those in the moderate to profound range differ in significant ways from their cognitively unaffected peers. In addition to more significant cognitive deficits, many also suffer from physical and/or neurological handicaps. This combination of impairments has significant ramifications for adaptive functioning and self-sufficiency. These children are often unable to live independently.

1.1. *History of intellectual disability definition*

Historically, more pejorative terms have been used to describe intellectual disability and its subtypes (*e.g.* feeble mindedness, idiocy, imbecility, and mental deficiency). The current terminology of mental retardation reflects efforts to lessen the negative undertone of the diagnosis. However, the term still has a somewhat negative connotation. Efforts to create a less stigmatizing term for this disability include the use of terms such as intellectual disability in the DSM-V proposed revision[1] and the recent name change of the American Association on Mental Retardation (AAMR) to the American Association on Intellectual and Developmental Disabilities (AAIDD). For the purposes of this chapter, the term intellectual disability will be used interchangeably with our current terminology of mental retardation, as described in both the International Classification of Diseases — 10th revision and *Diagnostic and Statistical Manual of Mental Disorders* — 4th edition, Text Revision (DSM-IV-TR).[2]

Changes in the definition of intellectual disability in the United States over the past 50 years have served to emphasize the relative rather than categorical nature of this impairment and our system of classification. The AAIDD, an organization of professionals who have the primary responsibility for defining intellectual disability and advocating for individuals with intellectual disabilities, has changed the definition used by the organization over 10 times since 1908.[3] For example, in 1959, the Heber Committee of the AAIDD defined intellectual disability as including any individual with an IQ score at least one standard deviation below the mean, thus including 16% of the population within the range of intellectual disability. In 1973, the definition changed, to include only those with IQ scores at least two standard deviations below the mean. This change (a 15-point difference) excluded almost 26 million previously classified individuals. In 1983, the Grossman committee recommended that clinical judgment be used when determining whether individuals whose IQ falls within a few points of the cut-off be diagnosed with intellectual disability or not. These shifts in the definition of intellectual disabilities highlight the fact that decisions about diagnosis are often administrative and somewhat arbitrary, rather than in accordance with an absolute standard.

2. Epidemiology

Intellectual disabilities are the most common and widely known of the neuropsychiatric disorders. Estimates of prevalence based on a normal distribution of intelligence, range from one to three percent of the general population in the United States. It has been suggested that the overall prevalence rate for intellectual disabilities in the United States is approximately three percent of the population when IQ scores alone are used. However, when adaptive behaviors are considered, the rate is likely to be closer to one percent. Furthermore, these rates, independently from the definition used, might be on the increase with the advances in medicine allowing fragile individuals with ID and multiple medical problems to live longer.

Prevalence of intellectual disabilities varies by age, sex, and socioeconomic status. Rates are thought to increase with age until early adulthood, at which point there is a decrease. The increase through childhood is attributed in part to the fact that children are assessed and diagnosed during the school years, when they begin to demonstrate difficulty mastering academic skills at the expected level. Individuals with mild intellectual disability are often able to successfully adapt to the demands of adulthood, including adjustment to work, community, and social expectations, offering one explanation for the decline in prevalence in adults previously diagnosed with an intellectual disability. Additionally, it is projected that the rates of intellectual disability will increase in light of the technical and therapeutic progress allowing medically ill compromised individuals, such as premature babies and children with multiple disabilities, to survive with intensive and state-of-the-art treatment.

For all levels of intellectual disabilities, the ratio of males to females is estimated at approximately 1.6:1. Explanations include overidentification in males or higher rates of biological causes of intellectual disabilities in males (*e.g.* X-linked disorders). The highest male-to-female ratio (1.94:1) is seen in individuals with mild intellectual disability, with a somewhat smaller ratio of male-to-female (1.5:1) in the severe to profound range. Studies have also indicated that mild intellectual disabilities are overrepresented in lower socioeconomic groups, while moderate to profound intellectual disabilities appear to be more equally distributed among the socioeconomic strata. This pattern is probably related to a social drift observed in individuals with limited cognitive abilities having the tendency to associate with each other.

3. Diagnosis

3.1. *Definition*

The ICD-10 defines mental retardation as "a condition of arrested or incomplete development of the mind, which is especially characterized by impairment of skills manifested during the developmental period, which contribute to the overall level of intelligence; *i.e.* cognitive, language, motor, and social abilities." In the

DSM-IV-TR, the American Psychiatric Association[2] identifies three criteria that must be present for a diagnosis of mental retardation to be made: "significantly subaverage intellectual functioning," accompanied by "significant limitations in adaptive functioning in at least two areas," with an onset during the developmental period (*i.e.* prior to age 18). No considerable changes are being suggested for DSM-V with the exception of a definition that is no longer based on IQ.[1] The AAIDD similarly defines mental retardation as "a disability characterized by significant limitations both in intellectual functioning and in adaptive behavior as expressed in conceptual, social, and practical adaptive skills" which must be present prior to age 18.[3] While the above definitions are helpful in characterizing individuals with limited cognitive abilities, it is expected that new versions of classifications of disorders such as ICD-11 and DSM-V, will refine their descriptions, but conclusions cannot be made before the final drafts are published.

Intellectual functioning is typically determined through administration of standardized intellectual testing (IQ), and "significantly subaverage" is defined as scores falling at least two standard deviations below the mean. Using a deviation IQ standard score (mean 100, standard deviation 15), scores of 70 and below would fall in the mentally retarded range.

The inclusion of adaptive behavior deficits refines the definition of intellectual disability beyond IQ to reflect the pervasive impairment in functioning which is considered a defining characteristic of individuals with an intellectual disability. The purpose of considering adaptive behavior formally is to insure that children are not classified by cognitive testing alone. Low scores can be the result of a variety of extraneous variables, such as school maladjustment, lack of educational opportunity, primary language, or cultural deprivation, in addition to situational factors. Such factors could lead to low scores on cognitive testing but might not affect adaptive functioning in developmentally appropriate psychosocial domains (home, neighborhood, school, peer group, *etc.*).

According to the AAIDD,[3] adaptive behavior is "the collection of conceptual, social, and practical skills that people have learned so they can function in their everyday lives." Conceptual skills include abilities such as expressive and receptive language, reading and writing, and self-directions. Examples of social skills include interpersonal skills, responsibility, and abiding by community rules and laws. Practical skills include activities of daily living (ADLs) like eating, dressing, and toileting, as well as instrumental activities, such as preparing meals, taking medication, using the telephone, managing personal finances, accessing transportation, and job skills. The standards of personal independence expected for a particular individual differ by age, sociocultural background, and community setting, and a person's level of adaptive functioning can be influenced by a variety of biopsychosocial factors, including motivation, personality/temperament, level of education, social and job opportunities, and comorbid psychiatric and medical issues.[2] Adaptive skills deficit is defined in the ICD-10 as a "diminished ability to adapt to the daily demands of the normal social environment." Specific areas of deficit are identified in the DSM-IV-TR to include "communication, self-care, home living, social/interpersonal skills, use of community resources, self-direction, functional academic skills, work, leisure, health, and safety."[2]

In addition to information obtained from educational, developmental, and medical histories, adaptive behavior is typically assessed using standardized measures of adaptive functioning, which are usually in the form of semistructured caregiver or teacher interviews. Adaptive functioning must be assessed within the context of social and cultural differences. Significant deficits in adaptive functioning are measured by domain of functioning (*e.g.* communication, daily living skills, socialization, motor), and significant deficits are also defined as scores falling at least two standard deviations below the mean. According to ICD-10 diagnostic guidelines, a diagnosis of mental retardation must be considered a provisional estimate if standardized assessment of intellectual and adaptive functioning was not conducted.

3.2. *Diagnostic categories*

Intellectual disability is divided into four specific diagnostic categories or subtypes that depict the severity of the disorder. Subtypes are based on IQ score, but a person's adaptive functioning must be either equivalent to what is expected of a given IQ or lower than expected. In cases where IQ scores and adaptive behavior scores are quite discrepant, both must be reported and clinical judgment used to determine subtype classification. Appropriate subtype classification can, in many instances, impact level of services and treatments received.

3.3. *Psychiatric comorbidity*

The presence of comorbid psychopathology in individuals with intellectual disability is estimated to be three to four times greater than the general population.[2] Children and adolescents with intellectual disability have a decreased ability to understand and respond adaptively to life demands and stresses, and have more emotional and behavioral problems than their typically developing peers. All types of psychiatric disorders can be present. Difficulty expressing needs and interpreting life events, societal nonacceptance and other issues related to being "different," as well as other biopsychosocial factors can all increase a child's susceptibility to behavioral disturbance and psychopathology. For example, communication deficits can increase aggression and disruptive behavior as a substitute for language or out of frustration. Additionally, individuals with intellectual disabilities are at risk for being exploited by others, and being physically or sexually abused. The lower the child's IQ, the greater the prevalence of behavioral problems and psychopathology. In individuals in the mild range, psychiatric and behavioral issues are also elevated, but the problems present similarly to cognitively unimpaired individuals. In children and adolescents with mild intellectual disabilities, there is a somewhat greater risk for psychopathology in boys than girls.

Estimates indicate that anywhere from 27 to 71% of individuals with intellectual disabilities may present with comorbid psychiatric and behavioral disorders. Symptoms may be expressed somewhat differently from those commonly observed in the specific conditions, due to the degree of cognitive abilities and associated deficits, and poor communication skills. Additionally vulnerabilities are related to the tendency of children with intellectual disabilities to communicate dysphoria, anxiety, anger, and frustration in more primitive forms, such as self-injurious behavior, stereotyped rocking, aggression, and self-stimulation.[2] Furthermore, associated deficits, particularly communication and cognitive impairments, may make it difficult to obtain reliable information about symptoms from the individual; therefore, diagnosis is often made using objectively observable symptoms that can be reported by collateral sources.

Although all psychiatric disorders can be represented in individuals with intellectual disabilities, the rates and patterns of specific disorders vary compared to the general population. In individuals with mild intellectual disabilities, the pattern of disorders seen is not significantly different from that of the general population. However, in individuals with moderate to profound intellectual disabilities, there is more evidence of pervasive developmental disorders, behavior disorders, and psychosis, and fewer cases of substance use. In general, commonly diagnosed psychiatric disorders in children and adolescents with intellectual disabilities include: autism and other pervasive developmental disorders, attention-deficit/hyperactivity disorder (ADHD), mood disorders, anxiety disorders, oppositional defiant disorder, intermittent explosive disorder, post-traumatic stress disorder, stereotypic movement disorder with self-injury, Pica, Tourette's disorder, and mental disorders due to a general medical condition.[2]

While a wide variety of psychiatric disorders can be observed in individuals with intellectual disabilities, certain genetic conditions are associated with specific behavioral and emotional symptoms. For example, hyperphagia and other compulsive behavior have been associated with Prader-Willi syndrome. In children and adolescents with Down syndrome, the most common comorbid psychiatric conditions include ADHD, oppositional defiant disorder, and conduct disorder, with females evidencing fewer problems than males. Autism-spectrum disorders also can be present.[4] Individuals with DS are also at increased risk for development of Alzheimer's disease later in life, with the prevalence of dementia by age 65 estimated to be between 30 and 75%, and the average age of onset between 50 and 55 years. In individuals with Fragile X (FraX), behavioral and psychiatric features can include hyperactivity, gaze aversion, shyness and social anxiety (especially in females), and motor stereotypies. In addition, autistic symptomatology has been reported in 5 to 40% of males with FraX, with specific symptoms of stereotyped motor mannerisms, unusual non-verbal interactions, and more difficulty with peer versus adult interactions.

Several challenges are usually encountered in the diagnoses and treatment of comorbid psychiatric disorders in individuals with intellectual disabilities. Diagnostic overshadowing refers to a tendency to consider all abnormal behavior observed in individuals with intellectual disabilities as secondary to the cognitive deficits. This common tendency among clinicians can lead to underdiagnosis of comorbid mental disorders and inappropriate minimization of the mental and affective life of individuals with intellectual disabilities. Even more damaging, diagnostic overshadowing can further lead to a denial of appropriate treatments, as well as premature reliance on pharmacotherapy or more mechanistic behavioral approaches, rather than adequately exploring underlying psychosocial contributions to the symptoms or the benefit of interpersonal psychotherapeutic treatments. A second common pitfall is assuming that all emotional or behavioral problems in children and adolescents with intellectual disabilities are the result of brain damage or dysfunction. A distinctive and painful array of psychosocial stressors and stigmatizations are encountered in children with intellectual disabilities that alone increase the risk of psychiatric disorders. Third, it is often the assumption that, because of their cognitive deficits, children diagnosed with intellectual disabilities are unable to provide useful diagnostic information during a clinical interview. However, children with mild intellectual disabilities, in particular, are often able to provide valuable clinical information, including information about precipitating factors known only to them, subjective distress, fears and fantasies, and affective symptoms. The psychiatric assessment of children with mild intellectual disabilities should therefore always include a clinical interview. Finally, communication between the psychiatric team and primary care providers, such as pediatricians, should occur on a continuous basis to allow the optimal management of acute and chronic medical illnesses that are frequently observed in individuals with intellectual disability, and especially in those individuals with more impairment.

While most mental disorders can be observed in typically developing individuals, PICA and stereotypic motor disorder (SMD) appear to be almost exclusively described in people with intellectual or developmental disabilities. PICA is defined as persistent eating of non-nutritive substances for at least one month. It is much more frequently observed in young children than in adults with prevalence rates of 10 to 32% in children between one and six years of age. Several factors have been implicated in the pathogenesis of this disorder but no clear etiologies have been identified. A higher than expected incidence of PICA seems to occur in the relatives of people with this disorder. Additionally, a history of parental neglect and deprivation has been associated with cases of PICA. SMD is defined as a repetitive, non-functional motor behavior that seems to be compulsive. The behavior can lead to self-inflicted bodily injuries severe enough to require medical attention. The exact prevalence of SMD is unknown but estimates have reported rates of 10 to 20% in children with ID. Similar to PICA, several etiological factors have been implicated with genetic, developmental, biological, and environmental factors playing a role in the genesis of these behaviors.

4. Clinical Description

4.1. *Mild mental retardation*

Approximately 85% of individuals diagnosed with intellectual disability have impairments in the mild range. Individuals scoring in this range are able to acquire social and job skills allowing successful independent functioning in many cases. Children in this range may not appear different from their typically developing peers in preschool, but may exhibit more apparent difficulties when academic demands increase. Therefore, they are often diagnosed at a later age than children with moderate to profound level of intellectual disability.[5] Children with mild mental retardation typically do not have dysmorphic features or medical conditions related to their cognitive disability, unless one of a number of genetic etiologies underlies their condition. They are generally able to attain academic skills up to about the sixth grade level, or up to about a 9-to-12-year-old level. As adults, most individuals with mild intellectual disability are able to live either independently or with some minimum supervision and assistance.[2] They are often more capable in jobs that do not emphasize academic skills, such as unskilled or semiskilled positions, and in this context their cognitive deficits may be less salient. However, when under social or economic stress, they may require additional support.

4.2. *Moderate mental retardation*

Of individuals diagnosed with intellectual disability, approximately 10% fall into the moderate range, or about 0.2% of the general population. These individuals typically attain adequate communication during childhood, and are able to learn personal care skills, although both are delayed and compromised. Academically, they are slow learners, but may be able to advance to approximately a second grade level (6-to-9-year-old level), and are able to learn basic reading, writing, and counting skills. They can also benefit from vocational, social, and occupational training. Social deficits become more of a problem beginning in later childhood, with difficulty recognizing the more complex social rules of adolescence, leading to problems in peer relationships. As adults, these individuals are often able to hold unskilled or semiskilled jobs with structure and supervision. They usually require some degree of supervision rather than living completely independently.[2]

4.3. *Severe mental retardation*

Severe intellectual disability occurs in about 3 to 4% of all individuals diagnosed with intellectual disability, and in about 0.13% of the general population.[2] These individuals have more significant deficits in learning functional language skills, and may not learn to speak until the school-age years. In addition, a significant degree of motor impairment is common, as are medical conditions and dysmorphic features. Training in basic self-care is possible, but these individuals benefit less from standard academic instruction. They are, however, often able to learn simple counting and recognition of some words. As adults, these individuals have a mental age of approximately 3 to 6 years, and are able to perform simple unskilled job tasks with close supervision in sheltered workshops. Individuals with severe mental retardation are typically unable to live independently, and often live in group homes or with their families.[2]

4.4. *Profound mental retardation*

The prevalence rate for profound intellectual disability is around 1 to 2% of all individuals with intellectual disability, and approximately 0.04% of the general population. These individuals function at a mental age of under three years. They have significant limitations in the ability to communicate, and in childhood have sensorimotor impairments and restricted mobility. They are unable to care for most of their personal needs and develop only simple non-verbal communication. Most have an identified neurological condition, as well as other related medical conditions and dysmorphic features.

5. Pathogenesis

Genetic advances have increased our understanding of the underlying etiology of specific syndromes associated with intellectual disabilities. To date, there are over

750 identified genetic causes of intellectual disability.[6] Approximately one-half of the population with intellectual disabilities has a known biologic etiology. Specific genetic etiologies are more likely to exist in individuals with moderate to profound levels of intellectual disabilities than in mild ones.

A majority of cases of mild intellectual disabilities are idiopathic or multifactorial in etiology, although this subgroup is gradually shrinking due to increasing identification of specific genetic or other specific causes. Multifactorial etiology refers to a combination of genetic and psychosocial factors. Estimates of the "reaction range" (*i.e.* IQ variations due to environmental versus genetic causes) suggest that benign or enriched environments have the potential to raise cognitive and adaptive functioning from the mild range into the normal ranges.

Known biologic etiologies can be divided into three broad categories: prenatal, perinatal, and postnatal. Examples of prenatal factors that may lead to intellectual disabilities include infection (*e.g.* rubella, toxoplasmosis, cytomegalovirus, herpes simplex, hepatitis, human immunodeficiency virus, syphilis), X-ray exposure, substance use (*e.g.* alcohol, heroin), prescribed drug treatments (*e.g.* anticonvulsants, thalidomide, chemotherapy), maternal mercury poisoning, genetic abnormalities (*e.g.* chromosomal, specific single-factor inheritance, unfavorable polygenic combinations), metabolic abnormalities (*e.g.* low T4), and maternal illness (*e.g.* diabetes, malnutrition, anemia, emphysema). Common perinatal factors include hypoxia, prematurity, and mechanical birth injury. Examples of post-natal factors include bacterial infections (*e.g.* hemophilus influenza, diplococcus pneumonia, viral encephalitis), head trauma, and lead intoxication.

5.1. *Fetal alcohol syndrome*

FAS is the most common example of the widespread and negative effects of an exogenous agent on central nervous system development. In FAS, intellectual disability is often present, occurring from prenatal exposure to high levels of alcohol at critical periods.[5] It is the leading cause of intellectual disability in the United States, with an incidence of approximately 6 to 7 out of 10,000 newborns. Associated physical symptoms include pre- and post-natal growth retardation, distinctive facial anomalies (*e.g.* thin upper lip, epicanthal folds, indistinct philtrum), and central nervous system dysfunction, with resultant cognitive deficits and behavioral problems. Average IQ for children with FAS is approximately 70, with a range of anywhere from 20 to 100. Children who were exposed to alcohol prenatally but do not meet criteria for FAS may also show low IQ scores, as well as symptoms of hyperactivity and inattention, impairments in learning and memory, and less consistently, in language function, motor abilities, and visuospatial skills.[7]

5.2. *Genetic disorders*

Genetic disorders can be divided into four types: chromosomal, single gene, multifactorial (polygenic), and nontraditional (Table 1). These disorders have been the focus of recent investigations applying cutting-edge state-of-the art imaging methodologies to help elucidate the neurobiology of developmental disabilities and consequently contributing to the field of neuroscience.[8] This path of deciphering the neurobiologic underpinning of specific ID will allow a better understanding of the pathophysiology of these disorders and help in the development of more specific treatments. However, this research interest in individuals with identifiable genetic disorders have led to limited focus on the study of people with idiopathic etiology (ies), the most common cause of intellectual disability.

Table 1: Genetic Disorders Associated with Intellectual Disability

Disorder	Description	Type
Angelman	15q11–13 microdeletion (usually on maternal chromosome 15)	Chromosomal microdeletion/contiguous gene syndrome, genomic imprinting defect
Chromosome 15q trisomy	Trisomy of the long arm of chromosome 15	Autosomal chromosomal abnormality
Cri du chat syndrome	5p deletion	Chromosomal deletion syndrome
Cornelia deLange syndrome	Mutations in NIPBL, SMC1A, SMC3 genes	Multifactorial/polygenic disorder
Down syndrome	Trisomy 21	Autosomal chromosomal abnormality
Fragile X	FMR1 gene mutation — triplet repeat expansion	X-linked recessive single gene disorder, anticipation disorder
Hunter syndrome	I2S gene mutation	X-linked recessive single gene disorder
Kearns-Sayre syndrome	Mitochondrial DNA mutations	Mitochondrial disorder
Klinefelter syndrome	47XXY	Sex chromosomal abnormality
Lesch-Nyhan syndrome	HPRT1 gene mutations	X-linked recessive single gene disorder
Multiple X	47XXX	Sex chromosomal abnormality
Neurofibromatosis type 1	Chromosome 17 mutation	Autosomal dominant single gene disorder

(*Continued*)

Table 1: (*Continued*)

Disorder	Description	Type
Noonan syndrome	Chromosome 12q24.1; PTPN11 gene mutation	Autosomal dominant single gene disorder
Phenylketonuria	Chromosome 12q23.2; PAH gene mutation	Autosomal recessive single gene disorder
Patau syndrome/ Trisomy 13	Trisomy 13	Autosomal chromosomal abnormality
Prader-Willi	15q11–13 microdeletion (usually on paternal chromosome 15)	Chromosomal microdeletion/contiguous gene syndrome, genomic imprinting defect
Rett syndrome	Xq28; MeCP2 mutation	X-linked single gene disorder
Smith-Magenis syndrome	17p11.2 microdeletion	Chromosomal microdeletion
Turner syndrome	45XO; complete or partial monosomy of the X chromosome	Sex chromosomal abnormality
Velocardiofacial syndrome	22q11.2 deletion	Chromosomal deletion syndrome
Williams syndrome	7q11.2 microdeletion	Chromosomal microdeletion, multifactorial/polygenic disorder
Wolf-Hirschhorn syndrome	4p deletion	Chromosomal deletion syndrome
18q deletion syndrome	18q deletion	Chromosomal deletion syndrome

5.2.1. *Chromosomal abnormalities*

Chromosome disorders include disorders of number (aneuploidy) and structure. Common autosomal chromosomal abnormalities include Down syndrome (trisomy 21), and trisomy 13, 14, and 15. Examples of sex chromosome abnormalities include Turner syndrome (45XO), Klinefelter syndrome (47XXY), and Multiple X (47XXX). All of the above-named conditions are examples of aneuploidy. Disorders of chromosome structure can include disorders where there is a deletion or duplication on a chromosome. Examples of deletion syndromes include Cri du chat syndrome (5p deletion), Wolf-Hirschhorn syndrome (4p deletion), Velocardiofacial/DiGeorge syndrome (22q11 deletion), and 18q deletion syndrome. Microdeletion syndromes (contiguous-gene syndromes) include Prader-Willi (15q11–13 microdeletion), Angelman (15q11–13), Smith-Magenis syndrome (17p11 microdeletion), and Williams Syndrome (7q microdeletion).

The incidence of Down syndrome (DS) in the general population is approximately 1 in 1000,[9] and it is the most common genetic cause of intellectual disability. Most often, DS is the result of trisomy 21, occurring as a result of nondisjunction during gamete formation. Most cases result from full trisomy 21 of maternal origin. More uncommon forms are due to mosaicism (*i.e.* nondisjunction occurs after fertilization, resulting in both trisomic and euploid cell lines), and to partial or full translocation of chromosome 21 to another chromosome.[10] Individuals with DS typically have a characteristic appearance, including short stature, hyperflexibility of joints, hypotonia, and distinctive facial features such as a low nasal bridge, epicanthal folds, and protrusion of tongue. Average IQ score for children with DS is approximately 50, with relative strengths in visuospatial skills, and a particular weakness in facial recognition.

5.2.2. *Single gene disorders*

Single gene, or monogenic disorders, include autosomal dominant, recessive, and X-linked conditions. Neurofibromatosis type 1 (mutation on chromosome 17) and Noonan syndrome are examples of autosomal dominant monogenic disorders. Phenylketonuria is an example of an autosomal recessive disorder. Examples of X-linked disorders include Fragile X, Rett syndrome, Lesch-Nyhan syndrome, and Hunter syndrome.

Fragile X syndrome (FraX; Xq27.3) is the second most frequent chromosomal cause of intellectual disability after Down syndrome,[9] and the most common inherited cause of neurodevelopmental disability. Frequency is estimated to be approximately 1 in every 2000 to 4000 live births. In addition to being a sex chromosome abnormality, it is an example of a single gene disorder. However, despite its seemingly simple etiology, the absence of one protein in FraX has widespread consequences for brain development and functioning. The condition is also an important example of the genetic phenomenon of triplet repeat expansion. FraX is caused by the deficiency in expression of a single gene, *FMR1*. Characteristic physical features include long face, prominent ears, macroorchidism in males, various musculoskeletal problems, and mitral valve prolapse. Nearly all males with FraX have mild to severe cognitive disability, and about one-half of affected females have borderline intellectual functioning to moderate intellectual disability.

5.2.3. *Multifactorial/polygenic disorders*

Polygenic disorders include neural tube defects and Williams syndrome. In addition, de Lange syndrome is presumed to be caused by a polygenic mutation.

Williams Syndrome (WS), a rare disorder that occurs in about 1 out of 25,000 births, is caused by deletion of approximately 17–20 contiguous genes on chromosome 7.[9] Specifically, there is a contiguous microdeletion on band 7q11.23 of chromosome 7 that involves the gene encoding elastin and roughly 17–20 other genes.[11] Physical features include distinctive facial features (*i.e.* flat nasal bridge, prominent lips and wide mouth, malar flattening, full cheeks, long philtrum, small mandible, epicanthal folds, and periorbital fullness), cardiac problems such as supravalvular aortic stenosis resulting from the deletion of elastin, and other connective tissue symptoms, such as joint and skin laxity. Cognitively, individuals with WS usually fall in the mild to moderate range of intellectual disability (mean IQ of 55, range 40–90). Comparatively, certain aspects of language are intact, including a proclivity for the use of unusual words and great facility with affectively laden language.[7] In addition, individuals have generalized impairments in visuospatial processing, while demonstrating good facial recognition skills.

5.2.4. *Nontraditional disorders*

Examples of nontraditional forms of inheritance include mitochondrial disorders, such as Kearns-Sayre syndrome, mosaicism, genomic imprinting (*e.g.* Prader-Willi, Angelman syndromes), and anticipation (Fragile X syndrome).

5.3. *Associated medical disorders*

Physical, sensory, and neurological impairments are commonly identified in children with moderate to profound intellectual disabilities and usually require regular and at times frequent communication between the mental health team and the primary care group.[9] The frequency of associated physical disorders increases as severity of the intellectual disability increases. For example, seizure disorders are diagnosed in about 10% of children and adolescents with moderate intellectual disability, and in approximately 50% of children and adolescents with severe to profound intellectual disability. Sensory impairments, including blindness and deafness are increased in individuals with severe and profound levels of cognitive disability compared to the general population.

6. Clinical Instruments and Methods for Diagnosis

6.1. *Measuring intellectual functioning*

Administration of individual, standardized cognitive testing is required in the diagnosis of mental retardation (Table 2). These instruments should be normed

Table 2: Tests and Measures

Test	Age Range (age expressed as year–month)	Functions Assessed
Infant cognitive development		
Bayley Scales of Infant and Toddler Development, 3rd edition (BSID-III; Bayley, 2005)	0–1 to 3–6	Mental and psychomotor development
Mullen Scales of Early Learning (Mullen, 1995)	0–1 to 5–8	Visual reception, gross and fine motor, expressive and receptive language abilities
Intelligence tests		
Wechsler Preschool and Primary Scale of Intelligence — 3rd edition (WPPSI-III; Wechsler, 2002)	2–6 to 7–3	Verbal and non-verbal reasoning, processing speed, expressive and receptive vocabulary
Wechsler Intelligence Scale for Children — 4th edition (WISC-IV; Wechsler, 2003)	6–0 to 16–11	Verbal and non-verbal reasoning, processing speed, and working memory
Wechsler Adult Intelligence Scale — 3rd edition (WAIS-III; Wechsler, 1997)	16–0 to 89–11	Verbal comprehension, perceptual organization, working memory, processing speed
Stanford-Binet Intelligence Scale — 5th edition (SB:FE; Roid, 2003)	2–0 to 85+	Verbal and non-verbal fluid reasoning, knowledge, quantitative reasoning, visual-spatial processing, working memory
Differential Ability Scales, 2nd edition (DAS-II; Elliot, 2006)	2–6 to 17–11; separate preschool and school-age versions	Verbal and non-verbal reasoning, numerical reasoning
Kaufman Assessment Battery for Children, 2nd edition (KABC-II; Kaufman & Kaufman, 2006)	3 to 18	Sequential and simultaneous mental processing, planning, learning, knowledge, and non-verbal functioning
Leiter International Performance Scale-Revised (LIPS-R; Roid and Miller, 1996)	2–0 to 18–11	Non-verbal intelligence, including measures of fluid reasoning, fundamental visualization, and spatial visualization; no language required

(*Continued*)

Table 2: (*Continued*)

Test	Age Range (age expressed as year–month)	Functions Assessed
Adaptive behavior		
Vineland Adaptive Behavior Scales, 2nd edition (Vineland-II; Sparrow, Cicchetti, and Balla, 2005)	0–1 to 18–11, and low-functioning adults	Communication, daily living, socialization, motor skills
Scale of Independent Behavior-Revised (SIB-R; Bruininks, *et al.*, 1996)	Infant to 80+ years	Social, motor, communication, personal living, community living skills
AAMR Adaptive Behavior Scale — School, 2nd edition (ABS-S-2; Lambert, Leland, and Nihira, 1993)	3 to 21 years	Independent functioning, physical development, economic activity, language development, prevocational/vocational activity, numbers and time, self-direction, responsibility, socialization

on a population representative of the child's cultural and ethnic background. Raw scores are converted to standard scores that can be compared to the results of other children of the same age who have taken the test (the standardization sample) and who are representative of the general local population. Children are identified as falling in the mentally retarded range on intelligence tests when their scores (IQ) fall at least two standard deviations below the average. For most cognitive tests, the average standard score is 100, and the standard deviation is 15; thus, scores of 70 and below would fall in the mentally retarded range. However, the standard error of measurement should be taken into account when determining whether a score falls in the appropriate range for a diagnosis. IQ scores typically have a measurement error of approximately five points, although this varies by age and test; therefore, a child scoring 75 on an IQ test might still qualify for a diagnosis of mental retardation if there are accompanying deficits in adaptive functioning.

Intellectual testing typically provides broad information about a child's overall level of cognitive functioning (often referred to as the "full scale IQ" score), in addition to providing information about abilities in different cognitive domains. Most traditional intellectual assessment measures provide information about a child's verbal and non-verbal reasoning skills separately. How these abilities are measured and described depends upon the theoretical basis of the specific measure. For example, in the Wechsler tests, full scale IQ is further divided into four broad domains: verbal comprehension, perceptual reasoning, processing speed, and working memory.[12] For a diagnosis of intellectual disability, however, a child's abilities should be impaired across cognitive domains. If a child has an overall IQ score below 70, but examination of specific cognitive domains reveals scattered skills, then domains should be interpreted separately rather than using the overall IQ score, which would not accurately reflect the variability of the child's skills. Children who have deficits in one area but not in others would not be considered to have an overall intellectual disability.

In the United States, the most commonly administered intellectual tests are the Wechsler scales. For preschoolers, the *Wechsler Preschool and Primary Scale of Intelligence* — 3rd edition (WPPSI-III)[13] is employed; for school-aged children the *Wechsler Intelligence Scale for Children* — 4th edition (WISC-IV)[12] is used; and for adults the *Wechsler Adult Intelligence Scale* — 3rd edition (WAIS-III) is chosen. Some of the other cognitive tests available include the *Differential Abilities Scale* — 2nd edition (DAS-II) and the *Kaufman Assessment Battery for Children* — 2nd edition (KABC-II).[14] A possible difficulty when using these measures to assess the presence of intellectual disability is the potential lack of adequate sensitivity to accurately assess the skills of individuals with more severe cognitive deficits. In these instances, the *Stanford-Binet Intelligence Scale*, 5th edition (SB5)[15] may be selected instead, as it allows for a slightly lower basal level than the Wechsler tests do. The KABC-II is also useful for this purpose. However, few, if any standardized cognitive measures are very good at assessing children with severe to profound intellectual disabilities. Accurately measuring IQ at the most extreme ends of the scale is quite difficult and often imprecise with any standardized instrument. Consequently, the importance of accurately assessing adaptive behavior increases in these children.

For children with sensory impairments, limited proficiency in the language of the test or administrator, autism, communication disorders, and other neurological conditions affecting speech, a non-verbal intelligence test may be substituted for the general cognitive test battery. Either selecting the non-verbal portion of tests such as the SB5 or KABC-II, or using a non-verbal battery may be appropriate. The Leiter International Performance Scale-Revised (Leiter-R) is one such non-verbal battery. Items are administered without the use of language by the examiner, and language is not required to complete any part of the test.

In some instances, a child cannot be assessed with standardized cognitive testing, thus an IQ score is not obtained. Children who are extremely impaired, have physical limitations, sensory deficits (*e.g.* visual or hearing impairment), or behavioral disturbance may be difficult or impossible to assess. In addition, in younger children it can be particularly difficult to establish basal levels on cognitive testing, and it is sometimes necessary to drop to developmental tests that do not measure IQ *per se*. In infants, intelligence cannot be validly measured, and instead developmental tests are designed to measure early learning and acquisition of developmental skills (*e.g.* verbal, motor, cognitive). Examples of developmental measures for infants, toddlers, and preschool children include the *Bayley Scales of Infant and Toddler Development*, 3rd edition (BSID-III)[16] and Mullen Scales of Early Learning.

When there is a clinical judgment that an individual's cognitive development is significantly delayed but formal cognitive testing cannot be achieved, the diagnosis of "mental retardation, severity unspecified" can be given[2] The ICD-10 provides a category for "other mental retardation" in this situation, and also has a category for "unspecified mental retardation" for situations in which an intellectual disability is clearly evident but there is not enough information to make a decision about severity.

6.2. *Measuring adaptive functioning*

An IQ score alone is not enough for a diagnosis of an intellectual disability; there must also be demonstrated adaptive skills deficits in at least two areas of functioning. Determining the presence of adaptive behavior deficits required for intellectual disability diagnosis has been proven to be a complex and often unreliable process. Unlike intellectual assessment, which attempts to measure optimal potential, adaptive behavior scales attempt to assess an individual's day-to-day functioning — what a child actually does on a daily basis rather than what he or she can do under the best circumstances. Adaptive functioning information is usually collected through semistructured interview of collateral sources, such as caregivers and teachers. The most commonly used measure in most European and North American countries is the *Vineland Adaptive Behavior Scales*, 2nd edition[17] developed from the Vineland Social Maturity Scale created by Edgar Doll in the 1930s (Table 2). Standard scores for domains as well as overall adaptive behavior are derived, and significant impairment can be generally defined as skills falling at least two standard deviations below the mean. Domains include communication (expressive, receptive, and written language), daily living skills (personal, domestic, and community), socialization (interpersonal relationships, play and leisure, and coping skills), and motor skills (gross and fine). Other measures of adaptive functioning are also available, such as the *Scales of Independent Behavior-Revised* (SIB-R), and the *AAIDD Adaptive Behavior Scale-School*, 2nd edition (ABS-S-2). All adaptive functioning measures should be used only if appropriate for the individual's cultural background.

7. Role of Primary Care Physicians

Primary prevention involves routine screening for treatable etiologies such as thyroid dysfunction and phenylketonuria. This step is routinely implemented at birth in developed countries but not in poor countries where pediatrician play a crucial role in the identification of early signs of developmental delay that should prompt a comprehensive assessment including testing for preventable diseases. Primary prevention aims also at eliminating or reducing the conditions that lead to the development of disorders associated with intellectual disabilities. These efforts include public education, adequate health professional training, free maternal and child health care, and eradication of known disorders that cause brain damage. Secondary preventions is also essential in alleviating the burden of intellectual disabilities through early identification of developmental delays which usually occurs in pediatricians' and family doctors' offices who routinely examine toddler and young children who are suspected of being delayed developmentally. Early identification is crucial in developed and underdeveloped countries to facilitate appropriate referrals for assessments. Therefore, training primary care providers in the identification of any red flags should be part of their educational programs so early interventions are implemented. Therapeutic interventions for individuals with intellectual disabilities involve the implementation of strategies that target a multitude of factors, ranging from primary prevention to the treatment of associated psychiatric disorders.

8. Treatment

The treatment of ID and associated psychiatric disorders is complex and typically requires a combination of psychosocial and pharmacological interventions. For children with intellectual disabilities, educational programming is typically the central component in the overall intervention plan, largely because educational services provide the necessary level of intervention intensity.

8.1. *Educational programs*

For individuals from birth to age 21, a significant portion of their intervention services are conducted through state agencies, including early intervention programs and the public school system. The federal government regulates the provision of early intervention and special education services for children with intellectual disabilities under the Individuals with Disabilities Education Act of 2004 (IDEA).[18] Each state provides early intervention services to children with special needs from birth to three years of age. Once these children are over the age of three years, the public education system becomes responsible for providing adequate services.

8.2. *Educational rights*

When working with children and families around developing an appropriate educational intervention program, parents must become informed about their child's rights to special education services and about what services are included in an adequate program. Services can be delivered either in inclusive or self-contained class settings, depending on the needs of the child and the available staff in the program. Special education law dictates that children are entitled to be educated in the "least restrictive environment" (*i.e.* a child should be placed in the least restrictive setting necessary for their educational success). Many children with intellectual disabilities are adequately educated in regular education classrooms with one-to-one paraprofessional support in addition to other specialized services (*e.g.* behavior support, resource specialist programming, speech therapy, *etc.*). However, some children are best served in the highly supportive environment provided by the self-contained special education classroom, where there is usually a low student-to-teacher ratio and fewer children. As such, when working with families around issues of educational placement, it is important to educate them about their options and the child's educational rights.

8.3. *Psychosocial interventions*

8.3.1. *Components of treatment*

Comprehensive treatment of intellectual disabilities should include interventions that address all problem behaviors, as well as goals for the development of functional skills. Treatment should facilitate supported participation in socially inclusive environments, such as preschool, child care, and other community settings, and be applied across a full range of routines, times of day, and conditions that the individual encounters. There should also be a focus on broad-based family support. Finally, interventions should be driven by functional behavior assessment, be appropriate to the context, and blend multiple procedures. It is important in the development of a treatment program that interventions and identified goals are developed and evaluated collaboratively, and that the treatments match the individual's current needs. Goals should be meaningful and contribute toward attainment of optimal outcomes. It is also critical that goals be monitored and reevaluated frequently, and that program modifications are made accordingly.

8.3.2. *Treatment goals*

Areas to target in intervention with individuals with intellectual disabilities may include the development of functional communication skills, social engagement, social and play skills, cognitive and academic skills, self-help skills (adaptive functioning), behavioral challenges, and motor skills. These goals are facilitated through a variety of services provided in multiple settings. For example, services may include special education services and an Individualized Educational Plan (IEP), family support and involvement, behavioral support services (based on a functional behavior assessment), speech-language therapy, occupational therapy, social skills interventions, pharmacological interventions, and ongoing monitoring and reevaluation by a psychologist or other professional. When possible, treatment should be conducted in settings in which skills will need to be demonstrated. For instance, school, home, and community settings are all environments where children will need to apply social communication skills and demonstrate appropriate behavior. Therefore, these settings should be included in treatment to increase generalization, maintenance, functional use of skills, and social validity. Parents and other caregivers should communicate regularly with professionals so goals can be practiced and applied outside therapy sessions. Treatment goals should have social validity (*i.e.* be important to children and families) and skills taught should be functional and strive to enhance the individuals' cognitive skills, social interactions, communication skills, independence, and quality of life. Goals should also embrace high expectations for individuals and should foster independence as much as possible.

8.3.3. *Positive behavior support*

Psychosocial therapies are used to shape and promote social behaviors and reduce aberrant as well as aggressive behaviors. For children and adolescents, psychosocial interventions often occur across settings (e.g., home and school). Positive behavior support (PBS) is a specific psychosocial intervention often employed by behavioral specialists working with children and adults with intellectual disabilities. PBS emerged from the fields of applied behavior analysis, social and organizational psychology, and the normalization and inclusion movements.[19] PBS places a focus on improving overall quality of life for individuals with disabilities and involving family and educational team members in this process.[19]

PBS intervention is based upon a principle of valued outcomes; *i.e.* PBS seeks to make meaningful changes in quality of life both for individuals with behavioral difficulties and the people involved in their lives. In contrast to traditional behavioral models, PBS places focus on making changes in the individual and the supporting environment to teach meaningful skills, enhance quality of life, and modify systems such that they more adequately support individuals with intellectual disability. This model relies on the application of behavior modification principles and realistic ways that skills can be maintained outside clinic settings.

The focus on quality of life, lifespan perspectives, stakeholder perspectives, and systems change in a PBS model means that intervention is based on more than just an assessment of discrete behaviors in individuals, as is seen in traditional behavioral intervention models. Rather, there is a focus on systemic assessment and change so that systems may better support individuals over time.

It has been noted in the literature that PBS brings changes in the "who," "where," "what," and "when" of intervention. Specifically, the "who" indicates that PBS includes the extended circle of people involved in the individual's life as active intervention agents (parents, teachers, friends, community members, *etc.*), as opposed to reliance on intervention provided solely by experts. The "where" emphasizes intervention that occurs in naturalistic community-based settings, as opposed to clinics and labs. The "what" of intervention brings the focus to comprehensive lifestyle change and quality of life issues, as opposed to developing one intervention to target one specific problem behavior. Finally, the "when" calls for interventions that are implemented proactively to prevent challenging behavior, with a focus on building strengths and creating supportive living environments, as opposed to the traditional focus on treating problem behaviors after they develop or using a crisis intervention approach.

8.3.3.1. Challenging behavior

Children with intellectual disabilities often engage in high levels of disruptive behavior. As a result, behavior support is of primary importance when working with this population. As disruptive behaviors can occur for many reasons, functional analysis or functional behavioral assessment (FBA) procedures are typically necessary to assess problem behavior prior to devising behavior plans. These procedures allow intervention providers to determine the communicative function of the behavior prior to deciding on an intervention plan. FBA places the focus on environmental events and considers carefully the role that such events play in eliciting, reinforcing, and maintaining problem behavior. Using functional assessment and analysis insures that the behavior plan will address the function of the disruptive behavior so it will be reduced and a positive replacement behavior can be taught in its place. Behavior plans not based on functional assessment and analysis are typically ineffective, as they do not address the need the child was trying to have met by using the disruptive behavior. Functional assessment and analysis of problem behavior involves taking systematic data on the setting events, antecedents, behaviors, and consequences (a.k.a., the "A-B-C's" of behavior) to determine relevant patterns of behavior. Once behavioral functions have been determined, intervention can be tailored accordingly.

Children with intellectual disabilities may engage in a variety of challenging behaviors for different reasons. The nature of their cognitive deficits is such that these children may have difficulty communicating with others, occupying their time constructively (*e.g.* by playing), complying with demands, following routines, making transitions, *etc.* Some of the most common causes of disruptive behaviors in children with intellectual disability may include: (1) Task avoidance (*i.e.* frustration with demands, whether seemingly easy or hard, due to the nature of the intellectual disability); (2) To obtain items (*i.e.* children who have difficulty communicating and who also have a low frustration tolerance may engage in challenging behaviors to obtain preferred items); (3) During transitions (*i.e.* they may not have the cognitive capacity to predict when transitions are approaching); and (4) When limits are set (*i.e.* children with intellectual disabilities may have a low frustration tolerance and may not have the cognitive capacity to predict when a limit may be set). Repetitive behaviors are also commonly seen in individuals with intellectual disability, although they are most commonly associated with autism spectrum disorders. These children may engage in body rocking, hand mannerisms, repetitive verbal behaviors, *etc.* Unlike the behavioral functions discussed above, which are typically maintained by environmental variables, self-stimulatory behaviors are typically maintained by automatic reinforcement. These behaviors are often quite concerning for children and families, as they cause the child to stand out from others and are often stigmatizing. They may also increase social isolation.

8.3.3.2. Strategies for reducing challenging behaviors

Once the functions of behaviors have been determined, an intervention plan can be developed. This plan should take two variables into account: (1) environmental changes that can decrease the likelihood of disruptive behavior, and (2) skills the person may need for use in place of disruptive behavior. Environmental changes may include modification of antecedents (*e.g.* giving a 5-min warning to an individual who has difficulty with unforeseen transitions), consequences (*e.g.* following through with demands rather than removing them when disruptive behavior occurs), or the environment (*e.g.* placing a child who becomes overwhelmed with task demands in a location where he or she will not become distracted).

In addition to these changes in the environment and how individuals react to behaviors, the child may also benefit from learning replacement behaviors based on the behavioral function. For example, if a child hits to obtain items, he or she can be taught to ask instead. The child will learn and maintain this behavior if intervention providers insure he or she only receives the item when he or she has asked, but not when hitting has occurred. Similarly, when behaviors occur for task avoidance, children can be taught to ask for breaks when they begin to feel overwhelmed. Children can also be taught to self-manage their disruptive behaviors in order to earn rewards. For example, children can be taught that if they do not engage in self-stimulatory behavior for a specified period of time they will earn a reward. While this type of intervention requires some up front training in the use of the procedures, self-management can be very effective in motivating decreases in disruptive behaviors and increases in more positive alternatives.

Strategies that are used in the reduction of inappropriate behaviors include reinforcement as well as punishment procedures. These procedures should only be applied once behavioral functions are determined to insure the behavior plan addresses the child's specific needs. Reinforcement procedures may include intermittently reinforcing more positive behaviors when they occur in natural environments and/or specific behavior plans whereby the child earns reinforcement when specific target behaviors are performed. Punishment is also sometimes used, such as time out for inappropriate behavior and removing points or tokens that the child has earned in working toward a larger reinforcer (*i.e.* response cost). Time out is one example of a procedure that must be carefully used based on behavioral functions, because children who engage in disruptive behaviors for task avoidance will inadvertently be reinforced by time out. Overcorrection is another punishment procedure whereby the child engages in restitution after engaging in a disruptive behavior, such as cleaning up a mess made during a tantrum and then being required to clean other related messes. Similarly, in positive practice, the child is required to excessively practice the adaptive behavior that should have been used in place of a disruptive behavior (*e.g.* having to walk back and forth from the scene of a toileting accident to the toilet five times after wetting occurs).

8.4. *Psychopharmacological interventions*

To date, there are no specific medication treatments that aim at targeting the underlying etiologies of intellectual disabilities. Therefore, the available interventions attempt to treat comorbid mental disorders while applying the same strategies and agents used with typically developing individuals. In the absence of well-designed, double-blind, and placebo-controlled studies, the current use is based on extrapolating from the use of medications in typically developing individuals. In fact, several behavioral syndromes, such as aggression and attention

Table 3: Behavioral Principles Commonly Used in Treatment of Individuals with Intellectual Disabilities

Technique	Description	Example
Reinforcement to increase behaviors		
Token economy	Reinforcing target behavior with "tokens" (*e.g.* stickers) that can then be traded in for reinforcers once multiple tokens have been earned.	The child receives points for each completed step in the morning routine. Before leaving for school s/he receives a reinforcer if enough points were earned.
Differential reinforcement of other behaviors	Reinforcing specific appropriate behaviors while ignoring inappropriate behaviors that serve the same function.	Attending to appropriate verbaliza tions while alternately ignoring whining.
Shaping	Reinforcing gradual approximations of a behavior.	Providing reinforcement for saying, "ba" and reinforcing better approximations until "ball" is said.
Punishment to decrease behaviors		
Overcorrection	Applied consequence that involves engaging in a series of retribution steps that are related to the inappropriate behavior	Washing soiled clothes after toileting accident.
Response cost	Removal of previously earned reinforcers as consequence of negative behavior.	Typically used in conjunction with token economy when "tokens" are removed.
Time out	Removing all sources of reinforcement for allotted period of time.	Involves placing the individual in a location where access to reinforcing activities, including social attention, is not available.
Extinction to decrease behaviors		
Extinction	Removing previous reinforcement to decrease the probability that the behavior will occur in the future.	Ignoring a child's cries when s/he is placed in bed to train the child to fall asleep independently.
Other terms related to behavioral teaching methods		
Prompting	Providing the child with a clear command about what behavior is expected.	Stating, "Come to the table and sit down" in reference to dinner being ready.
Prompt fading	Making prompts less explicit over time, such that the child more independently engages in a behavior.	First, manually prompting a child to come when called followed by teaching the child to respond to the command "come here."

(*Continued*)

Table 3: (*Continued*)

Technique	Description	Example
Positive practice	Repeatedly practicing positive behaviors immediately after a negative behavior.	Repeatedly practicing the steps in toilet training immediately after a toileting accident occurs.
Task analysis	Breaking a complex task down into its simpler parts and reinforcing the child for performing each step.	Teaching making the bed by reinforcing the child after each step.
Backwards chaining	Teaching a complex behavior by starting with reinforcement for correct performance of the last step and working successively backwards to the beginning until the child is being reinforced for performing the whole behavior.	Teaching dressing by first reinforcing the child for snapping the pants (the final step in the process), while helping with the preceding steps, then requiring the child to pull up the pants, place legs in the holes, *etc.* until he completes the sequence from the beginning without help.

deficit/hyperactivity disorder, have been treated based on studies conducted in typically developing individuals.

8.4.1. *Aggression*

Evidence from controlled and uncontrolled studies indicates that antipsychotics are very helpful in targeting these behaviors.[20,21] Double-blind placebo controlled studies and open clinical trials in children and adults with intellectual disabilities have indicated that the atypical antipsychotic risperidone is efficacious in decreasing aggression.[20] Some evidence from studies examining the efficacy and safety of lithium points to the usefulness of this agent in the treatment of violent behaviors in this population.[22] Carbamazepine and valproic acid have also been beneficial in decreasing the frequency and severity of aggression.[22] Interestingly, the above mentioned agents have also been found to be beneficial in the treatment of self-injurious behaviors.[22]

8.4.2. *Attention-deficit/hyperactivity disorder (ADHD)*

While there are several agents available on the market to treat typically developing children with ADHD, only methylphenidate has been examined in individuals with intellectual disabilities.[23] Studies of this medication in this population have shown clear efficacy of this agent when compared to placebo in targeting inattention and hyperactivity. However, no improvements were noted in social skills and learning, and more importantly, rates of side effects were higher than what is observed in typically developing children. Consequently, alternative agents should be considered and investigated, including atomoxetine, to determine whether tolerability can be improved with other compounds.

While several syndromes and target behaviors can be the subject of discussion, the limited evidence is alarming especially in light of the high rates of medications that are given to individuals with intellectual disabilities. In a recent survey, up to 45% of individuals with intellectual disability had received at least one psychotropic medication.[24] This number is too high in light of the limited evidence supporting the use of these medications in this population and warrants caution in the use of pharmacological treatment in individuals with intellectual disabilities.

Despite the limited scientific evidence available, prevalence rates of psychotropic medications use in individuals with intellectual disabilities range from 12 to 40% in institutions, from 19 to 29% in the community and over 50% in hospitalized individuals. Prescribing patterns appear to be stable across settings and over time, with a recent study reporting similar rates (22.8%) in individuals residing in group homes.[24] Interestingly, individuals with lower IQ tend to receive more medications than higher functioning individuals, and adults with intellectual disabilities more so than children. In light of these high prevalence rates, randomized controlled trials are needed to assess the safety and efficacy of different psychotropics in this patient population. This is particularly important taking into consideration the available data suggesting that persons with intellectual disabilities tend to have a poorer response to psychotropics and experience more side effects.[22]

While treatment studies have focused to date on the use of psychotropic medication to target associated behavioral problems, there is an increased interest in the development of disease specific interventions.[9] The use of ampakines in individuals with Fragile X illustrates this strategy.[25] The "ampakines" are a family of compounds that act as positive modulators at the glutamatergic α-amino-3-hydroxy-5-methylisoxazile-4-propionic acid (AMPA) receptor complex by increasing the peak of glutamate-induced AMPA receptor gated inward currents. These receptors play an important role in synaptic transmission and recent studies of the Fragile X mental retardation 1 (FMR1) knock-out mouse indicate that AMPA receptors are reduced significantly in number and activity. Accordingly, a human trial of the ampakine compound CX516 was recently described in individuals with FraX but no clear improvement was observed with agents.[25] Despite this negative finding, disease-specific interventions provide innovative strategies allowing the transition from agents targeting associated symptoms to compounds treating the underlying pathophysiology.

8.5. *Treatment outcome*

Long-term follow-up studies are lacking in the field on intellectual disabilities. However, it is clear that specific factors play an important role in the prognosis. First, individuals with severe cognitive deficits do have considerable comorbid medical conditions that will limit the success of interventions. Second, specific disabilities presents with particular trajectories with individuals with Fragile X develop in a pattern that is different than those with Williams' syndrome. Finally, intellectual disabilities with known etiologies can carry risk for specific disorders such as the association of early onset Alzheimer's disease in Down syndrome.

9. Approaches to Treatment at Stanford's Developmental Disabilities Clinic

9.1. *General approach*

The focus of the Stanford's developmental disabilities clinic is to provide diagnostic evaluation, psychoeducational testing, as well as behavioral and pharmacological treatment services to individuals with intellectual disabilities. The clinic population consists of children, adolescents, and some adults who are experiencing a wide range of comorbid psychopathology including ADHD, anxiety disorders, and mood disorders. A large number of patients are receiving services in the clinic with an average of 150 new evaluations and more than a 1000 treatment visits per year.

The treatment of children with intellectual disability in the clinic involves a multilevel approach, in order to allow the development of a comprehensive and successful treatment plan. There is an emphasis on providing pharmacological treatment, as well as behavioral support services, family guidance, and support in the attainment of educational and other services (*i.e.* social security benefits, vocational rehabilitation services, state support services, *etc.*). This is often accomplished *via* a team approach, including attending psychiatrists and psychologists, as well as fellows and other trainees. There is also a strong commitment to collaboration with the many other professionals involved in a child's care. For any given child, this can include working with the primary care physician, genetics, neurology, educational staff, case workers, speech-language therapists, occupational and physical therapists, advocates, and others. Finally, individuals are followed across the lifespan in many cases, and there is coordination with adult services for individuals transitioning from childhood to adulthood.

Once an intellectual disability has been suspected, the clinic provides psychological assessment to confirm diagnosis and level of impairment. Assessment includes evaluation of cognitive and adaptive functioning at a minimum. In addition, attempts are made to identify specific genetic or biologic etiologies for the intellectual disability by completing a medical workup that can include a referral for genetic testing and/or a neurological evaluation. Finally, assessment of associated neuropsychiatric symptoms is conducted to recognize any psychiatric disorders that will necessitate the implementation of specific interventions. However, this is not possible at times in light of the level of cognitive abilities of a child, and how that affects the expression of symptoms. Consequently, target symptoms are identified and non-specific interventions are implemented. While not ideal, this strategy is helpful in curbing disruptive or aggressive behaviors, although success rates are not elevated.

9.2. *Summary of our clinical approach*

With increased availability and possible effectiveness of pharmacological agents, there has been a decrease in reliance on psychosocial interventions in the field of psychiatry, with more individuals receiving medications before comprehensive and adequate behavioral and psychotherapeutic interventions have been considered or applied. Consequently, the primary role of the treatment team at the time of the initial evaluation in our clinic is to assess the quality and the effectiveness of any previous psychosocial interventions in general, and behavioral ones more specifically. The emphasis in the Stanford clinic, very early on in the course of treatment, is that non-pharmacological treatments are crucial and essential to a balanced strategy. These interventions can themselves be very effective in decreasing the rates of target behaviors, with high success rates observed when behavioral strategies are consistently implemented. Despite intense efforts, however, a considerable number of individuals with intellectual disabilities continue to be treated with medications in the absence of adequate and updated behavioral plans. Possible explanations for this observation include the time commitment required for the implementation of psychosocial interventions at home and in school, the absence of qualified and well-trained behaviorists in the community, and the availability of multiple medications. Our clinic focuses on educating new clinicians on the application of behavioral interventions, working with parents and school professionals in the use of behavioral approaches, providing psychoeducation to parents and other key individuals in the child's life, working with families on educational service attainment, and providing support in obtaining services.

In conclusion, the treatment of individuals with intellectual disabilities requires the availability of qualified professionals who work collaboratively to optimize the patient's adaptive and social functioning. The task of coordinating these efforts is usually challenging to members of the treatment team. Parents are strongly encouraged to play a significant role in their child's treatment. Family members and caregivers are the best advocates for a child's academic, emotional, medical, and vocational needs. Therefore, providing comprehensive psychoeducation is a primary goal in our clinic, to allow parents to have an active part in making informed decisions about their child's treatment. Optimizing these needs is the main mission of every individual being treated at Stanford.

10. Future directions

While limited progress has been made to date in the treatment if individuals with intellectual disabilities, the future is promising with the development of disease-specific interventions. Previously implemented treatments have not been specific to any disorders, with behavioral strategies and pharmacological agents being used independently of the underlying disorder. However, over the last decade several investigations have been completed using compounds that have been developed for specific disorders. This step is due to our increased understanding of the genetics and the neurobiology of these disorders that have led to the identifications of targets and in some instances to animal models. With this progress, a major breakthrough in one or several disorders is probable over the next decade which will probably revolutionalize our treatment approaches.

References

1. American Psychological Association. *Publication Manual of the American Psychological Association* 6th edn. Washington, DC, 2010.
2. American Psychiatric Association. *Diagnostic and Statistical Manual of Mental Disorders*, 4th edition, Text Revision. Washington, DC: American Psychiatric Association, 2000.
3. American Association on Mental Retardation. *Definition of Mental Retardation.* Washington DC: American Association on Mental Retardation, 2002.
4. Rasmussen P, Borjesson O, Wentz E, Gillberg C. Autistic disorders in Down syndrome: Background factors and clinical correlates, *Dev Med Child Neurol* 2001; **43**: 750–754.
5. Volkmar FR, Dykens E. Mental retardation. In: Lewis M, Ed. *Child and Adolescent Psychiatry: A Comprehensive Textbook*, 3rd edition. Philadelphia, PA: Lippincott Williams & Williams, 2002, pp. 603–611.

6. Opitz JM. Heterogeneity and minor anomalies, *Am J Med Genet* 2000; **91**: 254–255.
7. Bellugi U, Lichtenberger L, Jones W, Lai Z, St. George MI. The neurocognitive profile of Williams syndrome: A complex pattern of strengths and weaknesses, *J Cogn Neurosci* 2000; **12**: 7–29.
8. Gothelf D, Furfaro JA, Penniman LC, Glover GH, Reiss AL. The contribution of novel brain imaging techniques to understanding the neurobiology of mental retardation and developmental disabilities, *Ment Retard Dev Disabil Res Rev* 2005; **11**: 331–339.
9. Hardan AY, Reiss AR. The neurobiology of intellectual disabilities. In Charney DS, Nestler EJ. Eds. *Neurobiology of Mental Illness*, 3rd edition Oxford University Press, 2009.
10. Capone GT. Down syndrome: Advances in molecular biology and the neurosciences, *J Devl Behav Pediatrics* 2001; **22**: 40–59.
11. Korenberg JR, Chen XN, Hirota H, *et al*. Genome structure and cognitive map of Williams syndrome, *J Cogn Neurosci* 2000; **12**: 89–107.
12. Wechsler D. *Wechsler Intelligence Scale for Children*, 4th edition. San Antonio, TX: Psychological Corporation, 2003.
13. Wechsler D. *Wechsler Preschool and Primary Scale of Intelligence*, 3rd edition. San Antonio, TX: Psychological Corporation, 2002.
14. Kaufman AS, Kaufman NL. *Kaufman Assessment Battery for Children*, 2nd edition. *Manual*. Circle Pines, MN: AGS Publishing, 2004.
15. Roid GH. *Stanford-Binet Intelligence Scales*, 5th edition. Itasca, IL: Riverside Publishing, 2003.
16. Bayley N. *Bayley Scales of Infant and Toddler Development*, 3rd edition. San Antonio, TX: Harcourt Assessment, Inc., 2006.
17. Sparrow SS, Balla DA, Cicchetti DV. *Vineland Adaptive Behavior Scales*, 2nd edition. Circle Pines, MN: AGS, 2005.
18. U.S. Congress IDEA 2004 Public Law 108–446 *Individuals with Disabilities Education Improvement Act of 2004*. Washington, DC: Government Printing Office, 2004.
19. Carr EG, Dunlap, G, Horner, *et al*. Positive behavior support: Evolution of an applied science, *J Posit Behav Intervent* 2002; **4**: 4–16.
20. Aman MG, De Smedt G, Derivan A, Lyons B, Findling RL. Risperidone disruptive behavior study group. Double-blind, placebo-controlled study of risperidone for the treatment of disruptive behaviors in children with subaverage intelligence, *Am J Psychiatry* 2002; **159**: 1337–1346.
21. Handen BL, Hardan AY. Open-label, prospective trial of olanzapine in adolescents with subaverage intelligence and disruptive behavioral disorders. *J Am Acad Child Adolesc Psychiatry* 2006; **45**: 928–935.
22. Handen BL, Gilchrist R. Practitioner review: Psychopharmacology in children and adolescents with mental retardation, *J Child Psychol Psychiatry* 2006; **47**: 871–882.

23. Jou R, Handen B, Hardan A. Psychostimulant treatment of adults with mental retardation and attention-deficit hyperactivity disorder, *Australas Psychiatry* 2004; **12**: 376–379.
24. Ulzen TP, Powers RE. A review of empirical evidence of somatic treatment options for the MI/DD population, *Psychiatr Q* 2008; **79**: 265–273.
25. Berry-Kravis E, Krause SE, Block SS, *et al*. Effect of CX516, an AMPA-modulating compound, on cognition and behavior in Fragile X syndrome: A controlled trial, *J Child Adolesc Psychopharmacol* 2006; **16**: 525–540.

Chapter 17

Sleep Disorders in Children

Rafael Pelayo

1. Introduction

Your nighttime sleep affects your daytime behavior, no matter if you are a child or an adult. Sleep disorders mimic behavioral and psychiatric conditions. Sleep disorders encompass a wide range of disturbances including, sleep-related disordered breathing (obstructive sleep apnea), insomnia, parasomnias, and restless leg syndrome, There are over 90 recognized sleep disorders.[1]

Pediatric sleep medicine has evolved into a major field of study. Both the American Academy of Pediatrics and the American Academy of Sleep Medicine have published relevant clinical practice parameters.[2–4] Sleep disorders should be considered whenever a child is being evaluated for any behavioral problem. Insufficient quality or quantity of sleep may be associated with learning difficulties and attention problems. When a child does not sleep well it can impact the entire household leading to significant stress for the family. Unrecognized and under treated sleep disturbances can carry over into adulthood.

A question commonly posed by parents is, "How much sleep does my child need?" However, in the author's opinion, the focus should not be solely on the timing or quantity of sleep; ultimately, the overall quality must be considered. If a child is getting enough good-quality sleep at an appropriate circadian time, he or she should awaken spontaneously feeling refreshed. "Good sleep" can be simply described as the ability to fall asleep easily, sleep through the night, and wake feeling refreshed, without relying on hypnotics.

Sleep disorders in children are relatively common and readily treatable. This chapter reviews the various sleep disorders common in children and the management of these sleep disorders.

Perhaps, nowhere else in this text does modern neuroscience and psychiatry merge as naturally as in a discussion of sleep disorders. Sleep and dreams are at the core of the mystery (and wonderment) of the relationship between the brain and the mind. Seeking an understanding of sleep has been influential in the development of our culture. In prehistoric societies, attempts to understand the imagery of nighttime dreams and nightmares might have given rise to concepts of the spiritual world and religion. In medieval times, the phenomena of sleep paralysis, night terrors, and sleepwalking may have been interpreted as supernatural events.

Three hundred years ago the recurring nighttime afflictions of restless leg syndrome were thought to be a curse until Dr. Thomas Willis (of circle of Willis fame) accurately described it as a neurological disease. In the late 19th century, sleep was viewed as a passive state, which occurred in the absence of brain stimulation. Thomas Edison thought that the invention of the light bulb would allow us to avoid sleeping. The interest of a young neurologist named Sigmund Freud in sleep and dreams opened a new chapter in psychiatry. Years later, a medical student, William Dement, was interested in finding a neurological basis to understand Freud's dream theories. In 1952, he helped discover the relationship between electroencephalographically measured rapid eye movements in sleep and dream recall. Infants and small children were an early part of Dement's research into rapid eye movement (REM) sleep.

Dement joined the department of psychiatry at Stanford University and studied the relationship of sleep and dreams to mental illness. In 1972, he along with Christian Guilleminault, established the first clinic devoted exclusively to the treatment of sleep disorders. Not surprisingly, children were among the first patients seen at the new clinic.[5]

This landmark sleep clinic served as a worldwide model for the comprehensive multidisciplinary care of sleep disorder. The spread of clinical sleep medicine knowledge eventually led to the American Council of Graduate Medical Education recognizing it as a unique medical specialty. Stanford supports the largest ACGME training program in sleep medicine in the country. In 2009, the historic clinic was relocated to a state-of-the-art 24 bedroom facility at the Stanford outpatient campus. Thousands of patients are seen every year of which approximately 25% are children. The synergy of neuroscience and psychiatry was essential in establishing this new field. The study of normal sleep and sleep disorders in children is an integral part of the development of modern sleep medicine.

2. Epidemiology

It would seem self-evident from speaking to parents that sleep problems are common among children. The National Sleep Foundation yearly surveys of sleep in

America confirms parents are unsatisfied with their child's sleep habits. In 2004, the NSF reported that America's children sleep less than experts recommend for their age group, but parents do not always know how much sleep their child needs. More than two-thirds of all children experience one or more sleep problems at least a few nights a week according to parents. The NSF found that nearly one-third of children aged 10 and younger wake up at least once a night needing attention. In addition, about one-quarter of infants, toddlers, and preschoolers appear sleepy or overtired during the day, according to their parents/caregivers. About 26% of children between the ages of 3 and 10 drink at least one caffeinated beverage a day. In 2006, the NSF reported that over 25% high school students fall asleep in class at least once a week. Many of the high school students reported falling asleep doing homework and arriving late for school because they overslept.

In this chapter, we briefly review the most common sleep disorders starting with sleep disordered breathing. Sleep disordered breathing is the most common reason polysomnograms are performed in children. Narcolepsy is reviewed, which is a condition that commonly begins in childhood but is not diagnosed until adulthood. Insomnia is perhaps the most common sleep complaint in primary care and psychiatric practices. Restless leg syndrome is often not considered in the evaluation of sleep disorders in children but seems to be more common than previously thought.

3. Normal Childhood Sleep

Prior to discussing specific sleep disorders it is important to review normal sleep in children. Sleep needs and patterns differ with age. The basic principles of normal sleep are similar for children and adults. Normal sleep can be simply described as the ability to fall asleep easily, sleep through the night, and wake up feeling refreshed. A certain degree of serenity is needed to sleep well.

Long-term longitudinal data has been published by Iglowstein and colleagues to illustrate the developmental course and age-specific variability of sleep patterns.[6] They followed 493 children for 16 years. Total sleep duration decreased from an average of 14.2 h (SD: 1.9 h) at six months of age to an average of 8.1 h (SD: 0.8 h) at 16 years of age. Between 1.5 years and 4 years of age, there was a prominent decline in napping habits. At age 1.5 years, 96.4% of children had naps; by four years of age only 35.4% napped. However, napping behavior must be put into a cultural context. It would be less concerning if napping or "siestas" are part of the child's cultural environment.

In adults and most children, REM periods occur in cycles of approximately 90 min throughout the night. At the end of every REM cycle, there is usually an arousal or brief awakening. In infants, REM cycles are shorter (approximately

40–60 min). Parents maybe concerned that their infant seems to "wakes up every hour." These brief awakenings may be part of the child's normal rhythm but an overly attentive parent may inadvertently reinforce and prolong the awakenings. On the other hand, it is possible that child awakenings are due to a condition that is exacerbated by REM sleep such as obstructive sleep apnea. The percent of the total sleep time spent in REM decreases from birth when it may takes up 50% of the total sleep time to approximately 20% for three years. It remains at this percent throughout most of adulthood.

During drowsiness or light sleep (stage 1) children may not realize they are asleep and think they were awake. They may also have fragments of auditory or dream-like imagery called "hypnagogic" hallucinations. Similar episodes upon awakening are called hypnopompic hallucinations. These episodes occur more commonly with sleep deprivation and in conditions such as narcolepsy. They should not be confused with psychosis.

Delta or slow-wave sleep represents our deepest sleep as measured by the arousal threshold (amount of stimulation needed to wake up the sleeper). Delta sleep obeys homeostatic principles, it increases in duration and intensity in response to sleep deprivation. The amount of delta sleep is about 20% of the total sleep time in children and decreases after adolescence. Delta sleep clusters in the first third of the night. During delta, it is extremely difficult to arouse children. For example, smoke alarms will not reliably wake up a child during slow wave sleep. If aroused, they often appear disoriented and cognitively slowed. Parasomnias, such as sleepwalking and sleep terrors, usually emerge from slow wave sleep and in children commonly occur in the first third of the night.

The circadian modulation of alertness and sleepiness is an important part of sleep physiology. Part of our circadian physiology is our tendency to have decreased alertness in the afternoon and to have a surge of alertness ("second wind") in the evenings. This process is modulated by the suprachiasmatic nucleus and is referred to as clock-dependent alerting.[7] If a child is having trouble falling asleep, the imposition of an earlier bedtime or start of the nighttime routine may make the problem worse by creating greater frustration. The circadian system and normal adolescent sleep patterns are further discussed below in Sec. 8.

4. General Clinical Considerations

One of the characteristic idiosyncrasies of pediatric training is starting a medical presentation with short blurb on the birth history. For example, "the patient is 15-year-old girl born NSVD to a G2 P2 mother with a chief complaint of …." If the clinician taking the history of a chief complaint in a child uses the birth history as a starting point he/she has started too late. The history should begin with the history of parents' sleep habits and patterns (or other caretaker) before they were parents. Being a parent is arguably one of the most rewarding experiences for many adults; however, there is little argument that being a parent is one of the most impractical things for many adults. The only opportunity for many adults to have a semblance of what their preparenthood life was like is while their child is sleeping. Knowing what the parents' expectations are for their own sleep has to be taken into consideration when evaluating a child with a putative sleep disorder. As a simple example, if an infant who sleeps seven hours in a row without requiring the parents' assistance is born to a woman that, before she was mother used to be happy with getting six and half hours at night. That mother will proudly tell all who will listen what an easy baby she has and by inference, what a wonderful mother she is. Take that same seven hour sleeping infant and the mother was in the habit of sleeping nine hours at night before she was a mother, she will bitterly complain her baby does not sleep enough. Another example is a parent, say the father, had a subclinical case of obstructive sleep apnea. The sleep apnea may become unmasked with additional night time requirements of taking care of an infant. Financial factors may influence the parents' sleep. If both parents were receiving outside income before they were parents and one of them gives up that income to stay home with the infant. There will be greater pressure on the parent still receiving income not to lose that income source. The parent that gives up the income source to stay with the infant may fall into a trap of trying to quiet the infant immediately at night so as not to disturb the sleep of the parent that still has to leave the house in the morning to go to work. It is easy to conceptualize how resentment and increased stress can develop if the infant is perceived as not sleeping well. Given the near endless variations on what constitute a family factored in within the different cultural backgrounds of the individual family members the importance of understanding the family's sleep expectations should be self-evident as part of the evaluation of a pediatric sleep disorder.

When taking a history, it is important to keep in mind that the need for sleep is biological; however, the way someone sleeps is learned. All of us have been taught to sleep. It is analogous to food. All newborns have the same diet, milk. But five year olds throughout the world have different diets. The need for food is biological, but what you eat is cultural. Sleep is the same way. There are biological factors and learned or cultural factors. I illustrate this to parents by pointing out that as a couple they usually sleep on the same side of the bed every night. When they travel and have to sleep in an unfamiliar bed they still will typically pick the same side of the bed. A family can only place a child in a crib in a separate room if they can afford a crib in a separate room. As far as we know, early humans did not place their infants in separate caves or huts. Having an infant sleep in a crib in a separate room is clearly a cultural phenomenon. But for that matter so is wearing shoes. The clinician should avoid the temptation to make value judgments over cultural differences.

Sleep clearly fulfills some biological need (or needs) and has some homeostatic properties. In general, the longer you stay awake, the stronger the desire to sleep; the better you sleep the better you are able to stay awake. At the same time, it is intuitive that, in theory, a person could be vulnerable to being attacked while sleeping, so therefore there must be mechanisms present to allow us to sleep and be safe at the same time. We, like other animals, sleep differently depending on which circumstances we find ourselves. A woman in the last few days of her pregnancy may perceive her sleep to be of poor quality due to multiple factors fragmented her sleep. When the baby (or babies) finally arrives, will she then be able to regularly sleep soundly for eight hours in a row? How can we be supposedly 8-h sleeping diurnal mammals if our newborns have to nurse every 2–4 h? It is essential for our survival as mammals to have mechanisms hard wired into our brains to allow us to do without sleep under certain circumstances. All of us sleep best when we go to sleep feeling safe and comfortable. We learn feel this way by forming associations with our sleeping environment. These associations are formed starting from infancy. Just like in adults, these associations maybe maladaptive which can lead to sleep difficulties. When evaluating school-age children for a sleep problem, it is important to directly ask the children if they are scared of the dark or of being alone. The parents may previously have minimized these concerns and the children may be too embarrassed to volunteer the information. It is crucial in any evaluation to keep in mind the interaction between the physiology (the need for sleep) and the psychology of sleep.

When evaluating a sleep problem it is crucial to realize what wakes a patient up may not be what keeps the patient awake. For example, you could be awoken at night because of the sudden loud noise coming from a party next door. The fact that you were not invited to the party could bother you and keep you awake! It is not uncommon in a clinical situation to have two or more sleep disorders interacting in the same patient. A child may have an awakening due to difficulty breathing from sleep apnea, but then be unable to return to sleep because the child has not learned to settle back down without the parents' intervention.

Since the person who is being evaluated cannot provide us with information about their sleep once they are asleep, it is important to get as much information as possible from not only the child but also all the adults that are part of the household. When parents bring in a child for evaluation, a common question asked is the sleep problem due to a physical or behavioral cause. Although many times it is a combination of both, a useful rule of thumb is that a behavioral sleep problem, such as fear of the dark, may improve when the parents share sleeping space with the child and while a physical condition such as obstructive sleep apnea will not improve.

5. Sleep Disordered Breathing

Sleep disordered breathing (SDB) is a clinical syndrome ranging from simple snoring to potentially life threatening obstructive sleep apnea (OSA). This clinical spectrum can occur at any age. Many clinicians learn that OSA emerged from the study of Pickwickian syndrome. However, it is important to point out that in Charles Dicken's first novel, *The Posthumous Papers of the Pickwick Club*, the classic description of snoring with arousals and excessive daytime sleepiness was not in Mr. Pickwick (although he probably did have OSA too) but instead it was of a boy, Joe, who constantly falls asleep in any situation. The first medical description in English of children with abnormal breathing in sleep is attributed to William Osler in 1892. Osler wrote, "Chronic enlargement of the tonsillar tissue is an affection of great importance, and may influence in an extraordinary way the mental and bodily development of children... At night the child's sleep is greatly disturbed, the respirations are loud and snorting, and there is sometimes prolonged pauses, followed by deep, noisy inspiration. The child may wake up in a paroxysm of shortness of breath. In long-standing cases, the child is very stupid looking, responds slowly to questions, and may be sullen and cross."

In the modern era, there has been a realization that patients may be symptomatic in the absence of frank apneas.[8] This has led to use of the terms "sleep-disordered breathing" to better describe the clinical spectrum which includes snoring, upper airway resistance syndrome (UARS,) and obstructive hypopnea syndrome.

The most obvious nocturnal symptom is snoring. Snoring indicates turbulent airflow and is not normal in children.[9–12] The American Academy of Pediatrics has recommended all children showed be screened for snoring as part of well child care.[2] Not all snoring is due to obstructive sleep apnea. It may be due to other forms of obstruction such as nasal allergies or a cold.[13,14]

Many of these children's mouth breath. Regular mouth breathing should always lead to suspicion of SDB.[15] Children with disordered breathing may avoid going to bed at night due to hypnagogic hallucinations. Upon awakening, these children may report morning headaches, dry mouth, confusion, or irritability. As mentioned, daytime sleepiness may not be obvious depending on the age. It may translate only as a complaint of daytime tiredness.

Clinical signs include increased respiratory efforts with nasal flaring, suprasternal, or intercostal retractions, abnormal paradoxical inward motion of the chest may occur during inspiration and sweating during sleep. Information regarding the sleep position is helpful. Typically, the neck is hyperextended and the mouth is open.

A physical finding that may be overlooked in a child with SDB is a narrow and high-arched palate. Interestingly, the DSM IV's description of attention-deficit disorder mentions that minor physical anomalies such as high arch palates maybe present. Since both conditions may have similar daytime behavior in the same age group, a child with SDB could be misidentified as having attention deficit disorder. The possibility of a sleep disorder being present should be considered in any child being evaluated for attention deficit disorder. This is particularly important since treatment of SDB may improve behavior and academic performance.

Parasomnias maybe triggered or exacerbated by SDB. Individuals identified with SDB have a much higher incidence of nightmares, with reports of "drowning," "being buried alive," and "choking." SDB leads to sleep fragmentation or disruption. Any condition that disrupts slow wave sleep may lead to sleep terrors and sleepwalking in children.[16] SDB should be included in the evaluation of any child with parasomnias.

5.1. *Epidemiology*

The prevalence of SDB in children was studied by Rosen *et al.* who performed a cross-sectional study of school-aged children in a Cleveland cohort.[17] The cohort consisted of 829 children, 8-to-11-years old all of whom have unattended in-home overnight cardiorespiratory sleep recordings. SDB was found in 20% of the cohort. The remaining 80% had neither snoring nor OSA. Functional outcomes were assessed with two parent ratings scales of behavior problems: the Child Behavioral Checklist and the Conners Parent Rating Scale-Revised:Long. Children with SDB had significantly higher odds of elevated problem scores in the following domains: externalizing, hyperactive, emotional liability, oppositional, aggressive, internalizing, somatic complaints, and social problems. The authors concluded that children with mild SDB, have a higher prevalence of problem behaviors, with the strongest, most consistent associations for externalizing, hyperactive-type behaviors. An interesting finding in this study was that only 55% of the parents of children diagnosed with a polysomnogram with obstructive sleep apnea (OSA) reported loud snoring. If pediatricians and surgeons screen for OSA by asking the parents/caregiver if the child snores loudly, they may miss close to half of the cases.[18]

5.2. *Pathogenesis*

The pathogenesis of sleep disordered breathing is based on the inherent complexity of the throat. The throat is an area of the body where food and air mix. We need a rigid enough structure such that the negative pressure of the lungs allows the passage of air. It also has to be able to have the muscular strength to close and allow us to swallow food. In addition, it has to allow for the intricate movements of speech, singing, and laughter. There is clearly conflicting activity occurring in a relatively small space. When we fall asleep, throat reflexes relax causing the throat to be more collapsible. Any fixed obstruction in the throat such as enlarged tonsils will narrow the throat. Since the lungs need to obtain the same amount of air through a smaller passage, the work of breathing will increase by generating more negative pressure. This increase in negative pressure may further collapse the airway with resultant turbulent airflow. The result will be the ubiquitous snoring sound being generated. If the patient is sleeping supine, the tongue can slip back further occluding the airway. This can result in partial or complete obstruction called a hypopnea or apnea, respectively. These events can result in multiple either partial arousals or full awakenings from sleep throughout the night.

5.3. *Relevance in psychiatry and primary care*

While sleep-disordered breathing in children has many important similarities to the adult version of this disease, there are also marked differences in presentation, diagnosis, and management. The abnormal daytime sleepiness maybe recognized more often by school teachers than by parents of young children. An increase in total sleep time or an extra long nap may be considered as normal by parents. Non-specific behavioral difficulties are mentioned to the pediatrician such as abnormal shyness, hyperactivity, developmental delays, rebellious, or aggressive behavior.[19] Chervin *et al.* found conduct problems and hyperactivity are frequent among children referred for sleep-disordered breathing SDB during sleep. Bullying and other specific aggressive behaviors were generally two to three times more frequent among children at high risk for SDB.[20] Other daytime symptoms may include speech defects, poor appetite, or swallowing difficulties. Nocturnal enuresis or bedwetting accidents should raise suspicion of possible SDB.[21]

An important similarity is that both morbidly obese adults and children are at risk for obstructive sleep apnea.[22,23] Children do not need to be overweight to have SDB. Children with sleep apnea tend to be of normal weight. Very young children and infants may actually be underweight. OSA may be a risk factor for overall growth failure. The increased work of breathing through the narrow airway, along with the increased total sleep time in children and possible disruption of nocturnal growth hormone secretion from sleep fragmentation may all factor in to difficulty gaining weight. Ironically, children have become obese after being treated for obstructive sleep apnea.[24] Behavioral problems in children with obstructive sleep apnea seem to be independent of obesity. The clinician should not assume that a child with SDB must be overweight.

A study from Israel found that children with SDB had lower scores on neurocognitive testing compared to controls but the scores improve after treatment.[25]

This prospective study of 39 children aged five to nine years underwent a battery of neurocognitive tests. Children with SDB had lower scores compared with healthy children indicating impaired neurocognitive function. Further, six to ten months after adenotonsillectomy, the children demonstrated significant improvement in sleep characteristics, as well as in daytime behavior. Their neurocognitive performance improved considerably, reaching the level of the control group. The authors concluded that neurocognitive function is impaired in otherwise healthy children with SDB. Most functions improve to the level of the control group, indicating that the impaired neurocognitive functions are mostly reversible. An abrupt and persistent deterioration in grades must also raise the question of abnormal sleep and SDB.[9,26–28]

In schools, the tiredness and sleepiness may be labeled as inattentive or daydreaming.[29,30] The association between SDB, learning problems, and attention deficit disorder has been established.[9,29–36]

5.4. *Diagnosis*

The diagnostic criteria used for adults with OSAS cannot be used reliably in children.[8,37,38] The diagnosis of sleep-disordered breathing is based on the history, physical findings, and supportive data. Laboratory testing should be, ideally, tailored to the clinical question.

The polysomnogram in a child uses the same technology and the same type of information is recorded as in adults. Airflow, respiratory effort, and pulse oximetry make up the breathing measurements usually monitored.

Along with the absence of controlled studies, another problem with understanding pediatric sleep-disordered breathing is that definitions for key terms vary. Obstructive sleep apneas are defined as lasting at least 10 s in adults. However, since children have faster respiratory rates clinically significant apneas can occur in less time. Apneas as brief as 3 or 4 s may have oxygen desaturations. There is no universally accepted definition of hypopneas in children. The clinician needs to know how apneas and hypopneas are defined and scored when interpreting a polysomnogram report. The most recent edition of the *International Classification of Sleep Disorders* defines sleep apnea in children as having an apnea-hyponea index (AHI) > 1.[1] In adults, a higher AHI of 5 is required.

Controversy exists over whether a diagnosis of OSA, or the larger spectrum of sleep-disordered breathing, should be routinely made without a formal polysomnogram. Some have suggested that this diagnosis can be made in patients using either the history and physical examination alone, or in combination with an audio or videotape of the child sleeping, others have found an inability of clinical history alone to distinguish primary snoring from OSAS in children. A sleep study is the most definitive test for SDB.[39] Currently, some otolaryngologists who treat sleep-disordered breathing children may make the surgical recommendation based on clinical findings of airway obstruction, sometimes reviewing an audio or video tape.[40,41] Further controversy exist about the value of doing the sleep study in an attended sleep lab setting or allowing the child to sleep in their own bed with a home setting. The clinicians must be aware of the potential pitfalls to these different options. If the sleep study is done in an attended in-lab setting the staff must be trained how to work with children. The bedroom must be able to accommodate a parent or other adult that will accompany the child. SDB events tend to cluster during REM sleep in the last third of the night or early morning. The child should be allowed to awaken spontaneously. If, on the contrary, the sleep study is terminated abruptly and the child is forced to wake up earlier than usual then the true severity of the SDB may be underestimated.

SDB may occur more often in special populations.[42–46] Any condition or syndrome associated with cranial facial anomalies may be associated with SDB. Pierre-Robin, Apert's and Crouzon's are among these syndromes. Approximately, half of all children with Down syndrome have SDB. However, symptoms of daytime sleepiness and sleep disruptions at night may be due to non-neurological factors such as maxillofacial abnormalities, large tonsils or adenoids, small jaw, or other abnormalities. Such factors often lead to sleep fragmentation and daytime sleepiness. Sleep disorders often occur in patients with neuromuscular disorder because of associated weakness in respiratory muscles, which is further exacerbated by hypotonia during sleep. Diagnosis and treatment of sleep-disordered breathing in these patients can be an important part of comprehensive management.

5.5. *Treatment*

Not only are the diagnostic criteria different in children from adults but also the treatment. SDB in adults has different treatments options, which may be combined. Sleep specialist and ENT surgeons typically provide treatment. As the technology improves, the treatment may be provided by a wider range of healthcare providers. The most common treatment is continuous positive airway pressure (CPAP) to help splint open the upper airway. When CPAP is used correctly, snoring should be absent during sleep. There are several sophisticated surgical options with a wide range of success. As a conservative measure, adults with SDB are advised to sleep off their backs, lose weight, and avoid alcohol before sleeping.

Unlike adults, surgery in children is the most common treatment for SDB. Adenotonsillectomy is the most common initial treatment for SDB in children.

This procedure can be extremely effective and result in dramatic improvements (and very grateful parents). When surgery is being entertained, as a general rule, the adenoids and tonsils should both be removed during the same surgery. It is tempting in very small children to only remove the adenoids if the tonsils do not appear overly enlarged since this allows for less post-operative pain and lower risk of adverse events such as bleeding. This practice should be discouraged since even though the tonsils to do seem enlarged the surgeon must keep in mind that they are examining a child that is awake and sitting. If only the adenoids are removed there is the risk of residual breathing difficulties remaining needing further surgery.

The anesthesiologist should be familiar with sleep apnea since post-operative pulmonary complications can occur. Children with sleep apnea are often thinner than expected. This is may be due to multiple factors including the greater caloric demand of breathing through a narrow airway and possible disruption of growth hormone secretion. Children after sleep apnea surgery may unexpectedly increase their weight.[24]

Surgery does not always completely cure the child's SDB. If surgery is not a viable option for the child then continuous positive airway pressure (CPAP) therapy should be considered.[47–49] CPAP uses a small air compressor attached to mask via hose. CPAP is effective but can be cumbersome to use. Over time, the CPAP devices have become smaller and quieter. The masks have also been improved with many more styles and sizes available. A trial of newer CPAP masks specifically for small children is underway at Stanford.

The most recent advance in positive airway pressure has been the development of machines which can adjust the pressure required to keep the airway open on a breathe-by-breathe basis. These so-called "smart CPAP" units are promising but are not part of the mainstream treatment of children at this time.[47]

An alternative to CPAP for residual SDB is the use of orthodontics for rapid maxillary expansion.[50–54] The general concept is that expansion of the maxilla will allow more space for the tongue in the hard palate. The tongue is then less likely to fall back into the throat and cause obstruction. This treatment option is promising but not yet readily available. It does bring the orthodontist into the increasing large sleep medicine tent further demonstrating the multidisciplinary nature of sleep.

In summary, it is important for clinicians to be aware that SDB and snoring are not normal. Difficulty breathing while asleep may impact the daytime behavior of children. SDB is readily treatable.

6. Narcolepsy

Narcolepsy is a chronic autoimmune neurological disorder in which the boundaries between the awake, sleeping, and dreaming brain are blurred. The awake narcoleptic will feel sleepy. The sleeping narcoleptic will have disturbed sleep due to arousals. The neuropeptide hypocretin, also called orexin, is often dysfunctional. The cardinal features of narcolepsy are daytime somnolence, cataplexy, sleep paralysis, and hypnagogic hallucinations.[55]

6.1. *Clinical presentation*

Narcolepsy is characterized by abnormal sleep, including excessive daytime sleepiness with often disturbed nocturnal sleep later in life and pathological manifestations related to rapid eye movement sleep (REM sleep). REM sleep-related abnormalities include early REM sleep onset and cataplexy. The cardinal symptoms are cataplexy, hypnagogic hallucinations, excessive daytime sleepiness, sleep paralysis, and sleep attacks (a helpful mnemonic is CHESS).

Cataplexy is an abrupt and reversible decrease or loss of muscle tone, most frequently provoked by emotion particularly laughter. Consciousness typically remains intact. It may involve only certain muscles or the entire voluntary musculature. Most typically, the jaw sags, the head falls forward, the arms drop to the side, and the knees buckle. The severity and extent of cataplectic attacks can range from a state of absolute powerlessness, which seems to involve the entire body, to no more than a fleeting sensation of weakness. Cataleptic attacks can involve a complete loss of muscle tone, resulting in falls with subsequent injuries. The attacks may also be so subtle as not to be noticed by an observer. Laughter and anger seem to be the most common triggers. Cataplexy may be induced merely by remembering a funny situation.

Hypnagogic hallucinations are dream imagery that occurs just prior to sleep onset while the person still feels awake. A similar phenomenon is hypnopompic hallucinations that occur upon awakening. The hallucinations may be visual or auditory. Excessive daytime sleepiness in children with narcolepsy may persists despite the use of stimulants. Sleep paralysis can be a terrifying experience that occurs when the narcoleptic falls asleep or wakes up. Children find themselves suddenly unable to move the limbs, to speak, or even to breathe deeply. The episodes usually last only a few seconds. Hypnagogic hallucinations and sleep paralysis can occur to anybody who are acutely sleep deprived and are therefore not sufficient symptoms to diagnosis narcolepsy.

6.2. *Epidemiology*

The prevalence of narcolepsy has been calculated at about 1 per 2000 of the general population.[56] Age at onset varies from early childhood to the fifth decade, with a peak in the second decade. It is important to consider narcolepsy, especially in young patients, because it can take up to 20 years between the initial onset of the first symptom, commonly sleepiness, and development of the full clinical syndrome. During this lapse of time, the patient may be mislabeled with wide variety of diagnoses. The patient may be considered lazy, or depressed. Prior to being correctly diagnosed, the patient may turn to illegal drugs such as "crank" amphetamine to combat the sleepiness.

6.3. *Diagnosis*

Unless cataplexy is unequivocally witnessed by the examiner, polysomnogram and Multiple Sleep Latency Test, MSLT will be necessary to obtain an accurate diagnosis of narcolepsy. Clinical EEG and MRI studies are normal. The polysomnogram will be characterized by a short REM sleep latency. The MSLT consists of five 20-min nap opportunities which are done every 2 h spread throughout the day. After each nap, the patient must stay awake until the following scheduled nap. The MSLT records the sleep latency for each nap, and the presence or absence of REM sleep in any of the naps. If a subject falls asleep within the 20 min nap period, the nap is extended an additional 15 min to measure any sleep onset REM periods. Typical REM latency is usually about 90 min, so the presence of REM within 15 min is considered abnormal.

The maximum mean MSLT score obtainable is 20 min which corresponds to a subject staying awake during all naps. The diagnosis of narcolepsy requires a mean MSLT scores under 8 min and the presence of two or more sleep onset REM periods.[1]

6.4. *Pathogenesis*

The cause of narcolepsy was unknown for many years and treatment was based on empirical trials. Evidence now supports that narcolepsy is an autoimmune disorder. Hypocretin producing cells in the lateral hypothalamus are damaged in this condition. Absence of hypocretin is critical in the pathophysiology of most human narcoleptics. Hypocretin can be measured in cerebrospinal fluid. This is useful in diagnostic situations when the diagnosis is uncertain.[57,58]

6.5. *Relevance in psychiatry and primary care*

Narcolepsy is underrecognized. Since the symptoms may begin gradually in childhood, it may be several years before the diagnosis is made. The clinician's lack of suspicion may cause the symptoms to be misidentified as manifestations of psychosis or other mental disorder. These experiences are so frightful that the child may resist going to bed to sleep or talking about them. Primary care providers and psychiatrist will often see these patients before the sleep specialists and therefore should consider the possibility of narcolepsy being present in a child with new onset of either sleepiness or hallucinations.

6.6. *Treatment strategies*

If a primary care provider or psychiatrist suspects a child has symptomatic narcolepsy, they may consider initiating empirical treatment while awaiting a consultation with a sleep specialist if the clinical situation warrants it. However, most medications would be discontinued prior to formal diagnostic testing. Successful treatment for narcolepsy needs include both behavioral and pharmacological treatments. The situation is analogous to juvenile diabetes mellitus where a combination of diet with medication can control the condition. Treatment strategies must include conservative behavioral treatment such as usage of short naps, emotional support to parents and child, and education of school authorities. Children with narcolepsy should be encouraged to take one to two brief naps, typically less than 30 min, every day. Brief naps are typically refreshing. Only after the importance of naps and proper sleep habits is emphasized should medication be discussed.

Narcolepsy is a lifelong illness, and this must be taken into account when considering drug therapy along with possible side effects. No double-blind placebo controlled trials of medication have been specifically conducted for children with narcolepsy. Central nervous system stimulants have been the drugs most widely used.[59] Amphetamines were first proposed in 1935. However, a number of side effects including irritability, anxiety, nervousness, headache, psychosis, tachycardia, hypertension, nocturnal sleep disturbances, tolerance, and drug dependence, may arise. The use of methylphenidate was later encouraged because of a shorter half-life and lower incidence of similar side effects.

The American Academy of Sleep Medicine practice parameter for the treatment of narcolepsy recommends modafinil as a first-line treatment.[60] However, there are no guidelines for the use of this medication in children with narcolepsy.

A novel agent to treat both the excessive sleepiness and cataplexy symptoms of narcolepsy is sodium oxybate, also referred to as gamma-hydroxybutyrate (GHB). In the popular media, it has the infamous name of the "date rape drug." Illegal use of this substance for recreational purposes has been of great concern. Sodium oxybate has powerful central nervous system depressant effects and can increase slow wave sleep. The medication is a liquid preparation taken twice at night. Sodium oxybate should be taken at bedtime and again 2.5 to 4 h later. The recommended starting dose in adults is 4.5 g/day divided into two equal doses of

2.25 g. The starting dosage can then be increased to a maximum of 9 g/day in increments of 1.5 g/day (0.75 g per dose). The product's package insert does not recommend using the medication in patients younger than 16 years.

7. Behavioral Insomnia of Childhood

The symptom of insomnia is defined as "repeated difficulty with sleep initiation, duration, consolidation, or quality that occurs despite adequate time and opportunity to sleep and results in some form of daytime impairment."[1] The clinician must distinguish between insomnia symptoms and insomnia syndromes. The International Classification of Sleep Disorders lists several different insomnia syndromes but there are dozens of other conditions listed that may have insomnia symptoms.[1]

7.1. *Clinical presentation*

Behavioral insomnia of childhood is a relatively new term that combines two previously described pediatric sleep disorders: sleep onset association disorder and limit setting sleep disorder. Both of these disorders have in common inconsistent enforcement of bedtime routines. In normal infants, brief awakenings throughout the night are common. In reality nobody, neither adult or child, sleeps through the night. Awakenings lasting several seconds occur at the end of every REM period accompanied by large muscle movements. Small arousals lasting for only approximately 3 s may occur up to 10 times per hour. These awakenings and brief arousals are all part of normal sleep. The child and the parent are unaware of most of these, and unbeknownst to the parents, the child may simply drift back to sleep. The concern should not be the awakenings or arousals *per se*, the real problem for parents is does the child need their assistance to return to sleep. It is only when the child's awakenings disturb the parents sleep that a problem arises. If a brief awakening is followed by a full arousal in an active, alert child, and the child is unable to fall asleep, the child may simply become agitated. The child might only return to sleep after being comforted by the caregiver.

Although the need for sleep has a biological basis, the way we sleep is learned and influenced by the cultural environment. This is analogous to eating. All newborns first drink milk, but the diet of older children is different throughout the world. The child will learn or form associations with regard to sleep. As the child is readied for bed, the child may associate sleep onset with particular events. The child may associate this process with increased attention and activity rather than getting ready for bed. If continued, the child may then develop an association with parental activity that requires persistent parental involvement in order to fall asleep. The awakenings in the middle of night often necessitate similar actions. What initially were brief awakenings may develop into lengthy struggles. What wakes up the child may not be what is keeping the child awake. Now, the parental actions became the focus of the problem. If returning the child to sleep requires frequent parental assistance the parents' sleep may be very disturbed. The entire family may start to dread the nighttime instead of looking forward to going to sleep. The nighttime routines are no longer pleasurable but become a source of frustration. A vicious cycle may form which is exacerbated by middle-of-the night awakenings. Parents may report the infant wakes up crying every hour. The normal sleep cycle length in an infant is approximately 1 h and is followed by a brief arousal prior to initiating the next sleep cycle. Therefore, when a parent complains of hourly awakenings with prompt return to sleep with the parents' intervention the possibility of a sleep-onset association disorder should be considered.

Limit-setting sleep disorder is the term used to describe stalling behaviors or refusal to go to bed at the desired time associated with inadequate limit setting for a child's behaviors. This sleep disorder is usually seen in a child who is sleeping apart from the parents and is old enough to get out of bed or climb out of the crib the child may come to the parents' bedroom and disrupt the parents sleep. Usually, there is no enforcement of consistent bedtime rules. There may be possible recurrence of behaviors after nighttime awakenings. When the child does sleep, it is usually of normal quality and duration. The parents may lack an understanding of the importance of setting limits and inadequate knowledge of limit-setting techniques. There may be underlying psychosocial factors limiting the parents' ability to set limits. The limit-setting difficulties may also manifest in the child's daytime behavior such as tantrums.

7.2. *Relevance in psychiatry and primary care*

Insomnia characteristics fluctuate with age. With infants, the problem usually involves troubling settling to sleep without the parents' assistance. In toddlers, the problem may also involve inconsistent limit setting with regard to bed time expectations. By the time children are eight or nine years old, they seem to have fewer problems with insomnia. When problems with sleep are present at this age, there may be some unresolved fear of being alone at night. This might be expressed as a "fear of the dark." This fear may not be initially volunteered during the clinical interview but a description of the sleep routine and environment may reveal a need for nightlights or hallway lights to be left on at night. Adolescents have a characteristic insomnia pattern associated with sleep onset insomnia without sleep maintenance insomnia called delayed sleep phase syndrome (DSPS). DSPS is such a common sleep disorder among adolescents that it is discussed in a separate section below.

All of these insomnia types may merge in different ways in a given individual. In addition to this clinical heterogeneity, there are children who are described as being lifelong poor sleeper without any apparent cause. This condition is referred to, for lack of a better term, as idiopathic insomnia and fortunately is considered to be rare.

7.3. *Treatment*

These insomnia patterns are of a behavioral nature and usually do not need to be treated with medication.[61] Antihistamines and clonidine may be tried in some of these children but there is little evidence to suggest that these preparations provide anything but short-term sedation.[62] In particularly difficult situations, medication can be used as part of a comprehensive treatment program with behavior modification at its core.

Behavioral techniques have been helpful and applied to a variety of clinical situations.[4] The first issue to be addressed in a behavioral sleep problem in an infant or small child is where do the parents want the child to sleep. The child will typically prefer to sleep with the parents; the question is what the parents' preference is. There are many variations possible to where a child will sleep such as in a crib in a separate room, a crib in the parents' room, in the same bed with the parents, in the same bed or bedroom with a different relative. The sleep situation may change based on multiple factors such as new siblings or change in the size of the home. Cultural issues will also play a part in this situation. Once all parents and caretakers agree, then a plan to teach the child what to expect can be developed.

Perhaps, the best known behavioral approach was popularized by Dr. Richard Ferber at Harvard.[63] This approach has not been without some controversy and the clinician needs to be familiar with it since undoubtedly the parents will be. In essence, a "progressive" approach to helping the child fall asleep and stay asleep is advocated. Parents are advised once the child is in bed, to leave the room. If the child cries, wait a certain amount of time before checking in on the child. The suggested waiting time should be based on how comfortable the family is in the situation and can be charted to help track the progress. When the parent returns to the child's room, soothe the child verbally but avoid picking up, rocking, or feeding the child. Gradually increase the amount of time that passes between parental interventions. The time interval should be predetermined and not shortened during the night. Ideally within a week, the child will learn to sleep without the parents' help.

This method is not desired or effective for all families. A discussion of different approaches and counter arguments about helping a child sleep at night are beyond the scope of this chapter. Suffice is to say that parents will typically seek professional help only after they have tried one or more of the different popular approaches. The relationship between these parents may be suffering due to frustration and sleep deprivation. Given this situation, a pragmatic approach that takes into account the individual situation is appreciated by the family. A judgmental or patronizing attitude from the healthcare provider will not be appreciated. From the author's personal experience at Stanford usually when an infant or child is brought in for a behavioral insomnia of childhood the parents are often isolated without the assistance to extended family members such as the child's grandparents. In some families, grandparents may have taken the role of helping the infant or child sleep and decrease the pressure on the parents. In other families, there may be a conflict with extended family members that are playing a role in this behavioral pattern. When getting a history of a putative behavioral problem, it is important to obtain a history of how the child sleeps with other caretakers or environments such as nannies or daycare centers.

The clinician should keep in mind physical causes for the poor sleep. Obstructive sleep apnea, food allergies, or gastrointestinal reflux may mimic behavioral insomnia of childhood. As a rule of thumb, if the child sleeps better when they share a bed (*e.g.* while traveling) with the parents a behavioral component is likely. If the child sleeps poorly even when given the opportunity to sleep with the parents from the beginning of the night, then a physical factor needs to be explored. This may require a polysomnogram.

The parents may need additional direction to be able to implement firm limits for the child. For example, reassure the parents that they have not abandoned the child if they decide to sleep separately or that they are spoiling the infant if they decide to share their bed with the infant. If the child has learned to sleep in the parents' bed and the parents want to change this arrangement, they need to realize that the infant has no incentive to change. One approach is for the parents to start the night sleeping in the child's room. The amount of time that the parent spends with the child in bed could be decreased gradually until the child learns to sleep alone. These gradual interventions are not meant to be punitive, and require patience, persistence, and reassurance to both the parents and the child.

8. Delayed Sleep Phase Syndrome

DSPS is a circadian rhythm sleep disorder characterized by chronic sleep-onset insomnia and an inability to rise at a time in the morning that is appropriate, given the individual's commitments. Once the DSPS patient is able to fall asleep, he or she sleeps soundly and for a normal duration of approximately 8 h. When not required to maintain a strict sleep schedule (for *e.g.* at weekends, or during vacations and holiday periods) patients will awaken spontaneously, albeit late in the morning or early in the afternoon.[3]

DSPS can be conceptualized as resulting from a clock for which the time can only be readily adjusted in one direction, as it is intrinsically easier for patients to fall asleep later than usual, rather than earlier. People susceptible to DSPS may have more difficulty adjusting to an earlier sleep time than others.[64,65]

DSPS seems to be particularly common among adolescents. Sleep problems in teenagers can present a challenging situation, both for the family and the primary care provider (PCP). The PCP may have limited training in pediatric sleep disorders.

8.1. *Clinical features*

The main feature of DSPS is sleep-onset insomnia, a common disorder among teenagers, and DSPS should be included in the differential diagnosis whenever an adolescent is evaluated for these symptoms. After the initial description of DSPS, the clinical features of the syndrome were described in a case series of 22 adolescents by Thorpy *et al.* in 1988.[66] The ability to experience refreshing sleep is a key factor in a pure case of DSPS; if a teenager does not report waking refreshed after sleeping for several days on a stable schedule of his or her own choosing, a comorbid condition should, in the author's experience, be suspected. Sleeping late at a weekend may not provide sufficient time to establish whether or not sleep is truly refreshing. Furthermore, it is crucial for everybody, but teenagers in particular, to realize that chronic sleep restriction over five weekday nights cannot, be "made up" for over a two-day weekend.

8.2. *Epidemiology*

The sleep patterns of teenagers differ from those of children and adults. Younger children may nap prior to bedtime and are unlikely to stay awake after their parents have gone to sleep, whereas teenagers may be allowed to remain up after their parents have retired for the night and frequently spend hours awake in their bedroom. In the author's clinical experience, it is very unusual for a younger child to sleep late at weekends; they tend to have similar bedtimes and rising times on weekdays compared with weekends, often varying by <1 h. A similar pattern is seen in adults.

In contrast, teenagers may have large differences between their bedtimes and rising times depending on the day of the week. Sleeping in and getting out of bed several hours later at weekends seems, in the author's experience, to be common practice. This may be due to a combination of external societal influences and physiological changes. Extensive research on adolescent sleep has been undertaken in the United States, and the external influences on a teenager's sleep are numerous and pervasive.[67,68]

For example, parents may not be teaching children to value sleep sufficiently. Parents may consider children well behaved if they remain quietly in their own bedroom. When children are small they may be punished by being sent to their bedroom early, or as a reward they may be allowed to stay up later; late bedtimes are worn as "badges of honor." In the author's experience, even small children may realize that their parents have later bedtimes than they do. As the child gets older, a later bedtime on weekends may be allowed, perhaps reinforcing the message that staying up at night is good.

When children enter their teenage years, the levels of school work and extracurricular activities expected of them increase. The teenager is generally given more autonomy and the bedtime schedule is often further relaxed. Sleep is simply less of a priority. Since the teenager is becoming more adult, parents may incorrectly assume that he or she needs less sleep. It is increasingly apparent that adolescence may be a time of heightened sleep need coupled with a natural tendency to stay awake later.[69,70] As they get older, teenagers may stay up after their parents are in bed, therefore being allowed to set their own bedtime. Teenagers often want greater freedom, and what better opportunity when they are in their homes than when their parents are asleep? Therefore, teenagers have a number of incentives to stay awake later.

8.3. *Relevance in psychiatry and primary care*

DSPS is associated with depression and should be considered when evaluating teenagers with this disorder. Patients with DSPS manifested increased nervousness, depression, and difficulty regulating emotional displays when compared with a control group without insomnia or psychiatric symptoms, and were defensive, compulsive, introspective, and overly abstract in their thinking.[71]

Broad generalizations made from the results of a single study should be avoided; however, it is important to consider any factors that may influence the motivation of DSPS patients to modify their behavior. Changing sleeping habits can be challenging, and, in the author's experience, the incentive to improve sleep patterns may not be as profound in patients with DSPS compared with those without the condition. As with most chronic conditions, a vicious circle is often constituted.

8.4. *Treatment*

Once a clinician suspects DSPS, diagnosis is not difficult; however, there can be many problems in obtaining a satisfactory response to treatment. Both behavioral and pharmacological methods have been employed, either separately or in combination, to treat DSPS, but attempts to correct the sleep schedule will not be effective unless the patient chooses to alter lifestyle factors influencing the delayed bedtimes, particularly on weekends.[72] The importance of motivation cannot be overemphasized.

One of the benefits of a behavioral treatment approach is the ability of an individual to gain control over his or her sleep, with greater autonomy acquired as the condition improves. A mnemonic this author finds helpful in explaining a behavioral approach is "SELF correction." SELF is an acronym for social interactions, exercise, light, and food. By controlling these four variables on a regular schedule, the circadian pattern will stabilize over time. The term "zeitgerbers" is used for these givers of time in circadian research.

Chronotherapy was originally suggested for the treatment of DSPS. Chronotherapy resets the patient's sleep cycle using a series of consecutive, 3 h delay adjustments of bedtime and wake time over several days. To maintain the readjusted sleep pattern, the patient is encouraged to strictly adhere to the new sleep onset and wake times every day of the week, including weekends. However, this treatment can be impractical, as the progressive forward bedtime shifts will involve the patient temporarily sleeping in the daytime, and constant supervision must be ensured to prevent him or her sleeping at the wrong time. This treatment, although physiologically sound, therefore presents difficulties in its execution.

Another technique, phototherapy, resets the sleep–wake rhythm using bright morning light combined with evening light restriction to phase-advance the patient's sleep time.[73,74] Phototherapy is based on the principle that bright light in the morning, at the end of the habitual sleep period, can phase advance the circadian clock and hence wake onset, while bright light in the evening can phase delay the circadian clock and sleep onset. Different phototherapy protocols have been used with varying success, and a pragmatic approach for the individual patient must be developed in each case. However, the technique should not be used in patients who are bipolar, as it may aggravate mania.[72]

It has been suggested that patients with DSPS are particularly susceptible to the effects of evening light. A study by Aoki *et al.* reported that the suppressive effect of light on melatonin concentration was significantly greater in patients with DSPS than in control subjects.[75] The results indicate a hypersensitivity to nighttime light exposure in the condition, and further reinforce the importance of evening light restriction in patients with DSPS.

The practice at the Stanford Sleep Disorders Center (Stanford, CA, USA) is to use a light intensity of 10,000 lux for 30–45 min immediately after awakening, over a period of several weeks. In addition, bright lights should be minimized in the last 2 h before the expected sleep time, including restricting the use of computer monitors. A practical compromise in teenagers may be to minimize or restrict the use of computers before bedtime, but to allow their use promptly after awakening, therefore serving as an incentive for the adolescent to get up on time or early.

Treatment of patients with insomnia using melatonin has been described in a number of studies.[76–79] Melatonin is a hormone secreted by the pineal gland and its primary function appears to be the conveyance of information concerning the changing length of the night over the course of the year. According to Arendt *et al.* this information is used by photoperiodic animals to "ensure the correct timing of seasonally variable functions such as reproduction, coat growth, and probably the duration and organization of sleep."[80]

Melatonin has been used to treat poor sleep in a variety of conditions, including Asperger syndrome.[75,81] The timing of the dose must be individually determined, based on the subject's core body temperature rhythm. Melatonin is an over-the-counter product and therefore does not have the same degree of regulation as prescription pharmaceuticals. This lack of regulation may cause the quality of over-the-counter melatonin to be highly variable.[82]

9. Restless Leg Syndrome

9.1. *Clinical presentation*

Restless legs syndrome is a chronic autosomal dominant neurological disorder characterized by leg discomfort, most common in the evening, that makes the patients want to move their legs.[1] Discomfort is relieved with movement. The sensation may also be present when the patient is sitting still such as seated on an airplane or in a movie theater. The leg discomfort maybe hard to describe and in children may be characterized as "growing pains." In patients with restless legs syndrome, sleep maybe disrupted by hundreds of involuntary kicking movements of the legs during sleep called periodic limb movements of sleep.

Restless legs syndrome can result in significant daytime drowsiness as a result of poor sleep quality, which may lead to daytime behavior that mimics attention-deficit/hyperactivity disorder.[33,83] Children with RLS may present with non-specific symptom such as growing pains, restless sleep, insomnia, and daytime sleepiness, but most often these issues go unnoticed by their parents.[84,85]

A dysregulation of iron metabolism may play a role in the pathophysiology of restless legs syndrome. Iron is a cofactor in the production of dopamine. Allen *et al.* reported that decreases in iron concentration in nigrostriatal areas correlated with severity of restless legs syndrome.[86]

9.2. *Treatment*

Non-drug treatments may temporarily help counteract the sensations of restless legs syndrome. Patients may find that walking, stretching, taking a hot or cold bath, massaging the affected limb, applying hot or cold packs, using vibration, performing acupressure, and practicing relaxation techniques (such as biofeedback, meditation, or yoga) may help reduce or relieve the symptoms. In addition, some find that find that keeping their mind actively engaged through activities such as reading an interesting novel, or playing video games helps during times that they must be stay seated, such as when traveling.

Dopamine precursors and agonists have been effective in relieving restless legs syndrome. Dopamine class medications are effective and recommended by the American Academy of Sleep Medicine. However, specific guidelines for children were not reviewed.

No medication has a pediatric FDA indication for periodic limb movement disorders or restless leg syndrome. The use of any medications for these conditions is off label. Selective dopamine agonists are potent treatments for periodic limb movement disorders and restless leg syndrome. They tend to have fewer side effects than carbidopa/levodopa. Pramipexole, ropinirolole, and pergolide are the most commonly used medication in this category.[87]

10. Parasomnias

According to the International Classification of Sleep Disorders, parasomnias are groups of clinical disorders in which undesirable events or experiences occur during entry into sleep, within sleep, or during arousals from sleep.[1] The ICSD describes over a dozen different parasomnias, the majority of which can occur in children. In medieval times, the phenomena of sleep paralysis, night terrors, and sleepwalking may have been interpreted as supernatural events.

The arousal parasomnias are more common in children and include the clinical spectrum of confusional arousals, sleep terrors, and sleepwalking. These conditions are thought to arise from impaired arousal from sleep, typically slow wave sleep. Since slow wave sleep (stages 3 and 4) dominate in the first third of the night, the arousal parasomnias also occur at that time. Anything that increases the amount of slow wave sleep, such as recovery from sleep deprivation, may increase the likelihood of these parasomnias occurring in susceptible individuals. If necessary, clonazepam may help decrease these arousal parasomnias but should be avoided in the presence of sleep-disordered breathing.[61]

Confusional arousals may be partial manifestations of sleep terrors and sleep walking events. The episodes are described, as name implies, confusion during and following arousals, usually in the first third of night. The individual is disoriented, speech and mentation are slowed, and response to questioning is confused.[1] These behaviors usually last only a few minutes in children and can be precipitated by forced awakenings out of slow wave sleep. The condition is benign and tends to decrease over time. However, a child with a tendency to have these events may also be at risk for sleepwalking, and parents/caretakers should be warned of this possibility. The events can be minimized by avoiding situations that can increase slow wave sleep or sleep disruption.

Sleep terrors are characterized by a sudden arousal from slow wave sleep with a characteristic "blood-curdling" scream accompanied by intense fear. Pronounced autonomic nervous system discharge may occur with tachycardia and sweating. The child may be described as wide eyed with an intense look of fear staring past the parents. The prevalence of sleep terrors in children is 3% in children and decreases with age to about 2% in adults.[88] Arousal is difficult, and if successful, the patient may be confused and disoriented. The child may try to describe fragments of images with poor coherence. These images will not have the rich detail of a nightmare. Waking the child 15 min after they have fallen asleep has been a popular treatment. Awakening the child at the point that they would be expected to be entering slow wave sleep seems somehow to decrease the tendency for these parasomnias to occur. When the child returns to sleep, the homeostatic mechanism driving slow wave sleep may raise the arousal threshold and decrease the likelihood of the recurrence of the sleep terror. The parents should be warned that the child with sleep terrors might also sleepwalk.

Sleepwalking is also called somnambulism.[1] The term sleepwalking may be a misnomer, perhaps "sleepfleeing" would better characterize the dramatic behavior witnessed. The range of behaviors witnessed may range from simply sitting up in bed to running out of the home and driving an automobile. During the sleepwalking episode, the pain thresholds are elevated.[89] The child will be hard to awaken and may be confused and disoriented. The motor activity may terminate spontaneously or the child may simply return to bed without reaching alertness. Sleeptalking may occur during this event. The treatments mentioned above for the other arousal parasomnias may be helpful. Safety precautions should always be taken. Specifically, the child should sleep on a ground floor if possible to avoid injury while negotiating stairs. If the child has a bunk bed they should use the lower bunk. Drapery should be kept over the bedroom windows to protect the hands of the child in case the child tries to punch a window. A door alarm is helpful to warn the parents if the child walks out of the home. Weapons should be kept away from adults who may sleepwalk. It is helpful to keep precipitants of sleepwalking at a minimum. Thus, sleep deprivation should be avoided. Obstructive sleep apnea may be an occult aggravator and should be treated if present.[16]

Parasomnias such as sleepwalking and sleep terrors need to be distinguished from nocturnal seizures. The timing of seizures is different from sleepwalking and sleep terrors. Nocturnal seizures do not cluster during slow wave sleep in the first third of the night. The motor activity of generalized tonic-clonic seizures is very different from these parasomnias. Tongue biting and urinary incontinence are not characteristically seen in sleepwalking and night terrors. Patients with generalized nocturnal seizures have a low risk of daytime seizures.[90] The motor activity of a partial complex seizure may be more difficult to distinguish from parasomnias and may be resemble a confusional arousal.[91] Usually, the overall clinical picture can help with the diagnosis. If a patient has been injured during an apparent parasomnia, a comprehensive neurological evaluation should be considered including a sleep deprived electroencephalogram.

Some forms of epilepsy may be misidentified as a benign parasomnia and as narcolepsy in children.[92] Frontal lobe epilepsy is poorly understood and often unrecognized by health care workers dealing with children. Age of onset varies from infancy to adolescence. Seizures are typically brief (30 s to 2 min), stereotypic, nocturnal, and can occur several times during the night. They have an explosive onset, characterized by screaming, agitation, stiffening, kicking or bicycling of the legs, and incontinence. The interictal electroencephalogram is usually normal. Long-term video electroencephalographic monitoring is required to demonstrate the frontal epileptic discharges. This condition may be misdiagnosed as a sleep disorder or psychiatric problem. The movements are not symmetrical. Seizures control is difficult and may require epilepsy surgery.[93]

11. Children and Hypnotics

Children with pervasive developmental disorders and mental retardation may be particularly prone to an irregular sleep–wake rhythm type of circadian sleep disorder. It is important to keep in mind that waking up is a biological process but getting out of bed is a volitional event. Ask any person why they got out bed on a particular morning and they will almost inevitably say, "because I had to." But what happens when there is no incentive to get out bed? For many of our more impaired children, there may not be any motivation to get out of bed in the morning. The principal reason to attempt to regulate their sleep is to help the other members of the family sleep better. The importance of helping other family members sleep better cannot be minimized. If the child's caretakers are exhausted due to frequent interruptions of their own sleep they will not be able to provide optimal care. If the patient's sleep patterns disrupt their sibling's sleep it will further exacerbate a very difficult situation. Before embarking on any pharmacological approach, it is important to determine that subacute OSA is not present since many sedatives can worsen sleep apnea.

There is relatively little information available on the pharmacological management of sleep disorders in children.[94] Most pharmacological guidelines were developed for sleep disorders in adults and must be empirically extrapolated to children. The medications are typically neither FDA approved for the specific sleep disorder nor for the pediatric age range. The physician is often forced to prescribe medications as an "off label" indication. This may result in frustrating insurance reimbursement delays or denials for the family. These reimbursement problems may affect the availability of a specific medication, the family's compliance with the medication or force the physician to prescribe a less desirable alternative medication. The medication may not be available commercially in an easily administered format. Certain age range children may not be able to swallow pills, or ingest chewable tablets, which would require the local pharmacist to compound the medication into a suspension. In addition, due to the natural aversion among both parents and physicians to use medications for pediatric sleep disorders, medications are usually prescribed as a last resort or in the most refractory situations.

At times, a decision to use medication in a child may be made not necessarily to assist the child as much as to help the parents or other family members sleep better. It is not unusual that parents may finally seek help for a child's long-standing sleep problem when the parents feel they can no longer put up with interruptions to their own sleep.

Further complicating the pharmacological treatment of sleep disorders in children is the general lack of specialized training in sleep disorders available to the health care providers who are working with these children. Failure to consider or properly apply non-drug treatments as part of the comprehensive management of the child may also lead to unsatisfactory results for the patient and the family. These factors result in children with sleep disorders that are not properly managed due to either underdosing, or overdosing of medication or incorrect medication selection.

There maybe an overreliance on medications by both the parents and health-care provider without adequate application of behavioral techniques to help improve the child's sleep. A common scenario in clinical practice is a parents' complaint of a child's paradoxical reaction to a hypnotic medication. "It made it worse" or "he became hyper" may be the parent's complaint. This may occur because the timing or the dose provided was incorrect. The parents may expect that once a medication has been finally prescribed to help their child sleep that it will "knockout" the child. It is important that the healthcare provider advising this family take into account the circadian modulation of alertness. Humans will typically experience an enhanced alertness in the evening, which is often referred to as a "second wind." During this circadian phase, it is harder to fall asleep. If the hypnotic medication is given during this circadian time window, the medication may not work or the child may be frightened by hypnagogic hallucinations. If a medication has been previously shown to shorten sleep latency by only 20 or 30 min, giving this medication 2 or 3 h prior to the usual falling asleep time could elicit this common scenario. This same medication given at a more appropriate circadian time could be effective. A similar lack of efficacy or paradoxical reaction could occur if the medication dose is inadequate.

12. Future Directions

Perhaps the most important future direction of pediatric sleep medicine is to answer the basic questions of why do we sleep and dream. Nowhere in this extensive chapter are these questions addressed. How would the reader feel if after reading a cardiology or nephrology chapter the function of the heart or kidneys was never explained? The answers to these questions will be likely be revealed within most of our lifetimes. Research is pointing sleep and dreams as having multiple functions. In particular, sleep and dreams are important in memory and learning.[95,96] Sleep is also important in the overall homeostatic maintenance of the cerebral synapses.[97]

Clinical sleep medicine only became an official ACGME subspecialty in 2005. With this recognition, it is expected that sleep medicine will have greater importance within academic medical centers. This should allow the field to attract more trainees and improve the quality of research. A candidate for sleep training should have completed a prior residency in family medicine, internal medicine, neurology, otolaryngology, pediatrics, or psychiatry. Currently, applicant for sleep medicine training is dominated by pulmonologists. Psychiatry residents in particular should be encouraged to consider pursuing fellowships in sleep medicine given the comorbidity of psychiatric conditions and sleep disorders. Despite all of the progress made, the field of pediatric sleep disorders needs much more research. We lack sufficient normative and epidemiological data in children. There is a paucity of therapeutic clinical trials and health policy outcomes research.

With greater awareness of sleep disorders and their impact in the daytime behavior of children it is crucial that the field progress in a direction that allows non-sleep specialist to recognize and treat these children. There are simply not enough sleep specialists available to treat all these children. The reader is encouraged to learn more about sleep and look for these conditions. They are so common that if a primary care provider or psychiatrist is not routinely identifying sleep disorders in their clinical population they are probably being missed. If you are not identifying these children in your community, then who, if anybody, is? Sleep disorders in children are common and fairly easy to treat. You will find the positive impact made with successful treatment to be very rewarding to the patient and their family.

References

1. *International Classification of Sleep Disorders*. 2nd edition. Westchester, Illinois: American Academy of Sleep Medicine, 2005.
2. Clinical practice guideline: Diagnosis and management of childhood obstructive sleep apnea syndrome, *Pediatrics* 2002; **109**: 704–712.
3. Morgenthaler TI, Lee-Chiong T, Alessi C, *et al*. Practice parameters for the clinical evaluation and treatment of circadian rhythm sleep disorders. An American Academy of Sleep Medicine report, *Sleep* 2007; **30**: 1445–1459.
4. Morgenthaler TI, Owens J, Alessi C, *et al*. Practice parameters for behavioral treatment of bedtime problems and night wakings in infants and young children, *Sleep* 2006; **29**: 1277–1281.
5. Pelayo R, Hodgson N, Guilleminault C. The history of sleep medicine. In: *Handb Clin Neurol* 2009; pp. 547–556.
6. Iglowstein I, Jenni OG, Molinari L, Largo RH. Sleep duration from infancy to adolescence: Reference values and generational trends, *Pediatrics* 2003; **111**: 302–307.
7. Wurts SW, Edgar DM. Circadian and homeostatic control of rapid eye movement (REM) sleep: Promotion of REM tendency by the suprachiasmatic nucleus, *J Neurosci* 2000; **20**: 4300–4310.
8. Carroll JL. Obstructive sleep-disordered breathing in children: New controversies, new directions, *Clin Chest Med* 2003; **24**: 261–282.
9. Kennedy JD, Blunden S, Hirte C, *et al*. Reduced neurocognition in children who snore, *Pediatr Pulmonol* 2004; **37**: 330–337.
10. Montgomery-Downs HE, Gozal D. Snore-associated sleep fragmentation in infancy: Mental development effects and contribution of secondhand cigarette smoke exposure, *Pediatrics* 2006; **117**: e496–e502.
11. Halbower AC, Mahone EM. Neuropsychological morbidity linked to childhood sleep-disordered breathing, *Sleep Med Rev* 2006; **10**: 97–107.
12. Gozal D, Kheirandish L. Oxidant stress and inflammation in the snoring child: Confluent pathways to upper airway pathogenesis and end-organ morbidity, *Sleep Med Rev* 2006.
13. Montgomery-Downs HE, O'Brien LM, Holbrook CR, Gozal D. Snoring and sleep-disordered breathing in young children: Subjective and objective correlates, *Sleep* 2004; **27**: 87–94.
14. Tauman R, O'Brien LM, Holbrook CR, Gozal D. Sleep pressure score: A new index of sleep disruption in snoring children, *Sleep* 2004; **27**: 274–278.

15. Guilleminault C, Li K, Khramtsov A, Palombini L, Pelayo R. Breathing patterns in prepubertal children with sleep-related breathing disorders, *Arch Pediatr Adolesc Med* 2004; **158**: 153–161.
16. Guilleminault C, Palombini L, Pelayo R, Chervin RD. Sleepwalking and sleep terrors in prepubertal children: What triggers them? *Pediatrics* 2003; **111**: e17–e25.
17. Rosen CL, Storfer-Isser A, Taylor HG, Kirchner HL, Emancipator JL, Redline S. Increased behavioral morbidity in school-aged children with sleep-disordered breathing, *Pediatrics* 2004; **114**: 1640–1648.
18. Pelayo R, Sivan Y. Increased behavioral morbidity in school-aged children with sleep-disordered breathing, *Pediatrics* 2005; **116**: 797–798.
19. Ivanenko A, Crabtree VM, Gozal D. Sleep in children with psychiatric disorders, *Pediatr Clin North Am* 2004; **51**: 51–68.
20. Chervin RD, Dillon JE, Archbold KH, Ruzicka DL. Conduct problems and symptoms of sleep disorders in children, *J Am Acad Child Adolesc Psychiatry* 2003; **42**: 201–208.
21. Weissbach A, Leiberman A, Tarasiuk A, Goldbart A, Tal A. Adenotonsilectomy improves enuresis in children with obstructive sleep apnea syndrome, *Int J Pediatr Otorhinolaryngol* 2006; **70**: 1351–1356.
22. Wing YK, Hui SH, Pak WM, *et al.* A controlled study of sleep related disordered breathing in obese children, *Arch Dis Child* 2003; **88**: 1043–1047.
23. Ievers-Landis CE, Redline S. Pediatric sleep apnea: Implications of the epidemic of childhood overweight, *Am J Respir Crit Care Med* 2007; **175**: 436–441.
24. Roemmich JN, Barkley JE, D'Andrea L, *et al.* Increases in overweight after adenotonsillectomy in overweight children with obstructive sleep-disordered breathing are associated with decreases in motor activity and hyperactivity, *Pediatrics* 2006; **117**: e200–e208.
25. Friedman BC, Hendeles-Amitai A, Kozminsky E, *et al.* Adenotonsillectomy improves neurocognitive function in children with obstructive sleep apnea syndrome, *Sleep* 2003; **26**: 999–1005.
26. O'Brien LM, Gozal D. Neurocognitive dysfunction and sleep in children: From human to rodent, *Pediatr Clin North Am* 2004; **51**: 187–202.
27. Archbold KH, Giordani B, Ruzicka DL, Chervin RD. Cognitive executive dysfunction in children with mild sleep-disordered breathing, *Biol Res Nurs* 2004; **5**: 168–176.
28. Chervin RD, Clarke DF, Huffman JL, *et al.* School performance, race, and other correlates of sleep-disordered breathing in children, *Sleep Med* 2003; **4**: 21–27.
29. O'Brien LM, Holbrook CR, Mervis CB, *et al.* Sleep and neurobehavioral characteristics of 5- to 7-year-old children with parentally reported symptoms of attention-deficit/hyperactivity disorder, *Pediatrics* 2003; **111**: 554–563.
30. O'Brien LM, Ivanenko A, Crabtree VM, *et al.* Sleep disturbances in children with attention deficit hyperactivity disorder, *Pediatr Res* 2003; **54**: 237–243.

31. Gottlieb DJ, Vezina RM, Chase C, *et al.* Symptoms of sleep-disordered breathing in 5-year-old children are associated with sleepiness and problem behaviors, *Pediatrics* 2003; **112**: 870–877.
32. Crabtree VM, Ivanenko A, Gozal D. Clinical and parental assessment of sleep in children with attention-deficit/hyperactivity disorder referred to a pediatric sleep medicine center, *Clin Pediatr* 2003; **42**: 807–813.
33. Chervin RD, Archbold KH, Dillon JE, *et al.* Associations between symptoms of inattention, hyperactivity, restless legs, and periodic leg movements, *Sleep* 2002; **25**: 213–218.
34. Mulvaney SA, Goodwin JL, Morgan WJ, Rosen GR, Quan SF, Kaemingk KL. Behavior problems associated with sleep disordered breathing in school-aged children — the Tucson children's assessment of sleep apnea study. *J Pediatr Psychol* 2006; **31**: 322–330.
35. Mitchell RB, Kelly J. Behavior, neurocognition and quality-of-life in children with sleep-disordered breathing, *Int J Pediatr Otorhinolaryngol* 2006; **70**: 395–406.
36. Kurnatowski P, Putynski L, Lapienis M, Kowalska B. Neurocognitive abilities in children with adenotonsillar hypertrophy, *Int J Pediatr Otorhinolaryngol* 2006; **70**: 419–424.
37. Uliel S, Tauman R, Greenfeld M, Sivan Y. Normal polysomnographic respiratory values in children and adolescents, *Chest* 2004; **125**: 872–878.
38. Rosen CL. Obstructive sleep apnea syndrome in children: Controversies in diagnosis and treatment, *Pediatr Clin North Am* 2004; **51**: 153–167, vii.
39. Schechter MS. Technical report: diagnosis and management of childhood obstructive sleep apnea syndrome, *Pediatrics* 2002; **109**: e69.
40. Guilleminault C, Pelayo R. And if the polysomnogram was faulty? *Pediatr Pulmonol* 1998; **26**: 1–3.
41. Messner AH. Treating pediatric patients with obstructive sleep disorders: An update, *Otolaryngol Clin North Am* 2003; **36**: 519–530.
42. Shott SR, Amin R, Chini B, Heubi C, Hotze S, Akers R. Obstructive sleep apnea: Should all children with Down syndrome be tested? *Arch Otolaryngol Head Neck Surg* 2006; **132**: 432–436.
43. Pavone M, Paglietti MG, Petrone A, Crino A, De Vincentiis GC, Cutrera R. Adenotonsillectomy for obstructive sleep apnea in children with Prader-Willi syndrome, *Pediatr Pulmonol* 2006; **41**: 74–79.
44. Onodera K, Niikuni N, Chigono T, Nakajima I, Sakata H, Motizuki H. Sleep disordered breathing in children with achondroplasia. Part 2. Relationship with craniofacial and airway morphology, *Int J Pediatr Otorhinolaryngol* 2006; **70**: 453–461.
45. Monfared A, Messner A. Death following tonsillectomy in a child with Williams syndrome, *Int J Pediatr Otorhinolaryngol* 2006; **70**: 1133–1135.
46. Suresh S, Wales P, Dakin C, Harris MA, Cooper DG. Sleep-related breathing disorder in Duchenne muscular dystrophy: Disease spectrum in the paediatric population, *J Paediatr Child Health* 2005; **41**: 500–503.

47. Palombini L, Pelayo R, Guilleminault C. Efficacy of automated continuous positive airway pressure in children with sleep-related breathing disorders in an attended setting, *Pediatrics* 2004; **113**: e412–e417.
48. Malow BA, Weatherwax KJ, Chervin RD, *et al.* Identification and treatment of obstructive sleep apnea in adults and children with epilepsy: A prospective pilot study, *Sleep Med* 2003; **4**: 509–515.
49. Marcus CL, Rosen G, Ward SL, *et al.* Adherence to and effectiveness of positive airway pressure therapy in children with obstructive sleep apnea, *Pediatrics* 2006; **117**: e442–e451.
50. Villa MP, Malagola C, Pagani J, *et al.* Rapid maxillary expansion in children with obstructive sleep apnea syndrome: 12-month follow-up, *Sleep Med* 2007; **8**: 128–134.
51. Rose E, Schessl J. Orthodontic procedures in the treatment of obstructive sleep apnea in children, *J Orofac Orthop* 2006; **67**: 58–67.
52. Pirelli P, Saponara M, Attanasio G. Obstructive sleep apnoea syndrome (OSAS) and rhino-tubaric disfunction in children: Therapeutic effects of RME therapy, *Prog Orthod* 2005; **6**: 48–61.
53. Guilleminault C, Li KK. Maxillomandibular expansion for the treatment of sleep-disordered breathing: Preliminary result, *Laryngoscope* 2004; **114**: 893–896.
54. Cistulli PA. Rapid maxillary expansion in obstructive sleep apnea — hope on the horizon? *Sleep* 2004; **27**: 606–607.
55. Guilleminault C, Pelayo R. Narcolepsy in children: A practical guide to its diagnosis, treatment and follow-up, *Paediatr Drugs* 2000; **2**: 1–9.
56. Silber MH, Krahn LE, Olson EJ, Pankratz VS. The epidemiology of narcolepsy in Olmsted County, Minnesota: A population-based study, *Sleep* 2002; **25**: 197–202.
57. Mignot E, Lammers GJ, Ripley B, *et al.* The role of cerebrospinal fluid hypocretin measurement in the diagnosis of narcolepsy and other hypersomnias, *Arch Neurol* 2002; **59**: 1553–1562.
58. Mignot E, Chen W, Black J. On the value of measuring CSF hypocretin-1 in diagnosing narcolepsy, *Sleep* 2003; **26**: 646–649.
59. Littner M, Johnson SF, McCall WV, *et al.* Practice parameters for the treatment of narcolepsy: An update for 2000, *Sleep* 2001; **24**: 451–466.
60. Morgenthaler TI, Kapur VK, Brown T, *et al.* Practice parameters for the treatment of narcolepsy and other hypersomnias of central origin, *Sleep* 2007; **30**: 1705–1711.
61. Pelayo R, Chen W, Monzon S, Guilleminault C. Pediatric sleep pharmacology: You want to give my kid sleeping pills? *Pediatr Clin North Am* 2004; **51**: 117–134.
62. Owens JA, Rosen CL, Mindell JA. Medication use in the treatment of pediatric insomnia: Results of a survey of community-based pediatricians, *Pediatrics* 2003; **111**: e628–e635.
63. Ferber R. Childhood sleep disorders, *Neurol Clin* 1996; **14**: 493–511.

64. Takahashi Y, Hohjoh H, Matsuura K. Predisposing factors in delayed sleep phase syndrome, *Psychiatry Clin Neurosci* 2000; **54**: 356–358.

65. Watanabe T, Kajimura N, Kato M, *et al.* Sleep and circadian rhythm disturbances in patients with delayed sleep phase syndrome, *Sleep* 2003; **26**: 657–661.

66. Thorpy MJ, Korman E, Spielman AJ, Glovinsky PB. Delayed sleep phase syndrome in adolescents, *J Adolesc Health Care* 1988; **9**: 22–27.

67. Carskadon MA, Acebo C, Jenni OG. Regulation of adolescent sleep: Implications for behavior, *Ann N Y Acad Sci* 2004; **1021**: 276–291.

68. Fallone G, Seifer R, Acebo C, Carskadon MA. How well do school-aged children comply with imposed sleep schedules at home? *Sleep* 2002; **25**: 739–745.

69. Jenni OG, Achermann P, Carskadon MA. Homeostatic sleep regulation in adolescents, *Sleep* 2005; **28**: 1446–1454.

70. Taylor DJ, Jenni OG, Acebo C, Carskadon MA. Sleep tendency during extended wakefulness: insights into adolescent sleep regulation and behavior, *J Sleep Res* 2005; **14**: 239–244.

71. Shirayama M, Shirayama Y, Iida H, *et al.* The psychological aspects of patients with delayed sleep phase syndrome (DSPS), *Sleep Med* 2003; **4**: 427–433.

72. Chesson AL, Jr., Littner M, Davila D, *et al.* Practice parameters for the use of light therapy in the treatment of sleep disorders. Standards of Practice Committee, American Academy of Sleep Medicine, *Sleep* 1999; **22**: 641–660.

73. Hori T, Watanabe T, Kajimura N, Kato M, Sekimoto M, Takahashi K. Effects of phototherapy on the phase relationship between sleep and body temperature rhythm in a delayed sleep phase syndrome case, *Psychiatry Clin Neurosci* 2000; **54**: 371–373.

74. Cole RJ, Smith JS, Alcala YC, Elliott JA, Kripke DF. Bright-light mask treatment of delayed sleep phase syndrome, *J Biol Rhythms* 2002; **17**: 89–101.

75. Aoki H, Ozeki Y, Yamada N. Hypersensitivity of melatonin suppression in response to light in patients with delayed sleep phase syndrome, *Chronobiol Int* 2001; **18**: 263–271.

76. Paavonen EJ, Nieminen-von Wendt T, Vanhala R, Aronen ET, von Wendt L. Effectiveness of melatonin in the treatment of sleep disturbances in children with Asperger disorder, *J Child Adolesc Psychopharmacol* 2003; **13**: 83–95.

77. Smits MG, van Stel HF, van der Heijden K, Meijer AM, Coenen AM, Kerkhof GA. Melatonin improves health status and sleep in children with idiopathic chronic sleep-onset insomnia: A randomized placebo-controlled trial, *J Am Acad Child Adolesc Psychiatry* 2003; **42**: 1286–1293.

78. van der Heijden KB, Smits MG, van Someren EJ, Boudewijn Gunning W. Prediction of melatonin efficacy by pretreatment dim light melatonin onset in children with idiopathic chronic sleep onset insomnia, *J Sleep Res* 2005; **14**: 187–194.

79. Sack RL, Hughes RJ, Edgar DM, Lewy AJ. Sleep-promoting effects of melatonin: At what dose, in whom, under what conditions, and by what mechanisms? *Sleep* 1997; **20**: 908–915.
80. Arendt J, Middleton B, Stone B, Skene D. Complex effects of melatonin: Evidence for photoperiodic responses in humans? *Sleep* 1999; **22**: 625–635.
81. Nagtegaal JE, Laurant MW, Kerkhof GA, Smits MG, van der Meer YG, Coenen AM. Effects of melatonin on the quality of life in patients with delayed sleep phase syndrome, *J Psychosom Res* 2000; **48**: 45–50.
82. Williamson BL, Tomlinson AJ, Mishra PK, Gleich GJ, Naylor S. Structural characterization of contaminants found in commercial preparations of melatonin: Similarities to case-related compounds from L-tryptophan associated with eosinophilia-myalgia syndrome, *Chem Res Toxicol* 1998; **11**: 234–240.
83. Picchietti DL, Underwood DJ, Farris WA, *et al.* Further studies on periodic limb movement disorder and restless legs syndrome in children with attention-deficit hyperactivity disorder, *Mov Disord* 1999; **14**: 1000–1007.
84. Picchietti D, Allen RP, Walters AS, Davidson JE, Myers A, Ferini-Strambi L. Restless legs syndrome: Prevalence and impact in children and adolescents — the Peds REST study, *Pediatrics* 2007; **120**: 253–266.
85. Walters AS, Silvestri R, Zucconi M, Chandrashekariah R, Konofal E. Review of the possible relationship and hypothetical links between attention deficit hyperactivity disorder (ADHD) and the simple sleep related movement disorders, parasomnias, hypersomnias, and circadian rhythm disorders, *J Clin Sleep Med* 2008; **4**: 591–600.
86. Allen RP, Barker PB, Wehrl F, Song HK, Earley CJ. MRI measurement of brain iron in patients with restless legs syndrome, *Neurology* 2001; **56**: 263–265.
87. Stiasny K, Wetter TC, Winkelmann J, *et al.* Long-term effects of pergolide in the treatment of restless legs syndrome, *Neurology* 2001; **56**: 1399–1402.
88. Ohayon MM, Guilleminault C, Priest RG. Night terrors, sleepwalking, and confusional arousals in the general population: Their frequency and relationship to other sleep and mental disorders, *J Clin Psychiatry* 1999; **60**: 268–276; quiz 77.
89. Cartwright R. Sleep-related violence: Does the polysomnogram help establish the diagnosis? *Sleep Med* 2000; **1**: 331–335.
90. D'Alessandro R, Guarino M, Greco G, Bassein L. Risk of seizures while awake in pure sleep epilepsies: A prospective study, *Neurology* 2004; **62**: 254–257.
91. Lahorgue Nunes M, Ferri R, Arzimanoglou A, Curzi L, Appel CC, Costa da Costa J. Sleep organization in children with partial refractory epilepsy, *J Child Neurol* 2003; **18**: 763–766.
92. Kotagal P. The relationship between sleep and epilepsy, *Semin Pediatr Neurol* 2001; **8**: 241–250.
93. Sinclair DB, Wheatley M, Snyder T. Frontal lobe epilepsy in childhood, *Pediatr Neurol* 2004; **30**: 169–176.

94. Pelayo R, Dubik M. Pediatric sleep pharmacology, *Semin Pediatr Neurol* 2008; **15**: 79–90.
95. Walker MP. The role of slow wave sleep in memory processing, *J Clin Sleep Med* 2009; **5**: S20–S26.
96. Walker MP. The role of sleep in cognition and emotion, *Ann N Y Acad Sci* 2009; **1156**: 168–197.
97. Tononi G. Slow wave homeostasis and synaptic plasticity, *J Clin Sleep Med* 2009; **5**: S16–S19.

Author Index

Subject Index